Recovery from Schizophrenia

Recovery from Schizophrenia
An International Perspective

A Report from the WHO Collaborative Project,
The International Study of Schizophrenia

Edited by

Kim Hopper

Glynn Harrison

Aleksandar Janca

Norman Sartorius

OXFORD
UNIVERSITY PRESS

2007

OXFORD
UNIVERSITY PRESS

Oxford University Press, Inc., publishes works that further
Oxford University's objective of excellence
in research, scholarship, and education.

Oxford New York
Auckland Cape Town Dar es Salaam Hong Kong Karachi
Kuala Lumpur Madrid Melbourne Mexico City Nairobi
New Delhi Shanghai Taipei Toronto

With offices in
Argentina Austria Brazil Chile Czech Republic France Greece
Guatemala Hungary Italy Japan Poland Portugal Singapore
South Korea Switzerland Thailand Turkey Ukraine Vietnam

Published by Oxford University Press, Inc.
198 Madison Avenue, New York, New York 10016
www.oup.com

Library of Congress Cataloging-in-Publication Data
Recovery from schizophrenia : an international perspective—results
from the WHO-coordinated international study of schizophrenia
(ISoS) / edited by Kim Hopper ... [et al.].
p. ; cm.
Includes bibliographical references.
ISBN-13: 978-0-19-531367-3
ISBN-10: 0-19-531367-4
1. Schizophrenia—Epidemiology. I. Hopper, Kim.
[DNLM: 1. World Health Organization. 2. Schizophrenia—therapy.
3. Follow-Up Studies. 4. International Cooperation. 5. Treatment
Outcome. WM 203 R3124 2007]
RC514.R385 2007
362.2'6—dc22 2006026433

1 3 5 7 9 8 6 4 2

Printed in the United States of America
on acid-free paper

Contents

Contributors

Sherryl Baker, Ph.D.
Former Research Scientist
Nathan Kline Institute for Psychiatric Research
Orangeburg, New York

Rheta Bank, M.A.*
Former Director, Educational Technology Department
Nathan Kline Institute for Psychiatric Research
Orangeburg, New York

Pavel Baudis, M.D.
Psychiatrist
Formerly with ISoS Collaborative Study
Prague Field Research Center
Prague, Czech Republic

Robert Cancro, M.D., Med.D.Sc.
Former Director
Nathan Kline Institute for Psychiatric Research
Lucius N. Littauer Professor of Psychiatry
New York University Medical Center
New York, New York

Changhui Chen, M.D.
Professor and Physician, Retired
Beijing Medical University
Beijing, China

Thomas J. Craig, M.D.
Chief Quality and Performance Officer
Department of Veterans Affairs
Washington, DC

Ate de Jong, Ph.D.
University Medical Center Groningen
Department of Psychiatry
University Medical Center
Groningen, The Netherlands

Barbara Digman
Formerly with ISoS Collaborative Study
Honolulu Field Research Center
Honolulu, Hawaii

Eva Dragomirecká, M.D.
Senior Researcher, Department of Social Psychiatry
Prague Psychiatric Center
Prague, Czech Republic

Christiana Drake, Ph.D.
Professor of Statistics
University of California, Davis
Davis, California

K.C. Dube, M.D.*
Former Professor of Psychiatrist and Senior Medical Superintendent
Mental Hospital
Agra, India

Aine Finnerty
St. Canice's Hospital
Kilkenny, Ireland

Amy S. M. Fung
Formerly with ISoS Collaborative Study
Hong Kong Field Research Center
Hong Kong

Kimon Ganev, M.D.
Clinical Director
Mental Health Centre Dinamika
Visiting Lecturer
New Bulgarian University
Sofia, Bulgaria

Robert Giel, M.D.
Emeritus Professor
University Medical Center Groningen
Department of Psychiatry
University of Groningen
Groningen, The Netherlands

Glynn Harrison, M.D., FRCPsych
Norah Cooke Hurle Professor of Mental Health
University of Bristol
Former Professor of Community Mental Health
University of Nottingham
United Kingdom

* Deceased.

Wolfram an der Heiden, Dipl.-Psych
Deputy Head
Schizophrenia Research Group
Central Institute of Mental Health
Mannheim, Germany

Keiko Hatada
Formerly with ISoS Collaborative Study
Nagasaki Field Research Center
Nagasaki, Japan

Sharon Holmberg, Ph.D., RN
Associate Professor of Nursing
Decker School of Nursing
Binghamton University
Binghamton, New York

Kim Hopper, Ph.D.
Research Scientist
Nathan Kline Institute for Psychiatric Research
Orangeburg, New York
Professor of Clinical Sociomedical Sciences
Mailman School of Public Health, Columbia University
New York, New York

Plamen Ivanov
Formerly with ISoS Collaborative Study
Sofia Field Research Center
Sofia, Bulgaria

Aleksandar Janca, M.D., FRCPsych, FRANZCP
Professor and Head, School of Psychiatry and Clinical Neurosciences
University of Western Australia
Director, World Health Organization Collaborating Center for Research & Training in Mental Health
Perth, Australia

A. Albert Joseph, MSc
Biostatistics, SCARF
Chennai, India

Martin M. Katz, Ph.D.
Past Director, Clinical Research Branch
National Institute of Mental Health
Bethesda, Maryland

Fiona Keogh
Researcher
Mental Health Commission
Dublin, Ireland

Bertram Krumm
Formerly with ISoS Collaborative Study
Mannheim Field Research Center
Mannheim, Germany

Narendar Kumar, M.D.
Deputy Director General
Indian Council for Medical Research
New Delhi, India

Julia Lam
Formerly with ISoS Collaborative Study
Hong Kong Field Research Center
Hong Kong

Eugene M. Laska, Ph.D.
Director, Statistical Sciences Laboratory
Nathan Kline Institute for Psychiatric Research
Orangeburg, New York

Peter W.H. Lee, M.D.
Professor in Clinical & Health Psychology
Department of Psychiatry
The University of Hong Kong
Hong Kong

Thomas Leland, M.D.
Chief Psychiatrist
Kalihi-Palama Mental Health Services
Clinical Professor, Department of Psychiatry
John Burns School of Medicine
Hawaii

Agatha León, Ph.D.
Director
Chiquitines
Cali, Columbia

Carlos A. León, M.D.
Professor Emeritus
Universidad del Valle
Cali, Columbia

Richard Levine, Ph.D.
Associate Professor
Department of Mathematics and Statistics
San Diego State University
San Diego, California

Felice Lieh-Mak, M.D.
Emeritus Professor
The University of Hong Kong
Hong Kong

Shang Lin, Ph.D.
Research Associate and Associate Professor
Department of Health Studies
University of Chicago
Chicago, Illinois

K.Y. Mak
Formerly with ISoS Collaborative Study
Hong Kong Field Research Center
Hong Kong

SAVITA MALHOTRA, M.D.
Professor of Psychiatry
Post Graduate Institute of Medical Education and Research
Chandigarh, India

ANTHONY J. MARSELLA, PH.D., D.H.C.
Emeritus Professor, Department of Psychology
University of Hawaii
Honolulu, Hawaii

PETER MASON, M.D.
Psychiatrist
Formerly with ISoS Collaborative Study
Nottingham Field Research Center
Nottingham, United Kingdom

MORRIS MEISNER, PH.D.
Research Scientist
Nathan Kline Institute for Psychiatric Research
Orangeburg, New York

HEATHER MORSE
Formerly with ISoS Collaborative Study
Honolulu Field Research Center
Honolulu, Hawaii

SABINE MÜLLER
Formerly with ISoS Collaborative Study
Mannheim Field Research Center
Mannheim, Germany

YOSHIBUMI NAKANE, M.D.
Professor and Chairman, Department of Neuropsychiatry
University School of Medicine
Nagasaki, Japan

FOKKO J. NIENHUIS, PH.D.
University Medical Center Groningen
Department of Psychiatry
University of Groninge,
Groningen, The Netherlands

ANNE O'GRADY WALSHE, M.D.
Consultant Psychiatrist
Tallaght Hospital
Dublin, Ireland

GEORGI ONCHEV, M.D., PH.D.
Senior Lecturer in Psychiatry, Department of Psychiatry
Medical University
Sofia, Bulgaria

S. RAJKUMAR, M.D.
Professor
Mid Western Area Health/University of Newcastle
Australia

NORMAN SARTORIUS, M.D., PH.D., FRCPSYCH
Previous Director, Division of Mental Health
World Health Organization
Professor of Psychiatry
University of Geneva, Switzerland
President, World Psychiatric Association
Scientific Director, Global Programme against Stigma and Discrimination Because of Schizophrenia

MARIANNE SCHÄFER
Formerly with ISoS Collaborative Study
Mannheim Field Research Center
Mannheim, Germany

ALICE SCHEURER
Formerly with ISoS Collaborative Study
Honolulu Field Research Center
Honolulu, Hawaii

BETTINA SCHWERD
Formerly with ISoS Collaborative Study
Mannheim Field Research Center
Mannheim, Germany

YUCUN SHEN, M.D.
Academician
The Chinese Academy of Engineering
Professor and Honorary Director
Institute of Mental Health, Peking University, China
Member; World Health Organization Expert Advisory Panel on Mental Health
China

CAROLE SIEGEL, PH.D.
Director, Statistics and Services Research Division
Nathan Kline Institute for Psychiatric Research,
Orangeburg, New York

CTIRAD SKODA, M.D.*
Former Psychiatrist and Director of ISoS Collaborative Study
Prague Field Research Center
Prague, Czech Republic

CEES J. SLOOFF, M.D., PH.D.
University Medical Center Groningen
Department of Psychiatry
University of Groningen
Groningen, The Netherlands

EDWARD SUAREZ, PH.D.
Director, Adult Patient Rehabilitation Services
Hawaii State Hospital
Hawaii

KOICHI TAKADA
Formerly with ISoS Collaborative Study
Nagasaki Field Research Center
Nagasaki, Japan

Dei-In Tang, Ph.D.
Research Scientist
Nathan Kline Institute for Psychiatric Research
Orangeburg, New York

R. Thara, M.D., Ph.D.
Director, Schizophrenia Research Foundation (SCARF)
Chennai, India

Sergey Tsirkin, M.D.
Research Institute of Clinical Psychiatry
National Mental Health Center
Moscow, Russia

Vijoy K. Varma, M.D.
Clinical Professor of Psychiatry
Indiana University School of Medicine
Retired Professor and Head, Department of Psychiatry
Post Graduate Institute of Medical Education and Research
Chandigarh, India

Dermot Walsh, M.D.
Psychiatrist
Health Research Board
Dublin, Ireland

Joseph A. Wanderling, M.A.
Research Scientist
Nathan Kline Institute for Psychiatric Research
Orangeburg, New York

Iris Weber
Formerly with ISoS Collaborative Study
Mannheim Field Research Center
Mannheim, Germany

Durk Wiersma, Ph.D.
University Medical Center Groningen
Department of Psychiatry
University of Groningen
Groningen, The Netherlands

M.C. Wong
Formerly with ISoS Collaborative Study
Hong Kong Field Research Center
Hong Kong

Lyman C. Wynne, M.D., Ph.D.
Research Professor, Emeritus, Department of Psychiatry
University of Rochester, New York
Rochester, New York

Kazuyasu Yoshitake
Formerly with ISoS Collaborative Study
Nagasaki Field Research Center
Nagasaki, Japan

Introduction

Since the early 1980s, a body of epidemiological evidence has taken shape (Huber, Gross, and Schuttler, 1975; Bleuler, 1978; Tsuang, Woolson, and Fleming, 1979; Ciompi, 1980; McGlashan, 1984; Ogawa et al., 1987; Shepherd, Watt, Falloon, and Smeeton, 1989; Johnstone, 1991) challenging the early Kraepelinian view (Kraepelin, 1893) that the long-term prognosis for schizophrenia was almost uniformly poor. Beginning with M. Bleuler's striking and, at the time, skeptically received, report on a cohort of 208 patients intensively followed for over 20 years (Bleuler, 1978), investigators have repeatedly documented patterns of long-term outcome at odds with the more pessimistic view. Nor are such findings restricted to less-developed countries of the world, although the evidence for more favorable outcome there is longstanding (Warner, 1985; Kleinman, 1988). Persisting diagnostic ambiguities aside, the European studies in the second half of the 20th century as a whole offer consistent evidence for generally better outcome (Angst, 1988). Swiss (Bleuler, 1978; Ciompi, 1985), German (Huber et al., 1975), and British studies (Shepherd et al., 1989), for example, document a more promising course for at least half of patients followed over time.

The North American record is less clear, owing perhaps to substantial variation in both study design and cohorts tracked. As early as 1975, researchers there were documenting a wide range of functioning in subjects assessed 5 years after entry into the study (Hawk, Carpenter, and Strauss, 1975). Long-term follow-up studies since then have compiled a record of inconsistency. Compare, for example, the picture of former hospital patients in rural Vermont (Harding, Brooks, Ashikaga, Strauss, and Breier, 1987) with that of subjects in the Chestnut Lodge study in suburban Maryland (McGlashan, 1984). Follow-up periods averaged 20 and 15 years, respectively. Over two thirds (68%) of the Vermont cohort were found to have few or no symptoms; an almost identical proportion (64%) of the Chestnut Lodge group was judged to be incapacitated or only marginally functioning.

As such findings illustrate, difficulties arise when comparisons are made across studies using different sampling frames, periods of follow-up, and measures for the complex domains of course and outcome (Harrison and Mason, 1993). The Vermont study, for example, followed up inpatients selected as good prospects for participation in an aggressive rehabilitation program. The Chestnut Lodge Study sampled cases admitted for long-term residential treatment, most of whom were young, persistently ill "treatment failures." In treated prevalence samples drawn from consecutive hospital admissions, too, readmissions and cases of longer illness duration tend to be overrepresented, further hedging the generalizability of the findings. Because such sampling biases can limit generalizability to such an extent, they ought to be given greater visibility when reporting outcomes for schizophrenia (Schwartz, Terkelsen, and Smith, 1992). The ideal situation for tracking course and outcome in such disorders would be incidence samples, identified in a number of "representative" settings, followed with minimum attrition and assessed with standardized measures of proven reliability. Few studies can meet that standard.

Notwithstanding these methodological caveats, the literature suggests that substantial heterogeneity in course and outcome remains the rule. Observed variation increases when subtypes of schizophrenia are considered (Fenton, 1996) and holds true even in prospective studies restricted to first-admission cohorts (Ram, Bromet, Eaton, Pato, and Schwartz, 1992). A meta-analysis of follow-up studies in the 20th century concludes that approximately half (48.5%) of patients followed between 1955 and 1985 improved significantly, as compared with just over a third (35.4%) of those followed in the half-century preceding that period (Hegarty, Baldessarini, Tohen, Waternaux, and Oepen, 1994). More optimistic readings of prognosis have also been voiced when separate domains of competency or recovery are considered, and the 32-year follow-up study by Harding and colleagues (Harding et al., 1987) posited that a substantial proportion of patients may show recovery late in the course of their illness. In the judgment of three leading researchers, it may well be time for chronicity to give way to the expectation of "slow, uphill returns to health" with allowances for "multiple levels of functioning in housing, occupational and social skills" (Harding, Zubin, and Strauss, 1992).

The International Study of Schizophrenia (ISoS) offers a singular opportunity to test the prospect of "slow, uphill" progress in cross-cultural cohorts of great diversity. The study encompasses a large number of treated incidence cohorts—chiefly from two earlier WHO studies, the Determinants of Outcome of Severe Mental Disorders, and the Reduction and Assessment of Psychiatric Disability—assembled from diverse catchment areas, using common case-finding techniques and inclusion criteria. To broaden the global representativeness of the follow-up study, these were supplemented by opportunistic cohorts from two additional centers, Chennai (Madras) and Hong Kong, where circumstances allowed the retrospective identification of broadly comparable incidence cases. It was possible, too, to include three prevalence cohorts from the original International Pilot Study of Schizophrenia, as well as an additional retrospective prevalence analysis cohort (Beijing), from which information about very long-term outcome may be gained. These additions not only ensured representation from China (the original IPSS center, Taipei, did not participate in ISoS), but also extended coverage of the Indian subcontinent to the south as well. In all, sufficient data for analysis were collected on 1043 individuals, from 18 study cohorts scattered across 16 field research centers. Follow-up times ranged from 12 to 26 years.

PLAN OF THE BOOK

This volume reports the findings of the ISoS, in aggregate and by individual Field Research Center. The five synoptic chapters address issues of methodology, overall course and outcome across the centers as a whole, mortality, diagnosis, and prediction of outcome. These are followed by 16 chapters, grouped by original substudy (except for Prague, which combines two), presenting the findings by individual center. A concluding chapter highlights findings and considers what might be gleaned about the role of culture in recovery from the evidence at hand.

A note on the tabulation of data is in order here. Readers will find three sets of tables at the end of the volume, displayed by center:

- Set A (4 tables) Baseline and Short-Term Follow-Up
- Set B (35 tables) Course and Outcome for the Alive Cohort
- Set C (6 tables) Deceased Subjects

The appendices contain additional data drawn upon in reporting findings in both synoptic and center chapters. We are in the process of creating an Internet website that will describe the ISoS study, provide the schedules used with accompanying instructions, and house the ISoS data in SAS and SPSS formats. The URL will be: http://csipmh.rfmh.org/isos.html.

POSTSCRIPT

This volume has had an unusually troubled publication history. The completed manuscript was delivered to our original publisher in the spring of 1999. For reasons never explained, production stalled and communication shut down, stranding the manuscript in a kind of limbo. Outside counsel and formal proceedings were required to recover copyright from the original publisher. In 2006, Oxford University Press formally took the book over and brought its production to fruition. We are grateful to Marion Osmun of Oxford for her commitment to expediting the publication process and to seeing this long-delayed project through to completion.

A word, too, about lapsed time: In the decade or so since ISoS data collection ended, globalization has extended its reach substantially and the pace of change has accelerated everywhere. That said, we have elected *not* to modify the area profiles with which each center chapter begins, for the simple reason that the portraits contained there—locked as they are in an "ethnographic present"—remain faithful descriptions of the local circumstances that prevailed at the time these subjects were interviewed. Updating the descriptions without re-examining the subjects would have been misleading. If context matters to the story of recovery recounted here, these profiles capture its dimensions for the long-term course of illness our research teams set out to track and assess.

By way of bringing the book's survey into the current era, however, we present here a brief summary of recent developments in the study of schizophrenia. Indeed, research into the course and outcome of schizophrenia, along with rigorous inquiry into interventions that can positively affect that trajectory, has made considerable progress since the early 1990s when the last of our studies' data were collected (Jablensky, 2000). Among notable findings and initiatives:

- Recent work has underscored the importance of cognitive impairments in schizophrenia, especially in the areas of verbal memory, executive functioning, and vigilance. Their effects on adaptive function and long-term course of illness may be substantial. Important as barriers to functioning in their own right, such deficits may also moderate the effectiveness of psychosocial interventions (Green, 1996; Velligan et al., 2000) and so may warrant specialized interventions (McGurk et al., 2003; Hogarty et al., 2004).
- Even with access to optimal medications, a host of disabling contingencies may apply, ranging from scarce jobs, to inadequate housing, poor social skills, clueless friends, and anxious and unsupportive families. Psychosocial interventions address such collateral difficulties. Careful studies confirm the wisdom of combining psychosocial with psychopharmacological interventions to enhance treatment outcomes in schizophrenia (Fenton and Schooler, 2000). These synergistic effects extend to the new atypical medications as well (Rosenheck et al., 1998). Some interventions are specifically targeted: resurgence of interest in designing supported employment prospects for persons with psychiatric histories, even in rapidly globalizing economies with tight labor markets, attests both to the importance of socially valued participation in the work of recovery and to the necessity of non-market approaches to this kind of integration (Becker and Drake, 2003; Marwaha and Johnson, 2004). Peer support groups, too, are a burgeoning force for both advocacy and recovery (Clay, 2005; Sayce, 2000; Davidson et al., 1999), and have vastly expanded their reach through the Internet (Haker et al., 2005; see, for example, Schizophrenia.org; PeopleWho.org; MindFreedom.org). Work with families has been shown to have positive effects on relapse prevention and social functioning (Leff, 2000). Building on WHO-initiated work in disability assessment (Janca et al., 1996; WHO, 2001), researchers are grappling as well with profound conceptual and measurement issues in assessing "quality of life" in psychiatry (Katschnig et al., 2005).
- After a period of relative neglect, clinical and epidemiological research has returned in recent years to document the frequency and severity of co-morbid physical disorders in persons diagnosed with schizophrenia, an association often missed in research studies where such conditions are reasons for exclusion. Commonly found conditions include diabetes, hyperlipidaemia, cardiovascular disease, and obesity, and there has been much debate about the possible contributory role of antipsychotic medications (Lambert et al., 2003; Lieberman et al., 2005). Even if their contribution to early mortality has been eased by the availability of modern treatments in countries where such statistics are routinely available, these conditions add to the disabling toll of impairment and suffering (Jeste et al., 1996; Goldman, 1999).
- More aggressive, effective, and insistently participatory approaches to reducing the stigma of severe mental illness have been mounted in an impressive range of settings. The World Psychiatric Association's *Open the Doors* program documents an array of effective approaches to combating stigma, ranging from organizing of stakeholder groups (people living with schizophrenia), to staged public events (plays, films, theater workshops), to targeted outreach to other sectors (police, high schools, judicial system); its coordinators stress that the program's durability will be essential to effectiveness. Social marketing approaches have been adapted to enlist institutional allies and shape interventions for specific audiences (Sartorius and Schulze, 2005; Warner, 2005). Other advocates stress the damage done by self-stigmatizing in a hostile and uncomprehending culture and place great importance on protest, education, and direct contact with first-person representatives (service users or family members) by any anti-stigma campaigns (Corrigan, 2005). Increasing attention is being paid, too, to the role of power in stigma and to its often structural nature, as when discriminatory laws and practices enforce social exclusion even in the absence of individuals acting in a prejudicial manner (Link and Phelan, 2001; Angermeyer and Schulze, 2001).
- Finally, drawing inspiration from follow-up studies showing the importance of social and cultural factors in shaping long-term outcomes of illness, a steadily mounting number of studies are pursuing

an "upstream" (or primary causal) role for psychosocial factors in the development of schizophrenia, likely to be interacting with genetic predispositions. Distressed groups, such as minority migrants in inhospitable settings exposing them to repeated instances of "social defeat," may be especially at risk (Harrison, 2004; Selten & Cantor-Graae, 2005).

Kim Hopper
Glynn Harrison
Aleksandar Janca
Norman Sartorius

REFERENCES

Angermeyer, M. C. & Schulze, B. (2001), Reducing the stigma of schizophrenia: Understanding the process and options for interventions. *Epidemiologia e Psichiatria Sociale* 10:1–7.

Angst, J. (1988), European long-term follow-up studies of schizophrenia. *Schizophr. Bull.* 14:501–513.

Becker, D. R., & Drake, R. E. (2003), *A Working Life for Persons with Severe Mental Illness*. New York: Oxford University Press.

Bleuler, M. (1978), *The Schizophrenic Disorders. Long-Term Patient and Family Studies*, tr. S. M. Clemens. New Haven, CT: Yale University Press.

Ciompi, L. (1980), Catamnestic long-term study on the course of life and aging of schizophrenics. *Schizophr. Bull.*, 5:606–618.

—— (1985), Aging and schizophrenic psychosis. *Acta Psychiatr. Scand.*, 71:93–105.

Clay, S. (2005), *On Our Own, Together*. Nashville: Vanderbilt University Press.

Corrigan, P. W., ed. (2005), *On the Stigma of Mental Illness*. Washington, D.C.: American Psychological Association.

Davidson, L., Chinman, M., Kloos, B., Weingarten, R., Stayner, D., & Tebes, J. K. (1999), Peer support among individuals with severe mental illness: A review of the evidence. *Clin. Psychol. Sci. Prac.*, 6 (2): 165–187.

Fenton, W. S. (1996), Longitudinal course and outcome in schizophrenia. In: *Handbook of Mental Health Economics and Health Policy*, Vol. 1, ed. M. Moscarelli, A. Rupp, & N. Sartorius. New York: Wiley.

Fenton, W. S., & Schooler, N. R., (eds.) (2000), Evidence-based psychosocial treatment for schizophrenia. Special Issue of *Schizophr. Bull.*, 26:1–155.

Goldman, L. S. (1999), Medical illness in patients with schizophrenia. *J. Clin. Psychiatry*, (Suppl.) 60, 21:15.

Green, M. F. (1996), What are the functional consequences of neurocognitive deficits in schizophrenia? *Am. J. Psychiatry*, 153:321–330.

Haker, H., Lauber, C., & Rösler, W. (2005), Internet forums: A self-help approach for individuals with schizophrenia? *Acta Psychiatr. Scand.* 112:474–477.

Harding, C. M., Brooks, G. W., Ashikaga, T., Strauss, J. S., & Breier, A. (1987), The Vermont longitudinal study of persons with severe mental illness. 1. Methodology, study samples, and overall status 32 years later. *Amer. J. Psychiatry*, 144:718–726.

—— Zubin, J., & Strauss, J. S. (1992), Chronicity in schizophrenia: Revisited. *Brit. J. Psychiatry*, 161(Suppl. 18): 27–37.

Harrison, G. (2004), Course and outcome in schizophrenia. Towards a new social biology of psychotic disorders. In: *Search for the Causes of Schizophrenia*, Vol. 5, ed. W.F. Gattaz & H. Hafner. Steinkopff Verlag Darmstadt.

Harrison, G., & Mason, P. (1993), Schizophrenia: Falling incidence and better outcome? *Brit. J. Psychiatry*, 163: 535–541.

Hawk, A. B., Carpenter, W. T., & Strauss, J. S. (1975), Diagnostic criteria and 5-year outcome in schizophrenia: A report from the International Pilot Study of Schizophrenia. *Arch. Gen. Psychiatry*, 32:343–347.

Hegarty, J. D., Baldessarini, R. J., Tohen, M., Waternaux, C., & Oepen, G. (1994), One hundred years of schizophrenia. A metaanalysis of the outcome literature. *Amer. J. Psychiatry*, 151:1409–1416.

Hogarty, G. E., Flesher, S., Ulrich, R., Carter, M., Greenwald, D., Pogue-Geile, M., Kechavan, M., Cooley, S., DiBarry, A. L., Garrett, A., Parepally, H., & Zoretich, R. (2004), Cognitive enhancement therapy for schizophrenia: Effects of a 2-year randomized trial on cognition and behavior. *Arch. Gen. Psychiatry*, 61:866–876.

Huber, G., Gross, G., & Schuttler, R. A. (1975), A long-term follow-up study of schizophrenia: Psychiatric course of illness and prognosis. *Acta Psychiatr. Scand.*, 52:49–57.

Jablensky, A. (2000), Epidemiology of schizophrenia: The global burden of disease and disability. *Eur. Arch. Psychiatr. Clin. Neuroscience*, 250:274–285.

Janca, A., Kastrup, M., Katschnig, H., Lopez-Ibor, J., Mezzich, J., & Sartorius, N. (1996), The ICD-10 Multiaxial System for Use in Adult Psychiatry: Structure and Applications. *J. Nervous & Mental Disease*, 184: 191–192.

Jeste, D. V., Gladsjo, J. A., Lindamer, L. A., & Lacro, J. P. (1996), Medical comorbidity in schizophrenia. *Schizophr. Bull.*, 22:413–430.

Johnstone, E. C. (1991), Disability and circumstances of schizophrenic patients—A follow-up study. *Brit. J. Psychiatry*, 159 (Suppl. 13):1–46.

Katschnig, H., Freeman, H., & Sartorius, N. (Eds.) (2005), *Quality of Life in Mental Disorders*, 2nd edition. New York: John Wiley.

Kleinman, A. (1988), *Rethinking Psychiatry*. New York: Basic Books.

Kraepelin, E. (1893), *Dementia Praecox and Paraphrenia*, tr. M. Barclay, ed. G. M. Robertson. Huntington, New York: Robert E. Kreiger, 1971.

Lambert, T. J. R., Velakoulins, D., & Pantelis, C. (2003), Medical comorbidity in schizophrenia. *Med. J. Australia*, 178 (9) (Suppl 5):S67–S70.

Leff, J. (2000), Family work for schizophrenia: practical application. *Acta Psychiatr. Scand.*, 102 (Suppl. 407):78–82.

Lieberman, J. A., Stroup, T. S., McEvoy, J. P., Swartz, M. S., Rosenheck, R. A., Perkins, D. O., Keefe, R. S. E., Davis, S. M., Davis, C. E., Lebowitz, B. D., Severe, J., & Hsiao, J. K. (2005), Effectiveness of antipsychotic drugs in patients with chronic schizophrenia. *N. E. J. Med*, 353:1209–1223.

Link, B. G., & Phelan, J. (2001), Conceptualizing stigma. *Ann. Rev. Sociology*, 27:363–385.

Marwaha, S., & Johnson, S. (2004), Schizophrenia and employment. *Social Psychiatry and Psychiatric Epidemiology*, 39:337–349.

McGlashan, T. H. (1984), The Chestnut Lodge follow-study. II. Long-term outcome of schizophrenia and the affective disorders. *Arch. Gen. Psychiatry*, 41:586–601.

McGurk, S. R., Mueser, K. T., Harvey, P. D., LaPuglia, R., & Marder, J. (2003), Cognitive and symptoms predictors of work outcomes for clients with schizophrenia in supported employment. *Psychiatric Services*, 54:1129–1135.

Ogawa, K., Miya, M., Watarai, A., Nakazawa, M., Yuasa, S., & Utena, H. (1987), A long-term follow-up study of schizophrenia in Japan—with special reference to the course of social adjustment. *Brit. J. Psychiatry*, 151: 758–765.

Ram, R., Bromet, E. J., Eaton, W. W., Pato, C., & Schwartz, J. E. (1992), The natural course of schizophrenia: A review of first admission studies. *Schizophr. Bull.*, 18: 185–207.

Rosenheck, R., Tekell, J., Peters, J., Cramer, J., Fontana, A., Xu, W., Thomas, J., Henderson, W., & Charney, D. (1998), Does participation in psychosocial treatment augment the benefit of clozapine? *Arch. Gen. Psychiatr.*, 55:618–625.

Schwartz, F., Terkelsen, K. G., & Smith, T. E. (1992), Long term outcome in schizophrenia. *Arch. Gen. Psychiatry*, 49:502–503.

Selten, J-P., & Cantor-Graae, E. (2005), Social defeat: risk factor for schizophrenia? *Brit. J. Psychiatry*, 187:101–102.

Sartorius, N., & Schulze, H. (2005), *Reducing the Stigma of Mental Illness: A Report from a Global Programme of the World Psychiatric Association*. New York: Cambridge.

Sayce, L. (2000), *From Psychiatric Patient to Citizen*. New York: Routledge.

Shepherd, M., Watt, D., Falloon, I., & Smeeton, J. (1989), The natural history of schizophrenia: A five-year follow-up study of outcome and prediction in a representative sample of schizophrenics. *Psycholog. Med.*, (Suppl.)15:1–45.

Tsuang, M. T., Woolson, R., & Fleming, J. (1979), Long-term outcome of major psychoses: 1. Schizophrenia and affective disorders compared with psychiatrically symptom-free surgical conditions. *Arch. Gen. Psychiatry*, 36:1295–1301.

Velligan, D. I., Bow-Thomas, C. C., Mahurin, R. K., Miller, A. L., & Halgunseth, L. (2000), Do specific neurocognitive deficits predict specific domains of community function in schizophrenia? *J. Nervous & Mental Disease*, 188:518–524.

Warner, R. (1985), *Recovery from Schizophrenia: Psychiatry and Political Economy*. London: Routledge & Kegan Paul.

———. (2005), Local projects of the World Psychiatric Association Programme to Reduce Stigma and Discrimination. *Psychiatric Services*, 56:70–575.

World Health Organization (2001), *International Classification of Functioning, Disability and Health*. Geneva.

Acknowledgments

This book is based on the data and experience obtained in the *International Study of Schizophrenia* (ISoS), a project sponsored by the World Health Organization, the Laureate Foundation (United States of America), and the participating centers.

The *International Study of Schizophrenia*, a transcultural investigation coordinated by WHO in 18 centers in 14 countries, was designed to examine patterns of long-term course and outcome of severe mental disorders in different cultures, to develop further methods for the study of characteristics of mental disorders and their course in different settings, and to strengthen the scientific basis for future international multidisciplinary research on schizophrenia and other psychiatric disorders seen in a public health perspective.

The chief collaborating investigators in the field research centers are: Aarhus, Denmark: A. Bertelsen; Agra, India: K. C. Dube; Beijing, China: Y. Shen; Cali, Colombia: C. León; Chandigarh, India: V. Varma and (since 1994) S. Malhotra; Dublin, Ireland: D. Walsh; Groningen, The Netherlands: R. Giel and (since 1994) D. Wiersma; Hong Kong: P. W. H. Lee; Honolulu, Hawai'i: A. J. Marsella; Chennai (Madras), India: R. Thara; Mannheim, Germany: H. Häfner and (since 1989) W. an der Heiden; Moscow, Russia: S. J. Tsirkin; Nagasaki, Japan: Y. Nakane; Nottingham, U.K.: G. Harrison; Prague, Czech Republic: C. Skoda; Rochester, NY: L. Wynne; and Sofia, Bulgaria: K. Ganev. Coordination of the data collection, experimental design, and data analysis were carried out by the WHO Collaborating Center at the Nathan S. Kline Institute for Psychiatric Research under the direction of E. Laska. At WHO Headquarters, Geneva, the study has been coordinated by N. Sartorius (until August 1993), by W. Gulbinat (September 1993–April 1996), and by A. Janca (since May 1996).

The views expressed in this book are the collective views of an international group of researchers and do not necessarily represent the views or policy of the World Health Organization.

Cross-cultural studies of this magnitude and range present obvious logistical and, for want of a better term, *momentum* problems. Standardization and coordination of data collection, transmission, cleaning, and analysis present huge problems whose resolution can be time-consuming and frustrating. Vast distances and time zones must be spanned, and although computer technology represents a substantial advance, its power is diminished in areas where the equipment itself is not readily available. And always, funds must be found, renewed when deadlines lapse, and their sources reassured of progress. Finally, political upheavals—in the interval between baseline and follow-up, the national boundaries and/or central governments of four of the participating centers were restructured—complicate matters further.

Throughout it all, Walter Gulbinat, formerly a senior scientist at the World Health Organization (WHO) and personally responsible for on-site troubleshooting for most of the project, and Dr. Eugene Laska, Chief of the Statistical Sciences and Epidemiology Division at the Nathan S. Kline Institute (NKI) and Director of the WHO Collaborating Center at NKI, provided the steady hands and clear vision needed to see the effort through to completion. The final report owes much to the individual directors of Field Research Centers. Special mention should be made of the long tenure of the late Dr. Ctirad Skoda.

The patience and steadfast support of the Laureate Foundation (now the Warren Medical Research Center, the William K. Warren Foundation, and Laureate Psychiatric Clinic and Hospital within the St. Francis

Health System, Tulsa, Oklahoma) are a model of what generous private funding can provide in pursuit of a public good. In particular, we acknowledge the late Dr. Robert Tompkins, then project officer at the Laureate Foundation, for his unfailingly courtly advice and watchful interest. The Laureate Foundation also sponsored a meeting of investigators at a critical juncture in October 1992, which clinched agreement on instruments.

Several other investigators hosted strategic meetings of investigators, providing the continuity needed to sustain a collaborative enterprise over time and through obstacles: Dr. F. Lieh Mak in Hong Kong, April 1991; Dr. Axel Bertelsen in Aarhus, Denmark, August 1991; Dr. Eugene Laska in Orangeburg, New York, United States, March 1996; Dr. Giovanni de Girolamo in Bologna, Italy, September 1995; and Drs. Dirk Wiersma and Fokko Nienhuis in Groningen, The Netherlands, November 1996.

A number of investigators played crucial enabling roles in the early stages of mounting the ISoS but, for various reasons, were unable to see the project through to closure. We thank Drs. Kathryn Abel, Axel Bertelsen, T. Baasher, O. Baiyewu, John Cooper, Martin Katz, Tsung-yi Lin, Alan Lipton, M. Olatawura, Steen Straarup, and E. Strömgren. Special thanks, too, are owed Dr. Ezra Susser, who initiated and led the study in its first two years, and Sarah Conover for her early work on research design and instrumentation.

The names of several NKI staff recur throughout this report, but such mention is a poor index of services rendered. David Bertollo designed the computer formatting for recording and transmitting ISoS data, greatly easing the task of further analyses. Special mention should be made, too, of the data cleaning, organizing, and analyzing work of Joe Wanderling and Dr. Sherryl Baker; they were responsible for preparing the tables and shepherding the computer runs that made possible the analyses in the pages that follow. For stalwart secretarial support, we thank the late Mary Stebbins and Evelyn Rand Whalen. Finally, no longitudinal project worth its salt can succeed without an institutional memory. For ISoS, the late Rheta Bank performed that function, faithfully serving as archivist, organizer, administrator, e-mail impressaria, and correspondent.

The Editors

Abbreviations

BII	Basic Information on Informants
BIS	Basic Information on Study Subject
BRS	Broad Rating Schedule
CART	Classification and Regression Trees
CIMH	Central Institute for Mental Health
CMH	Community Mental Health Clinic
CNS	Central Nervous System
DAS	Disability Assessment Schedule
DOSMeD	Determinants of Outcome of Severe Mental Disorders
DSM	Diagnostic and Statistical Manual of Mental Disorders
DSS	Diagnostic Schedule Scoresheet
EE	Expressed Emotion
FIS	Family Interview Schedule
FRG	Federal Republic of Germany
FTP	File Transfer Protocol
GAF	Global Assessment of Functioning
GAF-D	Global Assessment of Functioning—Disability
GAF-S	Global Assessment of Functioning—Symptomatology
GDR	German Democratic Republic
ICC	Intra-Class Correlation Coefficient
ICD	International Classification of Diseases
IMH	Integrated Mental Health
IOR	Information on Refusers
IPSS	International Pilot Study of Schizophrenia
IRB	Institutional Review Board
ISoS	International Study of Schizophrenia
LAP	Local Area Profile
LCS	Life Chart Schedule
MHTS	Mental Health Treatment System Survey
NKI	Nathan Kline Institute
PAR	Pairwise Agreement Ratio
PIRS	Psychological Impairments Rating Schedule
PPHS	Psychiatric and Personal History Schedule
PSE	Present State Examination
RAPYD	Reducation and Assessment of Psychiatric Disability
SANS	Scale for the Assessment of Negative Symptoms
SAS	Statistical Analysis Software
SAS	Substance Abuse Schedule
SDP	Schedule for Deceased Patients
SPSS	Statistical Package for the Social Sciences
WHO	World Health Organization

Part I

Background

Chapter 1

Twenty-five Years of WHO-Coordinated Activities Concerning Schizophrenia

Norman Sartorius

Some 20 million people in the world suffer from schizophrenia. The disease usually starts early and often has a chronic, disabling course. Treatment, unless rationalized, can be expensive, and the losses in terms of working capacity are staggering. Family members of patients experience disadvantages because of the stigma attached to both the diseased person and his or her relatives. Schizophrenia is a major public health problem.

Despite advances in our knowledge about schizophrenia in the past few decades, nothing allows us to surmise that the causes of schizophrenia will soon become known, or that the prevention of the disorder will become possible in the immediate future. Nor is it likely that it will become easier to help people with schizophrenia: The increasing complexity of human society and the disruption of social networks often accompanying economic growth raise the probability that despite progress in treatment, schizophrenia will continue to result in disability and in diminished quality of life. In addition, the increased life expectancy at all ages in most countries and the consequent increase in the numbers of young adults—the population group at highest risk for schizophrenia—allows the prediction that the prevalence of schizophrenia will grow significantly over the next few decades.

These facts were among the reasons that made the World Health Organization (WHO) pay special attention to the problem and launch or stimulate studies seeking a better understanding of schizophrenia and more effective ways to deal with it. These investigations aim at: (1) advancing understanding of the nature of schizophrenia—its form, course, and outcome in different sociocultural settings; (2) improving methods of treatment of schizophrenia; and (3) determining how health and other social services can best apply knowledge about schizophrenia in the provision of care, in programs of rehabilitation, and in mental health education of the general population.

The basis for work in this area was laid in the early 1960s following the recommendations of an expert committee on the epidemiology of mental disorders (WHO, 1960). That committee urged WHO to (1) develop methods which would allow standardization of the assessment of psychiatric patients in different cultures; (2) promote the use of these methods in epidemiological studies and in training mental health workers; and (3) carry out comparative studies of mental disorders in different cultures.

A few years later, the first major WHO-coordinated study on schizophrenia was launched (WHO, 1973). The International Pilot Study of Schizophrenia (IPSS) was seen as preparing the ground for in-depth studies of schizophrenia and other mental disorders. Its aims were to address basic methodological problems and to answer questions about the nature and distribution of schizophrenia. The three major methodological questions the study set out to answer were:

1. Is it feasible to carry out a large-scale international psychiatric study requiring the coordination and collaboration of psychiatrists and mental health workers from different theoretical backgrounds and from widely separated countries with different cultures and socioeconomic conditions?
2. Is it possible to develop standardized research instruments and procedures for psychiatric assessments that can be reliably applied in a variety of cultural settings?
3. Can teams of research workers be trained to use such instruments and procedures so that comparable observations can be made both in developed and developing countries?

The major questions about the nature and distribution of schizophrenia this study was intended to explore were:

1. In what sense can it be said that schizophrenic disorders exist in different parts of the world?
2. Are there groups of schizophrenic patients with similar characteristics present in every one of the countries studied?
3. Are there groups of schizophrenic patients whose symptoms differ in form or content from one country to another, and if so, are such differences the result of variations in diagnostic practice or are they true cultural differences in the manner of presentation of the various types of schizophrenia?
4. Do the clinical course and social outcome of schizophrenia in one country or group of countries differ from those in other countries?
5. How do the characteristics of schizophrenic patients compare with those of patients with other psychoses in various countries?
6. Do the courses of other psychoses differ from country to country?

To answer the questions outlined above, a comparative prospective study was designed. A series of psychotic patients was selected from among those contacting psychiatric services in nine countries. These patients were examined in a systematic and standardized fashion, and as many as possible were followed up 2 and 5 years after the initial examination. The field research centers that participated in this study were in Cali (Colombia), Taipei (China), Prague (Czech Republic), Aarhus (Denmark), Agra (India), Ibadan (Nigeria), Moscow (Russia), London (U.K.), and Washington, DC (United States). Each field research center assessed all patients contacting specified mental health facilities with two screens (demographic and psychosis) that were designed to select patients with functional psychoses who would likely be available for long-term follow-up. The psychosis screen identified all patients who passed the demographic screen, who did not meet any of the exclusion criteria, and who met at least one of the inclusion criteria. Exclusion criteria screened out chronic patients and patients whose conditions may have been caused or significantly influenced by an organic condition. Inclusion categories were divided into symptoms whose presence automatically qualified the patient regardless of degree of severity (i.e., delusions, hallucinations, gross psychomotor disorder, and definitely inappropriate and unusual behavior), and those which would qualify a prospective subject only if present in severe degree (i.e., social withdrawal, disorders of form of thinking, overwhelming fear, disorders of affect, self-neglect, and depersonalization).

In all, the study population consisted of 1202 patients, divided approximately equally over the nine centers. Of these, 811 had a center diagnosis of schizophrenia, 164 affective psychosis, 29 paranoid psychosis, 73 other psychoses, 71 neurotic depression, and 54 had other diagnoses. Although IPSS was not designed to select patients who were representative of all schizophrenic patients, or of all patients with functional psychoses seen at the centers, it is nevertheless of interest to know to what extent IPSS patients are typical of all patients seen. The collaborating investigators were asked, therefore, to give their impressions about the typicality of the series of patients from their centers. It was the general impression that, taking into consideration that very young, very old, and chronic patients were excluded by design, the schizophrenic patients and the patients with affective psychoses included in the IPSS were, for the most part, typical with regard to clinical characteristics of all such relatively acute patients within the stated age range admitted to the centers.

Each of the 1202 patients received an intensive, lengthy (about 5 hours) initial evaluation at the field research centers, resulting in the accumulation of some 1600 items of information. Data were elicited with eight standardized instruments developed or adapted for the study. A full description of the instruments and reliability data about their use is presented in Volume 1 of the IPSS Report (WHO, 1973) and in the review of WHO instruments for the assessment of mental illness (Sartorius and Janca, 1995, 1996).

The study provided answers to the three methodological questions that it set out to explore: that (1) it is possible to carry out effectively a large-scale cross-cultural investigation of psychiatric disorders; (2) transculturally applicable instruments for psychiatric research can be produced; and (3) teams of research workers can be trained to use standardized research instruments and procedures so that comparable observations can be made in both developed and developing countries.

Questions about the nature and distribution of schizophrenia were approached by analysis of the psychopathology of patient groups, application of computer-simulated diagnosis, cluster analysis, and the identification and description of a concordant category of schizophrenia on which three methods of classification agree.

The results of the analysis of the psychopathology of patient groups and the application of computer-simulated diagnosis indicated that the major functional psychoses were present in each of the centers, and that there were some groups of schizophrenic patients who had center-specific characteristics. A follow-up study conducted in all nine centers aimed to determine the feasibility of tracing patients suffering from schizophrenia and other functional psychoses and of examining the course and outcome of patients living in the different cultures. This latter study demonstrated that it is feasible, in many different cultures, to reinterview, to assess the mental status of, and to collect psychiatric and social history data about a high percentage of patients with functional psychoses 2 years after an initial evaluation. It also showed that there were sharp differences in the course and outcome of schizophrenia in the different centers (WHO, 1979).

When seen at the time of the second-year follow-up, 37% (202 of 543) of schizophrenic patients followed up were psychotic; 31% (169 of 543) were symptomatic but not psychotic; and 32% (172 of 543) were asymptomatic. Ibadan patients clearly had the best course and outcome: 57% fell into the best overall outcome group, while only 5% fell into the worst overall outcome. Agra patients had the next best course and outcome for most of the factors considered, including overall outcome. Aarhus patients had the worst course and outcome: 50% were still in the episode of inclusion at the time of the second-year follow-up; 31% fell into the worst overall outcome group, and only 6% into the best group. The other centers varied according to the factor being assessed. In general, Cali and Moscow patients had an intermediate outcome, and Washington, DC, Taipei, and Prague patients a relatively poor outcome.

For all variables considered, the schizophrenic patients in Ibadan, Agra, and Cali (all centers in developing countries) tended to have a better outcome on average than the schizophrenic patients in the other six centers. Furthermore, it was shown that no single variable and no combination of a few "key" variables could explain a large proportion of the variation of any of the course and outcome measures in schizophrenia; in other words, no characteristics of the patient, of the environment, or of the initial manifestations of the disorder considered in isolation would be an effective predictor of the subsequent course and outcome of the illness.

In view of the great potential significance of the IPSS finding, WHO decided to undertake a new study focused more sharply than the IPSS on the frequency of occurrence, the natural history of schizophrenic illness, and the factors associated with differences in course and outcome in representative patient samples in different cultures (Sartorius et al., 1986; Jablensky et al., 1992). The case-finding strategy designed for the new study consisted of: (1) a prospective surveillance of specified psychiatric, other medical, and social services in a given catchment area in each setting; and (2) identification of all individuals making a first lifetime contact with such services who exhibited signs and symptoms of a possible schizophrenic illness.[1] By extending the case-finding network to include a variety of "helping agencies" in the community (e.g., religious institutions, traditional healers), this strategy was expected to result in better coverage of the incident cases of the disorder than the first admission method, although persons who never contact any agency would still be missed.

Several research techniques used in other studies that had earlier thrown light on specific facets of the course of schizophrenia were also used. These included ascertainment of stressful life events prior to the onset of psychotic episodes, measurement of "expressed emotion" in a key relative, assessment of the perception of psychotic symptoms by the patient's family, and evaluation of functional impairment and social disability. It was hoped that the application of these techniques might help to obtain data that could contribute to an explanation of the extraordinary finding of the IPSS that patients in developing countries on the whole have a better outcome than those living in more developed countries.

The total population included in this second major study consisted of 1379 subjects (745 men and 634 women), most of whom were urban residents. With the exception of Ibadan, Cali, and the rural area of

1. The alternative design of a cross-sectional community survey, in which a representative Prevalence sample of cases is identified first and Incidence is then estimated by attempting to date retrospectively the onset of the disorder, was rejected because of (a) low yield of cases per 1000 persons who have to be interviewed; (b) certainty of missing patients who either died early after the onset of a psychotic illness or migrated out of the area; and (c) exposure of the patients to periods of treatment of varying length and to psychosocial environmental influences that might alter the presenting features of the disorder.

Chandigarh where most patients came from very poor neighborhoods, in the majority of cases the socioeconomic status of the patients' neighborhoods and households in the other centers was rated as "average" in comparison with local standards. The great majority, 86% of the 1218 cases in whom the beginning of the psychotic illness could be dated, had been identified by the case-finding network and assessed within 12 months of the onset of the disorder; in 61%, this had occurred within 3 months. With regard to the proportion of patients with length of previous illness less than 6 months and with 6 months and over, there was no significant difference between the centers in developed and those in developing countries.

The study permitted the calculation of incidence of schizophrenia with a "broad" diagnostic definition of the condition (i.e., all included cases except 34 for whom insufficient data were available) and with a "restrictive" definition based only on the presence of an initial clinical picture satisfying the criteria for CATEGO class S+ (Wing, Cooper, and Sartorius, 1974). The annual rates were obtained by halving the number of cases identified over 2 years of continuous case-finding and dividing them by the denominator value. The analysis of incidence was carried out using data from eight catchment areas in which satisfactory coverage of all potential "helping agencies" that might have been contacted was achieved. For the "broad" definition of schizophrenia and related illnesses, the combined rates for males and females amounted to 3.7 and 4.8 per 10,000, respectively. The lowest rates for males (1.8) were found in Aarhus and Honolulu; for females, the lowest rate (1.2) was in Aarhus. Differences across the areas were statistically significant for both males and females.

The application of the "restrictive" definition of the CATEGO S+ class resulted in lower combined rates for males and females, ranging from 0.7 in Aarhus to 1.4 in Nottingham. In males, the lowest rate of 0.8 was in Chandigarh (urban area) and the highest rate of 1.7 was in Nottingham. In females, the lowest rate (0.5) was found in Aarhus and the highest rate (1.4) in Moscow. The differences in the incidence rates of disorders meeting the CATEGO S+ criteria were not statistically significant in males and only marginally significant in females. The change in range occurring with the application of the "restrictive" definition cannot be explained simply as a loss of the statistical significance of the differences because of a drop in the statistical power to detect such differences in smaller samples: The *actual* values of the incidence rates in the different centers do indeed become more similar, contrary to what might be expected as the result of a mere decrease of individual sample sizes in diagnostically heterogeneous populations. This lends support to the notion that the "central" schizophrenic syndrome may be occurring with approximately equal probability in different populations.

Follow-up examinations of patients, with the full battery of research instruments (including follow-up versions of the Psychiatric History schedule, Social Description and Diagnostic Assessment schedules), were carried out twice, at 1 and 2 years following the baseline assessments. In addition to two cross sections of symptomatology and one assessment of social disability, the longitudinal, month-by-month ratings and narrative notes on symptoms and behavior provided the basis for an evaluation of the 2-year (24 ± 6 months) pattern of course of the disorder. Complete follow-up data were available on 1014 (74%) of the original 1379 patients; 600 subjects were assessed in developed countries (76% coverage) and 414 in centers in developing countries (71% coverage).

A significantly higher percentage (56%) of the subjects in developing countries exhibited "mild" patterns of course, compared to their counterparts in developed countries (39%). At the same time, a significantly higher percentage (40%) of the cases in developed countries had "severe" patterns of course, compared to the cases in developing countries (24%). The proportions falling into the "intermediate" group were almost identical in the two groups.

The other studies mentioned above—on the frequency of life events (Day et al., 1987), emotional interaction in families of schizophrenic patients (Leff et al., 1987), and the perception of schizophrenic patients by their families (Katz et al., 1988)—were also successfully completed. Each of these studies made a methodological contribution and produced new knowledge about schizophrenia. They involved a large number of investigators and centers in a variety of countries. The collaboration among these centers established in the course of these studies continued after the studies were terminated and is undoubtedly a most valuable achievement of this work. Among the noteworthy findings of these studies were:

1. The study on the association of life events and schizophrenia provided substantial evidence that there is a temporal association between stressful life events and the onset of episodes of

schizophrenia. It could not, however, determine the precise nature and extent of the causal effect, and so concluded only that stressful life events are among the risk factors associated with the onset of schizophrenia.

2. The series of studies dealing with expressed emotions and schizophrenia in different cultures demonstrated that the methods used in the assessment of expressed emotions can be used in cultures that are very different from those for which they were originally developed. In the comparison of components of expressed emotion among two samples of relatives of first-contact patients from Aarhus (Denmark) and Chandigarh (India), it was shown that the Danes were very similar in most respects to samples of British relatives, whereas the Indian relatives expressed significantly fewer critical comments, fewer positive remarks, and less overinvolvement. Within the Chandigarh sample, city dwellers were significantly more expressive than villagers in all expressed emotion (EE) components except overinvolvement.

   In the one-year follow-up of schizophrenic patients in Chandigarh, a statistically significant relationship between relatives' hostility (using the same criteria as in the Anglo-American studies for "high EE") and relapse was found. This relationship was not explained by other factors often associated with higher relapse rates. The conclusion of that study was that the significantly better outcome of Chandigarh first-contact patients compared with a London sample was largely due to the significantly lower proportion of high-EE relatives in the North Indian sample.

3. The study of the manner in which psychosis was perceived in different cultures showed that Indian patients diagnosed with schizophrenia were described by family members as manifesting a more affective and "self-centered" orientation; the Nigerian patients were described as being highly suspicious, bizarre in their behavior, and anxious. The main features of pathology were in general accord with the descriptions of indigenous psychiatrists. The special qualities of the psychosis in the two cultures were interpreted against the background of traditional psychopathological and anthropological theories concerning the psychodynamics and the influence of differing social conflictual themes in the two cultures.

Another international study, the Reduction and Assessment of Psychiatric Disability (1978), was launched by WHO in 1978 to explore possibilities for the reduction of behavioral impairments and social disabilities in schizophrenic patients with recent illness onset. Five hundred and twenty patients in seven countries were examined initially and again 1 and 2 years later (Jablensky, Schwarz, and Tomov, 1980). In addition to the schedules, which were used in the previous WHO studies of schizophrenia, two additional schedules were developed: the WHO Disability Assessment Schedule (DAS) and the Psychological Impairments Rating Schedule (PIRS). The PIRS was designed to record impairment, while the purpose of the DAS was to elicit and rate social role performance and identify environmental factors influencing such performance. This work permitted the study of the 2-year course of schizophrenia in terms of disability. A specific pattern in the occurrence of disabilities was demonstrated in the sense that performance in some social roles was impaired before others: Specifically, family relationships tended to suffer first, followed by work performance. Self-care, which had initially been preserved, became dysfunctional only when the majority of the other social roles had been impaired. Negative symptoms, such as inactivity, loss of interest and initiative, and poverty of speech, were the best predictors of outcome at the 2-year follow-up.

As such findings illustrate, many similarities have emerged in patients from geographically dispersed centers in terms of frequency of diagnostically important syndromes, the nature and severity of psychological and behavioral impairments, and the pattern of development of social role dysfunction. Taken together, these studies have resulted in a large pool of data about patients in many countries, in some of which the WHO investigations were the first systematic attempt to gather knowledge about the form, course, and outcome of schizophrenia. The various methods developed for these studies have since been used in research in these and other countries, a legacy that makes it fair to say that the cluster of WHO studies has made an important contribution to the improvement of mental health research technology worldwide.

There were, however, some questions posed when these studies were first contemplated that were not answered from the data collected. One might ask, for example, whether there are people suffering from schizophrenia whose symptoms are very different from those set as meriting inclusion for the WHO studies. This seems unlikely owing to the painstaking tracking of all cases that were reported to be sufficiently severe to require medical help in all of the cultures in which the studies were done; nevertheless, it is possible that such cases exist, even if they are very rare. Some of the explanatory studies undertaken to investigate the possible reasons for differences in the short-term course and outcome of schizophrenia in different cultures have produced valuable results, while failing to deliver definitive answers to the hypotheses that they were designed to explore. It would undoubtedly have been valuable to explore the implications of such results for the prediction of long-term course and outcome. For a variety of reasons, such an exploration was not possible. Finally, it seems plausible that other questions might have been posed, explicitly or implicitly, by some of the investigators at the beginning or during the course of the studies in the different centers, for which answers are yet forthcoming.

By and large, however, the group of WHO studies have addressed most of the original questions in a satisfactory manner. The results of the studies allow us today to state categorically that cases of schizophrenia with a well-defined clinical picture exist in different cultures; that multicenter studies—even of great complexity and involving investigators from different cultures—are possible, providing the centers and the collaborators are well selected, a modicum of material support is available, and continuous and appropriate institutional and individual leadership is provided; and, finally, that it is possible to develop instruments with cross-cultural applicability that yield valid and reliable results. These are achievements well worth the investment of time, money, and effort by the individuals who participated in the study, and by WHO, NIMH in the United States, and the institutions in the various countries.

At the same time, the results of these studies have opened new vistas and posed new questions. Accordingly, the most recent WHO-Collaborative Study, ISoS, was designed to:

- Describe the long-term (15–26 year) natural history of schizophrenia and related psychoses in a highly varied, multinational cohort;
- Determine which features of the short-term course and outcome of schizophrenia and related disorders are of significance in predicting the medium- (15 years) and long- (26 years) term course and outcome of these disorders;
- Examine the efficiency of diagnostic strategies in predicting long-term course and outcome, and explore possibly distinctive aspects of outcome for different diagnostic subgroups;
- Determine whether short-term differences in course and outcome between developing and developed countries are borne out in the long run;
- Identify contextual variables that might account for such differences (if borne out) as well as for certain anomalous findings (e.g., centers that fail to align with their assigned grouping), and to propose hypotheses for further causal inquiry; and
- Document the consequences of, and methods for coping with, episodes of schizophrenia in the lives of both sufferers and their families in different cultural settings.

The answers to such questions are of considerable practical and theoretical importance. Exploration of the differences in long-term course and outcome of severe mental disorder, both within and between developing and developed countries, would not only indicate directions for future research but also help in the planning of services for mentally ill people in different countries. Similarly, more informed choices with respect to individual therapy and rehabilitation, as well as techniques for supporting families, could come from better knowledge of the long-term consequences of falling ill.

The set of long-term follow-up studies described in this volume was undertaken to obtain data that would help to give an empirical answer to the questions listed above. Investigators in the centers that had taken part in the original WHO studies were approached first and invited to consider participating in the study; most replied positively. Next, investigators from several other centers were invited to ensure that at least some comparable answers were obtained from areas that were not covered by the original studies; here again it was possible to enlist the participation of several outstandingly well-qualified groups. The methods used to make the data that these new centers were to contribute comparable to the data gathered previously in the WHO studies are described in the relevant chapters. Still, the fact that a larger set of centers was recruited for this study in no way obviates the need to carry out similar studies in other settings and on other cultures—preferably using similar methods and striving to obtain results comparable with those obtained in this study.

This most recent effort to follow up persons diagnosed with severe mental disorder has several characteristics that distinguish it from previous WHO studies. First, the long-term follow-up study took place in a climate of increasing stringency of resources and thus required much more effort on the part of the investigators (e.g., to find resources for their work), all the more so since "central" funds provided by WHO or donors were insufficient to cover the study's expenses. Second, the collaborating centers have played a more important role in this study than in previous studies. The data analysis for the study as a whole, for example, has been entrusted to the Nathan Kline Institute, a center outside of WHO, and many of the activities in the course of the study (e.g., the organization of meetings) were taken on by the collaborating investigators without continuing technical or financial input by WHO. Third, the increasing commercial cooperation between countries has not been paralleled by enthusiasm or facilitation for international collaborative scientific work, particularly that involving developing countries. That the long-term follow-up study described in this volume was nevertheless a success is therefore all the more remarkable.

The chapters that follow rejoin the attempt, begun three decades ago by WHO, to chart the clinical course and social outcome of schizophrenia in its cross-cultural complexity. Much remains to be documented, but the broad plot lines, points of convergence and divergence, and overall narrative thrust are, we trust better understood for the efforts recounted here.

Acknowledgments Parts of this text were included in N. Sartorius (1988), "Solving the Conundrum of Schizophrenia: WHO's Contribution." In: *Schizophrenia: Recent Biosocial Developments*, ed. C. N. Stefanis & A. D. Rabavilas. New York: Human Sciences Press, pp. 23–28.

References

Day, R., Nielsen, J. A., Korten, A., Ernberg, G., Dube, K. C., Gebhart, J., Jablensky, A., León, C., Marsella, A., Olatawura, M., Sartorius, N., Stromgren, E., Takahashi, R., Wig, N., & Wynne, L. C. (1987), Stressful life events preceding the acute onset of schizophrenia: A cross-national study from the World Health Organization. *Cult., Med. & Psychiatry*, 11(2):123–205.

Jablensky, A., Sartorius, N., Ernberg, G., Anker, M., Korten, A., Cooper, J. E., Day, R., & Bertelsen, A. (1992), Schizophrenia: Manifestations, incidence and course in different cultures: A World Health Organization ten-country study. *Psycholog. Med.*, 20(Monogr. Suppl.):1–97.

——Schwarz, R., & Tomov, T. (1980), WHO collaborative study on impairments and disabilities. *Acta Psychiatr. Scand.*, (Suppl) 285:62–152.

Katz, M. M., Marsella, A., Dube, K. C., Olatawura, M., Takahashi, R., Nakane, Y., Wynne, L. C., Gift, T., Brennan, J., Sartorius, N., & Jablensky, A. (1988), On the expression of psychosis in different cultures: Schizophrenia in an Indian and in a Nigerian community: A report from the World Health Organization project on determinants of outcome of severe mental disorders. *Cult., Med., & Psychiatry*, 12:331–355.

Leff, J., Wig, N. N., Gosh, A., Bedi, H., Menon, D. K., Kuipers, L., Nielsen, J. A., Thestrup, G., Korten, A., Ernberg, G., Day, R., Sartorius, N., & Jablensky, A. (1987), Expressed emotion and schizophrenia in North India: III. Influence of relatives' expressed emotion on the course of schizophrenia in Chandigarh. *Brit. J. Psychiatry*, 151:166–173.

Sartorius, N. (1988), Solving the conundrum of schizophrenia: WHO's contribution. In: *Schizophrenia: Recent Biosocial Developments*, eds. C. N. Stefanis & A. D. Rabavilas. New York: Human Sciences Press, pp. 23–28.

——Jablensky, A., Korten, A., Ernberg, G., Ander, M., Cooper, J. E., & Day, R. (1986), Early manifestations and first contact incidence of schizophrenia in different cultures: A preliminary report on the initial evaluation phase of the WHO collaborative study on determinants of outcome of severe mental disorders. *Psycholog. Med.*, 16(4):909–928.

——Janca, A. (1995), The World Health Organization's recent work on the lexicography of mental disorders. *Eur. Psychiatry*, 10:321–325.

——, ——(1996), Psychiatric assessment instruments developed by the World Health Organization. *Soc. Psychiatry & Psychiatric Epidemiol.*, 31:55–69.

World Health Organization (WHO) (1960), *Epidemiology of Mental Disorders*. 8th Report of the Expert Committee on Mental Health, Technical Report Series No. 185. Geneva: World Health Organization.

——(1973), *The International Pilot Study of Schizophrenia*, Vol. 1. Geneva: World Health Organization.

——(1979), *Schizophrenia: An International Follow-up Study*. New York: Wiley.

Wing, J. K., Cooper, J. E., & Sartorius, N. (1974), *Present State Examination*. Cambridge, U.K.: Cambridge University Press.

CHAPTER 2

Study Methodology

Carole Siegel, Eugene M. Laska, Joseph A. Wanderling, Sherryl Baker, Glynn Harrison, Rheta Bank, and Morris Meisner

GENERAL DESIGN

ISoS is a follow-up study on the course of illness and outcomes of a subset of subjects who had been in previous WHO-coordinated research studies of schizophrenia—the International Pilot Study of Schizophrenia (IPSS), the study on the Determinants of Outcome of Severe Mental Disorders (DOSMeD), and the study on Reduction and Assessment of Psychiatric Disability (RAPyD or Disability)—and additionally, subjects who had been in studies conducted locally at three other centers (Retrospective Analysis or Invited). Throughout this volume, these four distinct long-term follow-up cohorts (IPSS, DOSMeD, RAPyD, and Retrospective Analysis) are referred to as the "subsamples" of ISoS.

International committees were convened to participate in developing the methodology for study design, instrument selection/modification/development, project coordination and management, reliability, diagnosis, and data analysis. Participants included: Sherryl Baker, Ph.D., Rheta Bank, Aksel Bertelsen, M.D., Sarah Conover, Thomas Craig, M.D., Walter Gulbinat, Glynn Harrison, M.D., Kim Hopper, Ph.D., Waguik Ishak, M.D., Assen Jablensky, M.D., Aleksandar Janca, M.D., Stacy Lane, M.D., Eugene Laska, Ph.D., Peter Mason, M.D., Morris Meisner, Ph.D., Norman Sartorius, M.D., Carole Siegel, Ph.D., Ezra Susser, M.D., and Joseph A. Wanderling, M.A. In addition, principal investigators from all participating centers met throughout the study, five meetings in total (1991–1996), for purposes of training, instrument development, and data analysis.

Inclusion Criteria

The original selection criteria for the subsamples were different:

IPSS

Selected subjects all had functional psychosis and were at various stages of illness, some with prior exposure to treatment but none with severe psychotic symptoms continuously present for more than 3 years (WHO, 1973, 1979). The cohorts were comprised of consecutive admissions to psychiatric facilities in participating centers in nine countries between April 1968 and April 1969. The centers from IPSS in ISoS are Agra, Cali, and Prague.

DOSMeD

In this treated incidence study, subjects were selected for study entry as close as possible to the onset of their illness, between 1978 and 1980 (Sartorius et al., 1986). Specifically, subjects had experienced disturbing psychiatric symptoms (most commonly, odd behavior, appearance, or talk) within the prior 12 months and had their first contact with a "helping agency" within the prior 3 months. Special efforts were made to monitor all probable entry points into the treatment system of persons likely to meet study criteria, including traditional healers, local clinics, and the police. Success in case-finding was later checked through leakage studies. The centers from DOSMeD participating in ISoS are Chandigarh (urban and rural), Dublin, Honolulu, Moscow, Nagasaki, Nottingham, Prague, and Rochester.

RAPyD

The Reduction and Assessment of Psychiatric Disability study was initiated in 1976 to explore ways of evaluating behavioral impairments and social disabilities in subjects with schizophrenia and related disorders with recent onset and to chart their natural history through repeated assessments (Jablensky, Schwarz, and Tomov, 1980). Subjects with a recent onset of nonaffective psychotic illness (less than 2 years prior to screening of administrative files of participating institutions) were recruited over a 2-year period (1978 to 1979), within defined geographical areas in seven countries. The centers from the RAPyD study participating in ISoS are Groningen, Mannheim, and Sofia.

Retrospective Analysis

Three centers that had not participated in the previous WHO studies were invited to join ISoS because they had conducted epidemiological studies that were similar to the WHO sponsored studies. Entry criteria for these studies varied:

Beijing: During a 1982 epidemiological survey of mental disorders, 217 subjects with a diagnosis of schizophrenia (using ICD-9 criteria) were identified by community surveys (including residents of institutions) of a dozen districts with relatively stable and ethnically homogeneous populations. Heads of households and other key informants identified potential cases; clinical interviews then determined eligible study subjects (i.e., those whose symptoms had detectable effects on daily life; Cooper and Sartorius, 1996). All clinically diagnosed cases of schizophrenia from the eight urban districts (N=89) were selected for follow-up in ISoS.

Hong Kong: A random sample of 100 cases was drawn for inclusion in ISoS from case records of 797 first onset patients who contacted mental health services in Hong Kong between 1977 and 1978. An ICD-9 diagnosis of schizophrenia was confirmed through case reviews by participating investigators.

Chennai (Madras): A study in 1981 and 1982 assembled a cohort of 100 consecutive subjects who came to the Department of Psychiatry, Madras Medical College and Government General Hospital, and who fulfilled both ICD-9 and modified Feighner's criteria for schizophrenia. Ninety of the 100 were first episode cases making their initial contact with a treatment facility (Indian Council of Medical Research, 1988). All cases were followed up in ISoS.

Feasibility Study/Tracing Exercise

Prior to commencement of the formal study, the feasibility of locating subjects was assessed (Sartorius, Gulbinat, Harrison, Laska, and Siegel, 1996). All IPSS and DOSMeD ISoS centers participated in this exercise, as did two of the RAPyD centers. (Mannheim did not participate because it was engaged in its own follow-up study and therefore had already demonstrated its tracking capability.) The Retrospective Analysis centers did not participate in this exercise. For each participating center, 20 cases were randomly selected from the original cohorts. A Tracing Schedule was used to record efforts to locate these subjects. The percentage for whom data were available was high, ranging from 75 to 95%, and clearly demonstrated the feasibility of relocating subjects for the follow-up study.

Sample Size and Numbers to Follow-Up

With a few exceptions, all the participating centers attempted to trace all persons from the original cohorts for a long-term follow-up interview. (In Moscow, only persons who entered the study in the first year were followed up.) Additionally, in several DOSMeD centers, subjects who were not in the original cohorts but for whom baseline data were available were added, totaling 33 cases in all. Table 2.1 presents the number traced, whether alive with sufficient date for analysis, dead or lost to follow-up. The DOSMeD subsample of 810 was comprised of subjects from nine centers; the IPSS subsample of 392 from three centers; the RAPyD subsample of 213 from three centers; and the Retrospective Analysis (or Invited) subsample of 289 from three centers. Sample sizes in individual centers ranged from 55 in Chandigarh rural to 155 in Chandigarh urban.

Lost to follow-up in some cases was higher than anticipated from the tracing exercise. The percentage lost ranged from a low of 4% in Nottingham to a high of 58% for the Honolulu cohort. The overall percent lost to follow-up for the DOSMeD cohort was 31%; for the IPSS cohort, 29%; for RAPyD cohort, 10%; and for the Retrospective Analysis cohorts, 15%.[1]

Duration of Follow-Up

The time from study entry to the time of ISoS assessment (the follow-up period) varied across and within substudies. The mean follow-up period for

1. In DOSMeD, three centers (Honolulu, Nagasaki, and Rochester) all had "lost" rates above 40%, and together account for 47% of the total lost for that substudy. Of these centers, two—59% in Honolulu, 41% in Nagasaki—substantial percentages of subjects were lost soon after the initial episode. In Rochester, nearly half of those "lost" to follow-up had in fact been contacted and refused to participate.

TABLE 2.1 ISoS Cohorts

		ISoS Analysis Group						*Original Study Total*	*Follow-up Years*
		Alive[b]		*Dead*		*Lost*[c]			
		N	%	N	%	N	%	N	*Mean*
Subsample	Center								
Prevalence Cohort									
IPSS	Agra	61	43.6	43	30.7	36	25.7	140	26
	Cali	72	56.7	12	9.4	43	33.9	127	26
	Prague	43	34.3	46	36.8	36	28.8	125	26
	Total	176	44.9	101	25.8	115	29.3	392	
Invited	Beijing	58	65.2	20	22.5	11	12.4	89	12
Total Prevalence		234	48.6	121	25.2	126	26.2	481	
Incidence Cohort									
DOSMeD	Chandigarh Rur.	38	69.1	10	18.2	7	12.7	55	15
	Chandigarh Urb.	80	51.6	14	9.0	61	39.4	155	15
	Dublin	37	55.2	8	11.9	22	32.8	67	16
	Honolulu	26	36.6	4	5.6	41	57.7	71	16
	Moscow	52	72.2	10	13.9	10	13.9	72	15
	Nagasaki	57	49.6	7	6.1	51	44.3	115	15
	Nottingham	86	86.9	9	9.1	4	4.0	99	13
	Prague	79	66.9	11	9.3	28	23.7	118	15
	Rochester	33	56.9			25	43.1	58	16
	Total	488	60.2	73	9.0	249	30.7	810	
RAPyD[a]	Groningen	63	75.9	9	10.8	11	13.3	83	14
(Disability)	Mannheim	56	80.0	6	8.6	8	11.4	70	14
	Sofia	55	91.7	2	3.3	3	5.0	60	16
	Total	174	81.7	17	8.0	22	10.3	213	
Invited	Hong Kong	70	70.0	11	11.0	19	19.0	100	17
	Madras	77	77.0	9	9.0	14	14.0	100	13
	Total	147	73.5	20	10.0	33	16.5	200	
Total Incidence		809	66.1	110	9.0	304	24.9	1223	
Total ISoS		1043	61.2	231	13.6	430	25.2	1704	

[a] RAPyD—Included in original study total are prospective cases only.

[b] Alive category—Cases with sufficient follow-up data for analysis.

[c] Lost category—Includes cases alive with insufficient data for analysis, cases lost to follow-up for whom some ISoS data were supplied, and cases in original study totals for whom no ISoS forms were received.

alive subjects ranged from 12 years to 26 years. The modal mean follow-up time for the DOSMeD subsample was 15 years and for the RAPyD subsample was 14 years. The mean follow-up times for the Retrospective Analysis centers ranged from 12 (Beijing) to 17 (Hong Kong) years. The IPSS subsample had the longest mean follow-up time, 26 years, for each center.

Ethical Review and Government Approval

In all participating countries, Field Research Centers received approval for carrying out the study from relevant local ethical review boards and, where required, from governmental committees. Because such review bodies differed in their demands, ground rules regarding privacy of the subjects, confidentiality of the records, and informed consent were established, and their feasibility tested during the tracing exercise. These included:

- Information obtained during the interview should not be shared with providers, family members, or other persons without the study subject's explicit permission.
- The study subject's history of treatment for psychiatric disorder should never be revealed to persons who were not already aware of it.
- The study should be explained to the subject, and he or she should understand that participation is entirely voluntary.

A prototype informed consent form was developed and sent to all investigators, some of whom modified it for use as per the requirements of local review committees. The identity of the subjects remained with the centers; all records sent to WHO were identified only by an ISoS case number.

Study Instruments

A set of subject-focused instruments for assessing long-term course and outcome of schizophrenia was selected and/or adapted from established instruments; a few were also developed specifically for ISoS. Items included in every new scale were reviewed for cross-cultural relevance, with modifications made so as to ensure applicability in each center. In addition, two setting-level instruments were developed: one describing local area characteristics of the center settings, and the other the treatment systems in the setting available during the study time to persons with severe mental illness. The subject-focused instruments covered the domains of clinical functioning and daily living and adaptation; time frames covered current status as well as the entire follow-up period (the Life Chart and Substance Abuse Schedules). Instruments were pilot tested under field conditions and revised as necessary. New instruments were translated for local use, and back translating was used to verify accuracy (Sartorius and Kuyken, 1996).

CLINICAL ASSESSMENTS

Present State Examination (PSE)

For comparability with other studies, the Present State Examination (PSE) version 9, a semistructured clinical interview covering a broad range of psychiatric symptoms present over the previous 4 weeks (Wing, Cooper, and Sartorius, 1974), was chosen as the principal instrument for assessing mental state. The PSE had previously been used successfully in international studies including IPSS and DOSMeD; it had already been translated into many of the languages used in the Field Research Centers, including Bulgarian, Chinese, Czech, Hindu, Japanese, Russian, and Spanish. Most of the investigators were familiar with it, many having already been trained in its use. The reliability of the PSE in the hands of trained interviewers is well established (Jablensky, 1987).

Diagnostic Schedule Scoresheet (DSS)

The DSS, devised in collaboration with the Nottingham Field Research Center, records the consensus of the research team with respect to the subject's diagnoses using DSM-III-R (APA, 1986) and ICD-10 criteria. In addition, the schedule captures alternative and additional diagnoses and records changes in diagnosis over time. Thus research teams had to come to consensus on three diagnoses: First, the team has to rediagnose the subject using only the information available at the time of the subject's entry into the study; second, they had to agree upon a current diagnosis (most recent 2 years) using the information from PSE and other ISoS study instruments, as well as other records of the past 2 years; and third, they had to agree upon an overall lifetime diagnosis taking into account all of the information available.

Scale for the Assessment of Negative Symptoms (SANS)

The SANS records data on currently displayed "negative" symptoms of schizophrenia such as avolition, blunted affect, and anhedonia (Andreasen, 1989). It has been tested and used in several cultures and is available in several languages, including Spanish and Japanese.

Psychological Impairments Rating Schedule (PIRS-II)

The PIRS-II, an updating of the PIRS, records the behavior of the subject observed during the PSE interview. Interaction skills such as self-presentation, attention, initiative, affect, and communication skills are noted.

DAILY LIVING ADAPTATION

Disability Assessment Schedule (DAS)

The DAS was originally developed and tested by WHO for use in the RAPyD study. The modified version used here captures data for the past month on the subject's levels of social withdrawal and self-care, performance of social roles (e.g., household activities, marriage/sexual relationships, and work) and, if relevant, behavior in hospital. It also asks for an overall assessment of level of disability. Trained investigators are asked to make such ratings relying primarily upon interviews with key informants and subjects, but also drawing upon other clinical material, as available. Ratings take into account clinical assessment, applicable local cultural norms (e.g., regarding gender), and the subject's social background and status.

Substance Abuse Schedule (SAS)

The SAS collects data on the subject's use of alcohol, nonprescribed drugs, and psychoactive substances both in the most recent month and for the entire follow-up period. Raters used ICD-10 definitions of harmful use and dependency syndromes, and coding relied upon all available sources of information.

Family Interview Schedule (FIS)

The FIS records perceptions of family members on several familial and cultural factors and measurements of the relatives' perceptions of factors that may influence the outcome of schizophrenia. The subject's symptoms and social behavior were assessed for the past month. With reference to the last episode or overall course, additional questions sought to determine the informant's assessment of the stigma associated with the subject's psychiatric problems; his or her understanding of the source of the family member's difficulties and the various sources of supports relied upon; and the degree to which the informant has been involved in helping that family member during episodes of illness, and with what impact on the informant's own life. The development of this instrument entailed extensive consultation with experts, so that the FSI incorporates scales which have been used in many other studies and whose psychometric properties are established. Among those consulted were: Martin Katz (symptoms and social behavior from the Katz Adjustment Scale); S. R. Kay, L. A. Opler, and A. Fiszbein (items from the Positive and Negative Symptom Scale); Bruce Link (items from the Family Stigma Scale); and Richard Tessler (impact and support from the Continuity of Care Interview). The section on attribution of illness was taken from the Psychiatric and Personal History Schedule (PPHS) used in the DOSMeD.

GLOBAL ASSESSMENTS

Life Chart Schedule (LCS)

The LCS, a new instrument developed in collaboration with researchers at the Nathan S. Kline Institute for Psychiatric Research, is a semistructured "conversational" interview with the subject and with key informant(s), modeled after the work of Courtenay Harding and her colleagues (Harding, McCormick, Strauss, Ashikaga, and Brooks, 1989). Assisted by a visual aid, the "life chart," this participatory conversation covers work, residence, symptoms, and treatment for two time frames: the most recent 2 years and the entire period since the initial examination. After conducting interviews and consulting all other available sources of information, the interviewer completes a LCS synthesizing all the material.

Broad Rating Schedule (BRS)

The BRS records broad overall ratings in the domains of severity of symptoms and global assessment of functioning for alive subjects based on information available for the last month. For subjects lost to follow-up or dead, the severity of symptoms is rated for the period for which information is available. The BRS includes the Global Assessment of Functioning (GAF) scales for symptoms and for disability, modified from DSM-III-R, Appendix 12, and (a modified) Bleuler Severity of Psychotic Symptoms scale.

DESCRIPTIVE

Basic Information on Study Subject (BIS)

The BIS records basic social and demographic data on the study subject, including current living arrangements for the past month, marriage and children, migration, and behavior during the interview. To retain comparability, most items were selected from the Psychiatric and Personal History Schedule (PPHS) used in the DOSMeD.

Schedule for Deceased Patients (SDP)

The SDP records information surrounding the death of the subject including date, cause, and mental health status at the time.

Information on Refusers (IOR)

The IOR was used to document interaction with persons who, although eligible, declined to participate in all or part of the study. The IOR thus allowed investigators to distinguish subjects who refused to participate in only some aspects of the study; for example, some persons refused to be interviewed but gave permission for the use of clinical records; others agreed to be interviewed and allowed the use of clinical records, but would not give permission for interviews with informants. It also records total refusals.

Background Information on Study Subjects at Retrospective Analysis Centers

This instrument was used by the Retrospective Analysis centers to record data on key variables at the time of the subject's entry into the original study (and at the time of early follow-up). For comparability, the questions were taken from study instruments used in DOSMeD.

AREA DESCRIPTIONS

Local Area Profile (LAP)

The LAP collects information from key informants on selected characteristics of the catchment area served by the Field Research Center, as well as on changes in those characteristics that have occurred since the time that the subjects first entered the original study. Four specific areas are covered: economic activity, population and social organization, prevailing beliefs and practices, and events in local history that have had a significant impact on everyday life.

Mental Health Treatment System Survey (MHTS)

The MHTS collects information on features of the mental health treatment system available to the study subject, both at present and at the time of entry into the original study. Specific areas covered include past and current availability of hospitals, resources for living in the community, outpatient services, medications, traditional healing, and professional personnel. The survey also records information on the organizational structure of the mental health treatment system, on its financing and on the governmental authorities responsible for its administration.

DATA COLLECTION PROCEDURES

Information on the study subjects was derived from three sources: interview with the subject, interview with key informant(s), and records review including clinical records, mortality records, and previous study records. Some instruments were used during the interview with the study subject; some in interviews with the key informants; and others were completed subsequent to the interviews. Clinical interviews were carried out for the most part by psychiatrists; some centers also employed nonclinical research workers for interviewing informants. Consensus among the investigators is that the average length of the clinical and informant interviews was 90 minutes. The only instrument for which informant input (when available) was not sought was the PSE; likewise, only for the FIS was the subject excluded.

In addition, researchers sought out other sources of information to supplement knowledge of both the subject and the setting. These included review of available case notes, interviews with general practitioners, faith healers, and other community providers, as well as conversations with persons with long-standing relationships with the subject. Information on the setting was collected on descriptive instruments through consultation with local experts on various aspects of local life. Consultants included other researchers, professors in university departments of social science, clinicians, service providers, government/policy officials, and administrators.

TRAINING

Most of the principal investigators had extensive experience using the PSE (and several other ISoS follow-up instruments) from prior involvement in the IPSS, DOSMeD, and RAPyD studies, as well as subsequent research. Two of the three Retrospective Analysis centers had also collected PSE data at baseline. Because new instruments were introduced into the ISoS and inexperienced field workers who required additional training were recruited, training and reliability were approached in a systematic and comprehensive fashion.

The ISoS follow-up instruments were combined into a single instrumentation package, accompanied by procedural guidance for local training and implementation in fieldwork exercises. PSE training was arranged locally by seasoned trainers or by visiting trainers from other centers. The full complement of instruments was introduced at two training seminars for principal investigators, held in Hong Kong in April 1991 and in Aarhus, Denmark, in August 1991. Instruments were introduced by experienced users, and training made use of videotapes and/or case vignettes, a format that encouraged discussion and feedback. Additional guidance was provided for training local fieldworkers in the full range of follow-up instruments. A final meeting to winnow down an overly demanding package and further refine the reliability exercise was held in Tulsa, Oklahoma in October 1992.

RELIABILITY EXERCISES

The main statistical measures of reliability for grouped categorical data were the kappa statistic and the Pairwise Agreement Ratio (PAR, the ratio of the number of agreements to the total number of possible agreements). The Intra-Class Correlation Coefficient (ICC) for interval and ordinal data was also used. The results of the reliability exercises are summarized using the kappa statistic for variables with two outcomes (usually absence/presence of symptoms). One concern when using kappa is its lack of precision when there is little variation in the ratings for a variable. To overcome this, variables were divided into those with and those without sufficient variation of ratings. First for each variable, the percentage of ratings that were scored "absent"—meaning the symptom was not detected—was computed. The variable was put into the insufficient variation group if the percentage scored "absent" approached 0 or 100% (i.e., 0–10% or 90–100%). A percentage scoring "absent" that fell into the 10 to 90% range was considered sufficient variation. A kappa of 0.4 is generally considered to indicate acceptable reliability. The utility of the kappa statistic as a measure of interrater reliability is clear for the second group, but questionable for the first. The cutoff was chosen so as to optimize the separation of variables with a kappa of 0.4 or higher from those with a kappa rating lower.

Intracenter Reliability

For reliability in the use of the course and outcome measures within centers, the assessment method was rater-observers doing live interviews while other observers made independent ratings. For the Life Chart Schedule, reliability was examined for "best overall judgment" ratings, derived from both the subject interview and the supplementary case material. These exercises were done separately, prior to and during the collection of data on study subjects.

Prior to Actual Study

Reliability exercises done prior to the actual study were analyzed and the results were distributed to each center prior to the start of the data collection. Reliability assessments were done for the Present State Examination (PSE), Scale for the Assessment of Negative Symptoms (SANS), Psychological Impairments Rating Scale (PIRS), Life Chart Schedule (LCS), and the Disability Assessment Schedule (DAS). Some centers also assessed the Substance Abuse Schedule (SAS), the Broad Rating Schedule (BRS), and the Family Interview Schedule (FIS). Each center reviewed the results and instituted corrective measures for those items that showed poor reliability between raters.

Each center aimed to assess 10 patients. This target was met, with two or more investigators assessing at least 10 cases, in nine centers; another completed ratings for 5 cases; and one center with only a single clinician doing the actual study ratings did test-retest assessments. No ratings were done by Moscow where all study ratings were done by a single investigator, and none were done in Rochester, New York, and Honolulu where almost all ratings were done by a single clinician. Mannheim and Cali did not do within-center reliability using the ISoS instruments, since their data collection had been completed as part of existing studies before ISoS began. Mannheim did

TABLE 2.2A Intracenter Reliability Exercise Done Prior to Actual Study: Distribution of Kappa by Amount of Variation in Variable N (%)

	PSE		DAS		LCS	
kappa	*<10 >90%*	*10–90%*	*<10 >90%*	*10–90%*	*<10 >90%*	*10–90%*
<0.2	14(18.2)				4(28.6)	1 (3.2)
0.2–0.4	13(16.9)	1 (2.0)			2(14.3)	
0.4–0.6	23(29.9)	10(20.0)	1(100)		4(28.6)	2 (6.5)
0.6–0.8	22(28.6)	30(60.0)		11(37.9)	2(14.3)	20(64.5)
0.8–1.	3 (3.9)	9(18.0)		18(62.1)	1 (7.1)	8(25.9)
Constant*	2 (2.6)				1 (7.1)	
Total	77 (100)	50(100)	1(100)	29(100)	14(100)	31(100)

*All ratings for a variable are the same

reliability exercises using their own forms, and Cali had a rater very familiar with PSE.

The results are given in Table 2.2a for the PSE, DAS, and LCS. Variables are divided into two groups: those for which more than 90% or less than 10% of the ratings were scored "absent" and those for which the "absent" ratings range from 10 to 90%. Only two variables for the three schedules have a kappa less than 0.4 for those variables with sufficient variation, while 108 variables have a kappa greater than 0.4. This indicates that the reliability exercise showed sufficient agreement among the raters at each center even before additional training occurred.

During the Actual Study

During the actual study, multiple raters of the same study subjects were assessed to show that levels of reliability were maintained. Five centers (Agra, Beijing, Nagasaki, Nottingham, and Sofia) took part with a total of 42 subjects and an average of four raters were subject. Reliability assessments were done for the DAS, LCS, PIRS, PSE, SANS, and SAS.

Table 2.2b gives the results for these within-center reliability exercises during the actual study for the PSE, DAS, and LCS. The division for variability was again done at the 10 to 90% split. None of the 111 variables with sufficient variation for the three schedules had a kappa less than 0.4, and all but one were greater than 0.6. For these same centers, the prior to study analysis showed that 18 of the 108 variables were sufficient variation in the three schedules had a kappa less than 0.6, and six were also less than 0.4. This indicates that the review of the earlier reliability analysis and the additional training improved reliability among raters.

TABLE 2.2B Intracenter Reliability Exercise Done During Actual Study: Distribution of Kappa by Amount of Variation in Variable (%)

	PSE		DAS		LCS	
kappa	*<10 >90%*	*10–90%*	*<10 >90%*	*10–90%*	*<10 >90%*	*10–90%*
<0.2	3 (4.3)				4(21.1)	
0.2–0.4	4 (5.8)				2(10.5)	
0.4–0.6	7(10.1)			1 (3.6)	3(15.8)	
0.6–0.8	16(23.2)	11(19.01)		4(14.3)		3(12.0)
0.8–0.1.	29(42.0)	47(81.0)		23(82.1)	7(36.9)	22(88.0)
Constant*	10(14.5)		2(100)		3(15.8)	
Total	69(100)	58(100)	2(100)	28(100)	19(100)	25(100)

* All ratings for a variable are the same

Intercenter Reliability

To assess between-center reliability, videotapes that had been prepared at four centers and circulated to all centers were rated by one or more observers. The five videotapes were comprised of interviews with patients with a history of psychosis broadly comparable to the ISoS follow-up cases. The videotaped interviews were carried out in English with English-speaking subjects and were accompanied both by an English transcript of the interview and a structured case vignette (to enable raters to complete certain items requiring historical data normally available from case notes or an informant). Videotapes and vignettes were circulated to the FRCs for reliability assessments of the Present State Examination (PSE), Substance Abuse Schedule (SAS), Scale for the Assessment of Negative Symptoms (SANS), Psychological Impairments Rating Scale (PIRS), Life Chart Schedule (LCS), and the Disability Assessment Schedule (DAS).

The five cases were assessed by an average of 29 raters per case. The numbers of raters varied depending upon the number of fieldworkers involved in each center. All centers but one (Cali) completed at least one tape; the majority completed three or more.

Table 2.2c gives the results of the between-center videotape reliability analysis for the PSE, DAS, and LCS. Owing to the best split of kappa values at the 0.4 value, the range of sufficient variation was set at 25 to 75%. Eleven of the 60 variables with sufficient variation (i.e., between 25 and 75% of the ratings for a variable were scored "absent") had a kappa less than 0.4.

DATA HANDLING AND ANALYSIS

Data Entry

To create a study database, several computer data entry programs were supplied to the investigators. Most of the data were entered using Epi Info, a public domain program developed and supported by the U.S. Centers for Disease Control and the World Health Organization (Dean, Dean, Burton, and Dicker, 1990), which allows for the creation of data entry screens for epidemiological studies. A small menu-driven, front-end program was written by NKI to simplify the use of the data collection system, and a screen was created for each ISoS instrument. Values keyed into each field were checked for conformity with allowable values for the field. Free-form narrative was collected by a program specifically written by NKI for ISoS.

All collected data were combined into two compact archive files which were either placed on a floppy disk and mailed to NKI or sent electronically via either e-mail or Internet FTP (file transfer protocol). At NKI, the data were examined for duplications and/or for incorrect values in a few key fields (e.g., center identification number), and processed into one data set for each of the data collection instruments. Internal consistency checks for each instrument were then performed.

Descriptive Analysis

A series of meetings with experts was held to delineate from the huge volume of information collected

TABLE 2.2C Intercenter Reliability Exercise Done Throughout Study: Distribution of Kappa by Amount of Variation in Variable N(%)

	PSE		DAS		LCS	
kappa	*<25 >75%*	*25–75%*	*<25 >75%*	*25–75%*	*<25 >75%*	*25–75%*
<0.2	51(51.5)	1 (3.6)	3(50.0)	1(10.0)	14(60.9)	4(18.2)
0.2–0.4	11(11.1)	3(10.7)	1(16.7)	1(10.0)	5(21.7)	1 (4.5)
0.4–0.6	9 (9.1)	14(50.0)		5(50.0)	2 (8.7)	4(18.2)
0.6–0.8	7 (7.1)	8(28.6)	1(16.7)	1(10.0)	1 (4.3)	5(22.7)
0.8–0.1	1 (1.0)	2 (7.1)		2(20.0)		8(36.4)
Constant*	20(20.2)		1(16.7)		1 (4.3)	
Total	99(100)	28(100)	6 (100)	10 (100)	23 (100)	22 (100)

*All ratings for a variable are the same

a parsimonious but comprehensive set of variables that would be used uniformly to represent the clinical status and psychosocial functioning of the subjects. These included variables from baseline interviews on demographics, onset of illness and diagnosis, and from short-term follow-up, if available.

Multiple diagnoses have been used to describe study subjects. The diagnosis chosen for the basic descriptive analysis is the clinical diagnosis given to the subject at entry into the original study, converted to ICD-10 format. The relationship of this baseline diagnosis to lifetime diagnosis is discussed in Chapter 5 by Craig et al., this volume.

Domains for the follow-up assessment of the alive cohort included: *clinical status* described by recent course type, current symptomatology, and overall course of illness; *psychosocial functioning* including current disability, work experience, and living arrangements; *noteworthy events* such as suicide and assault; and *treatment* in terms of medications and hospitalizations, both current and over the entire period.

For persons who died, information was provided on the age, year, and nature of death and the mental health status at the time of death. Each center was provided with standardized mortality ratios, to enable comparison of the death experience of the center cohort with that of the general population.

References

American Psychiatric Association (1986), *Diagnostic and Statistical Manual of Mental Disorders*, 3rd ed. rev. (DSM-III-R). Washington, DC: American Psychiatric Press.

Andreasen, N. C. (1989), The scale for the assessment of negative symptoms (SANS): Conceptual and theoretical foundations. *Brit. J. Psychiatry*, 155(Suppl. 7):49–52.

Cooper, J. E., & Sartorius, N., Eds. (1996), *Mental Disorders in China*. Glasgow: Royal Scottish College of Psychiatrists.

Dean, A. G., Dean, J. A., Burton, A. H., & Dicker, R. C. (1990), *Epi Info, Version 5: A Word Processing, Database, and Statistics Program for Epidemiology on Microcomputers*. Stone Mountain, GA: USD.

Harding, C., McCormick, R. V., Strauss, J. S., Ashikaga, T., & Brooks, G. W. (1989), Computerised life chart methods to map domains of function and illustrate patterns of interactions in the long-term course trajectories of patients who once met the criteria for DSM-III schizophrenia. *Brit. J. Psychiatry*, 155(Suppl. 5):100–106.

Indian Council of Medical Research (1988), *Final Report of the Longitudinal Study of Functional Psychoses in an Urban Community*. New Delhi: Indian Council of Medical Research.

Jablensky, A. (1987), Multicultural studies and the nature of schizophrenia: A review. *Roy. Soc. Med.*, 80:162–167.

——Schwarz, R., & Tomov, T. (1980), WHO collaborative study on impairments and disabilities associated with schizophrenia disorders. A preliminary communication: Objectives and methods. In: Epidemiological Research as a Basis for the Organization of Extramural Psychiatry. Proceedings of Second European Symposium on Social Psychiatry. *Acta Psychiatr. Scand.*, 62(Suppl. 285):152–163.

Sartorius, N., Gulbinat, W., Harrison, G., Laska, E., & Siegel, C. (1996), Long-term follow-up of schizophrenia in 16 countries. A description of the International Study of Schizophrenia conducted by the World Health Organization. *Soc. Psychiatry & Psychiatric Epidemiol.*, 31(5):249–258.

——Jablensky, A., Korten, A., Ernberg, G., Anker, M., Cooper, J. E., & Day, R. (1986), Early manifestations and first contact incidence of schizophrenia in different cultures. *Psycholog. Med.*, 16:909–928.

——Kuyken, W. (1994), Translation of health status instruments. In: *Quality of Life Assessment: International Perspective*, ed. J. Orley & W. Kuyken. Berlin: Springer.

Wing, J. K., Cooper, J. E., & Sartorius, N. (1974), *Measurement and Classification of Psychiatric Symptoms: An Instruction Manual for the PSE (Present State Examination and CATEGO Program)*. London: Cambridge University Press.

World Health Organization (WHO) (1973), *International Pilot Study of Schizophrenia*, Vol. 1. Geneva: World Health Organization.

——(1979), *Schizophrenia: An International Follow-up*. Chichester, U.K.: Wiley.

Part II

Findings

Chapter 3

An Overview of Course and Outcome in ISoS

Kim Hopper, Glynn Harrison, and Joseph A. Wanderling

The International Pilot Study of Schizophrenia (IPSS) demonstrated that large-scale international studies in psychiatric epidemiology were feasible; that, for research purposes, a diagnostic entity ("schizophrenia") could be identified cross-culturally, using a standardized diagnostic interview (the Present State Examination); that assessment instruments of proven reliability could be used in settings as widely varying as Ibadan, Nigeria, Cali, Colombia, and Washington, DC; and that respectable proportions of the initial cohorts could subsequently be located and assessed (WHO, 1973). Two- and 5-year follow-up studies of those patients found that those living in nonindustrialized ("developing") settings had better social and symptomatic outcomes (WHO, 1979; Leff, Sartorius, Jablensky, Korten, and Ernberg, 1992). A second study, the Determinants of Outcome of Severe Mental Disorder (DOSMeD), was undertaken in 1978. This time, subjects were entered as close as possible to the onset of initial treatment (by a variety of local options) for a first-time disorder. Two-year assessment of outcome again favored subjects in the developing centers (Sartorius et al., 1986; Jablensky et al., 1992). Substudies of the DOSMeD further sharpened the picture of cultural variation with respect to the expression of psychoses, illuminated local differences in the pattern and impact of expressed emotion in the family, and explored the culturally specific relevance of stressful life events to relapse (Wig, Menon, Bedi, Ghosh et al., 1987; Wig, Menon, Bedi, Leff et al., 1987; Day et al., 1987; Leff, Katz et al., 1988; Leff et al., 1990). (For further details, see Sartorius, chapter 1 of this volume.)

The International Study of Schizophrenia (ISoS) was mounted to test the long-term durability of such findings. Researchers sought to overcome some of the methodological problems that have limited the generalizability of findings from previous studies.

Specifically, researchers aimed to:

1. Pursue intriguing suggestions from several European studies (e.g., Ciompi, 1985; Bleuler, 1978) that the long-term outcome of schizophrenia may be better than conventionally thought.
2. Revisit the "developing" versus "developed" distinction to determine whether short-term differences in course and outcome are borne out over time.
3. Examine the evidence for "late recovery" at 15 years in a multinational cohort.

Collaborating investigators completed follow-up interviews in three of the original seven IPSS cohorts (26 years after the episode of inclusion), nine of the original 13 DOSMeD cohorts (15 years after initial episode), Incidence cohorts from three centers of the Reduction and Assessment of Psychiatric Disability Study (RAPyD, from 1978–1980), and a mixed set (two treated incidence cohorts, one prevalence) from the three Retrospective Analysis centers.

METHODS

A detailed description of the research protocol and instruments used in ISoS has been published elsewhere (Sartorius, Gulbinat, Harrison, Laska, and Siegel, 1996), as have initial results for the Nottingham (Mason et al., 1995; Harrison, Croudace, Mason, Glazebrook, and Medley, 1996) and Groningen (Wiersma, Nienhuis, Giel, deJong, and Sloof, 1996; Wiersma, Nienhuis, Sloof, and Giel, 1998) cohorts. This report presents data for course and outcome in the ISoS

TABLE 3.1 Subjects with Baseline Psychotic Diagnosis by Center: Subjects with Nonpsychotic or Missing Diagnosis for Total

		ISoS Analytic Group						*Original Study Total*
		Alive[b]		*Dead*		*Lost*[c]		
		N	%	N	%	N	%	N
Subsample	Center							
Prevalence Cohort								
IPSS	Agra	60	43.5	43	31.2	35	25.4	138
	Cali	69	61.6	12	10.7	31	27.7	112
	Prague	42	34.1	45	36.6	36	29.3	123
	Total	171	45.8	100	26.8	102	27.3	373
Retro. Anal.	Beijing	58	65.2	20	22.5	11	12.4	89
Total Prevalence Psychotic		229	49.6	120	26.0	113	24.5	462
Incidence Cohort								
DOSMeD	Chandigarh Rural	38	69.1	10	18.2	7	12.7	55
	Chandigarh Urban	75	50.7	14	9.5	59	39.9	148
	Dublin	37	55.2	8	11.9	22	32.8	67
	Honolulu	24	35.8	4	6.0	39	58.2	67
	Moscow	45	72.6	10	16.1	7	11.3	62
	Nagasaki	56	50.5	7	6.3	48	43.2	111
	Nottingham	83	88.3	8	18.5	3	3.2	94
	Prague	70	66.0	11	10.4	25	23.6	106
	Rochester	33	58.9	0	0	23	41.1	56
	Total	461	60.2	72	9.4	233	30.4	766
RAPyD (Disability)[a]	Groningen	61	77.2	8	10.1	10	12.7	79
	Mannheim	53	79.1	7	10.4	7	10.4	67
	Sofia	54	91.5	2	3.4	3	5.1	59
	Total	168	82.0	17	8.3	20	9.8	205
Retro. Anal.	Hong Kong	70	70.0	11	11.0	19	19.0	100
	Madras	77	77.0	9	9.0	14	14.0	100
	Total	147	73.5	20	10.0	33	16.5	200
Total Incidence Psychotic		776	66.3	109	9.3	286	24.4	1171
Total ISoS Psychotic		1005	61.5	229	14.0	399	24.4	1633
Total ISoS Nonpsychotic		31	50.0	3	4.8	28	45.2	62
Total ISoS Missing		7	77.8	0	0.0	2	22.2	9

[a] Disability—Included in original study total are prospective cases only

[b] "Alive" includes cases with sufficient follow-up data for analysis

[c] "Lost" includes cases alive with insufficient data for analysis (sometimes because subjects refused to participate); cases not found but for whom some ISoS data were supplied; and cases in the original studies for whom no ISoS follow-up forms were received

cohort as a whole (N=1005),[1] subdivided into treated[2] Incidence (N=776) and Prevalence (N=229) groups. Table 3.1 shows the distribution of "alive" (cases with sufficient follow-up data for analysis), dead, and "lost to follow-up" subjects (cases with insufficient follow-up data for analysis, owing to a variety of reasons; see notes to Table 3.1).

The Substudy Cohorts

In the Incidence cohort, 461 subjects in participating DOSMeD centers were found alive with sufficient data for analysis. They had been originally selected as close as possible to the onset of illness and first contact with a local agency of assistance or control (clinical facilities, traditional healers, the police). The 168 subjects of the original 205 subjects from the RAPyD centers were originally ascertained by screening administrative records for recent onset of nonaffective disorder. In the retrospective analysis group, the 70 Hong Kong subjects (of 100 originally) were randomly selected through a record review of all first admissions for schizophrenia to local clinics, and the 77 Chennai (Madras) subjects (of 100 originally) were part of a longitudinal study of first-episode psychoses that met Feighner criteria for schizophrenia. In the Prevalence cohort, the 171 IPSS subjects were initially part of a one-year Prevalence study of consecutive admissions for functional psychoses in participating centers; the 58 Beijing subjects represent all cases meeting criteria for schizophrenia identified in a community epidemiological survey.[3]

Initial Assessments

Although details vary across the substudies, all subjects received extensive clinical examinations, using a standardized assessment of mental state (the then-current version of the Present State Examination), as well as social, familial, and functional evaluations (in the WHO studies, using the Disability Assessment and Personal and Psychiatric History Schedules). For almost all subjects, too, information on initial course of illness (2 years) was available, most commonly through direct interviews conducted as part of earlier follow-up studies.

Follow-Up Study

Investigations in all Field Research Centers were cleared through local institutional review committees (or their functional equivalents, where available), so as to meet prevailing standards for ethical research.

Methods of Relocation

Subject tracing methods varied considerably, depending chiefly upon the degree of ongoing contact local investigators (and/or their clinical collaborators) had had with the subjects over the intervening years. In a good number of instances, current records or the first-hand knowledge of clinicians sufficed to locate many subjects. In others (e.g., Cali, Chandigarh, Chennai [Madras], Mannheim, Nottingham, Rochester), the relocation effort was greatly facilitated either because psychiatric case registries were available or intervening follow-up studies had been conducted. In most cases, however, investigators began with the last known address (in some instances, the whereabouts of the subject at the time of study inclusion) and worked forward in time, consulting clinical records, address directories, death registries, family, and/or neighborhood contacts. Effective tracing could demand not only the dogged sleuthing of shoe-leather epidemiology (compounded in places that had seen significant social upheaval and residential mobility in recent years), but also the gentle art of discreet inquiry (to ensure observance of confidentiality), especially in cases where the subject's marital status had changed. Logistical obstacles were formidable at times, especially where communication facilities were primitive (2 hours travel to the village, 30 to 40 minutes to find the subject). Knowledgeable key informants were sometimes reluctant to pass on information about a subject's current status (even when favorable), for fear of "opening old wounds" and reviving unpleasant memories. Owing to the length of the follow-up interview,

1. As Table 3.1 illustrates, 38 subjects passed the initial screen for psychoses but have been excluded in the analyses reported below: 31 were not given a primary ICD-9 diagnosis at entry, and 7 lacked diagnostic data.

2. In the DOSMeD study, "treated" included "cases in the early stages of the illness [evaluated] as closely as possible to the point of their first contact with any service or helping agency" (Jablensky et al., 1992, p. 6).

3. Mean year of birth for the Beijing cohort is identical to that of the IPSS cohort (1942), but the treatment histories of the two groups differ. Because of the way the sample was selected, all of the IPSS subjects were in treatment at the time they entered the study. Only 23 of the 58 Beijing subjects were in treatment prior to 1970; another 14 were in treatment by 1975. Thus, 64% (37 out of 58) of them might be considered to have early treatment history comparable to the IPSS group.

too, repeated visits were often necessary to complete the package of assessment instruments.

Follow-Up Assessments

The following instruments were used:

- The principal psychopathology assessment tool was the Present State Examination (PSE-9), supplemented in most cases by the Schedule for the Assessment of Negative Symptoms (SANS; Andreasen, 1989) and the Psychological Impairments Schedule (PIRS-II; WHO, 1992).
- Current functioning was assessed using both the Global Assessment of Functioning (Disability and Symptom scales; adapted from DSM-III-R) and a modified version of the WHO Disability Assessment Schedule (Jablensky, Schwarz, and Tomov, 1980).
- The course of illness—covering course of symptoms, engagement with treatment, residential status, involvement with work and kin—was constructed using the Life Chart Schedule, an instrument developed for the ISoS study that drew upon the earlier work of Harding and colleagues (Harding, McCormick, Strauss, Ashikaga, and Brooks, 1989).
- A global assessment of current clinical status, taking into account all information gathered with respect to course, symptoms, and functioning was made using a modified (past month only) version of Bleuler's criteria (Bleuler, 1978).
- The involvement of (and impact on) family members was investigated through a newly designed Family Interview Schedule (results to be reported elsewhere).

Training and reliability issues are reviewed in Siegel et al. (chapter 2, this volume). In the analyses below, results will be reported in summary form, using descriptive statistics (frequencies and percentages) and measures of statistical significance where pertinent.

RESULTS

Feasibility of Follow-Up and Success of Follow-Up Efforts

As Table 3.1 shows, attrition took its toll across all substudies of ISoS, ranging from an average of 30% in the DOSMeD group to 10% in the Disability centers. All told, 399 subjects, representing nearly a quarter of the original combined ISoS cohort, were lost to follow-up. Another 229 (or 14% of the original groups) died during the follow-up period. (For more detailed analysis, see mortality, Craig et al., chapter 6 of this volume.)

Bias in Tracing

The baseline variables gender, mode of onset, and short-term course of illness have all been cited in the literature as predictors of outcome. We compared their distribution in the alive groups versus those subjects lost to follow-up as a way of measuring potential bias in the follow-up cohort.

Incidence cases were divided into three subgroups for the main analyses (total psychoses, schizophrenia only, nonschizophrenia only). A significantly higher percentage of females in the alive groups compared with those subjects lost to follow-up was found for the total psychoses ($p < .10$) and schizophrenic ($p < .05$) groups (51.9 vs. 45.4%; 49.4 vs. 38.4%, respectively). The opposite occurs in the Prevalence cohorts, where a higher proportion of males appears in the traced-alive group in both analytic groups, although these were not significant. The percentages were almost equal for the nonschizophrenic group in both Incidence and Prevalence cohorts. Most published follow-up studies report an association between better outcome and female sex.

Mode of onset was grouped into sudden/acute and slow/insidious. No significant differences were found between alive and lost to follow-up cases, although in all six analytic groups there was a higher proportion of acute/sudden cases in the traced-alive group, and the power of our analysis may have been low. A more rapid mode of onset is generally thought to be associated with more favorable outcome.

The most favorable early course of illness (first 2 years) was defined as complete remission between psychotic episodes. These were compared with those cases in which remissions between episodes were incomplete or in which illness was continuous. Five of the six analytic groups showed a higher percentage of complete remissions in the alive group when compared with the lost group; none was statistically significant. The exception was the nonschizophrenic Incidence group where the percentages were essentially equal. A more favorable early course is also a prognostic factor for good outcome.

These attrition data require careful interpretation. They are informative concerning the likely biases in similar follow-up studies, given the consistency of these trends across a heterogeneous group of clinical service styles and cultural settings. Intuitively, we might predict that those with better outcome would more likely be lost to follow-up because of greater social and occupational mobility and reluctance to consent to interview about past events with strong negative associations. We found the opposite to be the case, although the differences did not reach statistical significance. Male patients with slow onset illness were more likely to be lost to follow-up, suggesting that, besides having higher risk of mortality, they are more likely to lose contact with services and/or to be more geographically mobile. This is a matter of potentially serious concern for the long-term care of patients who, by virtue of their negative prognostic profile, are conceivably most at risk.

The bias in follow-up also limits the generalizability of our findings (Schwartz, Terkelsen, and Smith, 1992). Even if not statistically significant, differential attrition rates for gender and early course type are sizable, and the generally positive findings for the alive group reported below should be interpreted with this in mind. At the same time, one incidence center (Nottingham) achieved an extremely high trace rate with only 4% missing cases. Global recovery rates for the Nottingham cohort are strikingly close to the global findings for ISoS as a whole, suggesting that differential attribution need not have severely biased our findings.

Diagnostic Process

The original IPSS and DOSMeD cohorts were identified before the widespread use of internationally accepted operationalized diagnostic criteria such as ICD-10 (WHO, 1994) and DSM-IV (APA, 1994). In addition, in the Retrospective Analysis centers samples were either identified retrospectively (relying upon case-note diagnosis) or by local diagnostic conventions. Ideally, we would have wanted to reassemble baseline and supplementary data for all ISoS cases, which would have allowed them to be rediagnosed in terms of current operationalized diagnostic criteria. Such an exercise would have involved a systematic assessment of original schedules, collateral history, and case records; diagnostic decisions would have had to have been blind to subsequent course and outcome. Candidate items for the diagnostic algorithms would have had to have been elicited in standardized format, and preferably accompanied by a reliability exercise. Resource constraints did not permit such a thorough program of assessment, and (apart from the retrospective diagnoses in the three added centers) we decided instead to rely upon the project diagnosis made at or close to the time of the baseline assessments for the three original studies (IPSS, DOSMeD, RAPyD). In most centers, the schedule was filled out by an individual investigator without further review by a research team. Diagnostic statements made in the format and terminology prevailing in each center had to be assigned an appropriate ICD-9 numerical code (ICD-8 in the case of IPSS) in accordance with the WHO glossary (WHO, 1978). The reliability of this process was investigated in the original DOSMeD study (Jablensky et al., 1992, pp. 15–16), where all field diagnoses were reviewed by a WHO team of experts, and found to be acceptable.

For purposes of analyses here, the original ICD-8 or ICD-9 diagnoses assigned at baseline were converted into ICD-10 diagnoses, as were the original case-notes or project diagnoses provided by the three Retrospective Analysis centers, using WHO cross-walk rules (WHO, 1994). This method provided the closest semblance of a standardized diagnostic system applied to symptoms at onset and remaining uncontaminated by knowledge of subsequent course and outcome. In the analyses reported below, outcome and course findings will be presented for total psychoses ("alive subjects") in Incidence and Prevalence groups, as well as for ICD-10 schizophrenia and nonschizophrenia[4] entry diagnoses separately. In the accompanying discussion, the different diagnostic categories are referred to as "analytic groups" (see Table 3.2).

OUTCOME

The most striking overall finding of ISoS is that the current global status of over half of these subjects—56% of the Incidence group and 60% of the Prevalence group—is rated as "recovered." Nearly half have

4. For the Incidence cohort, the last category (non-schizophrenia, N=274) is made up of the following ICD-10 diagnostic categories: one-third acute psychosis; one-third schizoaffective, depression, or bipolar; and one-third other psychoses; for the Prevalence cohort (N=87), it is one-third acute psychosis and one-quarter depression, with the remainder split evenly among schizoaffective, bipolar, and other psychoses.

TABLE 3.2 Analytic Groups

	All Psychoses		*Sz Only*		*Non-Sz*	
	Inc.	*Prev.*	*Inc.*	*Prev.*	*Inc.*	*Prev.*
N's	776	229	502	142	274	87
male/female	373/403	121/108	254/248	85/57	119/155	36/51

experienced no psychotic episodes in the last 2 years of follow-up. (Figures are somewhat lower for the schizophrenic subgroup, as we will see.) These percentages accord fairly well with ratings of both current symptoms and functioning (see Table 3.3). Equally noteworthy, even within the schizophrenic subgroup, over half the eligible subjects in the incidence group, and three-quarters of those in the prevalence group, had worked (either at a paid job or household activities) for the better part of the last 2 years of follow-up.

Measures of Current Symptomatic Status

1. *Bleuler's scale:* Severity of psychotic symptoms in the past month was rated for all alive subjects. Over half (56.2%) of all subjects in the Incidence group, and 60.2% of subjects in the Prevalence group, were rated as "recovered"; that is, they were virtually symptom-free or experienced only nondisabling residual symptoms. Comparable figures for the schizophrenic groups were slightly lower: 48.1% of Incidence schizophrenic patients and 53.5% of Prevalence schizophrenics were rated as recovered. Conversely, recovery rates for nonschizophrenic subjects in both Incidence and Prevalence groups were substantially higher (71.1% and 71.4%, respectively).
2. *Global Assessment of Functioning—Symptoms:* Comparable findings were obtained with this scale. Well over half (60.2% and 64.3%) of all subjects in the Incidence and Prevalence groups were rated as having either absent or mild symptoms (score 61 or higher). Again, rates were lower for the schizophrenic groups (54.0% I; 56.7% P), and higher for the nonschizophrenic groups (70.7% I; 77.1% P).

Measures of Current Disability

1. *Disability Assessment Scale:* For those for whom information was available, in global ratings of functioning over the past month at time of follow-up, 39.9% of all subjects in the Incidence group, and nearly half (49.3%) of those in the Prevalence group, were rated as "good" or "excellent." Figures for the schizophrenic subjects were somewhat lower: 33.4% and 47.7% for the two groups, respectively. Ratings were higher for the nonschizophrenic subjects: In each group, over half (52.1% of Incidence, 51.5% in Prevalence) were rated as good or excellent in their overall functioning.
2. *Global Assessment of Functioning Scale—Disability:* Over half (54.8%) of all subjects in the Incidence group, and nearly two-thirds (65.6%) of those in the Prevalence group, were

TABLE 3.3 Symptomatic State and Disability[a]

	All Psychoses		*Sz Only*		*Non-Sz*	
	Inc.	*Prev.*	*Inc.*	*Prev.*	*Inc.*	*Prev.*
Bleuler "recovered"	56.2	60.2	48.1	53.5	71.1	71.4
GAF-S (>60)	60.2	64.3	54.0	56.7	70.7	77.1
DAS ("Exc"/"Good")	39.9	49.3	33.4	47.7*	52.1	51.5*
[if add "Fair"]	64.9	78.9	56.0	77.9*	81.5	80.3*
GAF-D (>60)	54.8	65.6	50.7	60.3	62.1	74.7

[a] For table 3.3, except where indicated (*), all differences between schizophrenic and non-schizophrenic groups within Incidence or Prevalence cohorts are statistically significant at $p<.05$.

found to have either absent or mild disability (score 61 or higher). For schizophrenic subjects in the two groups, figures were 50.7 and 60.3%, respectively. For nonschizophrenic subjects, they were 62.1 and 74.7% (I and P). This score, which includes those with "some difficulty in social, occupational or school functioning," was higher than the DAS "good" or "excellent" ratings because subjects can achieve a GAF score of 61 or above while being assigned only a "fair" global rating in the DAS. In assessing the likely impact of persisting mild symptoms on quality of life, therefore, the overall DAS rating is a more conservative measure.

Measures of Current Living Arrangements

At the point of follow-up, the vast majority of subjects in both Incidence and Prevalence cohorts, in all three analytic groups, were currently living with friends or family. Figures range from 70% among schizophrenic subjects in the Incidence cohort to 85.9% of schizophrenic subjects in the Prevalence cohort. The local meaning of this arrangement and its association with independence are problematic, as we discuss below. A minority, ranging from 7% of Prevalence, cohort schizophrenic subjects to 20% of nonschizophrenic subjects in the Incidence cohort, were living alone. Smaller numbers still were to be found in hospital or supervised residences, ranging from 4.5% of nonschizophrenic subjects in the Prevalence cohort to 15.2% of schizophrenic subjects in the Incidence group.

Measures of Most Recent 2 Years of Follow-Up Period

1. *Life Chart Schedule—Course Type and Negative Symptoms:* Table 3.4 shows course of illness over the last 2 years of follow-up and presence of prominent negative symptoms by course type. Just over a quarter (26.8%) of all Incidence subjects were continuously ill over those last 2 years; that figure broke down to 33.6% of schizophrenic subjects and 14.6% of nonschizophrenic subjects. A pattern of continuous illness was more common in the Prevalence group, accounting for 37.5% of all subjects in that group, and nearly half (46.4%) of schizophrenic subjects. Negative symptoms were prominent in upwards of half the subjects with continuous illness, across all analytic groups except Incidence nonschizophrenic; they were relatively infrequent in those subjects with episodic or never psychotic courses. Approximately one-sixth of Incidence subjects in the three analytic groups experienced some psychotic episodes in the last 2 years; there was more variation in the Prevalence subjects, ranging from 8.5% in the schizophrenic group to 15.3% among nonschizophrenics. As noted earlier, almost half of all ISoS subjects have had no psychotic episodes in the last 2 years of follow-up, a percentage that falls somewhat when we examine schizophrenic subjects only (42.8% Incidence, 40.8% Prevalence). Nonschizophrenic episodes in those last 2 years were relatively infrequent in the Prevalence co-

TABLE 3.4 Last 2 Years Course of Illness (and percentage of that group with prominent negative symptoms)

	All Psychoses		*Sz Only*		*Non-Sz*	
	Inc.	*Prev.*	*Inc.*	*Prev.*	*Inc.*	*Prev.*
A. Course Type						
Episodic	16.6(14)	11.0(3.6)	16.6(17)	8.5(0)	16.9(8.9)	15.3(7.8)
Continuous	26.8(45)	37.5(46)	33.6(47.6)	46.4(47)	14.6(35)	22.4(42)
Neither (but psychotic in period)	6.9(10)	3.5(0)	6.9(0)	4.2(0)	7.0(0)	2.4(0)
Never Psychotic	49.4(6.1)	48.0(0.8)	42.8(9.1)	40.8(1.7)	61.5(2.4)	60.0(0)
B. Comorbidity						
% with nonpsychotic episodes	24.2	10.7	19.1	11.4	34.5	9.6

TABLE 3.5 Working (Paid or Household) (if eligible)

	All Psychoses		*Sz Only*		*Non-Sz*	
	Inc.	*Prev.*	*Inc.*	*Prev.*	*Inc.*	*Prev.*
Most of Last 2 yrs	61.3	75.9	56.8	73.9	69.2	78.8
Paid work	38.5	42.7	37.0	46.2	41.2	37.5
Male/female	50.0/28.0	65.0/20.2	45.4/28.4	64.8/18.8	59.5/27.4	65.5/21.6
Household activities	22.8	33.2	19.8	27.7	28.0	41.3
Male/female	1.8/42.0	3.0/63.6	2.2/37.8	1.4/66.7	0.9/48.6	6.9/60.8
% rated satisfactory (good or very good)[a]						
Paid work	89.0	91.0	88.3	94.1	90.0	85.2
Male/female	87.6/91.4	90.2/94.1	86.7/91.1	95.3/87.5	88.9/91.9	77.8/100.0
Household activities	80.4	84.1	68.6	81.3	94.4	87.1

[a]Performance rated for housework and full-time workers only (eliminates 11 subjects whose combined PT and FT work added up to more than 12 of last 24 months).

hort (averaging about 10%), but occurred in a quarter of the Incidence cohort subjects (19.1% of the schizophrenic group, 34.5% of the nonschizophrenic group).

2. *Life Chart Schedule—Employment:* For ratings of employment, subjects who were retired or jobless because of local economic circumstances were excluded. Work ratings for eligible subjects included both paid employment and housework.[5] As Table 3.5 shows employment figures for Incidence and Prevalence subjects across the three analytic groups range from 56.8% among schizophrenic subjects in the Incidence cohort to 73.9% or better in both schizophrenic and nonschizophrenic subjects in the Prevalence cohort. Quality of work was rated for full-time workers and those doing household work, and was found to be satisfactory in 80% or higher of all groups except the Incidence schizophrenic cohort doing household work, where it was satisfactory in two-thirds of the cases. Although men were much more likely to be employed at paid work, performance ratings for those women who did such work were comparable to those of men.

3. *Life Chart Schedule—Living Arrangements:* The majority of subjects in both Incidence and Prevalence cohorts, across all three analytic groups, had spent most of the past 2 years of follow-up period living with family or friends. Small percentages, ranging from 3.4% among nonschizophrenic subjects in the Prevalence cohort to 11.6% among schizophrenic subjects in the Incidence cohort, had spent the majority of those last 2 years in institutional settings. Twelve subjects (1.5%) in the Incidence cohort and four (1.7%) in the Prevalence cohort had been homeless (defined as living on the street or in a designated shelter) at some point in the last 2 years; in the Incidence cohort, three times that many (36 or 4.6%) had been homeless at some point during the entire follow-up period.

4. *Life Chart Schedule—Assaults:* Sixty-seven subjects (9.9%) in the Incidence cohort and eighteen (7.9%) in the Prevalence cohort were recorded as having committed assaults in the last 2 years of follow-up. Although the numbers are rather small, percentages were slightly higher for schizophrenic subjects in both groups (51 or 11.7%, and 16 or 11.3%, respectively). The majority of these were minor incidents, but in roughly a third of the cases overall (37.3% of Incidence, 33.3% of Prevalence), such assaults were rated as moderate ("causing some injury") or (in a single case) severe; for schizophrenic subjects in the Incidence cohort, the percentage was 45.1% versus 12.5% for nonschizophrenic subjects.

5. "Local economic circumstances" excluded only 20 subjects; another 56 were listed as "retired" although, arguably, the 35 in that group who were under 65 (men) or 60 (women) could have been included; and the situation of 19 was unknown. A total of 160 subjects known to be collecting disability pensions for most of the last 2 years were included, however, in the denominator. To be considered "working" in paid employment, a subject had to have held a full-time job at least some of that time; this excluded 33 subjects who worked most of the past 2 years, but only at part-time jobs.

5. *Life Chart Schedule—Suicide:* Five percent of subjects in the Incidence cohort across all diagnostic groups made at least one suicide attempt in the last 2 years. At least a third of the attempts (and up to a half in the nonschizophrenic group) were rated as serious. Analysis showed no gender differences in these results.
6. *Life Chart Schedule—Help-Seeking and Sources of Support:* A fifth (20.9%) of Incidence subjects had been hospitalized for psychiatric reasons at some point in the last 2 years; a considerably larger number (69.3%) had received some form of substantial psychiatric treatment (chiefly medication); a minority (23.8%) had received other professional help; and over half (52.9%) had been on neuroleptic medication for most of the last 2 years of follow-up. Percentages of all forms of treatment were smaller in the Prevalence cohort; 8.7% had been hospitalized; 53.7% had received some form of substantial care; 22.5% had sought other help; and 32.1% had been on neuroleptics for most of the last 2 years (although half had taken them at some point in that period) (see Table 3.6).

Stricter Senses of "Recovered"

Although roughly half of all ISoS subjects have experienced no psychotic episodes in the last 2 years of follow-up, some (6% in the Incidence group) continued to exhibit prominent negative symptoms, as shown in Table 3.4. If "end-state recovery" is defined as never psychotic in the last 2 years *and* exhibiting no residual symptoms, the never psychotic figures fall by 4.2 to 11.7% across the diagnostic subgroups. (Compare Tables 3.4 and 3.7.)

Negative symptoms, which are not rated as "prominent," may nevertheless exert subtle effects on functional disability and quality of life. If the threshold is therefore raised further, and the term applied only to those subjects who are asymptomatic, without significant disability and not in treatment (Mason et al., 1995), the number of "recovered" subjects falls substantially. In the ISoS group as a whole, only 23.2% of Incidence subjects and 27.5% of Prevalence subjects meet the stricter criteria, down from 56.2% and 60.2%, respectively, rated as recovered by the Bleuler

TABLE 3.6 Treatment Status Over Last 2 Years of Follow-up

	All Psychoses		*Sz Only*		*Non-Sz*	
	Inc.	*Prev.*	*Inc.*	*Prev.*	*Inc.*	*Prev.*
Ever Hospitalized	20.9	8.7	24.2	9.9	15.0	6.9
Substantial Psych. Care	69.3	53.7	76.0	52.8	57.1	55.3
Other Help	23.8	22.5	25.8	26.4	20.2	15.9
Any Neuroleptics	65.0	50.7	74.5	50.7	47.5	50.6
Neurolep. Most of Time	52.9	32.1	61.3	32.4	37.5	31.6

TABLE 3.7 "Recovered" by Stricter Criteria

	All Psychoses		*Sz Only*		*Non-Sz*	
	Inc.	*Prev.*	*Inc.*	*Prev.*	*Inc.*	*Prev.*
Never Psychotic in Last 2 years of Follow-up + No Residual Symptoms	39.0	41.9	31.1	36.6	53.1	50.6
Bleuler Rating of "Recovered" and GAF-D >60 and						
• not in treatment	23.2	27.5	16.3	25.4	35.8	31.0
• treatment +/ or hosp.	43.8	51.9	37.8	48.6	54.8	57.4

TABLE 3.8 Mixed Recovery: Percentages of Subjects Working Most of the Last 2 Years of Follow-up Who Continue to Experience Substantial Symptoms (Bleuler Rating of Moderate or Severe) and/or Significant Disability (GAF-D<61)

	All Psychoses		*Sz Only*		*Non-Sz*	
	Inc.	*Prev.*	*Inc.*	*Prev.*	*Inc.*	*Prev.*
Paid Work	19.0	21.2	18.6	21.8	19.8	20.0
(N's)	(273)	(85)	(167)	(55)	(106)	(30)
Developing[a]	18.1	23.6	15.4	23.6	23.7	23.8
Developed[a]	19.7	**7.7**[b]	21.3	**0**	17.7	**11.1**
Household Activities	30.9	35.9	36.7	51.5	23.6	19.4
(N's)	(162)	(64)	(90)	(33)	(72)	(31)
Developing	26.7	35.3	34.6	48.3	14.7	19.0
Developed	35.5	**38.5**	39.5	**75.0**	31.6	**22.2**

[a] "Developed" centers include Dublin, Honolulu, Moscow, Nagasaki, Nottingham, Prague, Rochester, Groningen, Mannheim, and Sofia; developed prevalence is Prague alone; "Developing" centers include Agra, Cali, Chandigarh rural and urban, Hong Kong, Madras, and Beijing.

[b] Figures in bold = for Prague only.

scale. Among schizophrenic subjects, the percentage falls to 16.3% in the Incidence group and 25.4% in the Prevalence group. The nonschizophrenic group fares better, with approximately one-third in both Incidence and Prevalence groups meeting strict criteria of recovered.

Alternatively, it could be argued that the concept of "treated recovery" should not be excluded because in many chronic or episodic disorders, patients are expected to take "maintenance" medication whilst achieving good quality of life. If we admit subjects who have received treatment or been hospitalized at any time in the last 2 years of assessed follow-up, but who are otherwise without symptoms or disability, the percentage of ISoS subjects considered recovered rises substantially to 43.8% in the Incidence group and to over half of the Prevalence group. The difference is especially marked for the Incidence schizophrenic group, where the percentage more than doubles, from 16.3% to 37.8%; in the Prevalence group, the percentage rises to 48.6%. By these modified criteria, too, over half of the nonschizophrenic group would be considered recovered.

Nor should we expect improvement in distinctive domains of recovery to proceed according to some integrated timetable. As suggested by the discrepant findings reported above for different measures of outcome, distinctive areas of outcome—symptoms, functioning, social role performance—may be affected by variables specific to that domain (Strauss and Carpenter, 1972). As Table 3.8 shows strikingly, roughly 20% of those working in paid employment for most of the last 2 years have suffered some significant symptomatology or disability (perhaps manifest in impaired social relationships) or both; for subjects doing household work, the figure was closer to a third. Moreover, the latter effect was generally stronger for subjects in the schizophrenic subgroup. Further analysis reveals no obvious center clusterings that would account for this result. Contrary to expectation, the percentage of subjects with significant psychiatric difficulties who were working (paid and household work) in developed centers is at least comparable to that in developing centers, especially in the Incidence schizophrenic groups.

COURSE

Overall Time Trends

Psychotic symptoms proved to be prominent only in the initial third of the follow-up period (first 5 to 8 years, depending upon length of period) for nearly two-thirds of ISoS subjects, across all analytic groups.

Disability was a prominent feature in the initial third of the course only for approximately half the subjects, and treatment with medication for a somewhat lower percentage (roughly 42%) of Incidence cohorts and somewhat higher percentage (roughly 58%) of Prevalence cohorts. For only a small percentage of ISoS subjects (5% or fewer) was there evidence of late improvement, with symptoms, disability, and/or medication prominent only in the first two-thirds of the follow-up period, and dropping off thereafter. Half or more of Incidence subjects across all analytic groups were rated by investigators as much or somewhat improved, as were approximately two-fifths of those in the Prevalence cohorts.

Course of Illness Over Entire Period

More detailed course of illness patterns were constructed using a modified version of Bleuler's typology (Bleuler, 1978), which combined mode of onset (acute vs. insidious), overall trajectory (simple vs. undulating course), and end state (recovered or mild impairment vs. moderate or severe impairment, as rated by the Bleuler scale). Table 3.9 displays the relative frequency of the eight resulting course types. With the sole exception of the Prevalence schizophrenia group (where the figure is 44%), episodic illness, whether of acute or insidious origin, accounts for favorable outcomes in well over half of all subjects. Of that group, at least 61% (and over two-thirds [68%] in the Incidence schizophrenic group) had at least two illness episodes.

Developed vs. Developing Centers

As Table 3.10 shows, findings for the ISoS Incidence cohorts also offer evidence for the durability of the differential course and outcome advantage enjoyed by developing centers. Whether using a strict (ICD-10) or a broad (spectrum) diagnostic classification, and whether considering overall clinical status, symptoms, disabilities, or social functioning (as indexed by work), subjects in the developing centers show a more favorable picture. Potential sources of bias were examined—differential loss to follow-up; arbitrary groupings of centers; diagnostic ambiguities (including the possible role played by "nonaffective acute remitting psychosis" [Susser and Wanderling, 1994]); selective outcome measures; and gender. These sources of bias were found inadequate to explain the differential (Hopper and Wanderling, 2000).

DISCUSSION

Comparison with Outcome and Course Findings of Other Longitudinal Studies

The ISoS results compare favorably with those found in other longitudinal studies of schizophrenia

TABLE 3.9 Modified Bleuler Course Types[a]

			All Psychoses		*Sz Only*		*Non-Sz*	
Course Type			*Inc.*	*Prev.*	*Inc.*	*Prev.*	*Inc.*	*Prev.*
1. Acute	Episodic	Good	39.4	20.3	29.4	17.7	57.4	24.7
2. Insidious	Simple	Poor	10.6	23.4	14.4	31.9	3.6	8.6
3. Acute	Episodic	Poor	5.0	1.4	4.9	1.4	5.2	1.2
4. Insidious	Simple	Good	7.7	12.6	10.4	14.9	2.8	8.6
5. Insidious	Episodic	Good	20.8	32.0	22.6	26.2	17.7	42.0
6. Acute	Simple	Poor	7.7	3.6	9.1	2.8	5.2	4.9
7. Insidious	Episodic	Poor	2.7	3.2	4.0	1.4	0.4	6.2
8. Acute	Simple	Good	6.1	3.6	5.3	3.5	7.6	3.7

[a] Pattern was constructed by combining mode of onset as rated by local investigator (with acute = ≤1 month, except for IPSS, where it was restricted to episodes that took shape precipitously, in a single day), overall course character (episodic vs. simple), and end state (Bleuler "recovered" or "minimal" symptomatology [good] vs. "moderate" or "severe" symptomatology [poor]). Note that for Bleuler and other investigators, the cut-off for acute mode of onset is longer, at least 6 months. Hence, an unknown number of cases classified as insidious here (those in the 1–6 month range) would have been classified as acute by Bleuler and others.

(Table 3.11). Judged by percentage of subjects considered recovered or without significant impairment (Bleuler "recovered" or "mild" impairment)—two-thirds of the Incidence schizophrenia group, slightly lower in the Prevalence group—the ISoS findings rank among the highest published to date.

The distribution of modified Bleuler course patterns constructed for the ISoS schizophrenic cohort can be compared with those found in three other longitudinal studies of schizophrenia (Table 3.12). If one allows for differences in the measurement of mode of onset, there are striking parallels between the Bleuler and Incidence ISoS cohorts, with approximately half of each group characterized by episodic courses with "good" outcomes. Simple courses with good outcomes account for another quarter of the Bleuler group, but

TABLE 3.10 Course and Outcome, "Developing" vs. "Developed" Centers,[a] Incidence Cohorts Only (percentages)

	Developed	*Developing*	*Odds Ratio (.95 confid. interval)*
A. ICD-10 Sz. N's	*319*	*183*	
Bleuler Scale Recovered	44	55	1.57 (1.09–2.27)
GAF-S (>60)	43	70	3.15 (2.12–4.70)
GAF-D (>60)	41	65	2.64 (1.79–3.90)
Global DAS (Excell/Good)	24	53	3.51 (2.27–5.41)
Never psychotic in last 2 yrs	37	53	1.97 (1.36–2.86)
Working most of last 2 yrs	46	73	3.13 (2.09–4.70)
B. Broad Spectrum Sz. (ICD-10+S/A+Sz.-like) N's	410	230	
Bleuler Scale Recovered	49	60	1.59 (1.15–2.21)
GAF-S (>60)	48	73	3.05 (2.13–4.38)
GAF-D (>60)	44	69	2.74 (1.93–3.89)
Global DAS (Excell/Good)	28	57	3.48 (2.38–5.08)
Never psychotic in last 2 yrs	40	58	2.07 (1.49–2.88)
Working most of last 2 yrs	49	77	3.61 (2.48–5.25)

(all differences significant at $p \leq .02$)

[a] See note[a] Table 3.8 above for classification of centers. Note that Incidence cohorts excludes subjects from Agra, Beijing, and Cali. Hence, "developing" here includes only Chandigarh (urban and rural), Chennai, and Hong Kong. Reclassifying Hong Kong as developed reduces the differential somewhat but not significantly (see Hopper and Wanderling, 2000, table 4).

TABLE 3.11 Comparison with Other Longitudinal Studies of Schizophrenia: End-Stage Outcome[d]

	Follow-Up Cohort Size	*Average F-U Period (yrs.)*	*% Recovered or Significantly Improved*	*Comments*
Bleuler (1978) (1st adm.)	208	23	53 66	Assessed for last 5 yrs.
Ciompi & Müller (1976)	289	37	57	Bleuler criteria
Huber et al. (1975)	502	22	56	"social recovery"
Tsuang et al. (1979)	186	35	46	Feighner criteria
Harding et al. (1987)	180	32	62–68	GAF-S > 60[a]
DSM-III Sz only	82	32	60	
DeSisto et al. (1995)	119	36	49	GAF-S > 60
Breier et al. (1992)	58	13[b]	21	GAF-S, work, social relations, BPRS, SANS
Marneros et al. (1992)	148	25	58 36	Full remiss, or non-Sz residual; DAS ≥ good
ISoS—ICD-10 Sz only				
Incidence	502	13–17	67/54	Recov. or mild/GAF-S
Prevalence	142	26[c]	63/57	>60 last mo.

[a] Described as "good functioning" (Harding et al., 1987) or "functioning at least 'pretty well'" (DeSisto et al., 1995, p.336).

[b] 13 years = average time since onset of illness; NIMH cohort described as "partially responsive" to neuroleptic medication.

[c] Beijing cohort (N = 58) was followed for an average of 12 years.

[d] Adapted from Harding, Zubin, and Strauss (1987), and updated.

only an additional 15% of the ISoS Incidence group. Episodic courses eventuating in poor outcomes, which account for nearly a third of the Vermont cohort (Harding, Brooks, Ashikaga, Strauss, and Breier, 1987), amount to only 9% of the Bleuler and ISoS Incidence cohorts. At this 15-year stage of follow-up, we observe only to a modest extent the "slow, uphill return to health" described elsewhere by Harding and colleagues (Harding, Zubin, and Strauss, 1992). Except for a small group of subjects,[6] we find the pattern of early course type to be strongly suggestive of the later pattern—a finding which underlines the potential long-term benefits of assertive intervention targeted on the early symptoms of the disorder.

Limitations of the Data

The rather hopeful picture embodied in these findings requires some qualification, however, in view of methodological constraints and selection bias. As discussed earlier, the alive ISoS cohort differs from those lost to follow-up in ways that could skew outcome for the former in a more favorable direction. Were findings adjusted to take this potential bias into account, this would reduce our percentage recovered scores somewhat, although they would remain among the most optimistic reported. Outcomes for the Prevalence cohort are most problematic in this respect. (But see Drake et al., chapter 7, this volume, for an analysis of lost-to-follow-up that suggests potential bias was negligible.) Still, those same findings nevertheless provide a window on the longer-term (25-year) perspective over and above that accorded by the 15-year follow-up period for the Incidence cohort. Our measures of social functioning, too, were crude at best and could be misleading. To take one example, living independently in the community turned out not to be a reliable proxy for needs assessment. Information on 200 subjects from a select group of centers (Beijing, Chennai [Madras], Hong Kong, Sofia), reveals that although three-quarters of the subjects were listed as living with family, for a substantial percentage (39.5%) this amounted to a surrogate institutional arrangement

6. The percentage of ISoS subjects with unremitting early course who go on to recover is 22 and 23% in the developing and developed groups of centers, respectively (Hopper and Wanderling, 2000).

TABLE 3.12 Comparisons with Other Longitudinal Studies of Schizophrenia: Course of Illness Typology (percentages)[a]

Course Type	*Ciompi/Müller*[b] (*n* = 228)	*Bleuler* (*n* = 208)	*Harding et al.* (*n*=82)	*ISoS*[c] (*n* = 539)
1. A/E/G	25.4	27 (mild)	7	29.4 Inc.
		22 (recov.)		17.7 Prv.
2. I/S/P	24.1	12	4	14.4
				31.9
3. A/E/P	11.9	9	4	4.9
				1.4
4. I/S/G	10.1	23	12	10.4
				14.9
5. I/E/G	9.6	0	38	22.6
				26.2
6. A/S/P	8.3	1	3	9.1
				2.8
7. I/E/P	5.3	0	27	4.0
				1.4
8. A/S/G	5.3	2	5	5.3
				3.5

[a] See studies for specific criteria used to determine diagnosis, rate onset (acute ≤ 6 months) and describe course (simple vs. episodic). The Swiss studies used same measures of end state—Bleuler "recovered" or "minimal" symptomatology (good) vs. Bleuler "moderate" or "severe" symptomatology (poor)—assessed (for most subjects) for a 5-year period. Harding used GAS and the Strauss-Carpenter Levels of Function Outcome Scale, finding 34% fully recovered and 34% significantly improved. ISoS used Bleuler criteria, but applied them to the most recent month assessed, rather than 5 years.

[b] Total cohort size = 289; course type could not be determined for 61 subjects.

[c] Incidence/Prevalence cohorts, converted baseline diagnosis of ICD-10 schizophrenia only.

at least some of the time. The burden of care on family could be considerable. Similarly, institutionalization rates (hospitalization and supervised residence) are problematic, reflecting administrative policy and resource availability as much as, if not more so, than need for care (Harrison et al., 1994; 1996). This figure was higher for centers within the developed world than for those within the developing world, with the exceptions of Hong Kong and Moscow. Finally, global ratings of recovery do not fully reflect subtle disabilities which may continue to exert a profound effect on the quality of life of subjects, caregivers, and families. Nor does recovery—if considered only as the absence of impairment—adequately capture lost potential in terms of sufferers' social, occupational, and personal development.

On other fronts, too, ISoS has been less successful than originally hoped. It has done little to lift the veil of persisting obscurity regarding the operant "cultural" or environmental factors that affect course of illness and restoration of function. Such putatively shaping forces remain, to steal a phrase from earlier critics, little more than "synonyms for unexplained variance" (Edgerton and Cohen, 1994). Data on the timing of "onset"—more precisely, on the emergence of early symptoms—that would have allowed us to determine the duration of untreated psychosis (DUP), were not reported consistently enough to permit analysis of the effects of early detection and treatment for the aggregated data, although this has been reported separately for some centers (e.g., Harrison et al., 1996). Preliminary inspection suggests, too, that insufficient numbers of key informants were interviewed to allow us to analyze the role of and impact on family caregivers, changes in vernacular notions of attribution, and felt weight and practical consequences of stigma. All such information is critical to the development of a comprehensive public health approach to severe mental illness.

CONCLUSION

Still, there is no gainsaying that this report amounts in the main, with qualifications, to a narrative of hope. This should not obscure the fact that for many patients, recovery is still a struggle, requiring long-term engagement with treatment services. The mixed nature of recovery—nowhere more apparent than in the 20% or better of subjects who managed to work regularly despite persisting symptoms and/or disabilities—highlights the need for a better understanding of the unevenness of restored function: the different "schedules" of recovery for different domains, running at varying paces, to disparate degrees of thoroughness (Strauss and Carpenter, 1972; Strauss, 1989; Davidson and Strauss, 1992). How are such discrepancies handled by subjects, and how do they infiltrate identity (Weingarten, 1994)? How are they supported or subverted by community-based programs? How should we best interpret, and explain to those prescribed it, "maintenance medication?" In short, ISoS adds to the evidence for the "open systems" (Strauss and Carpenter, 1972), or relatively autonomous, nature of domains of symptoms, functioning, and social performance, each requiring targeted interventions in treatment programs.

This overarching message—that schizophrenia is largely an episodic disorder with rather favorable outcome for a significant proportion of those afflicted—should be widely broadcast. Expectation, on the part of patient, family members, and treating clinicians, is a powerful factor in recovery. If anything, this report gives ample reason to hope. If it helps sustain the prospect of recovery, it will have served a purpose beyond the academic.

References

American Psychiatric Association (1994), *Diagnostic and Statistical Manual of Mental Disorders*, 4th ed. Washington, DC: American Psychiatric Press.

Andreasen, N. C. (1989), The scale for the assessment of negative symptoms (SANS): Conceptual and theoretical foundations. *Brit. J. Psychiatry*, 155(Suppl. 7):49–52.

Bleuler, M. (1978), *The Schizophrenic Disorders, Long-term Patient and Family Studies*, tr. S. M. Clemens. New Haven, CT: Yale University Press.

Breier, A., Schreiber, J. L., Dyer, J., & Pickar, D. (1992), Course of illness and predictors of outcome in chronic schizophrenia: Implications for pathophysiology. *Brit. J. Psychiatry*, 161(Suppl. 18):38–43.

Ciompi, L. (1985), Aging and schizophrenic psychosis. *Acta Psychiatr. Scand.*, 71:93–105.

——Müller, C. (1976), Lifestyle and age of schizophrenics: A catemnestic long-term study into old age. (In German) *Mongraphien aus dem Gesamtgebiete der Psychiatrie*. Psychiatry Series. 12:1–242.

Davidson, L., & Strauss, J. S. (1992), Sense of self in recovery from severe mental illness. *Brit. J. Med. Psychol.*, 65:131–145.

Day, R., Nielsen, J. A., Korten, A., Ernberg, G., Dube, K. C., Gebhart, J., Jablensky, A., Leon, C., Marsella, A., Olatawura, M., Sartorius, N., Stromgren, E., Takahashi, R., Wig, N., & Wynne, L. C. (1987), Stressful life events preceding the acute onset of schizophrenia: A cross-national study from the World Health Organization. *Culture, Med., & Psychiatry*, 11:123–205.

DeSisto, M., Harding, C. M., McCormick, R. V., Ashikaga, T., & Brooks, G. W. (1995), The Maine and Vermont three-decade studies of serious mental illness. II. Longitudinal course comparisons. *Brit. J. Psychiatry*, 167: 338–342.

Edgerton, R. B., & Cohen, A. (1994), Culture and schizophrenia: The DOSMD challenge. *Brit. J. Psychiatry*, 164:222–231.

Harding, C. M., Brooks, G. W., Ashikaga, T., Strauss, J. S., & Breier, A. (1987a), The Vermont longitudinal study of persons with severe mental illness. I. Methodology, study samples, and overall status 32 years later. *Amer. J. Psychiatry*, 144:718–726.

Harding, C. M., Brooks, G. W., Ashikaga, T., Strauss, J. S., & Breier, A. (1987b), The Vermont longitudinal study of persons with severe mental illness, II: Long-term outcome of subjects who respectively met DSM-III criteria for schizophrenia. *Amer. J. Psychiatry*, 144:727–735.

——McCormick, R. V., Strauss, J. S., Ashikaga, T., & Brooks, G. W. (1989), Computerized life chart methods to map domains of function and illustrate patterns of interactions in the long-term course trajectories of patients who once met the criteria for DSM-III schizophrenia. *Brit. J. Psychiatry*, 155(Suppl. 5):100–106.

——Zubin, J., & Strauss, J. S. (1987), Chronicity in schizophrenia: Fact, partial fact, or artifact? *Hosp. & Comm. Psychiatry*, 38:477–486.

——, ——, —— (1992), Chronicity in schizophrenia: Revisited. *Brit. J. Psychiatry*, 161(Suppl. 18):27–37.

Harrison, G., Croudace, T., Mason, P., Glazebrook, C., & Medley, I. (1996), Predicting the long-term outcome of schizophrenia. *Psycholog. Med.*, 26:697–705.

——Mason, P., Glazebrook, C., Medley, I., Croudace, T., & Doherty, S. (1994), Residence of incident cohort of pyschotic patients after 13 years of follow up. *Brit. Med. J.*, 308:813–816.

Hopper, K., & Wanderling, J. (2000), Revisiting the developed vs. developing country distinction in course and outcome in schizophrenia: Results from ISoS, the WHO-Collaborative Follow-up Project. *Schizoph. Bull.*, 26(4): 835–846.

——Huber, G., Gross, G., Schüttler, R., & Linz, M. (1975), A long-term follow-up study of schizophrenia: Psychiatric course of illness and prognosis. *Acta Psychiatr. Scand.*, 52:49–57.

Jablensky, A., Sartorius, N., Ernberg, G., Anker, M., Korten, A., Cooper, J. E., Day, R., & Bertelsen, A. (1992), Schizophrenia: Manifestations, incidence and course in different cultures: A World Health Organization ten-country study. *Psycholog. Med.*, 20 (Monogr. Suppl):1–97.

——Schwarz, R., & Tomov, T. (1980), WHO collaborative study on impairments and disabilities associated with schizophrenia. *Acta Psychiatr. Scand.*, 62(Suppl. 285):152–163.

Katz, M. M., Marsella, A., Dube, K. C., Olatawura, M., Takahashi, R., Nakane, Y., Wynne, L. C., Gift, T., Brennan, J., Sartorius N., & Jablensky, A. (1988), On the expression of psychosis in different cultures: Schizophrenia in an Indian and in a Nigerian community. *Culture, Med. & Psychiatry*, 12:331–355.

Leff, J., Sartorius, N., Jablensky, A., Korten, A., & Ernberg, G. (1992), The International Pilot Study of Schizophrenia: Five-year follow-up findings. *Psycholog. Med.*, 22:131–145.

——Wig, N. N., Bedi, H., Menon, D. K., Kuipers, L., Korten, A., Ernberg, G., Day, R., Sartorius, N., & Jablensky, A. (1990), Relatives' expressed emotion and the course of schizophrenia in Chandigarh. *Brit. J. Psychiatry*, 156:351–356.

——, ——Ghosh, A., Bedi, H., Menon, D. K., Kuipers, L., Korten, A., Ernberg, G., Day, R., Sartorius, N., & Jablensky, A. (1987), Influence of relatives' expressed emotion on the course of schizodphrenia in Chandigarh. *Brit. J. Psychiatry*, 151:166–173.

Marneros, A., Deister, A., & Rohde, A. (1992), Comparison of long-term outcome of schizophrenic, affective and schizoaffective disorders. *Brit. J. Psychiatry*, 161(Suppl. 18):44–51.

Mason, P., Harrison, G., Glazebrook, C., Medley, I., Dalkin, T., & Croudace, T. (1995), Characteristics of outcome in schizophrenia at 13 years. *Brit. J. Psychiatry*, 167:596–603.

Sartorius, N., Gulbinat, W., Harrison, G., Laska, E., & Siegel, C. (1996), Long-term follow-up of schizophrenia in 16 countries. *Soc. Psychol. Psychiatr. Epidemiol.*, 31:249–258.

——Jablensky, A., Korten, A., Ernberg, G., Anker, M., Cooper, J. E., & Day, R. (1986), Early manifestations and first contact incidence of schizophrenia in different cultures. *Psycholog. Med.*, 16:909–928.

Schwartz, F., Terkelsen, K. G., & Smith, T. E. (1992), Long-term outcome in schizophrenia. *Arch. Gen. Psychiatry*, 51:502–503.

Strauss, J. S. (1989), Mediating process in schizophrenia: Toward a new dynamic psychiatry. *Brit. J. Psychiatry*, 155 (Suppl. 5):22–28.

——Carpenter, W. T. (1972), Prediction of outcome in schizophrenia: I. Characteristics of outcome. *Arch. Gen. Psychiatry*, 27:739–746.

Susser, E., & Wanderling, J. (1994), Epidemiology of nonaffective acute remitting psychosis vs. schizophrenia. Sex and sociocultural setting. *Arch. Gen. Psychiatry*, 51: 294–301.

Tsuang, M., Woolson, R., & Fleming, J. (1979), Long-term outcome of major psychoses: I. Schizophrenia and affective disorders compared with psychiatrically symptom-free surgical conditions. *Arch. Gen. Psychiatry*, 36:1295–1301.

Weingarten, R. (1994), The ongoing process of recovery. *Psychiatry*, 57:369–375.

Wiersma, D., Nienhuis, F. J., Giel, R., deJong, A., & Sloof, C. J. (1996), Assessment of the need for care 15 years after onset of a Dutch cohort of schizophrenic patients and an international comparison. *Soc. Psychiatry & Psychiatric Epidemiol.*, 31:114–121.

——, —— Slooff, C. J., & Giel, R. (1998), Natural course of schizophrenic disorders. A 15-year follow-up of a Dutch incidence cohort. *Schizophr. Bull.*, 24:75–85.

Wig, N. N., Menon, D. K., Bedi, H., Ghosh, A., Kuipers, L., Leff, J., Korten, A., Day, R., Sartorius, N., Ernberg, G., & Jablensky, A. (1987), Expressed emotion and schizophrenia in North India. I. Cross-cultural transfer of ratings of relatives' expressed emotion. *Brit. J. Psychiatry*, 151:156–160.

——, ——, —— Leff, J., Kuipers, L., Ghosh, A., Day, R., Korten, A., Ernberg, G., Sartorius, N., & Jablensky, A. (1987), Expressed emotion and schizophrenia in North India. 2. Distribution of expressed emotion components among relatives of schizophrenia patients in Aarhus and Chandigarh. *Brit. J. Psychiatry*, 151:160–165.

World Health Organization (1973), *Report of the International Pilot Study of Schizophrenia*. Geneva: World Health Organization.

——(1978), Glossary. Geneva: World Health Organization.

——(1979), *Schizophrenia: An International Follow-up Study*. New York: Wiley.

——(1992), *Psychological Impairments Rating Scale*. Geneva: World Health Organization.

——(1994), *The ICD-10 Classification of Mental and Behavioral Disorders: Conversion Tables between ICD-8, ICD-9 and ICD-10, Revision 1* (WHO/MNH/92.16. Rev. 1). Geneva: World Health Organization.

Chapter 4

Predictors of Long-Term Course and Outcome for the DOSMeD Cohort

Carole Siegel, Joseph A. Wanderling, Shang Lin, and Sherryl Baker

An investigation of the predictors of long-term course and outcome for persons diagnosed with schizophrenia or a related psychosis was conducted using a subsample of subjects participating in ISoS who entered the study as Incidence cases.

Earlier analyses of 2-year outcomes in both the Determinants of Outcome of Schizophrenia (DOSMeD) study and the International Pilot Study of Schizophrenia (IPSS) concurred that both cultural and illness factors play a strong role in predicting outcome. Specifically, persons in developing countries had more favorable outcomes than persons in the developed countries, and insidious onset predicted poorer outcome. While some subsequent studies agreed with the WHO studies' finding on location (Karno and Jenkins, 1993), others questioned the prudence of the crude classification of centers according to the developing–developed dichotomy and the subsequent use of this categorization as a predictor of outcomes. Such an assignment, they argued, can mask differences both across cultures (Craig, Siegel, Hopper, Lin, and Sartorius, 1997) and within them, assuming as it does that cultures are relatively homogeneous (Hopper, 1991; Edgerton and Cohen, 1994).

Other studies in which the center categorization is not questioned have produced results that conflict with the finding of more favorable outcomes in the developing countries (Warner, 1994). Craig et al. (1997) reanalyzed data from the DOSMeD study in order to examine in greater depth the role that center locale plays as a predictor of course. A statistical approach was used in which the centers (as well as the categories of other variables) are not pregrouped; the method seeks to find subgroups defined by categorizations of variables that are homogeneous with respect to outcome. Their analysis confirmed earlier findings that the strongest predictor of "pattern of course" (defined in terms of the quality of remissions between episodes) was a grouping of centers. However, the grouping that emerged, while close to the developing—developed dichotomy, did not strictly adhere to it. Subjects in Nottingham and Prague joined those in the developing countries to form a subgroup in which greater proportions had more favorable outcome. As in the WHO monograph (Jablensky et al., 1992), type of onset was also a significant predictor of outcome for the group as a whole. But interaction effects were detected, and insidious onset did not predict poor outcome for all subgroups. In Nottingham and Prague, as well as in the developing countries, persons with insidious onset were equally likely to have good outcomes as they were to have poor outcomes, in contrast to persons from the other study areas in which insidious onset strongly predicted poorer outcome.

Recent studies have explored the role of factors predictive of short-term outcome in explaining longer-term outcome. Childers and Harding (1990) report on the relationship of gender and premorbid social functioning to outcomes of persons from the Vermont Longitudinal Research Project, subjects who were followed for more than 30 years after discharge from the hospital. Females had both better premorbid social functioning and better long-term outcomes than males, although the latter finding was not statistically different. In a 7-year follow-up study of persons treated for schizophrenia in Nigeria, the gender effect was reversed: Women had poorer outcome than men and were more subject to relapse. Insidious onset and poor early course of illness also predicted unfavorable long-term outcome (Ohaeri, 1993). In Madras, India, a 10-year follow-up study found that insidious onset, baseline symptoms of sexual, religious, and grandiose delusions, and flat affect all predicted poor outcomes for both men and women (Thara, Henrietta, Joseph, Rajkumar, and Eaton, 1994).

ISoS affords the opportunity for further investigation of the predictors of long-term outcome. By using the DOSMeD cohort participating in ISoS for whom short-term outcomes are known, we are able to include, in addition to factors of short-term course, early illness course itself in the list of predictors under consideration. Outcome is examined from three perspectives: current (last month of follow-up) symptoms, as well as disability and illness course over the follow-up period. A conceptual framework is introduced to guide the choice of factors expected to influence outcome, one that encompasses both illness and contextual variables.

METHODS

A detailed description of the research protocol and instruments used in the ISoS is presented in the chapter, "Study Methodology" (Siegel et al., chapter 2, this volume).

Sample

Sixty percent of those from the original DOSMeD cohort with a recorded diagnosis of psychosis at baseline, and who had short-term follow-up interviews (88% of the original cohort), were also available for the long-term follow-up interview of this study (30.6% were lost to follow-up, 9.4% had died). The study sample is comprised of these 461 alive DOSMeD subjects. A succeeding chapter examines the potential bias introduced by basing the analyses only on the alive cohort that was available for follow-up interviews, and concludes that it is negligible (Drake et al., chapter 7, this volume). The centers included in the study and the sample size of the alive, interviewed group for each is given in Table 4.1 The characteristics of the sample are described in

TABLE 4.1 Sample Size and Number (%) in Each Outcome Category by Center

		GAF-S			*GAF-D*			*Remission Over Entire Period*		
CENTER	*All (n)*	*Poor: 1–60*	*Good: 61–90*	*Missing*	*Poor: 1–60*	*Good: 61–90*	*Missing*	*Incomplete/ Continuous*	*Complete Remission*	*Missing*
Chandigarh Urban	75	18	57	0	19	56	0	31	40	4
		24.00	76.00	0.00	25.33	74.67	0.00	41.33	53.33	5.33
Chandigarh Rural	38	7	30	1	7	30	1	9	25	4
		18.42	78.95	2.63	18.42	78.95	2.63	23.68	65.79	10.53
Dublin	37	17	18	2	19	16	2	20	12	5
		45.95	48.65	5.41	51.35	43.24	5.41	54.05	32.43	13.51
Honolulu	24	13	11	0	11	13	0	14	8	2
		54.17	45.83	0.00	45.83	54.17	0.00	58.33	33.33	8.33
Moscow	45	12	33	0	13	32	0	21	23	1
		26.67	73.33	0.00	28.89	71.11	0.00	46.67	51.11	2.22
Nagasaki	56	30	26	0	34	22	0	40	15	1
		53.57	46.43	0.00	60.71	39.29	0.00	71.43	26.79	1.79
Nottingham	83	38	44	1	37	46	0	36	42	5
		45.78	53.01	1.20	44.58	55.42	0.00	43.37	50.60	6.02
Prague	70	26	40	4	35	31	4	42	24	4
		37.14	57.14	5.71	50.00	44.29	5.71	60.00	34.29	5.71
Rochester	33	18	13	2	19	11	3	17	11	5
		54.55	39.39	6.06	57.58	33.33	9.09	51.52	33.33	15.15
Total	461	179	272	10	194	257	10	230	200	31
		38.82	59.00	2.17	42.08	55.75	2.17	49.89	43.38	6.72

the introduction to the "Determinants of Outcome of Severe Mental Disorder (DOSMeD)" (Varma, this volume).

Outcome Measures

The analysis is based on two outcome measures of current status derived from the Global Assessment of Functioning Scale: one capturing symptoms (GAF-S) and the other disability (GAF-D). To measure course of illness over the entire follow-up period, type of remission over the entire period was obtained from the Life Chart Schedule, and dichotomized as complete versus incomplete remission or continuous psychosis. Complete remission is defined as single or multiple episodes with the subject showing virtually no symptoms and assuming his or her usual premorbid personality between episodes. Incomplete remission is defined as single or multiple episodes with residual psychotic symptoms or nonpsychotic symptoms that are not traits of the premorbid personality, or manifesting personality changes between episodes. This particular course variable is the same as that used by Jablensky et al. (1992) and Craig et al. (1997) so that comparisons can be made with the results from these 2-year outcome studies. Table 4.1 displays the number and percent of subjects in each outcome category.

Predictor Variables

The set of demographic and clinical predictor variables that were chosen are based on a conceptual framework that links environmental, predisposing, and clinical factors to outcomes, and includes factors that may mediate their impact. The framework is depicted in Figure 4.1. Predisposing and clinical factors came from the baseline interview and short-term follow-up assessment. In an attempt to open up the "black-box" of culture, macrolevel variables that characterize the available mental health services and the social context of an area over the follow-up period are included. Additionally, family involvement with treatment during the follow-up period is considered in its role as a possible mediator of outcome.

Selection of specific items within domains drew on those variables reported to be related to outcome in the prior DOSMeD study of short-term outcome (Craig et al., 1997), and on variables suggested in recent literature. From the prior DOSMeD study, these include age, gender, marital status, contacts with close

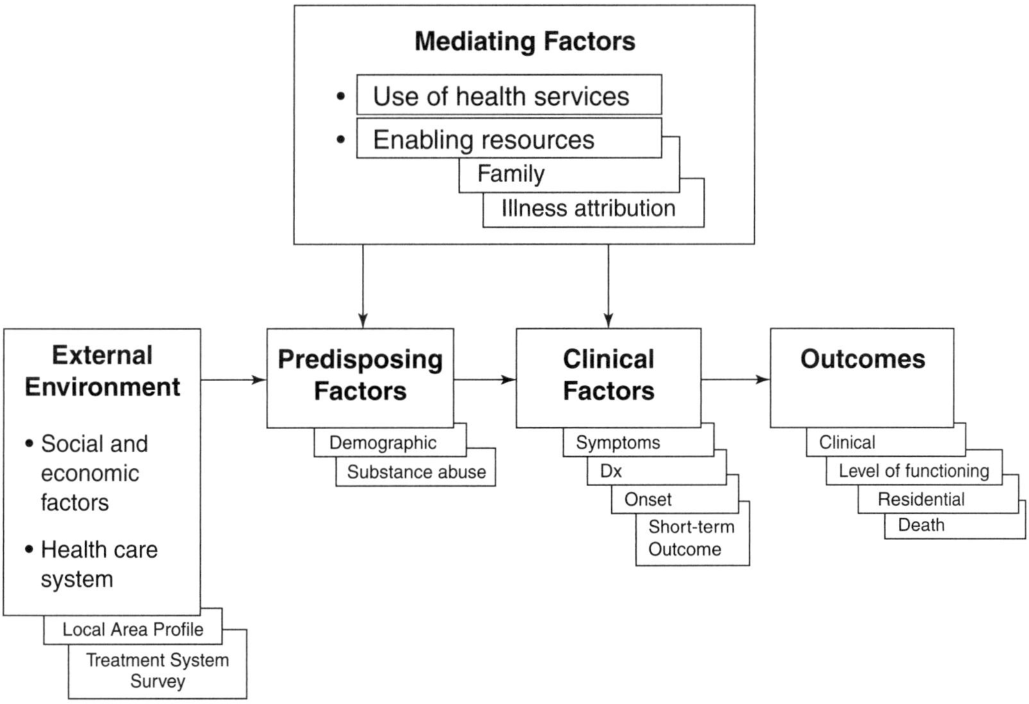

FIGURE 4.1. Conceptual Framework

friends, history of drug or alcohol use, type of onset, and diagnosis. The diagnosis is the baseline ICD-9 (converted to ICD-10) clinical consensus diagnosis, grouped into five categories: schizophrenia, schizoaffective disorder, acute schizophrenia disorder, bipolar disorders/depression, and other psychoses.

Some literature suggests that there is a clinically identifiable subgroup with a differential course that is defined by a constellation of symptoms and duration criteria known as deficit syndrome (Kirkpatrick, Buchanan, McKenney, Alphs, and Carpenter, 1989). While the DOSMeD protocol did not measure duration of symptoms, we include as predictors some of the defining symptoms of this syndrome. Assessments of these symptoms were made at baseline using the Present State Examination (PSE) and include: blunted affect, slowness and underactivity, restricted quantity of speech, loss of interest, and social withdrawal. We also considered using as a predictor baseline symptoms of hallucinations but did not, as it did not show even a weak univariate relationship to long-term outcome. Duration of untreated psychosis, cited by several researchers (e.g., Larsen, McGlashan, and Moe, 1996) as correlated with outcome, could not be included as it could not be operationalized by the data collected for all of the centers in the DOSMeD cohort.

A distinctive feature of our analysis of long-term outcome is that short-term outcome variables could be included as predictors. The short-term outcomes used are percent time psychotic and pattern of course for the initial 2 years.

Only one subject-level mediating variable is introduced in the models—family involvement with treatment over the follow-up period. The use of medications for psychiatric problems was also considered as a mediator of outcomes. However, in univariate analyses, we found that early on all subjects received medications, while later in the follow-up period, only the subjects with poor outcomes continued to receive medications. Therefore, medication use was not included in the prediction models, as it would have accounted for a large proportion of the variance in predictive models and diminished the ability to relate other variables to outcome.

Area-level mediating variables were based on information on the treatment system available to persons in the area and on the local social context during the follow-up period. These data were obtained from the area-level instruments of the ISoS package that were used to describe the external environment, as well as on information in the summary chapters describing each site's results. Key informants at each Field Research Center filled out these instruments—in most cases, the principal investigator at the center. Five research raters independently reviewed the semistructured qualitative information contained in these documents and the descriptions of the locales contained in the summary chapters. Using a Delphi-like procedure, the ratings were discussed at a group meeting, and the raters revised scores. The average of the revised scores is the item score. While extensively described in the Treatment System Survey, the health care system is covered in this analysis only by availability of inpatient services and by the type of health insurance available. Other variables related to health care turned out to be merely surrogate measures of the level of development of an area. To describe social context, variables were constructed to rate social stability, strength of nuclear and extended families, and local knowledge regarding the attribution of mental illness. Table 4.2 displays the scores for these variables by center.

Statistical Methods

A two-step statistical procedure was used for the two GAF outcome variables. First, stepwise linear regression model selection was applied to distinguish the variables most highly related to outcome. In these models, sample sizes are considerably reduced from the full cohort size because if data are missing for any regression variable, a subject is excluded from the analysis. Then, a second "fixed" model was fitted using only the variables distinguished in step 1. In these models, the sample size is considerably increased—to almost full sample size—because the set of regression variables is reduced and there are few missing data for these variables. Two sets of analyses are carried out. In one, center is included as a categorical variable; in the other, it is replaced by the set of descriptive locale variables. In the analysis that includes centers, Chandigarh urban was chosen as the contrast center. (This means that GAF scores for each center are compared to those of Chandigarh urban. The choice of the contrast center is arbitrary.) Tables 4.3a,b and 4.4a,b display the results of the fixed model regressions (i.e., the regression models based on the variables distinguished in the stepwise regressions) for symptom scores and disability scores, respectively.

Recursive partitioning was used to model the factors that impact on the course variable "complete remission vs. incomplete remission or continuously

TABLE 4.2 Area Variables by Center

	Inpatient Availability[a]	*Health Insurance Coverage*[b]			*Social Stability*[c]	*Kinship*[d]		*Attribution*[e]		
		Nations	*Private*	*Uninsured*		*Strength Nuclear Family*	*Strength Extend. Family*	*Med./ Biol.*	*Soc./ Psych.*	*Magi./ Relig.*
Chandigarh Rural	2	0	1	1	1	1.8	1.4	3	3	1
Chandigarh Urban	8	0	1	1	1.9	2	1.1	2	1	2.5
Dublin	2	1	0	0	1.9	1.2	2	1	3	3
Honolulu	6	0	1	1	1.7	2	2	2	2	2
Moscow	9	1	1	0	2.7	1.4	2	1.5	2	3
Nagasaki	5	1	1	0	1.3	1.8	1.4	1	2	2
Nottingham	12	1	0	0	1.3	1	3	1.5	2	2
Prague	2	1	1	0	2.9	1	2.3	2	1.5	3
Rochester	12	0	1	1	1.9	1	3	1	3	3

[a]1–12 = low-high
[b]1 = Yes; 0 = No
[c]1–3 = high-low stability
[d]1–3 = high-low strength
[e]1–3 = high-low attribution

TABLE 4.3a Multiple Regression with Dependent Variable: GAF-S: I. Center In, Moscow In, No Area Variables (N = 429)

Variable	*Variable Type*	*Entry Order*[a]	*Coefficient*	*Coef/SE*	*SIG* (P<.05)*
% Time Psychotic	Short-Term Follow-up	1	−0.25	−8.79	*
Center (Chandigarh Urban Contrast)		2			
Chandigarh Rural			5.17	1.39	
Dublin			−9.11	−2.40	*
Honolulu			−9.57	−2.13	*
Moscow			4.90	1.40	
Nagasaki			−4.98	−1.43	
Nottingham			−5.92	−1.95	*
Prague			−7.82	−2.39	*
Rochester			−16.27	−4.08	*
Constant			76.27		
$R^2 = 0.25$					

[a]Entry order based on stepwise regression (N = 211)

psychotic." One advantage of this method is the ability to detect interactive and subgroup effects without prespecifying the type of interactions that might occur; a second is that virtually the full sample is used, since no subject is excluded because of missing data on a predictive factor. (Surrogate variable splits are introduced for the cases in which the data for the predictor variables are missing.) The CART (Breiman, Friedman, Olshen, and Stone, 1986) method was used to conduct the partitioning. A category split of

TABLE 4.3b Multiple Regression with Dependent Variable: GAF-S II. Center Out, Area Variables In (N=419)

Variable	*Variable Type*	*Entry Order*[a]	*Coefficient*	*Coef/SE*	*SIG* (P<.05)*
Percent Time Psychotic	Short-term Follow-up	1	−0.23	−8.05	*
Diagnosis (Schizophrenia Contrast)	Baseline	2			
Schizoaffective			5.39	1.48	
Acute schizophrenia			7.08	2.85	*
Bipolar disorders/ depression			7.28	2.42	*
Other psychotic			−.94	−.24	
Age at Study Entry	Baseline	3	.20	2.13	*
Drug Use	Baseline	4	−6.16	−1.83	
Private Health Insurance	Area Mediator	5	4.05	1.92	
Constant			60.95		
$R^2=0.22$					

[a] Entry order based on stepwise regression (N=174)

a predictor variable is sought (e.g., for percent time psychotic, a split of ≤13.5% and >13.5%) that results at a particular juncture in the most accurate assignment of subjects into the outcome class in which they belong, as measured by a misclassification error. The predictor variable and its binary division that minimizes the misclassification error are chosen to start the process. All variables and all possible category splits within them are considered at each successive stage of a multistage process that branches at "nodes" resulting from prior stages of the procedure. The splitting process continues until a node is either too small to split further or is one at which all persons have the same outcome.

This large tree is then cut back progressively to form a sequence of nested subtrees. The pruning process is based on a cost–complexity measure, which is the misclassification error plus a "cost" per terminal node times the number of terminal nodes. Each subtree in the sequence is optimal in the sense that it has the smallest cost–complexity measure among all trees of the same size. While misclassification error on the full data set (resubstitution relative cost) can be used to choose a right-sized tree from the sequence, a cross-validation technique is preferred to obtain an "honest" estimate of the true misclassification error (see Breiman et al., 1986, for details). Unlike the resubstitution error, the cross-validation errors will reach a plateau after initial decreases (and in some cases, will begin to increase), as the tree size expands in contrast to the resubstitution error that continues to decrease. Cross-validation can be "n"-fold. For our analysis, the smallest node tree having close to the minimum 10-fold cross-validation error is selected as the best explanatory or predictive tree. This tree will be presented along with the larger tree for which resubstitution relative cost is reduced by 40% or more. The smaller tree gives the most robust predictive power. The larger tree, an exploratory tree, provides additional but weaker information on variables that might be related to outcome.

As in the regression analyses, in one set of the CART analyses the center is included and area variables excluded (Figure 4.2a). In a second set, the center is excluded in favor of area level variables (Figure 4.2b). The CART figures depict the splitting variables, the division of those at each split, and the percentage of subjects in the two outcome classes at each node. The first proportion in a node represents those who had poor course (incomplete remissions or

TABLE 4.4a Multiple Regression with Dependent Variable: GAF-D: I. Center In, No Area Variables (N=419)

Variable	*Variable Type*	*Entry Order*[a]	*Coefficient*	*Coef/SE*	*Sig** (*p*<.05)
Percent Time Psychotic	Short-term Follow-up	1	–.20	–7.06	*
Center (Chandigarh Urban Contrast)		2			
Chandigarh Rural			3.85	1.04	
Dublin			–9.44	–2.36	*
Honolulu			1.18	.23	
Moscow			2.79	.77	
Nagasaki			–6.53	–1.81	
Nottingham			–2.59	–.82	
Prague			–12.23	–3.49	*
Rochester			–16.93	–4.05	*
Diagnosis (Schizophrenia Contrast)	**Baseline**	3			
Schizoaffective			12.75	3.37	*
Acute Schizophrenia			6.65	2.55	*
Bipolar Disorders/ depression			6.83	2.21	*
Other Psychoses			6.13	1.56	
Drug Use	Baseline	4	–3.82	–1.00	
Constant			71.54		
R^2=26					

[a] Entry order based on stepwise regression (N=211)

TABLE 4.4b Multiple Regression with Dependent Variable: GAF-D (continued) II. Center Out, Area Variables In (N=325)

Variable	*Variable Type*	*Entry Order*[a]	*Coefficient*	*Coef/SE*	*Sig** (*p*<.05)
Percent Time Psychotic	Short-term Follow-up	1	–.18	–5.78	*
Diagnosis (Schizophrenia Contrast)	**Baseline**	2			
Schizoaffective			9.19	2.36	*
Acute schizophrenia			5.70	1.97	*
Bipolar disorders/depression			5.13	1.26	
Other psychoses			–2.28	–.50	
Blunted Affect	Baseline PSE	3	–3.79	–2.40	*
National Health Insurance	Area Mediator	4	–10.68	–3.65	*
Drug Use	Baseline	5	–10.33	–2.69	*
Family Involvement	Subject Mediator	6	–3.57	–2.56	*
Constant			80.53		
R^2=23					

[a] Entry order based on stepwise regression (N=174)

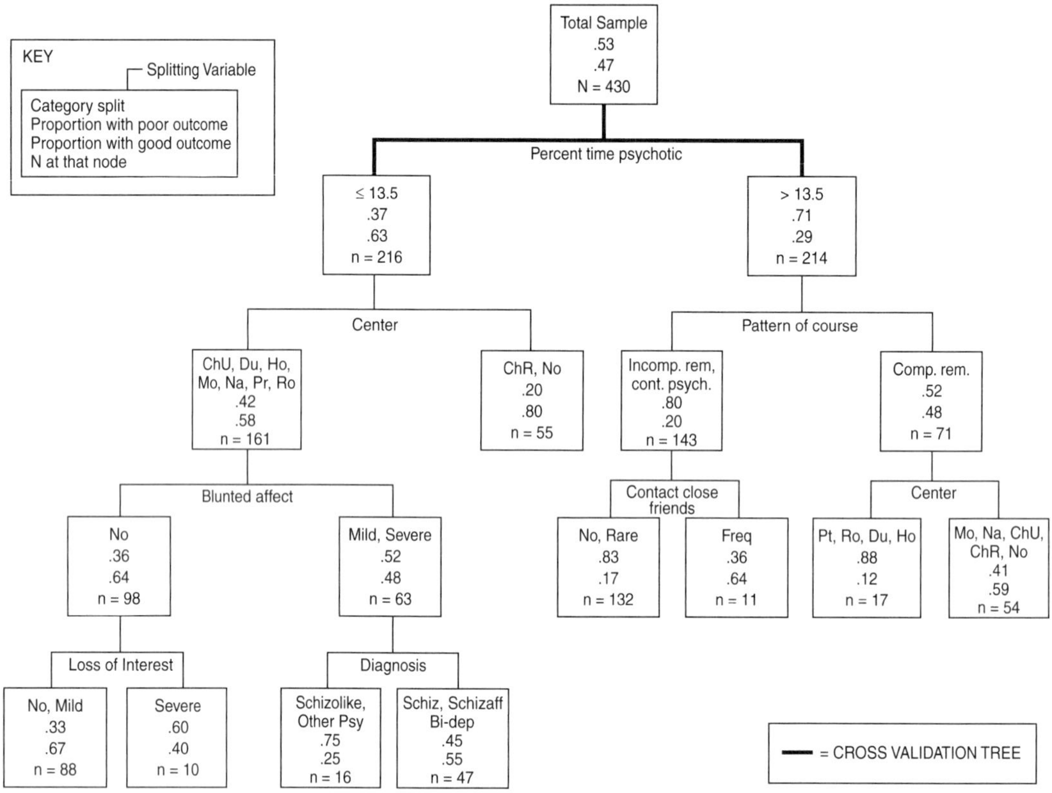

FIGURE 4.2a. CART Classification Tree: Remission Over Entire Period—Incomplete or Complete (Variables include center, exclude area descriptions)

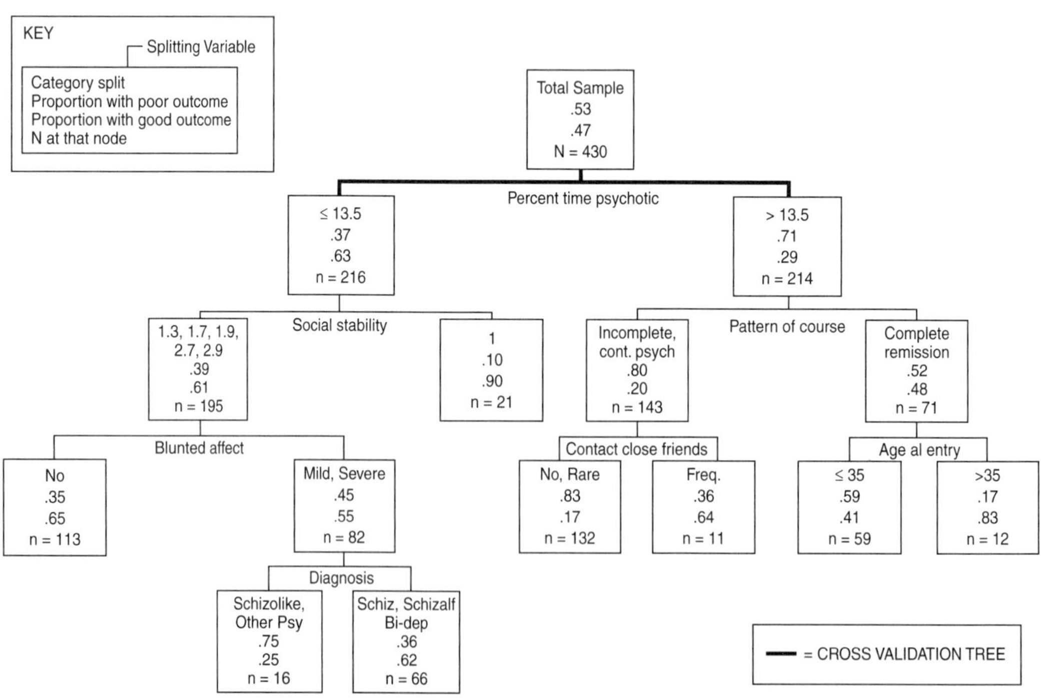

FIGURE 4.2b. CART Classification Tree: Remission Over Entire Period—Incomplete or Complete (Variables exclude Center, include area descriptions)

continuously psychotic) and the second, those with good course (complete remissions).

RESULTS

Regressions

GAF-S and GAF-D: In all regression models, percent time psychotic in the first 2 years is the strongest predictor (first to enter stepwise regression models) of both symptom and disability scores. For symptoms, the only additional variable that enters the model in which center is included (Table 4.3a) is the center variable. Subjects in Dublin, Honolulu, Nottingham, Prague, and Rochester had significantly poorer symptom scores than those in Chandigarh urban. Scores of those in Chandigarh rural, Nagasaki, and Moscow did not differ from those in Chandigarh urban. In the analysis that included area variables (Table 4.3b) *four* additional variables enter the model. By order of entry, they are baseline diagnosis, age at study entry, history of drug use, and private health insurance. Those with a baseline diagnosis of schizophrenia had significantly poorer symptom scores than those with acute schizophrenia or bipolar disorders/depression. Scores for those with other psychoses did not differ from those with schizophrenia. Persons who were younger at study entry also had poorer symptom scores. History of drug use and private health insurance were not significant in step 2.

For disability, in addition to percent time psychotic, the variables that enter the model in which center is included (Table 4.4a) are, in order of entry: center, diagnosis, and a history of drug use. In a comparison of all centers with Chandigarh urban, only those in Dublin, Prague, and Rochester had significantly poorer disability scores than those in Chandigarh urban. The finding on diagnosis is similar to that for the symptom score when center is excluded, except that those with schizoaffective disorder were also significantly better than those with schizophrenia, while drug use was not significant at step 2. In the analysis that included area variables (Table 4.4b), additional variables that enter the model are, by order of entry: diagnosis, blunted affect, national health insurance, history of drug use, and family involvement in treatment. The finding for diagnosis indicated that those with acute schizophrenia and schizoaffective disorders had better outcomes than those with schizophrenia. Those without national health insurance had better disability scores. Family involvement with treatment decisions, presence of blunted affect from the baseline PSE, and premorbid drug use were associated with poorer disability scores.

CART

In the analysis that includes center (Figure 4.2a), the optimal cross-validation tree (24% reduction in cross-validated relative cost) is based on the 2-year follow-up variable percent time psychotic. The nine-node exploratory tree (40% reduction in resubstitution relative cost) adds center, pattern of course, a premorbid adjustment variable ("contact with close friends"), presenting diagnosis, and the presenting symptoms of "blunted affect" and "loss of interest." Percent time psychotic, the first variable to enter the model and the only variable in the cross-validation tree, splits at 13.5%. For those with percent time psychotic less than or equal to 13.5%, center next enters the "exploratory" tree model. Good outcome occurs for 80% of those who live in Chandigarh rural or in Nottingham in contrast to the 58% of those in other areas. If at baseline the persons in the latter group of centers exhibited mild to severe blunted affect and were classified as having schizophrenia-like or other psychotic disorders, their chance of poor outcome increased to 75%.

For those with percent time psychotic greater than 13.5%, incomplete remission, or continuous psychosis in the 2-year period from baseline, and poor premorbid adjustment as indicated by no (or rare) contact with close friends, 83% had incomplete remission or were continuously psychotic over the 15-year follow-up. However, for those who had experienced a favorable 2-year course, nearly half continued to show complete remission over the entire period, in contrast to 20% in the group that had poorer short-term course. However, the few persons in Prague, Rochester, Dublin, and Honolulu who fell in this category (i.e., significant time psychotic coupled with remitting early course) were highly likely to have poor outcome (88%).

In the analysis in which area variables are included (Figure 4.2b), once again the cross-validation tree is based only on percent time psychotic (24% reduction in cross-validated relative cost). A 10-node exploratory tree (40% reduction in resubstitution relative cost) adds to the cross-validation tree the variables 2-year pattern of course, social stability of the area, blunted affect, contact with close friends, age at entry, and diagnosis. Percent time psychotic initially splits at 13.5%. For those with percent time psychotic less than or equal to 13.5%, Chandigarh rural (identified by the social stability variable equal to 1) is differentiated from all other centers in having a higher complete remission rate (91% versus 61%). In these latter centers, blunted affect further acts to distinguish course. Among those not having the symptom, 65% have good course in contrast to 55% among those with mild or severe blunted affect. Diagnosis provides some further but modest degree of discrimination.

For subjects with percent time psychotic greater than 13.5%, those who had 2-year incomplete remission or continuous psychosis were 80% likely to have poor longer-term pattern of course. This group was mainly comprised of those who had had no or rare premorbid contact with close friends. For those who had complete remission, those over 35 years had an 83% likelihood of good course versus 41% for the younger group.

DISCUSSION

The robust finding of this study is that among the variables considered to relate to long-term course and outcome, the strongest predictors are early illness course measures. Percent time psychotic in 2 years following onset is the most important predictor for all outcome measures: The lower the percent time psychotic, the better are long-term symptom and disability scores as well as overall course of illness. Pattern of course in the first 2 years is also related to long-term pattern of course. A presenting diagnosis of schizophrenia (in contrast to schizoaffective, acute schizophrenia, or bipolar disorders/depression) enhances the likelihood of having poor symptom and disability scores; those with other types of psychoses do not differ from those with schizophrenia. Baseline diagnosis played a smaller role in the prediction of course. Type of onset did not play an independent explanatory role for any study measures, but can be viewed as having a once-removed effect, since it was significantly related to percent time psychotic in the 2-year follow-up study of this cohort (Jablensky et al., 1992). In addition, baseline variables of age, lack of close contact with friends, history of drug use, and symptoms of blunted affect were somewhat related to an enhanced likelihood of poor course or outcome.

The regression models do suggest that cultural variables play a role in explaining outcome. Center entered the stepwise regression models for both symptoms and disabilities at the second step indicating that rates of recovery do vary by location. The two Indian centers and Moscow were always among the centers that had greater proportions of persons with good GAF scores, whereas Dublin, Prague, and Rochester had higher proportions of persons with poorer outcomes. A center grouping for the course variable emerged in the CART analysis distinguishing those in Chandigarh rural and Nottingham with better course from those in other centers, but this was only for those with percent time psychotic in the 2-year follow-up less than or equal to 13.5%. For subjects with percent time psychotic in the 2-year follow-up greater than 13.5%, but who were classified as having had complete remissions early on, center played a role for the few persons in Prague, Rochester, Dublin, and Honolulu falling in this category. They had substantially poorer course than those in other centers.

The finding that persons in areas with greater social stability have better disability scores did not hold for symptom scores, suggesting that the ability (or, perhaps, the necessity) to function at normal levels is more dependent on social climate than is symptomatology. Social stability entered a CART model for course, but merely distinguishes Chandigarh rural from all other centers.

In the 2-year follow-up, studies on the DOSMeD subjects report that those from Prague had outcomes as favorable as those in developing centers (Jablensky et al., 1992; Craig et al., 1997). Thirteen years later, the Prague cohort had consistently poor disability outcomes. As is well known, Prague (as well as other eastern European countries) has undergone significant political and social upheaval. In their report on the Bulgarian ISoS cohort, Ganev, Onchev, and Ivanov (1998) document that the sample has poorer outcomes on social disability and on symptoms than do samples from Chennai (Thara et al., 1994), Groningen (Wiersma et al., 1998), and Nottingham (Mason et al., 1995). Since Bulgaria underwent greater social upheaval than did these other areas, further credibility is lent to a hypothesis that the social stability of an area can impact levels of functioning. Acting as a counterpoint to this speculation, however, persons in the Moscow center—whose area had been ranked high on social instability—are among those with better symptom and disability outcomes.

The finding that areas in which there is national insurance are more likely than those without such insurance to have persons with lower GAF disability scores is less easily explained. While seemingly incongruous, the finding is most likely a surrogate effect, owing to the contribution made to the model by the proportionately larger samples from the two Indian centers than from other centers. The Indian areas have large uninsured populations, and are also the areas in which persons are more likely for unrelated reasons to have good GAF scores. Thus, little is learned from this finding regarding the value of national insurance.

The role of family in treatment emerged as an independent mediator of disability in the negative direction. But for this cohort, families were more likely to be involved in treatment in the case of a more severely ill family member, a finding also reported by Ganev et al. (1998).

Overall, the research suggests that early clinical features of the illness play a primary role in the prediction of long-term outcomes. Poor outcomes seen early on in illness sadly predict a continuation of incomplete remissions and poor long-term status on both symptom and disability assessments. Premorbid signs and symptoms related to poor social adjustment and deficit syndrome enhance the likelihood of poorer long-term outcomes. Yet for some, including those with a less favorable early clinical picture, living in certain areas improves chances of recovery. The characteristics of an area were only crudely measured in this study, but stability of the area appears to be related to disability outcomes. We continue to question the predictive value of the developing–developed dichotomy based on the CART model: Given good short-term outcome, subjects in Chandigarh urban had poorer long-term course than their rural Chandigarh counterparts. The challenge remains to open up further the black box of culture using both qualitative and quantitative methodologies that will allow us to explore the specific characteristics of an environment that promote greater recovery for those with severe mental illness.

References

Breiman, L., Friedman, J., Olshen, R., & Stone, C. (1986), *Classification and Regression Trees*. New York: Chapman & Hall.

Childers, S. E., & Harding, C. M. (1990), Gender, premorbid social functioning, and long-term outcome in DSM-III schizophrenia. *Schizophr. Bull.*, 16(2):309–318.

Craig, T. J., Siegel, C., Hopper, K., Lin, S., & Sartorius, N. (1997), Outcome in schizophrenia and related disorders compared between developing and developed countries. *Brit. J. Psychiatry*, 170:229–233.

Edgerton, R. B., & Cohen, A. (1994), Culture and schizophrenia: The DOSMD challenge. *Brit. J. Psychiatry*, 174: 222–231.

Ganev, K., Onchev, G., Ivanov, P. (1998), A 16-year follow-up study of schizophrenia and related disorders in Sofia, Bulgaria. *Acta Psychiatr. Scand.*, 98:200–207.

Hopper, K. (1991), Some old questions for the new cross-cultural psychiatry. *Med. Anthrop. Quart.*, 5:299–329.

Jablensky, A., Sartorius, N., Ernberg, G., Anker, M., Korten, A., Cooper, J. E., Day, R., & Bertelsen, A. (1992), Schizophrenia: Manifestations, incidence and course in different cultures. A World Health Organization ten-country study. *Psycholog. Med.*, 120 (Monogr. Suppl.):1–97.

Karno, M., & Jenkins, J. H. (1993), Cross-cultural issues in the course and treatment of schizophrenia. *Psychiatr. Clin. N. Amer.*, 16(2):339–350.

Kirkpatrick, B., Buchanan, R. W., McKenney, P. D., Alphs, L. D., & Carpenter, W. T., Jr. (1989), The schedule for the deficit syndrome: An instrument for research in schizophrenia. *Psychiatry Res.*, 30(2):119–123.

Larsen, T. K., McGlashan, T. H., & Moe, L. C. (1996), First-episode schizophrenia: 1. Early course parameters. *Schizophr. Bull.*, 22(2):241–256.

Mason, P., Harrison, G., Glazebrook, C., Medley, I., Dalkin, T., & Croudace, T. (1995), Characteristics of outcome in schizophrenia at 13 years. *Brit. J. Psychiatry*, 167:596–601.

Ohaeri, J. U. (1993), Long-term outcome of treated schizophrenia in a Nigerian cohort: Retrospective analysis of 7-year follow-ups. *J. Nerv. & Ment. Dis.*, 181:514–516.

Thara, R., Henrietta, M., Joseph A., Rajkumar, S., & Eaton, W. W. (1994), Ten-year course of schizophrenia—The Madras longitudinal study. *Acta Psychiatr. Scand.*, 90: 329–336.

Warner, R. (1994), *Recovery from Schizophrenia*, 2nd ed. New York: Routledge & Kegan Paul.

Waxler, N. (1974), Culture and mental illness. *J. Nerv. & Ment. Dis.*, 159:379–395.

Wiersma, D., Nienhuis, F. J., Sloof, C. J., & Giel, R. (1998), Natural course of schizophrenic disorders: A 15 year follow-up of a Dutch incidence cohort. *Schizophr. Bull.*, 24:75–85.

Chapter 5

Long-Term Diagnostic Stability in International Cohorts of Persons with Schizophrenia and Related Psychoses

Thomas J. Craig, Joseph A. Wanderling, and Aleksandar Janca

In the epidemiologic study of schizophrenia and related psychoses, it is most common that an initial cross-sectional diagnosis is derived using a structured interview instrument from which study diagnostic categories are created for longitudinal analysis of outcome. Only recently have such studies examined longitudinal diagnostic stability (Babigian, Gardner, Miles, and Romano, 1965; Kendell, 1974; Tsuang, Woolson, Winokur, and Crowe, 1981; Weeke, 1984; Jorgensen and Mortensen, 1988; Beiser, Iacono, and Erickson, 1989; Lenz, Simhandl, Tharu, Berner, and Gabriel, 1991; Marneros, Deister, and Rohde, 1991; Stanton and Joyce, 1993; Rabinowitz, Slyuzberg, Retsner, Mark, Popper, and Ginath, 1994; Fennig, Kovasznay et al., 1994; Fenning, Bromet, Craig, Jandorf, and Schwartz, 1995; Chen, Swann, and Burt, 1996) despite the fact that differential diagnostic change over time could have serious implications for the interpretation of outcome data. Relatively few in number, such studies had very different study designs which limit their comparability. Few studies have used the same structured diagnostic interview at baseline and follow-up, for example, relying instead on routinely collected baseline clinical data—for example, from case registries (Babigian et al., 1965; Kendell, 1974; Tsuang et al., 1981; Weeke, 1984; Jorgensen and Mortensen, 1988; Marneros et al., 1991; Stanton and Joyce, 1993; Rabinowitz et al., 1994; Fennig, Craig et al., 1994). This raises concerns about information variance (Deutsch and Davis, 1983; Fennig, Craig et al., 1994) in the interpretation of the observed diagnostic stability. While some recent short-term follow-up studies have examined first episode (or admission) samples (Jorgensen and Mortensen, 1988; Beiser et al., 1989; Lenz et al., 1991; Stanton and Joyce, 1993; Fennig, Kovasznay et al., 1994), the few longer-term studies have generally included more heterogeneous prevalence patient samples (Babigian et al., 1965; Kendell, 1974; Tsuang et al., 1981; Weeke, 1984; Marneros et al., 1991; Rabinowitz et al., 1994; Chen et al., 1996). Almost all prior studies have examined patients from a single cultural setting, generally from Western centers; for example, United States, Europe, New Zealand (Babigian et al., 1965; Kendell, 1974; Tsuang et al., 1981; Weeke, 1984; Jorgensen and Mortensen, 1988; Beiser et al., 1989; Lenz et al., 1991; Marneros et al., 1991; Stanton and Joyce, 1993; Rabinowitz et al., 1994; Fennig, Kovasznay et al., 1994; Chen et al., 1996), limiting generalizability to non-Western settings. Only one first admission study examined diagnostic stability over a period exceeding 7 years (Tsuang et al., 1981), and that study, using chart review at baseline, excluded a large proportion of the clinically diagnosed schizophrenic patients (Morrison, Clancy, Crowe, and Winokur, 1972).

Data from the International Study of Schizophrenia (ISoS) permit us to address a number of the deficiencies cited above. First, the study design for all but one patient sample included both baseline and follow-up interviews using the same structured interview, the Present State Examination (PSE) (Wing, Cooper, and Sartorius, 1974), thus minimizing the potential for information variance. Second, the four ISoS cohorts had differing selection criteria, including two prospective treated incidence samples (Jablensky, Schwarz, and Tomov, 1980; Jablensky et al., 1992), a prospective prevalence sample (Sartorius, Shapiro, Kimura, and Barrett, 1972), and one retrospective mixed sample, thus permitting the examination of the effect of varying selection criteria and study design on estimates of diagnostic stability. A third methodological advantage is the use of the same diagnostic criteria, ICD-10 (Sartorius, Kaelber et al., 1993; Sartorius, Ustun, Korten, Cooper, and Van Drinimelen, 1995) to express both baseline and lifetime diagnoses, the latter using the best estimate diagnostic procedure, which has been demonstrated to be reliable and valid in establishing a longitudinal diagnosis (Leckman, Sholomskas, Thompson, Belanger, and Weissman, 1982; Roy et al., 1997). Finally, this is the first long-term follow-up (12 to 26 years) to use a prospective diagnostic design and to include centers from a variety of cultural settings.

METHODS

The overall ISoS methodology is presented in the chapter on methods; its application to the present report is summarized here. The IPSS subjects were recruited by screening consecutive admissions to psychiatric facilities and included persons at various stages of what could have been long-standing illnesses. These subjects were then prospectively followed up in what would properly be termed a *longitudinal treated prevalence* study. The DOSMeD sample admitted patients as closely as possible to the onset of the illness but no more than 3 months after entry to treatment, while the RAPyD sample included patients with recent onset of nonaffective psychosis (both constituting *treated incidence* samples). The latter study was designed to explore behavioral impairments and social disabilities in schizophrenic patients. Finally, a group of three centers was invited to participate. Two had access to populations which had been examined through standardized instruments (the PSE in Beijing and detailed case notes in Hong Kong) that permitted the retrospective assessment of symptomatology and other characteristics at the time of initial examination; the third, Chennai, had built upon an ongoing research study. Two of these samples were also treated incidence samples—Hong Kong and Chennai (for 90% of the cohort); the third was a treated prevalence sample (Beijing). For our purposes, the three invited centers will be termed *retrospective analysis* cohorts.

For all but one of the study cohorts (Hong Kong), baseline diagnoses had been established using the same structured diagnostic assessment (the PSE) and coded in either ICD-8 (for the IPSS cohorts) or ICD-9 (for the others). For the Hong Kong cohort, retrospective application of ICD-10 criteria by the follow-up study team to detailed case notes available from 1977 were used to derive ICD-10 baseline diagnoses. Thus, for the three study samples other than the Retrospective Analysis centers, subjects were given a research diagnosis at study entry. For the IPSS and DOSMeD samples, some patients who did not meet research diagnoses of schizophrenia but who had received either clinical or computerized (CATEGO) diagnoses compatible with schizophrenia were also entered into the studies (Wing et al., 1974). Thus, some of these subjects had baseline nonschizophrenic diagnoses but had some clinical characteristics of schizophrenia at the time of study entry. Since the RAPyD sample was focused on disability, subjects were entered if they met criteria for a broad clinical diagnosis of schizophrenia or other nonorganic psychosis and tended to exhibit some degree of functional disability. For purposes of the present report, the baseline research diagnoses for the subjects in these three study samples were converted to ICD-10 diagnoses using a cross-walk algorithm developed by WHO (1994).

In contrast, the baseline diagnoses given to subjects from the Retrospective Analysis centers were retrospectively applied by the follow-up team using either PSE-generated data (Chennai and Beijing) or detailed case notes (Hong Kong). These baseline diagnoses were applied blind to subsequent course of illness, but the retrospective application of current criteria to these subjects permitted the exclusion of subjects from the initial study sample who may have been admitted to the other study samples because of the broader criteria for study entry. In this regard, the invited center methodology most resembles that used by Tsuang et al. (1981) in one of the few prior long-term follow-up studies of diagnostic stability.

For all study subjects, follow-up diagnostic assessment was based on the PSE-9 administered by research clinicians in the languages of the centers using methods recommended by WHO for this purpose (Sartorius et al., 1972). The PSE is a semistructured clinical interview covering a broad range of psychiatric symptoms present over the previous month (Wing et al., 1974), whose reliability in the hands of trained interviewers is well established and which has been used extensively in cross-cultural studies (Sartorius et al., 1972). A separate Diagnostic Schedule Scoresheet, developed in collaboration with the Nottingham Field Research Center, required the completion of the ICD-10 symptom checklist whose results were used to complete the Schedule. From this, a lifetime diagnosis using ICD-10 criteria was generated, taking into account available clinical information from all sources—including PSEs carried out at baseline and at follow-up points (1 and 2 years and long term), case notes (where available), and the Life Chart Schedule (LCS), which covers work, residence, symptoms, treatment, and relapse data over the entire period since the initial examination (Sartorius, Gulbinat, Harrison, Laska, and Siegel, 1996). The LCS was completed by the interviewer using all available sources of information to characterize both short- and long-term pattern of course in each of the above domains. These assessments were used to examine for this chapter the association between these domains and diagnostic stability.

Diagnostic stability was assessed by comparing the *baseline* ICD-10 diagnoses with the *lifetime* ICD-10 diagnoses. For three of the study samples, excluding the Retrospective Analysis sample, this comparison involved diagnoses generated at different time points by different research teams, although the lifetime diagnosis included data available from the baseline assessment. For the newly included centers, both baseline and lifetime diagnoses were generated at follow-up by the same research team, although baseline diagnosis was made prior to and blind to lifetime diagnosis. Diagnostic stability was assessed for six specific diagnoses (schizophrenia (F20.0–20.3, 20.5–20.9), schizoaffective disorders (F25.0–25.9), acute schizophrenia (F23.1, 23.2), affective disorders (F30.0–30.9, 31.0–31.9, 32.0–32.9, 33.0–33.9, 34.0–34.9, 39, 41.2), other psychotic disorders (F10.5, 15.5, 16.5, 19.5, 22.0–22.9, 23.0, 23.3–23.9, 24, 28.0–28.9, 29.0–29.9), and other nonpsychotic disorders (all other ICD-10 categories). In addition, the three schizophrenia diagnoses were combined into a schizophrenia spectrum diagnostic category which was compared to all other diagnoses (nonschizophrenia). These two summary diagnostic categories were used to assess the association between diagnostic stability and a number of demographic and clinical course categories (gender; age at study entry; type of remission; type of short- and long-term course [episodic/continuous]; overall trend of illness; percent of time receiving neuroleptic medicine; percent of time in independent living; percent of time in hospital or supervised residence; and prominence, over the last third of the follow-up period, of psychotic symptoms, disability, and hospitalization), using the chi-square or F statistics. Finally, the concordance between baseline and lifetime diagnoses of schizophrenia spectrum versus nonschizophrenia was assessed for the total ISoS sample and for each study subsample using the kappa statistic.

RESULTS

Table 5.1 presents a cross-tabulation of the baseline and lifetime ICD-10 diagnoses for the total sample (N=1043). The majority of subjects for both baseline and lifetime fell into the schizophrenia spectrum, which included ICD-10 categories of schizophrenia, schizoaffective disorders, and acute schizophrenia. Seven hundred twenty-six (87.7%) of the patients in this diagnostic grouping at baseline were also diagnosed in this category by lifetime diagnosis. However, patients within this category differed substantially in their subcategory diagnostic stability: 86.6% of those with a baseline diagnosis of schizophrenia retained the diagnosis at lifetime follow-up, compared to only 33.9% with baseline of schizoaffective disorder and 20% with baseline of acute schizophrenia. In both the latter cases, the majority of those experiencing diagnostic change moved into the lifetime diagnosis of schizophrenia (37.3% of all with baseline of schizoaffective disorder and 51.2% of all with baseline of acute schizophrenia), with almost 80% of both baseline diagnostic categories remaining in the schizophrenia spectrum at follow-up.

Among the patients with nonschizophrenia spectrum diagnoses at baseline, approximately three-fifths of those with other psychotic (58.4%) and other nonpsychotic (61.3%) diagnoses at baseline received schizophrenia spectrum diagnoses (mostly schizophrenia) at follow-up. This compares with only 13.6% of those with an affective disorder baseline diagnosis, almost 80% of whom retained the diagnosis at follow-up.

Cohort-Specific Diagnostic Stability

Table 5.2 compares the correlation between baseline and lifetime ICD-10 diagnoses for the total sample and for each substudy cohort, using the kappa statistic as a measure of statistical correlation. Four cells were examined in each comparison: (1) those cells in which baseline and lifetime diagnoses were in the same broad category, using the schizophrenia spectrum (S/S) and nonschizophrenia (N/N) as the two diagnostic categories; and (2) those cells where change occurred between baseline and lifetime diagnoses (either from schizophrenia spectrum to nonschizophrenia [S/N], or vice versa [N/S]). For the total sample, correlation between baseline and lifetime diagnoses was modest (kappa=0.463), with an approximately equal number of subjects experiencing diagnostic

TABLE 5.1 Cross-Tabulation of Baseline with Lifetime ICD-10: Diagnosis for Total Sample Alive at Follow-up

Baseline Diagnosis		Lifetime Diagnosis																		
		S		*SA*		*AS*		*SS*[a]		*AD*		*OP*		*ONP*		*M/U*		*Total*		*Baseline*
		N	%	N	%	N	%	N	%	N	%	N	%	N	%	N	%	N	%	%
Schizophrenia	(S)	558	(86.6)	19	(3.0)	4	(0.6)	581	(90.2)	27	(4.2)	22	(3.4)	8	(1.2)	6	(0.9)	644	(100)	61.7
Schizoaffective	(SA)	22	(37.3)	20	(33.9)	5	(8.5)	47	(79.7)	9	(15.3)	2	(3.4)		—	1	(1.7)	59	(100)	5.7
Acute Schizophrenia	(AS)	64	(51.2)	9	(7.2)	25	(20)	98	(78.4)	12	(9.6)	10	(8.0)	3	(2.4)	2	(1.6)	125	(100)	12.0
Schizophrenia Spectrum	(SS)[a]	644	(77.8)	48	(5.8)	34	(4.1)	726	(87.7)	48	(5.8)	34	(4.1)	11	(1.3)	9	(1.1)	828	(100)	79.4
Affective Disorder	(AD)	9	(10.2)	3	(3.4)	—		12	(13.6)	67	(76.1)	4	(4.5)	2	(2.3)	3	(3.4)	88	(100)	8.4
Other Psychotic	(OP)	40	(44.9)	4	(4.5)	8	(9.0)	52	(58.4)	9	(10.1)	23	(25.8)	2	(2.3)	3	(3.4)	89	(100)	8.5
Other Nonpsychotic	(ONP)	16	(51.6)	3	(9.7)	—		19	(61.3)	3	(9.7)	1	(3.2)	6	(19.4)	2	(6.5)	31	(100)	3.0
Missing/Unknown	(M/U)	5	(71.4)	0		—		5	(71.4)	2	(28.6)	—		—		—		7	(100)	.7
TOTAL		714	(68.5)	58	(5.6)	42	(4.0)	814	(78.1)	129	(12.4)	62	(5.9)	21	(2.0)	17	(1.6)	1043	(100)	(100)

[a] Schizophrenia Spectrum (SS) = Schizophrenia + Schizoaffective + Acute Schizophrenia

TABLE 5.2 Magnitude of Correlation (Kappa) of Baseline and Lifetime ICD-10: Diagnostic Categories for Total Alive Sample and Four Subsamples

			Diagnostic Categories (Baseline/Lifetime)									
			S/S		*N/S*		*S/N*		*N/N*			
Sample	*Total*		N	%	N	%	N	%	N	%	*Kappa*	*p value*
Total	1019	(100)	726	(71.2)	83	(8.2)	93	(9.1)	117	(11.5)	0.463	<.001
DOSMeD	469	(100)	315	(67.2)	35	(7.5)	60	(12.8)	59	(12.6)	0.425	<.001
IPSS	173	(100)	109	(63.0)	11	(6.4)	20	(11.6)	33	(19.1)	0.557	<.001
RAPyD	172	(100)	100	(58.1)	37	(21.5)	10	(5.8)	25	(14.5)	0.345	<.001
Invited	205	(100)	202	(98.5)		—	3	(1.5)				

S/S = Schizophrenia Spectrum at both times

N/S = Nonschizophrenia (Baseline)/Schizophrenia Spectrum (Lifetime)

S/N = Schizophrenia Spectrum (Baseline)/Nonschizophrenia (Lifetime)

N/N = Nonschizophrenia at both times

changes into or out of the schizophrenia spectrum; however, the four substudy cohorts showed substantial differences in correlation. The DOSMeD sample had somewhat lower concordance than the total sample, but almost twice as many patients' diagnoses changed from the schizophrenia spectrum to nonschizophrenia than the reverse. Likewise, the IPSS had twice as many patients moving to nonschizophrenia than to schizophrenia, while the RAPyD sample had almost four times as many moving to schizophrenia as to nonschizophrenia. Concordance for the Retrospective Analysis centers could not be assessed, owing to the absence of any patients with a baseline diagnosis other than schizophrenia spectrum and only three patients moving to a nonschizophrenia lifetime diagnosis.

Association Between Demographic and Course Variables and ICD-10 Diagnostic Change

Table 5.3 displays an analysis of the association between specific demographic and course variables and diagnostic change over time for the total living sample at follow-up. For each variable, the analysis examines the association for those subjects with information on the study variables. Thus, total sample size varies somewhat because of missing data for some variables. While there was no significant gender difference across diagnostic change categories, age at study entry did vary significantly: Those subjects with schizophrenia spectrum diagnoses for both baseline and lifetime assessment were significantly younger at study entry than the two subgroups whose lifetime diagnoses were nonschizophrenia, while those who changed to a lifetime schizophrenia spectrum diagnosis were intermediate between these extremes.

In terms of clinical course variables, complete remission during the first 2 years of follow-up and during the entire follow-up period, use of neuroleptic medication most of the time, percent time in hospital or supervised residence, and percent time in independent living status significantly separated those with a lifetime diagnosis of schizophrenia from those with a nonschizophrenia lifetime diagnosis, regardless of baseline diagnosis. In contrast, the long-term course since first episode and overall trend of illness differed significantly across the four diagnostic change groups, but showed a more gradual transition from those concordant for schizophrenia spectrum to those concordant for nonschizophrenia, suggesting a possible effect of baseline diagnosis.

DISCUSSION

Since most of our study samples have a treated incidence focus, perhaps the most appropriate literature comparison of our findings is to the few first admission diagnostic stability studies. As regards schizophrenia, our finding of 86.6% diagnostic stability is similar to the long-term follow-up study by Tsuang et al. (1981), which reported 92.5% diagnostic stability

TABLE 5.3 Association between Demographic and Course Variables and ICD-10 Diagnostic Change

	(Baseline/Lifetime) for the Total Alive Sample Diagnostic Change Categories					
	S/S	*N/S*	*S/N*	*N/N*	*Total*	*Statistical Association*
Demographic Variables	(N=726)	(N=83)	(N=93)	(N=117)	(N=1019)	
Gender (% Male)	49.5	49.5	54.8	47.0	49.7	(χ^2=1.34, df=3, p=.72)
Age at Entry (Mean±SD) S/S is significantly (p<.05) different from S/N and N/N	27.0±9.32	28.70±8.23	29.37±10.28	30.25±9.35	27.8±9.40	(F=5.41, p<.001)
Short Term Follow-up						
Pattern of Course	(N=627)	(N=73)	(N=80)	(N=102)	(N=882)	
(% of Complete Remission)	41.5	42.5	65.0	64.7	46.4	(χ^2=31.5, df=3, p<.001)
Last of Third Course Variables						
%Predominant Psychotic	(N=665)	(N=78)	(N=86)	(N=109)	(N=938)	
Symptoms	23.9	18.0	16.3	12.8	21.4	(χ^2=9.12, df=3, p=.03)
%Predominant Disability	(N=666)	(N=79)	(N=86)	(N=109)	(N=940)	
	33.2	40.5	24.4	23.9	31.9	(χ^2=8.66, df=3, p=.03)
%Predominant	(N=583)	(N=68)	(N=76)	(N=83)	(N=810)	
Hospitalization	17.5	14.7	11.8	13.3	16.3	(χ^2=2.41, df=3, p=.49)
Entire Period Since First Contact						
Neuroleptic Use	(N=720)	(N=83)	(N=91)	(N=112)	(N=1006)	
% Most of Time	56.5	45.8	25.3	24.1	49.2	(χ^2=64.9, df=3, p<.001)
%Time Independent Living	(N=723)	(N=83)	(N=93)	(N=117)	(N=1016)	
±SD S/S and N/S significantly (p<.05) different from S/N and N/N	89.1±21.7	89.6±19.2	97.4±5.1	95.6±11.1	90.7±19.8	(F=7.69, p<.001)
%Time Hospitalized or	(N=724)	(N=83)	(N=93)	(N=117)	(N=1017)	
Supervised Residence±SD S/S and N/S significantly (p<.05) different from S/N and N/N	10.2±20.7	10.3±19.1	2.4±4.6	4.4±11.0	8.8±18.9	(F=7.43, p<.001)
Course of Illness Since First Episode						
Type	(N=718)	(N=82)	(N=93)	(N=117)	(N=1010)	
%Episodic	51.1	65.9	73.1	70.9	56.6	(χ^2=43.0, df=6, p<.001)
%Continuous	29.9	19.5	9.7	9.4	24.9	
%Other	18.9	14.6	17.2	19.7	18.5	
Overall Trend of Illness	(N=624)	(N=74)	(N=83)	(N=94)	(N=875)	
%Better	49.0	55.4	68.7	69.2	53.6	(χ^2=22.8, df=6, p<.001)
%Same	28.2	24.3	20.5	18.1	26.2	
%Worse	22.8	20.3	10.8	12.8	20.3	

over a 30- to 40-year follow-up using a retrospective chart review-based baseline diagnosis and study-specific diagnostic criteria. As noted earlier, this study excluded a large number of patients who received clinical diagnoses of schizophrenia at baseline, but who failed to meet the authors' retrospectively applied inclusion criteria. Virtually all studies which used clinical (not research) baseline diagnoses reported lower temporal diagnostic stability (67–78%) for schizophrenia over shorter time frames, up to 10 years (Babigian et al., 1965; Kendell, 1974; Weeke, 1984; Jorgensen and Mortensen, 1988; Marneros et al., 1991; Stanton and Joyce, 1993; Rabinowitz et al., 1994; Chen et al., 1996). In contrast, shorter-term studies using structured interviews at baseline and follow-up (Tsuang et al., 1981; Beiser et al., 1989; Lenz et al., 1991; Fennig, Kovasznay et al., 1994) tended to report diagnostic stability comparable to our findings (range 86.4–90%). One such study, which examined schizophreniform disorder (similar to ICD-10 acute schizophrenia), found that 52.0% were rediagnosed as schizophrenic at 18 months (Beiser et al., 1989), which is virtually identical to our rate of 51.2% for acute schizophrenia. These similarities lend support to the validity of our findings despite the fact that our study included a much more heterogeneous patient population with respect to both study inclusion criteria and cultural settings. Thus, our findings suggest a remarkably uniform stability for the diagnosis of schizophrenia regardless of setting and despite using a variety of diagnostic schemes.

No earlier study has examined the broad schizophrenia spectrum diagnoses as we have. Lenz et al. (1991), using the PSE in a 7-year follow-up of an Austrian population, found a diagnostic shift from schizophrenia to schizoaffective disorder in 6.8% of baseline diagnoses, somewhat higher than our 3.0%. Fennig, Kovasznay et al. (1994) found 14.0% of subjects with baseline diagnosis of schizophrenia to be rediagnosed as schizoaffective at 6 months using a structured interview and DSM-III criteria (APA, 1980), although their short follow-up may have contributed to diagnostic instability. In summary, our findings replicate and expand those of earlier reports and suggest a remarkable stability to the schizophrenia spectrum as a whole, with 87.7% of baseline diagnoses retaining a spectrum diagnosis 12 to 26 years later. At the same time, we see a strong tendency for the subcategories of schizoaffective disorders (37.3%) and, especially, acute schizophrenia (51.2%) to shift to schizophrenia. The other notable shift for both these subcategories is to affective disorder (15.3% of those diagnosed as schizoaffective and 9.6% of those diagnosed with acute schizophrenia as compared to 4.2% of those diagnosed with schizophrenia). This finding is considerably different from those reported by Pope and Lipinski (1978) for follow-up studies prior to the use of specific diagnostic criteria, which found that a substantial number of those diagnosed with schizophrenia shifted to affective disorder diagnoses when specified criteria were used.

The broad diagnostic category of affective disorders including both bipolar and major depression diagnoses showed stability over the 12 to 26 years follow-up (76.1%), which is similar to earlier reports (range from 46 to 72.5% for retrospective chart reviews and 79 to 85.7% for studies using structured interviews over shorter follow-up periods). The one long-term retrospective follow-up (Tsuang et al., 1981) found 56.0% stability for bipolar disorder and 62.9% for unipolar depression. The only major shift in this category was to schizophrenia spectrum (13.6%), principally to schizophrenia (10.2%), similar to earlier studies (Kendell, 1974; Tsuang et al., 1981; Jorgensen and Mortensen, 1988; Lenz et al., 1991; Stanton and Joyce, 1993) that found a range of 1.3 to 17% of affective diagnoses switching to schizophrenia, including 8% of bipolar and 5.7% of unipolar in the long-term follow-up (Tsuang et al., 1981). Our findings are thus comparable to these earlier studies for this diagnostic category, again strengthening the case for relative long-term stability of these diagnoses.

Unlike most earlier studies that tended to focus primarily on the stability over time of the major functional psychoses, we included two other less specific diagnostic categories (other psychosis and other nonpsychosis) as permitted by the study entry criteria of the four subsamples. These criteria varied so that these findings relate most specifically to the DOSMeD and IPSS samples, which permitted inclusion of these subjects if they met either clinical diagnosis or CATEGO (Wing et al., 1974) criteria for psychosis. As noted in Table 5.1, these inclusion criteria were fortuitous to the extent that about three-fifths of both categories met schizophrenia spectrum criteria at follow-up (principally schizophrenia), and thus represent a subsample of patients with a lifetime schizophrenia diagnosis who would have gone unstudied if only patients meeting baseline research criteria for schizophrenia had been permitted study entry. In fact, these patients represent almost 10% of the lifetime schizophrenia spectrum sample. Another study (Fennig, Kovasznay et al., 1994), which followed a similar patient sample diagnosed as psychosis NOS, found a lower proportion of diagnostic shifts to schizophrenia (ranging from 26.5 to 33.3%) over shorter follow-up. It also found only 5.4% of patients diagnosed as not psychotic were rediagnosed as schizophrenic at 6 months, suggesting a need for longer follow-up of patients falling into these relatively nonspecific baseline categories.

Table 5.2 is unique to the literature in presenting the correlation between baseline and lifetime diagnoses for the total sample and four subsamples. Only one study listed earlier (Rabinowitz et al., 1994) examined diagnostic stability using the kappa statistic and found kappa of 0.74 for schizophrenia and 0.66 for other psychoses. However, this study examined only clinical admission and discharge diagnoses of a prevalence sample, which earlier reports have found to show much greater diagnostic stability than incidence samples (Fennig, Kovasznay et al., 1994; McGlashan, 1984). Since ISoS used the same diagnostic criteria and structured assessment at both baseline (for three of the four subsamples) and follow-up (for all samples), this analysis permits the comparison of diagnostic stability in relation to the methodological differences of the four study subsamples. With three exceptions, the DOSMeD and IPSS studies used virtually identical methodology: The former was a treated incidence and the latter a treated prevalence sample, IPSS had a longer (26- vs. 15-year) follow-up, and the initial diagnoses used ICD-9 and ICD-8, respectively. The proportion of diagnostic change was virtually identical for both samples, although there were somewhat more consistent schizophrenic diagnoses than consistent nonschizophrenic diagnoses in DOSMeD. This comparison suggests that if comparable methodology is used, a remarkably similar picture of diagnostic change emerges, regardless of whether an incidence or prevalence sample was studied.

In contrast, the RAPyD sample, while using similar methodology and being a longitudinal Incidence sample, appears to show the opposite diagnostic change compared to DOSMeD over a 15-year follow-up: Almost four times as many patients change to schizophrenia spectrum from nonschizophrenia than vice versa, and a lower overall concordance is seen. The major difference between this study and the DOSMeD sample is its focus on nonaffective psychosis and functional disability. This may have allowed the inclusion of a higher proportion of patients with a baseline nonschizophrenia diagnosis but evidence of functional disability, who may in turn have had a higher likelihood of receiving a schizophrenia spectrum diagnosis at follow-up. Were that the case, the findings would suggest that nonaffective psychosis with functional disability may predict an ultimate schizophrenia spectrum diagnosis (as emphasized by the DSM criteria which require evidence of 6 months of functional deterioration for that diagnosis). Conversely, when a functional decline criterion is added to an ICD-10 nonaffective psychosis diagnosis at baseline, the reverse will be true; that is, a greater number of baseline nonschizophrenics will receive a schizophrenia spectrum diagnosis at follow-up.

However, a simpler explanation—one deriving from prevailing clinical practice locally—may be at hand. For at least one of the centers making up the RAPyD cohort, an alternative account for the finding of a greater N/S than S/N movement was recently offered by the original investigators; namely, that "there was a certain reluctance to make the diagnosis of schizophrenia in the late 1970's" (Wiersma, Nienhuis, Sloof, and Giel, 1998). Indeed, that center accounted for 29 of the 37 N/S, and two of the 10 S/N. The remaining RAPyD centers have an equal number of S/N, and N/S, as compared with both IPSS and DOSMeD, which each have nearly a two to one ratio of S/N to N/S.

Finally, the Retrospective Analysis sample differed methodologically from the other three samples, resulting in 98.5% of the patients retaining their schziophrenia spectrum diagnosis at 15-year follow-up. As noted earlier, this finding may be confounded by the use of follow-up criteria to select only patients meeting these criteria at baseline, as suggested in one prior long-term study (Tsuang et al., 1981) which used similar methodology and found the highest diagnostic stability (92.5%) for schizophrenia of all studies reviewed. Thus, from these findings, it is clear that "diagnostic stability" is a function of the study sample, methodology, and criteria used, and cannot be seen as a universal phenomenon despite the relatively uniform findings from a variety of studies.

To examine which demographic and course variables are associated with diagnostic change, we looked at the association between sex, age, and several summary variables describing the short- and long-term course of the patient samples (Table 5.3). Age at study entry, but not gender, was significantly associated with diagnostic category in ascending fashion, with the patients concordant for schizophrenia spectrum having the lowest mean age at entry and those concordant for nonschizophrenia the highest, consistent with prior observations. However, the age difference from lowest to highest was only 3.25 years, raising questions as to the clinical significance of this finding. The absence of a significant gender difference across diagnostic change categories demands further investigation in view of the observed differences in gender ratios, especially among nonschizophrenic patients (e.g., affective disorders).

Regarding course variables, as noted in Table 5.3, at 2-year follow-up, those patients later given a lifetime schizophrenia spectrum diagnosis had a significantly different pattern of course from those later given a lifetime nonschizophrenic diagnosis: Regardless of baseline diagnosis, a significantly higher proportion of the latter achieved a complete remission early on. Over the entire course of the follow-up, patients whose baseline nonschizophrenic diagnosis changed to a lifetime schizophrenic diagnosis tended to have a more episodic course, resembling those with a lifetime nonschizophrenic diagnosis, with an intermediate proportion having a continuous course of illness over the entire study period. The fact that these course variables differed somewhat as regards their association with diagnostic change suggests that the lifetime diagnostic ratings were not merely reflections of course per se. In addition, the fact that many patients with lifetime schizophrenia spectrum diagnoses were rated as having relatively good outcomes (e.g., 90% of the time in independent living, 77% the same or better trend of illness) suggests that lifetime ratings were not unduly focused on poor outcome as a sine qua non of schizophrenia spectrum illness.

The latter observations are important since the key potential limitation of this study is the extent to which lifetime ratings may have been artificially influenced by prior knowledge of a poor course, especially the prominence of psychotic symptoms, disability, and hospitalization in the last third of the follow-up period. While two of these variables (psychotic symptoms and disability) had marginal significance associated with diagnostic change, the patterns of association were quite varied. For example, the prominence of psychotic symptoms separated the two concordant diagnostic groups, whereas those whose diagnoses changed (in both directions) were remarkably similar in percent of the sample with prominent psychotic symptoms in the last third of the follow-up. In contrast, prominent disability was worst among those whose diagnosis changed to schizophrenia spectrum. Finally, there was no significant difference across groups in proportion of patients with prominent patterns of hospitalization.

When the individual subsamples were examined with respect to the variables in Table 5.3, with the Retrospective Analysis centers excluded because of the lack of significant diagnostic change, the patterns observed in Table 5.3 were largely seen with a few exceptions. For the DOSMeD subsample, the proportion with prominent psychotic symptoms in the last third of follow-up was significantly associated with diagnostic change ($\chi^2=13.1$, df=3, p=.004); this is due chiefly to the concordant schizophrenia spectrum patients having 26.3% with the characteristic, whereas those who changed to this diagnosis were similar to those with a nonschizophrenic lifetime diagnosis. In contrast, diagnostic change showed no significant association with disability during this period for the DOSMeD group. In the IPSS subsample, none of the three variables of the last third of the follow-up was significantly associated with diagnostic change. For the RAPyD subsample, the proportion with prominent disability during the last third of the follow-up was significantly associated with diagnostic change ($\chi^2=12.6$, df=3, p=.006), with 70.6% of those concordant for the schizophrenia spectrum and 51.5% of those who changed to a lifetime schizophrenia spectrum diagnosis meeting the criterion, compared to 25 to 33.3% of those with a lifetime nonschizophrenic diagnosis. This reinforces the likelihood that the selection criterion for this subsample (functional disability) may have influenced diagnostic change indicated in Table 5.2.

In summary, our major overall study finding of a high degree of long-term diagnostic stability for schizophrenia and affective disorders extends those of earlier shorter-term studies. However, in addition, our findings suggest that a high proportion of patients with a number of diagnostic entities (e.g., schizoaffective disorder, acute schizophrenia, other psychoses, and even nonpsychotic disorders)—which meet broad clinical criteria but not research criteria for inclusion in a study of psychosis—will tend to move to a schizophrenic diagnosis over time, and that these changes will correlate with a course of illness similar to that of schizophrenia. The magnitude of these changes is also influenced by the study methodology and especially by the criteria used to select the initial study sample. Thus, future studies of diagnostic stability need to specify carefully their ultimate goals and to construct inclusion-exclusion criteria to meet these goals. For example, if the study goal is to identify, with maximum certainty, a core population of schizophrenic patients (e.g., for treatment trials), then the initial sample should be selected using narrowly defined criteria such as those of DSM-IV (APA, 1994) for schizophrenia. On the other hand, if the goal is to conduct a naturalistic study of schizophrenia outcome over time, the present results underscore the need to broaden the initial sample to include not only patients meeting initial schizophrenia spectrum diagnostic criteria but also those with other psychotic and even nonpsychotic diagnoses who meet some but not all of the criteria needed for a schizophrenia spectrum diagnosis.

References

American Psychiatric Association (1980), *Diagnostic and Statistical Manual of Mental Disorders*, 3rd ed. (DSM-III). Washington, DC: American Psychiatric Press.

——(1994), *Diagnostic and Statistical Manual of Mental Disorders*, 4th ed. (DSM-IV). Washington, DC: American Psychiatric Press.

Babigian, H. M., Gardner, E. A., Miles, H. C., & Romano, J. (1965), Diagnostic consistency and change in a follow-up study of 1215 patients. *Amer. J. Psychiatry*, 121: 895–901.

Beiser, M., Iacono, W. G., & Erickson, D. (1989), Temporal stability in the major mental disorders. In: *Validity of Psychiatric Diagnosis*, ed. L. Robins & J. Barrett. New York: Raven Press.

Chen, Y. R., Swann, A. C., & Burt, D. B. (1996), Stability of diagnosis in schizophrenia. *Amer. J. Psychiatry*, 153: 682–686.

Deutsch, S. I., & Davis, K. L. (1983), Schizophrenia: A review of diagnostic and biologic issues, I: Diagnosis and prognosis. *Hosp. Commun. Psychiatry*, 34:313–322.

Fennig, S., Bromet, E. J., Craig, T., Jandorf, L., & Schwartz, J. E. (1995), Psychotic patients with unclear diagnoses: A descriptive analysis. *J. Neru. & Ment. Dis.*, 183: 207–213.

——Craig, T. J., Tanenberg-Karant, M., & Bromet, E. G. (1994), Comparison of facility and research diagnoses in first admission psychotic patients. *Amer. J. Psychiatry*, 151:1423–1429.

——Kovasznay, B., Rich, C., Ram, R., Pato, C., Miller, A., Rubinstein, J., Carlson, G., Schwartz, J. E.; Phelan, J., Lavelle, J., Craig, T., & Bromet, E. (1994), Six-month stability of psychiatric diagnoses in first-admission patients with psychoses. *Amer. J. Psychiatry*, 151: 1200–1208.

Jablensky, A., Sartorius, N., Ernberg, G., Anker, M., Korten, A., Cooper, J. E., Day, R., & Bertelsen, A. (1992), Schizophrenia: Manifestation, incidence and course in different cultures. *Psychol. Med.*, 20 (Monogr. Suppl.): 1–97.

——Schwarz, R., & Tomov, T. (1980), WHO collaborative study on impairments and disabilities associated with schizophrenia. *Acta Psychiatr. Scand.*, 62 (Suppl. 285): 152–163.

Jorgensen, P., & Mortensen, P. B. (1988), Admission patterns and diagnostic stability of patients with functional psychoses in Denmark during a two-year observation period. *Acta Psychiatr. Scand.*, 78:361–365.

Kendell, R. E. (1974), The stability of diagnosis. *Brit. J. Psychiatry*, 124:352–356.

Leckman, J. F., Sholomskas, D., Thompson, W. D., Belanger, A., & Weissman, M. M. (1982), Best estimates of lifetime diagnosis: A methodological study. *Arch. Gen. Psychiatry*, 39:879–883.

Lenz, G., Simhandl, C., Tharu, K., Berner, P., & Gabriel, E. (1991), Temporal stability of diagnostic criteria for functional psychoses: Results from the Vienna follow-up study. *Psychopath.*, 24:328–335.

Marneros, A., Deister, A., & Rohde, A. (1991), Stability of diagnoses in affective, schizoaffective and schizophrenic disorders. *Eur. Arch. Psych. Clin. Neurosci.*, 241: 187–192.

McGlashan, T. H. (1984), Testing four diagnostic systems for schizophrenia. *Arch. Gen. Psychiatry*, 41:141–144.

Morrison, J., Clancy, J., Crowe, R., & Winokur, G. (1972), The Iowa 500, I: Diagnostic validity in mania, depression and schizophrenia. *Arch. Gen. Psychiatry*, 27: 457–461.

Pope, Jr., H. G., & Lipinski, Jr., J. F. (1978), Diagnosis in schizophrenia and manic—depressive illness: A reassessment of the specificity of "schizophrenic" symptoms in the light of current research. *Arch. Gen. Psychiatry*, 35:811–828.

Rabinowitz, J., Slyuzberg, M., Retsner, M., Mark, M., Popper, M., & Ginath, Y. (1994), Changes in diagnoses in a 9-year national longitudinal sample. *Comprehen. Psychiatry*, 35:361–365.

Roy, M. A., Lanctot, G., Merette, C., Cliche, D., Fournier, J-P., Bouten, P., Rodrigue, C., Charron, L., Turgeon, M., Hamel, M., Montgrain, N., Nicole, L. Pires, A., Wollot, H., Ponton, A-M., Garneau, Y., Dion, C., LaVallee, J-C., Potvin, A., Szatmari, P., & Maziade, M. (1997), Clinical and methodological factors related to reliability of the best-estimate diagnostic procedure. *Amer. J. Psychiatry*, 154:1726–1733.

Sartorius, N., Gulbinat, W., Harrison, G., Laska, E., & Siegel, C. (1996), Long-term follow-up of schizophrenia in 16 countries. *Soc. Psychiatr. Psychiatric Epidemiol.*, 31:249–258.

——Kaelber, C. T., Cooper, J. E., Roper, M. T., Rae, D. S., Gulbinat, W., Ustun, T. B., & Regier, D. A. (1993), Progress toward achieving a common language in psychiatry: Results from the field trial of the clinical guidelines accompanying the WHO classification of mental disorders in ICD-10. *Arch. Gen. Psychiatry*, 50:115–124.

——Shapiro, R., Kimura, M., & Barrett, K. (1972), WHO International Pilot Study of Schizophrenia: Preliminary communication. *Psychol. Med.*, 2:422–425.

——Ustun, T. B., Korten, A., Cooper, J. E., & Van Drimelen, J. (1995), Progress toward achieving a common language in psychiatry; II: Results from the international field trials of the ICD-10 diagnostic criteria for research for mental behavioral disorders. *Amer. J. Psychiatry*, 152:1427–1437.

Stanton, M. W., & Joyce, P. R. (1993), Stability of psychiatric diagnoses in New Zealand psychiatric hospitals. *Austral. N.Z. J. Psychiatry*, 27:2–8.

Tsuang, M. T., Woolson, R. F., Winokur, G., & Crowe, R. R. (1981), Stability of psychiatric diagnosis: Schizophrenia and affective disorders followed up over a 30- to 40-year period. *Arch. Gen. Psychiatry*, 38:535–539.

Weeke, A. (1984), Admission pattern and diagnostic stability among unipolar and bipolar manic—depressive patients. *Acta Psychiatr. Scand.*, 70:603–613.

Wiersma, D., Nienhuis, F. I., Sloof, C. J., & Giel, R. (1998), Natural course of schizophrenia disorders: A 15-year follow-up of a Dutch incidence cohort. *Schizophr. Bull.*, 24:75–85.

Wing, J. K., Cooper, J. E., & Sartorius, N. (1974), *The Measurement and Classification of Psychiatric Symptoms.* Cambridge, U.K.: Cambridge University Press.

World Health Organization (1994), *The ICD-10 Classification of Mental and Behavioral Disorders: Conversion Tables between ICD-8, ICD-9, and ICD-10, Revision 1.* (WHO/MNH/92.16.Rev.1). Geneva: World Health Organization.

Chapter 6

Long-Term Mortality Experience of International Cohorts of Persons with Schizophrenia and Related Psychoses

Thomas J. Craig, Dei-In Tang, Norman Sartorius, Eugene M. Laska, and Robert Cancro

The mortality experience of persons with schizophrenia and related psychoses has been a topic of research interest for over a century (Simpson, 1988; Allebeck, 1989; Newman and Bland, 1991; Simpson and Tsuang, 1996). Usually, the Standardized Mortality Ratio (SMR) is used to compare mortality rates in such individuals with those of the general population. Most recent studies, predominantly in industrialized countries (Lindelius and Kay, 1973; Weiner and Marvit, 1977; Ciompi, 1980; Black, Warrack, and Winokur, 1980; Herrmann, Baldwin, and Christie, 1983; Dube, Kumar, and Dube, 1984; Wood, Everson, Cho, and Hagan, 1985; Allebeck and Wisted, 1986; Seeman, 1986; Black and Winokur, 1988; Mortensen and Juel, 1990, 1993; Brown, 1997), have consistently found a twofold or greater SMR for schizophrenic samples compared to general population rates. Some of these studies have also found SMRs higher for the young male patients than for the old and for female rather than for male patients (Seeman, 1986; Simpson, 1988; Allebeck, 1989). Reported mortality ratios tend to decline with longer lengths of stay for inpatients or duration of follow-up for community patients (Simpson, 1988). Early in this century, deaths among such patients were attributed largely to infectious diseases such as tuberculosis and pneumonia, whereas more recent studies have found a preponderance of deaths to be due to unnatural causes, chiefly suicide and accidents. This not only reflects secular changes in causes of mortality over time, but also suggests a link with changes in the predominant locus of care from inpatient to outpatient settings (Haugland, Craig, Goodman, and Siegel, 1983; Simpson, 1988).

Despite the extensive literature on mortality among these patients, recent reviews (Simpson, 1988; Allebeck, 1989; Simpson and Tsuang, 1996) have identified a number of gaps in current knowledge. Simpson (1988) cites a lack of information about non-industrialized societies where cultural issues and differences in medical care availability might result in mortality patterns that are different from those in industrialized societies. In addition, most reported studies involve patients who died before the 1980s, when diagnostic criteria were less standardized and medical and psychiatric treatments less advanced. Simpson and Tsuang (1996) also point to the need for larger sample sizes in order to analyze mortality experience in population subgroups. It is remarkable, as Allebeck (1989) states, that despite the use of varying methodological and diagnostic techniques, similar results have emerged from studies which were conducted over half a century (i.e., the 1920s to 1970s). However, none of these studies examined the pattern of mortality across diverse national and cultural settings using comparable methodology. We attempt to do so in this chapter.

METHODS

Study Participants

This report includes data on patients from all participating centers of ISoS for which 15- to 25-year follow-up was completed by November 1996. These data include cohorts from three centers, Cali, Agra, and Prague, of the original International Pilot Study of Schizophrenia (IPSS; Sartorius, Shapiro, Kimura, and Barrett, 1972), followed up at 25 years. In addition, cohorts from nine of the original centers, Chandigarh rural, Chandigarh urban, Dublin, Honolulu, Moscow, Nagasaki, Nottingham, Prague, and Rochester, in the Determinants of Outcome of Severe Mental Disorders (DOSMeD) study (Jablensky et al., 1992); three of the original centers, Groningen, Mannheim, and Sofia, from the Reduction and Assessment of Psychiatric Disability (RAPyD) study (Jablensky, Schwarz, and Tomov, 1980); along with three Retrospective Analysis centers, Beijing, Hong Kong, and Chennai (Madras), were followed up at 15 years. Cause of death was determined from available data at each center (death certificates, autopsies, etc.). For our purposes, the decisive differences across the three substudies and the group of invited centers are: the age of the study cohort at entry, the state of vital statistics systems, and prevailing mortality rates.

Statistical Methods

Standardized mortality ratios (SMR) were used to quantify the mortality rates of a cohort of patients with schizophrenia and related psychoses to those of a standard or general population. The choice of the general population depended on the location of the centers. For all but the three centers in India, the general population comparison is the corresponding national population. For the centers in India, the standard population is the national population up to 1990 and the relevant state-specific populations thereafter. For most countries, the mortality rates contained in the WHO database were used (WHO, 1996); for some, recourse to other sources was also necessary (National Statistical Yearbooks [of Germany], 1977–1995; CDC-Vital and Health Statistics: Russian Federation and U.S., Selected Years 1980–93; Mari Bhat and Navaneetham, 1991; National Family Health Survey of India, 1993; Demographic Yearbook, United Nations, 1993; U.S. Bureau of the Census International Data Base [of Colombia], 1996; U.S. Bureau of the Census International Data Base [of Mainland China], 1996).

The general population mortality rates were used to compute the expected number of deaths (denominator) in each cohort based on the person-years lived during the study period by the cohort members. This number divided into the actual or observed (numerator) number of deaths in the cohort is the SMR. An SMR of 1 indicates that the mortality rate of the cohort and the general population do not differ. An SMR greater than 1 indicates that the cohort has a higher mortality rate than the general population. A statistical test of whether an SMR differs statistically from the value 1 was performed and a confidence interval for its value was constructed according to the method of Breslow and Day (1987). To study the effect of gender and age, we formed four subgroups for each center, males and females with study entry age younger and older than 30 years, for each of which an SMR was computed. Also, with the exception of Rochester (where no deaths were recorded), for each center a Kaplan–Meier survival distribution (Kaplan and Meier, 1958) was computed for deaths from any cause. The survival rates at 5, 10, and 15 years were compared among centers with no adjustment for multiple comparisons.

To investigate the influence on mortality of other possible factors including center, age, and diagnosis, proportional hazards regression models (Cox, 1972) were fitted for the DOSMeD centers. These models are multiplicative so that the combined mortality risk of two or more covariates is the product of the individual risks for total mortality. Two types of models were used: one that included an adjustment for the general population mortality rates and another than did not. When all (or total) deaths are considered, the adjusted model is essentially a means for comparing SMRs across centers. When only unnatural deaths are considered, the adjusted model cannot be computed, since the general population mortality rates for these causes were generally not available. The fitting of the adjusted model was nonstandard and followed the method described by Woolson (1981). The unadjusted model compares the mortality experience across centers directly. Thus, any differences in patient mortality rates may be due, in part, to unequal general population mortality rates. In these analyses, the covariates included in the model were selected by a stepwise procedure with the exception of the indicator "center," which was always present.

RESULTS

Total Mortality

Table 6.1 lists the sample size and mortality (total and by cause—unnatural [suicide, homicide, accident], natural, and unknown) for each of the participating centers. While differences in selection criteria among the four studies and in length of follow-up preclude drawing specific conclusions from this table (as discussed below), several general patterns emerge. First, almost two-fifths of the 231 deaths occurred in the three IPSS center samples (Cali, Agra, and Prague) which had the longest follow-up period (25 years).

TABLE 6.1 Death Counts by Center and Cause

Center	*No. of Subjects*	*All Cause*	*Natural Cause*	*Unnatural Cause*	*Unknown Cause*	*Expected All Cause*	*All C./ Exp AC*[a]	*Nat. C./ Exp. AC*
Agra	140	43[d]	26	7	10	22.55	1.86	1.15
Beijing	89	20	18	2	0	6.74	2.97	2.67
Cali	127[b]	12	8	2	2	9.18	1.31	0.87
Chandigarh Rural	55	10[d]	6	2	2	2.98	3.02	2.02
Chandigarh Urban	155	14	4	5	5	7.44	1.88	0.54
Dublin	67	8	3	5	0	1.95	4.10	1.54
Groningen	83	9	1	8	0	1.01	8.88	0.99
Hong Kong	100	11	2	9	0	1.91	5.76	1.05
Honolulu	71	4	1	3	0	1.28	3.13	0.78
Chennai	100[c]	9[c]	5	4[c]	0	4.21	1.90	1.19
Mannheim	70	6[e]	1	5	0	1.08	5.55	0.93
Moscow	72	10	2	4	4	7.07	1.41	0.28
Nagasaki	115	7	2	5	0	1.23	5.71	1.63
Nottingham	99	9	3	4	2	2.72	3.31	1.10
Prague DOSMeD	118	11	5	6	0	4.34	2.53	1.15
Prague IPSS	125	46	25	20	1	11.99	3.84	2.09
Rochester	58	0[f]	0	0	0	1.86	0.00	0.00
Sofia	60	2	0	2	0	1.93	1.04	0.00
All centers	1704	231	112	93	26	91.47	2.53	1.22

[a] This ratio is known as SMR.

[b] The year of birth of one patient, who remained alive, is missing; this case is deleted from analyses requiring this information.

[c] The year of birth of one patient, who died unnaturally, is missing; this patient is deleted from analyses requiring this information.

[d] One death time is unknown; the case is included in some analyses, as censored at the last known-to-be-alive time.

[e] One additional death was reported after analyses were completed, in which the mortality status of this case was considered missing.

[f] One suspected, but unconfirmed death.

Second, in centers in nonindustrialized countries, generally the majority of known deaths were listed as natural, whereas in centers in industrialized countries, the converse was true. The majority of deaths from unnatural causes were listed as suicides, although there were two homicides and one accidental death reported from the Agra center, one accidental death each from the Chennai and Prague IPSS samples, and one death listed as either suicide or accident from the Nagasaki center. In contrast to reports from other studies, our centers did not find that infectious diseases contributed disproportionately to the natural death toll. There was one listed case each of bronchopneumonia (Nottingham), pulmonary tuberculosis (Agra), and malaria (Agra), plus four deaths listed as caused by fever (three in Agra and one in Chennai), and two by diarrhea (both in Agra), while one death in Beijing was listed as caused by "infectious disease." Thus, with one exception, deaths attributed to infectious causes occurred in nonindustrialized centers, but were relatively infrequent.

Standardized Mortality Ratios

Table 6.2 provides a breakdown of the total SMR findings by the two demographic variables (gender and age at study entry). For total mortality, all but five of the centers had an SMR significantly greater than 1, indicating significantly higher mortality than the corresponding general population. Two of the four centers without a significantly elevated SMR are located in nonindustrialized countries (Cali and Chennai), two are in Eastern European countries (Sofia and Moscow); Rochester, recall, recorded no deaths. The

TABLE 6.2 SMR by Center, Gender, and Age

Center	All	Subgroup			
		Young[a] *Male*	*Old*[a] *Male*	*Young Female*	*Old Female*
Rochester	0.00	0.00	0.00	0.00	0.00
Sofia	1.04	2.14	0.00	0.00	1.47
Cali	1.31	1.22	2.39	0.56	0.99
Moscow	1.41	0.00	1.10	7.23	1.73
Chennai	1.90	1.57	1.92	2.08	2.21
Agra	1.86[b]	1.54	1.26	5.58[b]	1.56
Chandigarh Urban	1.88[b]	3.08[b]	1.02	1.35	1.96
Prague DOSMeD	2.53[b]	0.83	2.28	5.14[b]	2.99
Beijing	2.97[b]	0.00	3.53[b]	9.57	2.37[b]
Chandigarh Rural	3.02[b]	1.33	9.56[b]	0.00	3.14
Honolulu	3.13[b]	4.78	3.12	0.00	0.00
Nottingham	3.31[b]	3.72	1.99	0.00	6.71[b]
Prague IPSS	3.84[b]	1.23	1.98	7.03[b]	5.95[b]
Dublin	4.10[b]	13.48[b]	2.30	12.03	1.42
Mannheim	5.55[b]	7.52[b]	4.33	0.00	4.72
Nagasaki	5.71[b]	8.80[b]	0.00	5.53	7.88
Hong Kong	5.76[b]	10.21[b]	3.77	6.77	2.01
Groningen	8.88[b]	16.13[b]	3.82	4.70	5.99

[a] Young: age at entry <30; Old: age at entry ≥30.

[b] Statistically significantly different from 1 at 5% level.

eight highest SMRs were in industrialized countries, whereas 6 of the 10 centers with the lowest SMRs were in nonindustrialized countries.

A much more variable pattern was seen when the gender–age subgroups were examined. Young-entry male patients tended to have significantly elevated SMRs among the industrialized centers; the only two significantly increased SMRs for older-entry males were in nonindustrialized centers. In contrast, females showed no significant pattern of mortality risk by center type.

Mortality Risks: DOSMeD

Table 6.3 indicates that in DOSMeD only age at entry emerged as a significant risk factor for both total mortality and unnatural deaths in the analyses, without adjustment for the general population rates. After adjustment for the general population rates, none of the diagnostic subcategories was significantly associated with mortality risk.

Survival Probabilities—Total Deaths

Table 6.4 shows the survival probability estimates in the four studies for total mortality at years 5, 10, and 15 of the follow-up period. There were few significant differences in the survival probabilities among centers. Sofia and Cali experienced significantly higher survival probability than did 7 of the other centers, and Beijing and Prague IPSS experienced significantly lower survival probability than did 11 and 12, respectively, of the other 15 centers.

While the reason for the exceptionally high survival probabilities experienced by Sofia and Cali is not clear from the study data, the significantly lower survival probabilities experienced by the Beijing and Prague IPSS samples may be due to their significantly higher age at study entry, which was the only variable significantly associated with mortality risk in the DOSMeD subsample (Table 6.3). In this regard, Beijing had a significantly higher age at study entry (mean age, 42 years) than all other centers, while the mean age (31) of Prague IPSS was significantly higher than 13 of the 16 centers.

DISCUSSION

The chief potential limitation of this study is the degree of completeness with which subjects who entered the original studies were followed up at the study end points. For most centers, there were relatively few subjects whose follow-up status could not be ascertained. For the few in which a more substantial proportion were lost to follow-up, it is possible that the mortality risk might be somewhat overstated since it is likely that the status of deceased individuals could be ascertained more readily than that of living ones. This limitation is mitigated by the use of statistical methods that take into account censored follow-up. An additional potential limitation, relevant only to the specific cause of death analyses, is the possibility that there may have been cross-center variation in the reliability and validity of the listed causes of death as obtained from routinely completed death certificates. The major impact of such a limitation might have been to reduce, to some extent, the recording of unnatural

TABLE 6.3 Relative Mortality Risk[a] for All-Cause Death and Unnatural Death Estimated by Proportioned Hazards Regression Models

	All Causes Death		*Unnatural Death*
Variable	*Model Contains Pop. Rates Adjustment*	*Model Contains No Rates Adjustment*	*Model Contains No Rates Adjustment*
Reference[b]	4.37[c]	N[d]	N[d]
Center			
Chandigarh Urban	0.81	1.39	0.66
Chandigarh Rural	1.29	1.62	0.50
Dublin	2.09	1.13	1.46
Honolulu	1.32	1.03	1.17
Moscow	0.82	0.96	0.97
Nagasaki	2.46	0.61	1.03
Nottingham	1.71	1.25	1.12
Prague DOSMeD	1.00	1.00	1.00
Age at Entry	0.98	0.95[c]	0.94[c]
Diagnosis			
Schizo-spectrum	1.00	N	N
Bipolar/Depression	0.83	N	N
Other Psychotic	1.62	N	N
Other Nonpsychotic	0.38	N	N

[a] Each center is compared to Prague; each diagnosis category is compared to Schizo-spectrum; each age, say X (in years), is compared to the age X−1. The first model also gives the risk relative to the external general population for any set of values of the variables, by multiplying together the reference risk, the relative risk for the given center, the relative risk for the given diagnosis category and the relative risk for age raised to the power of the given age.

[b] The reference risk refers to the case when Center equals Prague, Diagnosis equals Schizo-spectrum and age equals 0.

[c] This estimate is statistically significantly different from 1 at level 5%.

[d] This variable is not included in the model.

causes of death, particularly in nonindustrialized centers. Indeed, Cali attributed eight deaths to natural causes when the cause of death could not be established with certainty.

With no deaths, the mortality experience of Rochester is at odds with that of the other centers. However, the cohort of this center included only 58 patients whose mean age at entry was 24.6. The expected mortality for this group was 1.86. Therefore, even if the true underlying SMRs were moderately higher than 1, it is not unlikely that there would be no deaths during the period. Indeed, the likelihood that there would be at least one such center is high when the fact that 18 centers participated in the study is taken into account.

The chief finding of these studies is that in developed and developing countries persons with the diagnosis of schizophrenia or related psychoses are at higher risk than their respective general population for premature death.

Mortality Risk vs. General Population

As regards total mortality, duration of follow-up was a factor in the number of deaths per center. In general, our findings confirm recent reports from industrialized countries that suggest that the main causes of death in people with schizophrenia are violent (chiefly

TABLE 6.4 Survival Probability Estimates[a]

Center	*Year 5*	*Year 10*	*Year 15*
DOSMeD Centers			
Chandigarh Urban	0.96	0.91	0.87
Chandigarh Rural	0.87	0.83	0.83
Dublin	0.95	0.86	0.86
Honolulu	0.97	0.92	0.92
Moscow	0.91	0.86	0.85
Nagasaki	0.99	0.93	0.92
Nottingham	0.98	0.94	0.92
Prague DOSMeD	0.95	0.94	0.90
IPSS Centers			
Agra	0.95	0.88	0.87
Cali	0.99	0.98	0.97
Prague IPSS	0.93	0.81	0.76
RAPyD Centers			
Groningen	0.94	0.89	0.89
Mannheim	0.99	0.94	0.91
Sofia	0.97	0.97	0.97
Retrospective Analysis Centers			
Beijing	0.94	0.79	0.79
Hong Kong	0.96	0.91	0.88
Chennai	0.98	0.91	0.91

[a] By the Kaplan–Meier method.

suicide and accidents). In the nonindustrialized countries, all but one center had a preponderance of natural deaths. Even in these centers, however, the predominant cause of death was no longer infectious diseases but chronic medical conditions (e.g., heart disease). These findings suggest that persons with schizophrenia and related psychoses are at increased risk for mortality from different causes depending on their setting. However, it should also be noted that these deaths occurred primarily during the early years of the current worldwide AIDS epidemic. Thus, it is possible that a similar cohort studied at the present time, especially in those settings most heavily affected by this epidemic (e.g., North America, Western Europe, Africa, and Southeast Asia) might again be subject to an increased mortality caused by infectious disease (Gottesman, 1997).

The SMR findings suggest that, whereas patients from centers in most industrialized countries experienced a threefold or greater mortality than their general populations, the mortality of patients from centers in nonindustrialized countries was much closer to that of their general population. In addition, young (at entry) male patients in industrialized settings are at greater risk for unnatural death whereas, in nonindustrialized settings, older entry male patients appear to be at increased risk of natural death. In contrast, female patients do not show a consistent pattern by age of entry or setting as regards specific mortality risks.

Mortality Risk Within Substudy Samples

Absolute mortality risks were remarkably similar across centers. In the DOSMeD proportional hazards risk analyses, only age at study entry significantly affected mortality risk. These data suggest that mortality risk was not significantly different across the centers or by diagnostic subgroup once adjustment was made for age at study entry.

In general, the survival probability analyses revealed two major findings. First, there were few significant differences in mortality risk among centers at the three time points. However, the differences seen in these cohorts should be examined with caution because the follow-up period was rather short (15 years) and more pronounced differences may appear later in a cohort's life. Still, these findings of remarkable similarity of survival patterns within the four studies suggest that, despite marked cultural differences and differences in mortality in the corresponding general population, mortality risk among patients with schizophrenia and related psychoses may be similar across settings and everywhere higher than the mortality risk of the general population. Thus, the high SMR findings for the centers in industrialized countries appear stable despite reduced mortality risk in the general population.

Since in the centers in industrialized countries the predominant causes of death were unnatural, these findings suggest that public health (or clinical) efforts toward reducing the causes of unnatural death (e.g., suicide prevention) could reduce the mortality risk in these patients, especially among young males. In some centers in nonindustrialized countries, the predominance of natural deaths may be due to differences in access to medical care between persons with schizophrenia and the general population, which suggests that health services should aim at earlier and better diagnosis and at treatment of comorbid medical conditions in people with schizophrenia.

Studies earlier in this century found a significant increase in deaths from infectious diseases among psychiatric patients, leading to suggestions of possible impairment of the immune system in these individuals. Our findings fail to replicate these data even in those centers with a relatively high proportion of natural deaths, casting some doubt on this hypothesis. In contrast, the marked preponderance of unnatural deaths in industrialized countries found here tends to confirm suggestions that the continued deinstitutionalization of severely mentally ill patients may have increased their risk for violent death (Brown, 1997).

In summary, our findings build on and expand the findings of earlier studies in populations from largely industrialized settings in a number of ways. First, despite marked variations in SMR across cultural settings, the absolute mortality risk for persons with schizophrenia and related psychoses is high and is remarkably similar in all the countries examined. Second, our findings do suggest differences between developed and nonindustrialized countries. Thus, while results for centers in industrialized countries tend to replicate some earlier reports from similar settings (e.g., increased mortality risk for unnatural death and for younger patients), those from nonindustrialized countries suggest different setting-specific risk factors, reinforcing the need for future studies to examine mortality in a broader range of cultural settings as suggested by Simpson (1988) and Simpson and Tsuang (1996). These findings should have direct consequences in the examination of health care for those suffering from mental illness.

As a final comment, several of the earlier reports from these and other samples have been interpreted as suggesting that schizophrenia has a better outcome in centers in nonindustrialized countries as compared to centers in industrialized countries (World Health Organization, 1973; Jablensky et al., 1992; Warner, 1994; Edgerton and Cohen, 1994). Examination solely of the SMR results (Tables 6.1 and 6.2) would seem generally to support this conclusion as regards mortality outcomes as well. However, the results of the survival analysis clearly demonstrate virtually no differences in mortality experience across centers in industrialized and nonindustrialized countries in this regard.

References

Allebeck, P. (1989), Schizophrenia: A life-shortening disease. *Schizophr. Bull.*, 15:81–89.

——Wisted, B. (1986), Mortality in schizophrenia: A ten-year follow-up based on the Stockholm County Inpatient Register. *Arch. Gen. Psychiatry*, 43:650–653.

Black, D. W., & Winokur, G. (1988), Age, mortality and chronic schizophrenia. *Schizophr. Res.*, 1:267–272.

——Warrack, G., & Winokur, G. (1980), The Iowa record-linkage study. III. Excess mortality among patients with "functional" disorders. *Arch. Gen. Psychiatry*, 42:82–88.

Breslow, N. E., & Day, N. E. (1987), *Statistical Methods in Cancer Research* for Vol. 2, *The Design and Analysis of Cohort Studies*, ed. E. Heseltine. (Tech. ed.: International Agency for Research on Cancer). Lyon, France: World Health Organization/International Agency for Research on Cancer.

Brown, S. (1997), Excess mortality of schizophrenia: A meta-analysis. *Brit. J. Psychiatry*, 171:502–506.

Ciompi, L. (1980), Catamnestic long-term study on the course of life and aging of schizophrenics. *Schizophr. Bull.*, 6:606–618.

Cox, D. R. (1972), Regression models and life-tables (with discussion). *J. Roy. Stat. Soc.*, Series B, 34:187–222.

Dube, K. C., Kumar, N., & Dube, S. (1984), Long term course and outcome of the Agra cases in the international pilot study of schizophrenia. *Acta Psychiatr. Scand.*, 70:170–179.

Edgerton, R. B., & Cohen, A. (1994), Culture and schizophrenia: The DOSMD challenge. *Brit. J. Psychiatry.*, 164:222–231.

Gottesman, I. I. (1997), HIV/AIDS risk as a consequence of schizophrenia. *Schizophr. Bull.*, 23:(4):675–684.

Haugland, G., Craig, T. J., Goodman, A. B., & Siegel, C. (1983), Mortality in the era of deinstitutionalization. *Amer. J. Psychiatry*, 140:848–852.

Herrmann, H. E., Baldwin, J. A., & Christie, D. (1983), A record-linkage study of mortality and general hospital discharge in patientsdiagnosed as schizophrenic. *Psychol. Med.*, 13:581–593.

Jablensky, A., Sartorius, N., Ernberg, G. G., Anker, M., Korten, A., Cooper, J. E., Day, R., & Bertelsen, A. (1992), Schizophrenia: Manifestation, incidence and course in different cultures. *Psychol. Med.*, 20(Monogr. Suppl.):1–97.

——Schwarz, R., & Tomov, T. (1980), WHO collaborative study on impairments and disabilities associated with schizophrenia. *Acta Psychiatr. Scand.*, 62(Suppl 285): 152–163.

Kaplan, E. L., & Meier, P. (1958), Nonparametric estimation from incomplete observations. *J. Amer. Stat. Assn.*, 53:347–481.

Lindelius, R., & Kay, D. W. K. (1973), Some change in the patterns of mortality in schizophrenia in Sweden. *Acta Psychiatr. Scand.*, 49:315–323.

Mari Bhat, P. N., & Navaneetham, K. (1991), Recent trends in agespecific mortality in India. *J. Inst. Econ. Res.*, 26(1 and 2).

Mortensen, P. B., & Juel, K. (1990), Mortality and causes of death in schizophrenic patients in Denmark. *Acta Psychiatr. Scand.*, 81:372–377.

——, ——(1993), Mortality and causes of death in first admitted schizophrenic patients. *Brit. J. Psychiatry*, 163:183–189.

National Center for Health Statistics (1995), Vital and health statistics: Russian Federation and U.S. selected years, 1980–93. *Vital Health Stat.*, 5(9).

Newman, S. C., & Bland, R. C. (1991), Mortality in a cohort of patients with schizophrenia: A record linkage study. *Can. J. Psychiatry*, 36:239–245.

Population Research Centre, Panjab University, Chandigarh (PRC, Chandigarh) and International Institute for Populations Studies (IIPS) (1995), *National Family Health Survey (MCH and Family Planning), Haryana 1993.* Bombay: PRC, Chandigarh and IIPS.

Sartorius, N., Shapiro, R., Kimura, M., & Barrett, K. (1972), WHO international pilot study of schizophrenia: Preliminary communication. *Psychol. Med.*, 2:422–425.

Seeman, M. V. (1986), Current outcome in schizophrenia: Women vs. men. *Acta Psychiatr. Scand.*, 73:609–617.

Simpson, J. C. (1988), Mortality studies in schizophrenia. In: *Handbook of Schizophrenia.* Vol. 3, ed. M. T. Tsuang & J. C. Simpson. Amsterdam: Elsevier, pp. 245–273.

——Tsuang, M. T. (1996), Mortality among patients with schizophrenia. *Schizophr. Bull.*, 22:485–499.

United Nations (1993), *Demographic Yearbook.* New York: United Nations.

U.S. Bureau of the Census International Data Base (1996), Web address: http://www.census.gov/ipc/www/idbprint.html

Warner, R. (1994), *Recovery from Schizophrenia,* 2nd ed. New York: Routledge, pp. 151–155.

Weiner, B. P., & Marvit, R. C. (1977), Schizophrenia in Hawaii: Analysis of cohort mortality risk in a multiethnic population. *Brit. J. Psychiatry*, 131:497–503.

Wood, J. B., Everson, R. C., Cho, D. W., & Hagan, B. J. (1985), Mortality variations among public mental health patients. *Acta Psychiatr. Scand.*, 72:218–229.

Woolson, R. F. (1981), Rank tests and a one-sample logrank test for comparing observed survival data to a standard population. *Bio-metrics*, 37:687–696.

World Health Organization (1973), *Report of the International Pilot Study of Schizophrenia.* Geneva: World Health Organization.

——(1996), *Statistical Information System: The Mortality Database.* Geneva: World Health Organization.

CHAPTER 7

Identifying Prognostic Factors That Predict Recovery in the Presence of Loss to Follow-Up

Christiana Drake, Richard Levine, and Eugene A. Laska

Typically, the identification of prognostic factors in longitudinal outcome studies is based on data from those individuals in the cohort who are not lost to follow-up (i.e., who have not been "censored"). Loss to follow-up is a common occurrence, and the longer the follow-up period the greater the chance it will occur. If the majority of subjects are uncensored, it is unlikely that estimates will be biased. But if the percentage of censored individuals is large, the likelihood of erroneous inference grows. Bias is not a problem if the mechanisms that govern loss to follow-up are statistically independent of the outcome measure. However, if this assumption does not hold, the possibility of bias must be considered.

In the context of ISoS, the possibility of bias cannot be ruled out a priori. Subjects who experience great improvement in the state of their illness after their index episode may subsequently have no further contact with the mental health care delivery system. Such individuals may move away or marry and change their names. Without further evidence, the possibility cannot be ruled out that subjects with better outcomes may be more likely to be lost to follow-up than those who remain ill and involved with caregivers. Similarly, the more seriously ill suicidal subjects may have higher death rates. Hence, outcomes and the reason for censoring may be related. If this is so, the distribution of outcome in the uncensored group may not be representative of the distribution of outcome in the entire cohort. Thus, it may be misleading or erroneous to assess the prognostic effects of variables measured at baseline on the basis of data from the uncensored group.

The epidemiological and statistical literatures have not produced a method to resolve this problem. Related phenomena, such as Simpson's Paradox in which stratum specific outcomes and overall outcomes are reversed, have been extensively considered. For example, Samuels (1993) derived conditions for Simpson's Paradox to occur. Testing to see if these conditions obtain in a given data set can only be accomplished if the outcome is known for all subjects. Unfortunately, it is not possible to use the method in follow-up studies with censored subjects. Therefore, one cannot be sure that the results observed in the uncensored stratum would be reversed in the whole population were outcomes in the censored group known. A new statistical method developed to evaluate this possibility is described below, followed by its application to some of the ISoS data.

To provide a conceptual basis for identifying prognostic factors in the presence of potential confounders, we adopted Rubin's model for causal inference (Holland, 1986). In this setting, we assume that the data on candidate baseline prognostic factors are available on all subjects in the study. (If there are subjects with some missing baseline data, it is not unreasonable to assume that these are missing at random.) Baseline information is used to gain some knowledge about outcomes of individuals in the censored group. Our approach is to use the baseline prognostic factors to predict whether a subject will be censored. Next, subjects are stratified so that similar outcomes are expected for those in the same stratum. In particular, the expected outcomes for censored individuals are the same as the expected outcomes for uncensored individuals in the same stratum. Therefore, we may perform analyses in each stratum using solely the outcome data of uncensored subjects. A global assessment of the importance of candidate prognostic factors may be made using all the data available by combining results across the stratum-specific analyses. If these results and the results of a similar analysis based totally on data from the uncensored subjects do not differ, then it may be concluded that the censoring mechanism had no impact on the outcome findings. One can then be confident about study conclusions based on analyses of those who were not lost to follow-up.

The propensity score, the probability of being censored given a vector of prognostic factors x and an outcome measure y, may be utilized to stratify subjects into outcome equivalent groups. The method is complicated because the censoring mechanism, outcome, and the prognostic factors are not statistically independent random variables. To overcome this difficulty, we developed a multistep procedure that begins by estimating the propensity score as a function of prognostic factors only. In the second step, the estimated outcome from the uncensored group (determined within strata in outcome equivalent groups) is incorporated into the estimate of the propensity score. The newly estimated propensity score is used to produce strata in which the relationship between outcome and prognostic factors is independent of censoring. In these groups, statistical analysis can be based on the uncensored group and the resulting estimates will be unbiased. In the next section is a detailed description of the method followed by the results of applying it to DOSMeD.

PROPENSITY SCORE STRATIFICATION

The method we have developed is based on the propensity score, introduced by Rosenbaum and Rubin (1983). In the present context, the propensity score is the probability of being censored given a set of covariates. Let y be an outcome variable, x a vector of covariates, and z an indicator of censoring status (censored=1, not censored=0). The propensity score is

$$e(x, y)=p(z=1 \mid x, y). \qquad (7.1)$$

Rosenbaum and Rubin (1983) showed that, conditional on the propensity score, the joint distribution of the covariates (y, x) is independent of censoring status. That is,

$$p\{x, y \mid z, e(x, y)\}=p\{x, y \mid e(x, y)\} \qquad (7.2)$$

which provides the basis for identifying outcome equivalent groups. In the usual application of Rosenbaum and Rubin's method, the propensity score is estimated from complete data sets. Typically, a logistic regression equation is used to relate the propensity score to covariates. Rosenbaum and Rubin (1983) showed that Equation 7.2 is asymptotically true for any consistent estimator of the propensity score. Simply put, estimating the propensity score does not introduce further bias. Unfortunately, in situations with loss to follow-up, the propensity score cannot be estimated directly since outcome is missing for some subjects. An estimated propensity score based only on prognostic factors is not a consistent estimator of the true probability of being censored since the probability depends on outcome as well. To overcome this difficulty, we have developed an iterative estimation procedure.

Denote the outcome of interest in the complete data by Y, which is comprised of outcomes from individuals not censored, Y_{nc}, and missing outcomes from censored individuals, Y_c. Thus $Y = \{Y_c, Y_{nc}\}$. The outcome measure can be either a discrete or continuous variable. The procedure:

a. Using only the baseline variables x, estimate the propensity score via a logistic regression model. That is, fit the model $e_c(x)=p(z=1|x)$ and denote the estimate by $\hat{e}_c(x)$.
b. Stratify the sample based on values of the estimated probabilities of being censored. That is, for each subject in the cohort, substitute the baseline value x into the propensity logistic regression to obtain the estimate $\hat{e}_c(x)$ and use these values to form strata.
c. Within each stratum, fit a model of the relationship between the outcome variable and the baseline covariate. That is, fit a regression model, $y(x)$, in each strata, using the data from the uncensored subjects in the strata. For discrete variables a logistic regression can be used.
d. For each censored subject, estimate the missing outcome value y_c, denoted $\hat{y}_c$, by substituting the baseline value x into the regression model $y(x)$ from the stratum in which the subject resides. For a discrete outcome measure, rather than estimating the outcome value itself, the result is an estimate of the probability of the outcome.
e. Reestimate the propensity score using a logistic regression model and both the baseline variables x and the known and estimated outcome variables. That is, fit the model $e(y_{nc}, \hat{y}_c, x) = p(z=1|y_{nc}, \hat{y}_c, x)$. For a discrete outcome measure the estimated probability of the outcome is used for both the known and missing outcome measures.
f. Repeat steps (b) and (c) using the new propensity score estimate.

Steps (d) through (f) should be repeated until the parameter estimates converge, i.e., they do not change by a significant amount with additional iterations.

g. Combine the estimated regression coefficients from step (f) across strata. One method that can be used is the Woolf estimator (Fleiss, 1981, section 10.2), a weighted average of the stratum-specific estimated regression coefficients. The weights are the inverse of the variances of the coefficients. Also note that the choice of stratum-specific regression models in step (c) is flexible; in fact, different regression models may be used in each stratum. The only requirement is that the same variables be utilized in the stratum-specific analyses.

A regression model, $y_{nc}(x)$ can be computed, without stratification, using the data from the uncensored subjects only. The estimated coefficients from this model can be compared with the coefficients from the combined regression estimates obtained in step (g) of the algorithm. If they are substantially different, the consequences of censoring on statistical inference may be considerable.

ANALYSIS OF PREDICTORS OF OUTCOME IN THE DOSMeD STUDY

The method was applied to the DOSMeD substudy. Subjects from nine centers (Chandigarh urban, Chandigarh rural, Dublin, Honolulu, Moscow, Nagasaki, Nottingham, Prague, and Rochester) were included in the analysis. A total of 694 subjects were considered. Of those, 233 (34%) were lost to follow-up. Another 10 were missing outcome for other reasons. Seventy-two subjects who had died were completely eliminated and not considered for inclusion in the data set.

The outcome measure was the Global Assessment of Functioning—Symptomatology (GAF-S) measured on a scale from 1–90, which was dichotomized into a binary variable (1–60 [poor], 61–90 [good]). Therefore, a logistic regression was used in step (c), and the probability of outcome is used in step (d) for both the censored and uncensored subjects. The variables that were considered potentially to be prognostic factors were:

1. Mode of onset (insidious [>1 month] versus noninsidious [≤1 month])
2. Center
3. Alcohol use (severe vs. none to moderate)
4. Drug use (severe vs. none to moderate)
5. Frequency of contact with close friends (frequent vs. not, including unknown)
6. Age at entry (older than 40 vs. 40 and younger)
7. Gender (male, female)
8. Marital status (married or cohabit vs. no)
9. Pattern of short-term follow-up course of illness (complete remission, incomplete remission, continuously psychotic)
10. Diagnosis (ICD-10 schizophrenia vs. all other psychoses)

If the *covariate* values are missing at random, the estimates of the probability of being censored should not be affected. If the missingness of covariate values is related to prognosis, then including the remaining data of such subjects should strengthen the estimate of the propensity score and also provide additional cases.

The method outlined above was used to form three strata defined by the 33rd and 66th percentiles of the estimated individual probabilities of being censored. Finally, the stratum-specific estimated coefficients and standard errors were combined via the Woolf estimator. Logistic regression models were fitted for the GAF-S using the complete cases only. We did some model fitting and variable selection at this point.

For the model found to best fit the data based on the algorithm, see Table 7.1. The center 1 and center 2 variables cluster subjects into two groups: (Dublin, Nottingham, Prague) and (Honolulu, Nagasaki, Rochester), respectively. The third or comparison group is comprised of the three remaining centers (Chandigarh urban, Chandigarh rural, Moscow). These combinations

TABLE 7.1 Estimated Coefficients, Standard Errors, and 95% Confidence Intervals for the Logistic Regression Model Fit to GAF-S Using the Propensity Score Algorithm

Coefficients	*Estimate*	*Standard Error*	*95% Confidence Interval*
Intercept	1.72	0.31	(1.12, 2.32)
Center 1 (D, Nott., P)	−1.00	0.37	(−1.72, −0.28)
Center 2 (H, Nag., R)	−1.12	0.39	(−1.89, −0.36)
Age Group	0.27	0.58	(−0.87, 1.40)
Close Friends	0.86	0.48	(−0.09, 1.81)
Incomplete Remission	−1.07	0.32	(−1.70, −0.43)
Continuously Psychotic	−2.07	0.56	(−3.16, −0.97)

TABLE 7.2 Estimated Coefficients, Standard Errors, and 95% Confidence Intervals for the Logistic Regression Model Fit to GAF-S Using Only the Uncensored Subjects

Coefficients	*Estimate*	*Standard Error*	*95% Confidence Interval*
Intercept	1.57	.25	(1.08, 2.06)
Center 1	−1.25	.28	(−1.79, −.70)
Center 2	−1.25	.32	(−1.88, −.62)
Age Group	.77	.36	(.06, 1.48)
Close Friends	1.39	.35	(.70, 2.08)
Incomplete Remission	−0.97	.25	(−1.46, −.48)
Continuously Psychotic	−1.86	.38	(−2.60, −1.11)

group the centers with similar outcomes together, as suggested by the model fits using uncensored subjects only. The variables *incomplete remission* and *continuously psychotic* are a recoding of short-term course of illness.

Notice that the *center* groupings, *incomplete remission* status and *continuously psychotic* status, are significantly related to the outcome GAF-S at the 5% level as evidenced by confidence intervals that do not contain the value zero (Table 7.1). The variables *age group* and *close friends* do not have statistical significance predictive of GAF-S, though the lower limit of the confidence interval for the regression coefficient of the latter variable is very close to zero.

Table 7.2 presents the estimated coefficients and 95% confidence intervals for a logistic regression model with the variables shown in Table 7.1, based on the outcomes of only the uncensored subjects. Notice that all of the variables in this model are related to GAF-S at the 5% level of significance. The estimated coefficients for the variables center groupings, *incomplete remission* status, and *continuously psychotic* status are similar to those displayed in Table 7.1 obtained by using the propensity score algorithm. Therefore, we conclude that censoring does not seem to be a problem for estimating the relationship between these variables and GAF-S.

The association between the outcome and the variables *close friends* and *age group* are significantly different from zero in one analysis but not in the other. Notice, though, that the standard errors in Table 7.1 are larger than the standard errors in Table 7.2. This difference is a consequence of the need for our algorithm to estimate outcome probabilities in the censored subjects. Consequently, the failure to find a significant association between outcome and the two variables *close friends* and *age group* may be a result of the increased error produced by incorporating the unknown outcome of censored individuals into the analysis. The estimated coefficients of the *close friends* and the *age group* variables in the two analyses are similar. Therefore, censoring does not appear to be a problem in estimating the relationship between these variables and GAF-S.

In summary, no variables in our model appear to be affected by censoring, thereby validating results obtained from analyses based solely on uncensored subjects. We can conclude that loss to follow-up did not systematically bias outcome.

References

Fleiss, J. L. (1981), *Statistical Methods for Rates and Proportions*, 2nd ed. New York: Wiley.

Holland, P. W. (1986), Statistics and causal inference. *J. Amer. Stat. Assn.*, 81:945–970.

Rosenbaum, P. R., & Rubin, D. B. (1983), The central role of the propensity score in observational studies for causal effects. *Biometrika*, 70:41–55.

Samuels, M. L. (1993), Simpson's paradox and related phenomena. *J. Amer. Stat. Assn.*, 88:81–88.

Part III

The Centers

INTERNATIONAL PILOT STUDY OF SCHIZOPHRENIA (IPSS)

Ctirad Skoda

In 1959, an expert committee on the epidemiology of mental disorders convened by the World Health Organization (WHO) recommended that WHO support and assist psychiatric epidemiology throughout the world and coordinate and initiate research in the field. High priority was placed on the development of methods necessary to carry out epidemiological research in cross-cultural settings. In 1965, an outline was produced for a long-term program of studies in this area, and an initial plan for the International Pilot Study of Schizophrenia (IPSS) was formulated. The IPSS was conceived as a pilot study in the sense that it was intended to lay scientific groundwork for future studies of schizophrenia and other psychiatric disorders. IPSS was to examine three major methodological questions:

1. Is it feasible to carry out a large-scale international psychiatric study requiring the coordination of psychiatrists and mental health workers from different theoretical backgrounds and widely differing cultures and socioeconomic conditions?
2. Is it possible to develop standardized research instruments and procedures for psychiatric assessment which can be reliably applied in a variety of cultural settings?
3. Can teams of research workers in different cultural settings be trained to use such instruments and procedures reliably?

In addition, IPSS set out to explore questions about the nature and distribution of schizophrenia in different parts of the world. For example, are there groups of schizophrenic patients whose symptoms differ in form or content from one country to another, and, if so, are such differences the result of variations in diagnostic practice or are they true cultural differences in the manner of presentation? Does the clinical course and social outcome of schizophrenia in one country or group of countries differ from that in others?

Nine international centers started case-finding for 12 months beginning April 1, 1968. Inclusion criteria were based on symptoms rather than on diagnostic labels; centers were required to include an adequate number of young patients across the range of functional psychoses of recent onset. A total of 1202 patients received intensive evaluations including the Present State Examination (PSE). The program demonstrated both the feasibility of cross-cultural epidemiological studies and the existence of schizophrenia disorders in all centers. Two- and 5-year follow-up studies found that patients living in nonindustrialized settings had better social and symptomatic outcomes. Three of the original IPSS Field Research Centers—Agra, Cali, and Prague—participated in ISoS and carried out a 26-year follow-up of their original cohorts.

Chapter 8

IPSS: Agra, India

K. C. Dube and Narendar Kumar

CULTURAL CONTEXT

Situated on the banks of the river Yamuna, 200 km southeast of Delhi, Agra is the third largest city (1.2 million population) in the northern province of Uttar Pradesh (UP), the largest Indian state with over 160 million population. The area lies in the fertile region of the Indo-Gangetic plains bounded on the north by the Himalayan mountains. In the 25 years since IPSS (1967), the city and other parts of the catchment area have had phenomenal growth and have developed industrially; the decennial growth rate between 1981 and 1991 was 25%. Consequently, Agra is very densely populated, and its narrow roads are choked with traffic of all sorts—automotive vehicles, rickshaws, scooters, cycles, bullock carts, horse-drawn carriages, and stray cattle, all with their various pollutants. The nearby town of Mathura has one of the biggest petroleum refineries in India, and the agricultural sector of the area is undergoing a green revolution with farmers converting to modern methods. Agra has two universities and scores of colleges and has become a tourist center.

Among major historical events occurring in this region during those 25 years were the murders of two former Prime Ministers, Indira Gandhi and her son Rajiv, and the destruction of Babri Masjid (Mosque) by Hindus, resulting in nationwide tension between Hindus and Muslims. Political awareness has reached the village level where women hold 30% of the positions as heads of village councils.

Ethnicity and Language

The ethnic makeup of the residents is mixed. An orthodox Hindu majority and a large minority community of Muslims predominate; but there are also Jains, Sikhs, and small minorities of Christians and Buddhists. All the groups are intensely religious but manage to live (most of the time) in harmony. Hindi, the national language, is the main spoken language of the region; the other is Urdu. Many dialects of Hindi are used in rural areas, but people have no difficulty understanding one another. English is the medium of instruction in most universities and colleges and is freely spoken in secondary schools.

Gender

Gender differences persist, but a strong movement for the emancipation of women has meant their progression in every sphere. At the same time, women are still underprivileged; in Indian society, a male child is preferred. Girls do not get the same attention and, in the lower stratas of society, have less chance of receiving education, attention, and care.

Mental Health Issues in Society

Regardless of religious affiliation, mental illness is viewed variously as a curse inflicted by providence, as fate, as a consequence of being possessed by evil spirits or jinns, as the result of a magic spell or rituals performed by enemies, as coming from bad atmospheric influences, or from potions or poison mixed in food or drink. Some Hindus believe that mental illness is a consequence of sins committed in a previous life and that a person is reborn to atone for these sins. In such cases, the afflicted person is taken to a religious site reputed to cure mental illness, there to pay obeisance and to pray for recovery.

Competition, a slow breakdown of family ties, a spurt in criminality, more social awareness, and other changes in the way of life may have resulted in a greater need for psychiatric help. Minor mental illness is often ignored, particularly in joint families where responsibility is shared, when demands are few, and when the person keeps working at a simple, routine job. Abnormality in a male is the common knowledge of all nearby, so despite the stigma, the illness cannot be hidden. Nor is there much effort to feel ashamed, because it hardly matters in the family's social life. In the case of a girl, it is a different story. She is kept confined to the precincts of the house, and her illness is hidden because if she is known to be mentally ill (or possessed), her chances of marrying are diminished.

MENTAL HEALTH SYSTEM IN THE AREA

Health is a joint responsibility of the central government and of the state. The original law relating to mental patients was the Indian Lunacy Act of 1912, replaced in 1987 by the Indian Mental Health Act, which simplified admission and discharge procedures, outlined commitment procedures, and defined the rights and privileges of mental patients.

Only when symptoms become too difficult to handle by the family is there explicit realization that a person might be mentally ill, and only then is treatment sought. The traditional healers or faith-healers (fakirs) are the first line of the treatment, and their services are either inexpensive or free. Two important traditional systems, the Ayurveda and Unani, provide treatments using herbal medicines, particularly in distant villages where no other treatment is available. The faith healers can, at least, allay family anxieties and, in some cases, are successful in relieving minor or psychoneurotic symptoms with mere suggestion. Also, a recurring illness may abate, in which case the faith healer gets the credit. Homeopathy and naturopathy are also practiced. Other unorthodox methods (such as "Grandmother's homemade remedies") are also used. Needless to say, there are also quacks who do much harm and who fleece the subjects. Should a person seek the services of modern medicine—a psychiatrist or a hospital—the expenses for treatment, for travel for himself and a family member/guardian, and for medicines can impose a considerable burden on the family. These costs are often a deterrent to seeking such treatment.

The 1980s saw a marked increase in the number of psychiatrists and an expansion of psychiatric services in public and private general hospitals. Still, mental hospitals continue to attract increasing numbers of patients, a trend likely to continue as the traditional family support system changes. After the introduction of psychiatric units into most general hospitals in India, the role of the mental hospital became unclear since both provide similar services (Sharma and Chadda, 1996, p. 1). Departments of psychiatry opened where none had existed; departments in centrally run colleges were upgraded; hospitals became postgraduate institutes of psychiatry; clinics were established; and research was encouraged. Although more state funds are now available in general, mental health remains a low priority.

In the catchment area during the beginning of the IPSS study (1968), the only facility serving severely mentally ill patients needing inpatient care was the Agra Mental Hospital, established in 1958. Serving almost a third of the population of Uttar Pradesh, the hospital consisted of a few trained psychiatrists, 718 inpatient beds, an outpatient department, and an active postgraduate education program. In 1960, a research center was established. In 1968, the Agra Mental Hospital Research Center became a training center for medical staff and for psychiatrists from other sites in India; for example, from the Medical College at Lucknow and from other parts of the world, particularly the Middle East. Less severe cases were treated at the outpatient facilities of Agra Mental Hospital, at the local medical college, and at Aligarh Medical College.

In 1974, administrative changes led to the hospital's decline, and in the early 1990s, the media filed a complaint before the Supreme Court of India. The landmark order of the Supreme Court on September 16, 1994, directed improvements to be initiated immediately: an overhaul of the administrative machinery; compulsory examination of patients by experts; employment of qualified staff; and improvements in the provision of food, living facilities, and such services as laundry, cooking facilities, bedding, and clothing. Since then, the hospital has become autonomous, removed from the control of the Director General of Health, and 20 million rupees have been appropriated for renovations.

Psychiatric Epidemiology

The existence of mental disorders has been known from ancient times. In Ayurvedic literature, mental illnesses have been described in detail in a nosology comparable to modern classifications (Dube, 1978). A large-scale epidemiological house-to-house census survey (1962–1964) revealed the prevalence of schizophrenia to be 2.2 per thousand, which was similar to the results of 12 other surveys conducted since 1929 (Dube, 1970, p. 358). Studies since 1964 also found similar prevalence rates for schizophrenia (Indian Council of Medical Research, 1987).

METHODS USED AT THE CENTER

The IPSS study was started in 1968 under the directorship of the then medical superintendent of Agra Mental Hospital. The team included two psychiatrists, a social scientist, a psychologist, a statistician, an office secretary, and a field assistant. The personnel underwent intensive training, and an intracenter reliability exercise was carried out on every tenth case. The center was equipped with a one-way mirror, a duplicating machine, an air-conditioned interview room with good lighting, video recording equipment, a soundproof conference room, a lecture room, and sufficient space for all staff. A number of videotapes were prepared for an intercenter reliability study. As a preclude to actual selection of the IPSS study cohort, 26 patients were selected for a trial. The center thus gained experience, trained staff, and tested the methodology. There was little or no change in method for the 2-, 5-, and 14-year follow-ups except that when a psychiatrist left, his or her replacement underwent rigorous training.

Defining the IPSS Cohort

The study cohort of 140 was selected from the patients attending the outpatient department of Agra Mental Hospital. The strictly adhered to inclusion criteria were: age between 15 and 45; sleeping in the catchment area for at least 6 months (and likely to be available for next 2 years); mental illness for no more than 5 years prior to inclusion; and presence of delusions, inappropriate or unusual behavior, hallucinations, gross psychomotor disorder, social withdrawal, thinking disorder, overwhelming fear, depersonalization, or self-neglect. The exclusion criteria were severe psychotic symptoms present for 3 years or more; hospitalization for 2 years or more; mental retardation; chronic brain syndrome; disease with toxic or organic causes; and hearing or language difficulties severe enough to impede the interview.

The 2-year follow-up posed no difficulty. Of all cases, 91.2% were seen either at the hospital or at their homes. At 5 years, 85% of the cases were traced, and at the 14-year follow-up 79% of the cases were traced. Visits often were made under very trying conditions, and so valuable experience in tracing subjects in the vast catchment area was gained. Most of the subjects live in villages not connected by proper roads; others live in dangerous, gangster-infested areas and could not be visited. The researchers traveled by bus and train, on bicycles, bullock carts, camel, and whatever other means of transport were available. At times, summer daytime temperatures surged up to 42°C. To illustrate the lighter side of the experience: A pair of team members sought a lift from a passing van and later came to realize that it was a hearse; in another instance, a team member was given a warm welcome and a feast, only to realize that his host was offering his daughter in marriage.

Tracing the Cohort at 25 Years (ISoS)

Twenty-five years is a long time for follow-up: The appearance of the area had changed, many new buildings had been constructed, and many political developments had taken place. Tracing subjects was challenging. The search was started in 1990 when letters were posted to subjects' addresses. Regular or registered letters were sent repeatedly to those who did not reply—in a few cases, as many as five times. Village headmen and post offices were also contacted. Visits to villages were undertaken, often in inclement weather and in inhospitable country. Unable to trace the location of one subject, for example, a psychiatrist visited the area, found four women with similar names, and finally, after much conversation, found the subject. In another instance, a young Muslim subject, whose parents' house had long been demolished and replaced by other buildings, was located through a conversation at a nearby mosque with an old *moulvi* and his wife who knew the address of a nephew 2 kilometers away. A female subject from a village of 800 residents that had since been merged into a nearby township where the local population had grown to 8,000, was traced by visiting a locality where other members of her caste were living. Another subject was found by inquiring of a general practitioner with the same family name.

At the 25-year follow-up, the original research team had dispersed. Assistance was secured at first from a psychiatrist who worked in his spare time and, subsequently, from a scientist at the Indian Council of Medical Research.

Use of Instruments

Previous experience with IPSS showed that translating instruments into Hindi was not worthwhile. A meeting of the original IPSS investigators approved the use of English versions of the ISoS instruments. Interviews took place in English with the English-speaking subjects and in Hindi with the Hindi-speaking individuals. There was little difficulty in conveying meaning, and interviews went smoothly. Intracenter reliability was carried out on every 10th case by two psychiatrists, each of whom interviewed the same subject; however, it was often not possible to repeat the family interview because of long distances, financial constraints, and disinterest on the part of the family member. In some cases, the subject came alone, so no family member was available. Cases who had moved some distance and who could not be traced were classified as lost to follow-up. As the catchment area is homogeneous with respect to language, culture, economic equivalence, and general way of life (mostly rural), there are no special groups to bias the outcome.

RESULTS

At 2 years, 46% of 92 cases of schizophrenia were asymptomatic; 34% spent less than one month in a psychotic episode. After dropping a few cases, 54.5% had the best outcome on a 5-point rating scale. At 5 years, 31 (42%) had the best outcome. At 14 years, of 62 schizophrenic subjects traced, 27 (43.5%) were asymptomatic. Forty-five (73.8%) of the 61 cases alive at the 25-year follow-up had been in complete remission at the initial 2-year follow-up, and 77% were currently asymptomatic (WHO, 1973, 1979; Dube, Kumar, and Dube, 1984).

Baseline and Short-Term Follow-Up

In the ISoS 25-year follow-up, 139 of the original inclusion cohort of 140 cases were earmarked for follow-up, one having been dropped at some earlier stage. This case has been included in the lost to follow-up group; thus, the number in the ISoS cohort remains 140. The breakdown of the cohort at 25 years is 61 alive, 43 dead, 36 lost to follow-up—three alive who refused to participate and 33 vital status unknown (9 absconders and 24 untraced).

Gender, Age, and Sociodemographic Characteristics

At inclusion, the cohort consisted of 55 females (39.3%) and 85 males (60.7%). At 25 years, the ISoS cohort had 61 alive cases—22 females (36.1%) and 39 males (63.9%). There was no difference in the mean birth age at inclusion and at follow-up, and no difference in the ages at follow-up in each decade of birth year from 1920 to 1959. Comparison of the sociodemographic characteristics of the 25-year ISoS cohort with the inclusion cohort showed no significant differences in marital status, type of family, residence, and diagnosis.

Type of Onset and Diagnosis

Similar rates of sudden and slow onset at inclusion were found in the living, dead, and lost to follow-up groups. Nor was much difference observed between sudden and slow onset in global evaluation at inclusion and at 25 years (ISoS) (about 50% in each category). In the vast majority of cases in Cali and Prague, slow onset was the rule. Since Cali resembles developed countries in some respects, slow onset is more likely to be of the same type as in the developed countries; in Agra, by contrast, the milder symptoms accompanying slow onset are often overlooked or are not recognized as symptoms of mental disturbance. Only when abnormal behavior erupts do relatives report sudden onset.

Information on missing or otherwise not available cases has been excluded. As observed, there was much lower overall severity of symptoms (Bleuler) in the Agra ISoS cohort than in the total IPSS sample, and recovery, too, was much better in the former.

During the 25-year course, change in diagnosis was observed in only five cases. Two schizophrenia cases and one neurotic changed to manic-depressive psychosis (MDP) while two MDP cases changed to schizophrenia. Of 101 cases of schizophrenia (including schizoaffective and acute schizophrenia-like) at inclusion, 39 were followed up; one-third were classed as "other schizophrenia," one-fifth as catatonic, and one-eighth as paranoid type. The 37 dead cases consisted of 35% who had been diagnosed as "other schizophrenia," 27% as catatonic, and 19% as paranoid. In Agra, unspecified schizophrenia was included in the category "other schizophrenia." In the lost to follow-up, there is an equal number of other schizophrenia and schizoaffective (eight each), and half that number (four) of catatonics; only three were paranoid.

Comparison of the alive cases in Agra with the other two IPSS centers shows that in Cali, acute schizophrenia was the most prominent ICD-8 schizophrenia diagnosis followed by hebephrenic, catatonic, and paranoid schizophrenia; in Prague, paranoid diagnosis took precedence with eight cases followed by schizoaffective and then by acute schizophrenia-like and other schizophrenia. Such differences could be due in part to the difficulty of distinguishing among different diagnostic categories in the unsophisticated population in and around Agra. The range of catatonic schizophrenia seen in Agra, from waxy flexibility to excitement, is quite rare in the West. The scant number of hebephrenic schizophrenia cases in the Agra cohort is due to strict adherence to the exclusion criteria—their symptoms were severe enough to impede an interview. (On the other hand, a substantial number of hebephrenics were found in Cali and in Beijing.) In ISoS, high percentages of catatonic schizophrenia were found only in four developing centers: Agra, Cali, Chandigarh rural, and Chennai (Madras).

Short-Term Course

Complete remission in the short-term follow-up for the alive cases in Agra (73.3%) was twice that in Prague and 2½ times that in Cali. The next best percentages of complete remission were found at Chandigarh rural, Chandigarh urban, Nottingham, Prague DOSMeD, and Chennai (Madras). Continuously psychotic cases made up 9.8% in Agra, while in Prague IPSS there were 1.25 times as many, and in the Cali center there were twice as many.

ALIVE SUBJECTS

Symptomatology

Rated according to the Bleuler Severity of Psychotic Symptoms Scale, 47 (77%) of the Agra ISoS cases were recovered, as against 72.5% in Prague and 56.9% in Cali. The other Indian centers (with briefer follow-up periods), Madras and both Chandigarh urban and rural cohorts had lower recovery rates than Agra. Symptomatically, the proportion of the Agra cohort having severe symptoms was 11.5%—near to that in Cali and Madras, but twice the percentage in Prague (IPSS) and Chandigarh urban. Interestingly, Chandigarh rural reported no subjects in the severe psychotic category, a finding inexplicably at odds with our own as most of the Agra cases were also rural. It is therefore concluded that although Agra had the highest proportion for the best outcome, there was also a high relative proportion for the worst outcome.

Over the course of the follow-up period, 19 (31.2%) patients remained asymptomatic for 21 to 25 years, four (6.6%) patients were asymptomatic for 16 to 20 years, two (3.3%) patients were asymptomatic for 11 to 15 years, three (4.9%) patients were asymptomatic for 6 to 10 years, and eight (13.1%) patients were asymptomatic under 5 years. Twenty-five (41%) patients had some symptoms throughout the entire period.

Course and Type, Last 2 Years of Follow-up

In Agra males, 21.1% had episodic illness and in the total IPSS, 10.8%. In females, the rate was the same as in the IPSS sample (13.6%). In Agra males, 15.8% had continuous illness, and in IPSS, 37.6%; in females, 9.1% had continuous illness, and in IPSS, 29.6%. Rates of episodic illness for those with sudden onset in Agra (16.1%) and IPSS (16.3%) samples were nearly the same. In Agra, 20.7% with slow onset had episodic illness while in IPSS, it was 10.6%. Overall, episodic illness occurs 1½ times more frequently in Agra than in IPSS. In Agra, 9.7% with sudden onset had continuous illness, while in IPSS it was 18.4%; 17.2% with slow onset had continuous illness versus 40.7% in IPSS. With respect to recent course of illness, Agra was equivalent to Prague, and both were much better than Cali. For the most recent 2 years, there was a higher percentage in Agra of never psychotic cases (63.3%) than in IPSS (52.9%).

Global Assessment of Functioning

The Global Assessment of Functioning for Symptomatology (GAF-S) in the last month showed that ratings between 81 and 90 were more frequent in both males (56.4%) and females (77.3%) for Agra, as compared to total IPSS (38.3% and 46.8%, respectively). The Global Assessment of Functioning for Disability (GAF-D) showed that there were more "better functioning" (ratings of 81 to 90) males (48.7%) and females (81.8%) in Agra than in the total IPSS sample

(36.2% for males and 45.5% for females). In total, the Agra cohort showed 1½ times better functioning for both GAF scores. Mode of onset, sudden or insidious, seems for most measures to play no role in the course and type of outcome. The GAF-S, in particular, gives no indication that mode of onset is related to clinical outcome.

Residential and Functional Status

Most subjects lived with families and friends. Note that independent living is a very confusing concept if it is equated to living with the family. Perhaps a person living with his nuclear family could be described as living independently; but in India, most people live with their joint or loosely joint families. "Living with the family" would have been a better category. In Agra, 3.3% lived alone, compared with 5.6% in Cali and 25.6% in Prague. In Cali and Agra in the last 2 years of follow-up, about 95% were in independent living for the entire period, but in Prague only 76.7%. The figure for Agra compared very well with the Indian centers, Chandigarh (rural and urban). Slightly lower rates were seen in Chennai, Beijing, and Hong Kong. These findings suggest that the developing centers, especially in the East Asian region, had more independent living. Most were also rated as "never in hospital." Vagrancy or living alone was infrequent in these centers, suggesting again that in developing countries, the dependence on the family is strong while in the more affluent, developed countries, welfare could obviate dependency on the family to the same extent. In almost all centers, very few subjects had been in prison.

Over 50% of subjects in Agra, Chennai, and Chandigarh rural were not employed in the last 2 years, rates that were similar to that of Prague. Forty-one percent were employed full time for the entire period. For those employed more than 12 months, work performance was rated good to very good in 84% of the subjects in Agra. High work performance is noted in most other centers. Of direct relevance is the fact that disability pensions are not available in India to persons suffering from mental disturbance. Work demands of patients in rural regions of the Agra catchment area were in routine, rustic jobs—such as taking cattle to graze and feed—tasks which family members judged them to be performing well. Of the 61 alive cases, 27 were employed, 21 were engaged in household activities, three had retired, six were unemployed, and for four there was no information.

Social Disability

The DAS global evaluation of excellent to good adjustment was found in over 50% of cases in Agra and Cali, but in far fewer cases in Prague (29%). The Agra Center scored this high rating in 36 cases (60%), while in most other centers, social disability ratings were lower. A score of 60 or more on the GAF-D scale is indicative of fairly good functioning; 79% of Agra ratings were above this, as compared with 62% in Cali and 77% in Prague.

Violence and Suicide

During the last 2 years of follow-up, 100% of subjects in Cali, 95.2% in Prague, and 91.7% in Agra reported no assaults. In the majority of other centers, no assaults were reported for over 90% of cases. In alive cases since the first inclusion, Cali reported no assaults for 100% of cases, Agra for 86.7%, and Prague for 83.7%. In the same last 2 years, no suicide attempts at all were reported in Agra, Chandigarh rural, and Prague IPSS, and no suicide attempts were reported in 98.6% of cases in Cali, 96.3% in Chandigarh urban, and 93.3% in Chennai. Since the study inclusion, no suicide attempts were made in 95.1% in Agra cases, 97.2% in Cali cases, and 97.7% in Prague cases. Suicide attempts were, therefore, very uncommon.

Treatment Status

In the last 2 years of follow-up, 72.7% of the Agra cases never used neuroleptic medication. The only other center showing such high nonuse was Chandigarh rural. Dublin, Nagasaki, and Hong Kong reported from 75 to 94% use most of the time. This phenomenon is better explained by a number of factors: better monitoring in the other centers, high cost of psychotropic drugs in India and their virtual unavailability in rural areas, and indifference to continuing medication after a patient improves, especially when laypersons consider it to be unnecessary. There is no understanding that medication maintains the patient's improved condition. Still, the fact that the recovery rates were so high suggests a much lower need for maintenance medication.

Hospitalization

While no subjects were currently in the hospital or in supervised nursing homes in Agra, one was hospitalized in Cali, and a small number in Prague. Within the last 2 years of follow-up, 96.7% of Agra cases and 97.2% of Cali cases had never been hospitalized. A similar trend was noticed in Chandigarh urban and rural, where 95% or more of cases were never hospitalized.

DECEASED PATIENTS

There was hardly any difference between the Agra and the total IPSS regarding the age at death. Similarly, no noticeable difference is found in males and females. Of the 43 dead at 25 years, 9.3% committed suicide. The other causes of death were 25 cases (60.4%) natural, two (4.7%) homicide, one (2.8%) accident, and 10 (23.3%) unknown. Nearly half (45.5%) of those with information not missing were well, 15.2% were in partial remission, and 39.4% were in an episode of illness or had been unwell continuously. The distribution of total IPSS cases was: well 33.8%; partially remitted 19.1%; and in episode 47.1%.

DISCUSSION

Interpreting the Status of Alive Subjects at Follow-Up

The disability assessments done at this center reveal that in all spheres—social withdrawal, self-care, participation in household activity, marital-affective role with spouse, and parental role—there was no dysfunction in over 60% of cases for whom information was available.

It is paradoxical that despite what might have been expected to be a continual need for treatment, most patients did not avail themselves of it, appeared not to need it in fact, and showed so much improvement. Subjects in this region get good family support and there are few demands on them—both of which may serve the cause of recovery. The fact that in India few families are nuclear may be another reason for better outcome. Also, there may be coping behaviors on the part of both family members and the subject.

Potential Bias in the Revaluation Diagnosis

The initial diagnosis was made using ICD-8, and converting these to corresponding ICD-10 diagnoses was difficult at times. For instance, no equivalent of category 295.9 in ICD-8 can be found in ICD-10. Because this study is an extension of a long WHO research program including intracenter and intercenter reliability methods, consultative visits to the participating centers, and a training program, the researchers are experienced enough so that local diagnostic practices present no significant problems.

Potential Cultural Influences on the Course of Recovery

Even though fissures have appeared, in India, the joint family still plays a very important role in caring for mentally ill persons, especially where close familial bonds exist. In rural areas, villagers too have developed affinity toward their co-villagers, and often when a mentally disturbed person comes to the hospital or to a psychiatrist for help, many villagers accompany him or her. Indeed, it is often the case that instead of the parents or a close relative coming to give information, a member of the village group poses as an important member of the family, although he might not even belong to the patient's caste. It is only after very close questioning that his real identity is revealed, and the validity of the proffered information assessed. Still, it is undeniable that villagers give help and show sympathy and concern for others who are disturbed. For example, a female patient who was participating in a center survey was found wandering aimlessly in a dilapidated condition in another village by someone from her own village. He felt that it was a slur on his village to see this woman roaming about and immediately took her back to his village, where everyone provided help in feeding, clothing, and caring for her. This story is typical of Indian culture and illustrates an important reason for better outcome.

From all the information that has been gathered, no one variable is seen to account for the outcome. It may be surmised that family affiliation, dependence, and strong family ties may play a role in ameliorating schizophrenic illness, but the conclusion that emerges from the study is that schizophrenia and MDP run a natural course, and time alone is mainly responsible for long-term positive outcome in cases of schizophrenic illness.

SUMMARY

After 25 years, it was possible to trace 81% of the original cohort of 140 patients. Examination of social and demographic variables such as age, sex, marital status, residence in urban and rural areas, and mean birth age showed no significant difference between the 61 ISoS living cases and the 140 cases at inclusion. Sudden and slow onsets in Agra cases were equally distributed and were similar to the distribution at inclusion. The diagnostic hierarchy was the same in both the ISoS cases and the cases at inclusion. Other schizophrenia was the largest schizophrenia subgroup, followed by catatonic type. Cases of hebephrenic schizophrenia at follow-up were conspicuous by their low occurrence, while in Cali acute schizophrenia-like illness was found in 28% of cases. In Prague, almost one-fifth of the living cases were diagnosed with paranoid schizophrenia. No explanation can be given for this except cultural variance (but see Chapter 10 for information regarding selective follow-up). Complete remission at short-term follow-up for the live cases in Agra was more than twice that in Prague and 2½ times that in Cali. In Agra, one-third of the alive were asymptomatic between 21 and 25 years and one-seventh had continuous illness. GAF-S ratings between 81 and 90 in Agra occurred in 56.4% of males and 77.3% of females, while in IPSS the figures were 38.3% and 46.8% respectively. GAF-D showed similar differences between Agra and the total IPSS. Global evaluation of disability from excellent to good adjustment was found in more than 50% of cases in both Agra and Cali, while in Prague it was much less.

Computation of the standardized mortality ratio (SMR) for the total cases of mental disturbance revealed that death among mentally ill persons was higher than that in the general population. In spite of the fact that use of neuroleptics is uncommon and hospitalization is not the usual treatment choice, global outcome in the final 2 years of follow-up was rated as much better. Examining various variables yielded no relationship that could be specifically related to outcome beside family care. It is therefore surmised that schizophrenia runs a natural course, and the longer the survival, the better the outcome.

References

Dube, K C. (1978), Nosology and therapy in Ayurveda. *Compar. Med. East & West*, 6(3):209–228.

——(1970), A study of prevalence and bio-social variables in mental illness in a rural and urban community in Uttar Pradesh, India. *Acta Psychiatr. Scand.*, 46(FASC 4): Appendix 2, 327–359.

——Kumar, N., & Dube, S. (1984), A long term course and outcome of the Agra cases in the IPSS cases. *Acta Psychiatr. Scand.*, 70:170–179.

Indian Council of Medical Research/Department of Science and Technology (1987), *Collaborative Study on Severe Mental Morbidity*. New Delhi: Indian Council of Medical Research/Department of Science and Technology.

Sartorius, N., Gulbinat, W., Harrison, G., Laska, E., & Siegel, C. (1996), Long-term follow-up of schizophrenia in 16 countries. *Soc. Psychol. Psychiatr. Epidemiol.*, 31:249–258.

Sharma, S. D., & Chadda, R. K. (1996), *Mental Hospitals in India: Current Status and Future Role in Mental Health Care*. Delhi: Shahadara/Institute of Human Behaviour and Allied Sciences.

World Health Organization (1973), *The International Pilot study of Schizophrenia*. Geneva: World Health Organization.

——(1979), *Schizophrenia: An International Follow-Up Study*. New York: Wiley.

Chapter 9

IPSS: Cali, Colombia

Carlos A. León and Agatha León

CULTURAL CONTEXT

The Cali World Health Organization (WHO) Collaborating Center for Research and Training in Mental Health originally selected the metropolitan district of the city as its catchment area for the IPSS. However, after June 1969, this area was expanded to include the neighboring town of Palmira. The city of Cali is the capital city of the Departamento del Valle and lies on one side of the long, fertile Cauca valley on the southwest side of Colombia, hemmed in by two of the three parallel ranges of the Andes mountains which edge the western coast of Colombia. Palmira lies across the valley, 25 km north of Cali; the Pacific Ocean is a mere 120 km to the west. Steep terrain and dense jungle vegetation to the west and high mountains to the east have effectively isolated Cali from the capital city of Bogotá. Although Cali lies just 3.5 degrees north of the Equator, its altitude of 1,000 meters insures a mild, semitropical climate all year round, with alternating rainy and dry seasons and small variations in temperature.

The Valle was colonized in 1536 by Spaniards who came from Ecuador and Peru after having accompanied Pizarro on his conquest of the Inca Empire. The Indians they encountered were subdued, killed, or died of infectious diseases introduced by the Spaniards during the first century of colonial rule. The survivors either intermarried or took refuge in the high mountains to the east; the latter have only gradually come into contact with Spanish-Colombian culture in the past 80 years. Spanish is spoken by all but a few Indian tribes.

Once they had settled, the conquistadores proceeded to parcel out vast tracts of land among themselves and, along with the land, the Indians who lived on it, creating a land-based aristocracy that ruled the Valle and most of Colombia for several centuries. As the Indian population diminished, African slaves were imported to work on cattle ranches, on sugar and tobacco plantations, and in gold mines. Because of the Spanish propensity toward intermarriage, the people of the Valle are largely a mestizo type, which now represents about 60% of the population; 20% are a mixture of black and caucasian or black and mestizo; approximately 14% are caucasians, 4% are pure black, and 2% are pure Indian. After 10 years of fierce struggle, Colombia became independent from Spain in 1820. Slavery was not formally abolished until 1850, but before that time slaves were often rewarded with their freedom, reducing the slave population to negligible proportions.

Over the past 50 years, the economy of the Valle has changed from predominantly cattle grazing to agriculture. Industrialization, which began right after World War II, lured thousands of peasants to the city with promises of higher wages and limited working hours. The population in Cali increased, and several industrial plants and multinational companies were established, especially during the late 1950s and early 1960s. Thus, Cali, which in 1810 had just over 7500 inhabitants and in 1946 had slightly above 104,000, suddenly grew into a large city; by 1968, it had almost a million inhabitants. According to the 1993 Census, Cali had a population of 1.84 million (Departamento Administrativo Nacional de Estadística, 1995), 70% of whom live in urban areas. Although Cali is the third largest city in Colombia, it is second to Bogotá in growth rate.

Another factor for increasing migration to Cali from the rural areas was the undeclared but very savage civil war, "La Violencia," that raged in the mountains around the Valle for about 15 years. It started in 1949 after the government tried to suppress the excesses and riots that took place in Bogotá, when a very popular political leader was murdered there during the Pan-American Conference of April 1948. This state of civil war ended officially in 1965, but was later complicated with the upsurge of violence related to organized crime and drug traffic. The period of La Violencia has been characterized as "the greatest destabilizing [effect] Colombian history has known since the nation became independent" (Lopez-Michelsen, 1987).

Shortly before this, the first guerrilla groups were already active in the countryside. After a series of struggles between two main leading political parties (liberal and conservative), and a military coup which was later toppled in 1957, the signing of a peace treaty and the agreement of the two parties to alternate in government brought some political stability. Yet the guerilla groups refused to lay down their arms and continued their bellicose activities, which gradually evolved into a kind of endemic banditry. Among the most notorious guerrilla groups over the past 30 years are the FARC (Fuerzas Armadas Revolucionarias de Colombia), ELN (Ejército de Liberación Nacional) and, until 1984, the group M-19 (Movimiento 19 de Abril). These groups have been active in kidnapping, murders, riots, sieges and, lately, drug trafficking as well.

The upsurge of organized crime on a grand scale in Colombia can be traced to a rising international demand for cocaine in the late 1960s and early 1970s. Smugglers, dealers, and intermediaries who had initially worked in isolation, merged, forming conglomerates such as the Medellín, Cali, and Bogotá cartels, trading in cocaine by the ton with annual profits of over $U.S. 8 billion. Attempts to eradicate drug trafficking provoked a series of crimes—the bombing of a passenger plane and the assassinations of a minister of justice, a liberal party presidential candidate in 1989, about 30 judges, several high-ranking police officers, and the director of one of the largest newspapers in the country. These crimes were intended not only as retaliation against legal action but also as gestures of "defiant bravado" to further intimidate an already terrorized community (León, 1992b).

The rise of the drug cartels in Cali brought improvement in economic conditions. During the late 1980s and 1990s, a boom in construction and other businesses was financed with laundered drug money and prompted a new wave of immigrants. In recent years, the persecution and imprisonment of notorious Medellín and Cali cartel leaders brought a relative respite in these activities, which was followed by the emergence of new and younger criminal groups.

Impact of Mental Health Issues on Society

A study conducted by León and Micklin (1971) focused on community opinions and attitudes regarding mental illness and its treatment using a stratified sample of 800 subjects obtained from the barrios (neighborhoods). In general, results suggested a considerable degree of confusion and uncertainty regarding the nature of mental disease. Results also showed a high degree of faith in the psychiatrist's professional ability and a tendency to place blind trust in the effectiveness of psychiatric treatments. Young informants belonging to the upper social classes had clearer notions about mental disorders and their treatment, emphasizing the physical dimensions of a mental disorder and showing lower levels of trust in psychiatrists. This study indicated that although it was necessary to increase the level of information, there was no evidence of hostility toward or rejection of psychiatrists and their activities.

Another study (Micklin and León, 1972) focused on attitudes toward mentally ill persons. The results suggested a lower level of rejection regarding social interaction when compared to studies in other countries. This may be interpreted as a higher level of tolerance for mentally ill persons in Cali and maybe in Latin America, or in developing countries in general.

MENTAL HEALTH SYSTEM IN THE AREA

Early Mental Health Policies and Changes Since IPSS

In the early 1960s, psychiatric resources, especially personnel, were scarce in Colombia, a situation aggravated by their concentration in metropolitan areas. Public psychiatric institutions were generally custodial. By the late 1960s, awareness of the lack of trained personnel and facilities for mental health care increased, but such priorities as the control of communicable diseases, combating malnutrition, and improving environmental sanitation absorbed most of the available public health resources. Nevertheless, government policies enabled the delivery of effective services by emphasizing prevention and treatment of family groups in urban and semirural areas by qualified auxiliary personnel.

In 1974, the Division of Mental Health was created within the Ministry of Health. A macrodiagnosis of the prevailing problems was followed by the design of specific mental health policies, objectives, subprograms and activities in research, promotion, prevention, personnel training, and delivery systems. The National Health Plan at the time (Olivares-Mora, 1974) aimed at a "more rational utilization of human-power and facilities." Within this plan, mental health activities were to become an integral part of the work of all health personnel through a system of delegated functions. Most of the mental health tasks were designed to be performed by general practitioners, nurses, auxiliary nurses, and health promoters; specialists would engage in consultation, supervision, and training.

Present Mental Health Policies

According to the 1991 Colombian Constitution, it is the state's obligation to protect especially those individuals who may be regarded as impaired because of their economic, physical, or mental condition. On this principle, a policy of social prevention, rehabilitation, and integration was implemented. The National Mental Health Plan presented by the Ministry of Health in 1991 proposed changes in the delivery of services at different levels: for example, the deinstitutionalization of the chronically mentally ill, who should be taken care of by their social network or the state, and the establishment of primary mental health care as a means to detect early mental disorders and to prevent chronicity. This plan also focused on the improvement of mental hospitals, as well as on "ethical, clinical, institutional and environmental aspects." At the same time, new community-based treatment strategies were implemented. Among the main objectives of the National Mental Health Plan is to offer "more effective referral practices, and the social reinsertion of patients with mental disorders in order to offer them more humane and technical treatment aimed at a better quality of life" (Gonzáles Posso, Agudelo Calderón, Mendoza Villalobos, and Cuadros Ferré, 1991).

Passed in 1993, Ley 100 (Law 100) places responsibility for health care on the individual citizen rather than on the state (Guzmán Cuevas, Albarez Giraldo, Vesga Sánchez, and Ruiz Echeverry, 1995). As of January 1995, the new health model expected "all families to obtain protection from disease" and to choose freely not only their "health promoting entity" (EPS), but also clinics, hospitals, laboratories, and physicians. However, the establishment of these policies has yet to produce positive results because of the prevailing economic and social conditions under which most Colombians live.

Structure of the Local Mental Health Services System

Founded in 1960, the San Isidro Psychiatric Hospital (HPSI) has since been the main public psychiatric facility not only in Cali but in the whole southwestern region of Colombia. A teaching hospital affiliated with the University of Valle School of Medicine, it is administratively and financially independent from the University and is supported through public funding. In 1961, the Department of Psychiatry at the University of Valle was officially appointed the scientific advisory body to the hospital, and began a vigorous and sustained effort on the part of the teaching staff to implement acceptable standards of patient care and to change ingrained attitudes on the part of nursing personnel, the administration, and the public. In the short span of 8 to 10 years, HPSI underwent changes representing 200 years in the evolution of psychiatry (León, 1979).

In 1968, institutional resources were divided among health centers, a public hospital, the social security system, and private clinics. Health centers scattered throughout the city cared for ambulatory patients almost exclusively, although some had oral rehydration units and a few beds for deliveries. The 40 health centers in the city of Cali and the three in Palmira offered inexpensive services to the poorest sectors of the community. Two of the health centers in Cali and one in Palmira ran psychiatric outpatient clinics. Of the five public hospitals in Cali, two were specialized: the San Isidro Psychiatric Hospital and a hospital for pulmonary diseases. In Palmira, there was one public general hospital. At the time, two facilities took care of nearly all psychiatric outpatients in Cali: San Isidro Psychiatric Hospital with about 9000 outpatient visits a year and the Social Security Outpatient Department with 8000 outpatient visits. General University Hospital also offered psychiatric outpatient services in Cali. In Palmira, the general hospital had only one psychiatrist for the outpatient service. About 40% of the outpatients seen at the San Isidro Hospital were first admissions. There was also a small private psychiatric clinic with 20 beds. The rate of new psychiatric admissions for the city was calculated as 80 per 100,000 inhabitants (Zambrano, 1967). As to the diagnostic distribution of the hospitalized population, in a 10-year study carried out between 1956 and 1965, schizophrenia was found to represent 40.2% of all psychiatric disorders (León and López, 1966).

Over the years, health facilities have increased in number and coverage. At the time of the ISoS follow-up there are 50 health centers, five public hospitals, and at least six large private clinics in Cali; however, the San Isidro Psychiatric Hospital has remained the main psychiatric facility in the region. Although social security has an outpatient clinic, the Mental Health Unit of the University Hospital has 15 beds, and there is a private mental health clinic, most hospitalizations are handled at the psychiatric hospital. During the late 1970s and early 1980s, HPSI was remodeled and enlarged, transforming wards and observation rooms into spacious modern areas. To raise revenues, the hospital offered the public supplementary services such as rehabilitation, pharmacy, and general medicine. At present, the hospital has 220 beds, and the average length of stay is 23 days. The Health Division of the University of Valle provides rotating interns who work at the outpatient clinics as well as medical students who do their internship at the hospital. During 1995, there were 18,300 visits to the outpatient clinic and 3200 hospitalizations. Psychotic disorders continue to be the most frequent pathology diagnosed in these services.

Financial Support

At the time of the study, all patients seen at HPSI were admitted using the following system: Any patient coming to the hospital for the first time, whether through the outpatient clinic or the emergency room, was taken to the Admissions Office where a social worker assessed socioeconomic status to determine the fees the patient should be charged. An indigent patient would be subsidized by the institution. Patients from high socioeconomic levels usually saw private psychiatrists or attended private clinics. The treatment of patients affiliated with social security was subsidized by the government.

During the late 1970s, an increase of private medical insurance, usually subscribed to by people from the upper-middle to the upper socioeconomic levels, brought about some changes. Although most insurance plans did not cover psychiatric hospitalizations, some allowed for up to 15 outpatient visits. According to Law 100, by 1995, all Colombians had to be affiliated with a Health Promoting Entity (EPS; Guzmán Cuevas et al., 1995). Those who were not were identified as either indigent (to be subsidized by the government) or "private" (to be charged full fees).

PSYCHIATRIC EPIDEMIOLOGY

Since its creation in 1955, the Department of Psychiatry at the University of Valle planned research activities aimed at exploring the characteristics, frequency, and distribution of mental disorders in the community. Initial efforts were limited to developing hospital statistics and to documenting the flow of patients at HPSI.

The first epidemiological studies conducted in the 1960s were designed to obtain basic information to be used for planning services and personnel training programs. Following a sequential plan, the research focused on such aspects as the prevalence of disorders (León, 1967), design of instruments for case finding (León and Climent, 1968), and community attitudes and notions with regard to mental illnesses, causes, and treatments (León and Micklin, 1971; Micklin and León, 1972).

Conducted in 1967, the first study of the prevalence of overt mental disorders in Cali found that the prevalence of overt psychoses was 4.8 per 1000 inhabitants of all ages; mental deficiencies 7.2 per 1000; and epilepsy 5.6 per 1000. Approximately three-fourths of the patients with overt psychoses in this sample were diagnosed as schizophrenic. About one-third of all the patients had not received any treatment at all, and half of them had previously been admitted to a psychiatric center. Because of the demographic socioeconomic characteristics of the sample of this study, it was assumed that at least one-third of the population of Cali could have similar rates (León, 1967).

In 1967, use of the Health Opinion Survey (HOS) as a case screening instrument showed a significant difference in the scores obtained by persons identified as cases vs. those free of disorder. The study also revealed that 21% of the individuals within the area were in need of treatment for mental disorders (León and Climent, 1968). An analysis of the content of delusions and hallucinations of patients cared for at the San Isidro Psychiatric Hospital during two different time periods showed significant differences in the content of the symptoms, which could be attributed to external factors operating in the two epochs (León, 1970).

To explore the relationship between readmission to the psychiatric hospital and socioeconomic and clinical variables, a retrospective study analyzing the behavior of two groups of patients seen in two different time periods was conducted (León and Alvarez, 1972). All cases admitted for the first time in 1956 were included as well as those admitted in 1964; the course of the disease during the following three consecutive years was observed. Among the most relevant findings are the following: In both groups, the predominant diagnosis was schizophrenia, amounting to 75% of all admissions in 1956 and 51% in 1964. The mean hospitalization period was 34 days in 1956 and 27 days in 1964 (a statistically significant difference). The readmission rate was 39% for those admitted in 1956 and 30% for those admitted in 1964 (not significant, but showing a decreasing trend). With regard to demographic variables, the likelihood of readmission was lower in persons older than 35 years hospitalized in 1964. No differences with regard to sex and a slight increase in readmission rates in single persons were also observed. The readmission rates for schizophrenic patients for both groups was similar: 45% in 1956 and 43% in 1964. Most of the readmissions were for cases identified as "chronic undifferentiated" schizophrenia, representing 29% in 1956 and 46% in 1964.

In the early 1970s, the Department of Psychiatry at the University of Valle launched the Social Psychiatry Pilot Project in an urban sector of Cali (Argandoña and Kiev, 1972; Leon, 1973, 1977). The project aimed at training health personnel in the delivery of primary mental health care, but was also an opportunity to study the natural history of mental disorders and to clarify the specific conditions and circumstances that surround the clinical picture in the community. Other objectives were to eradicate the stereotype of "crazy" people needing to be taken to an "asylum," to educate community leaders, and to create an awareness of how to handle people with mental diseases. Several community studies were conducted under this program, and most of them refer to schizophrenia in a specific or generic form.

A study of geographic and social mobility related to mental disorders (Micklin and León, 1978) showed very high scores for both men and women on the Langner scale (Langner, 1962), used as an estimator of the level of psychiatric disturbance. For both sexes, average scores rose as education levels fell. Contrariwise, ascending social mobility and higher social status were related to lower scores. Men older than 40 years of age had lower scores, and women older than 30 years had higher scores. In general, women and people with incomplete elementary education showed higher average scores.

Pilot studies on the use of primary health care workers for the care of psychiatric patients showed how an auxiliary nurse could successfully perform simple diagnostic and treatment functions (Climent, de Arango, Plutchik, and León, 1978; Climent and de Arango, 1980). Under the auspices of WHO, a multicenter project on Strategies for the Extension of Mental Health Care in Developing Countries was undertaken in 1975 (Harding et al., 1980). Among its objectives were: to evaluate alternative and innovative low-cost and highly effective mental health care methods in developing countries; to provide realistic support to improve and widen mental health care; and to prepare and assess training methods and manuals. A total of 1624 patients who attended public health centers in four countries were assessed. Among them, 225 were identified as mental disorder cases (13.9%). In Cali, the percentage was 10.8% (48 of 444 patients), with schizophrenia accounting for 3.1%. Results showed that primary health care workers handle patients with mental disorders in their daily tasks, but they can only identify a relatively small proportion of them. It was deemed necessary to improve their diagnostic abilities.

A project with similar objectives was designed to train community members in the detection of cases (León, 1981). A group of rural high school students, trained to identify mental disorders in the community, conducted a prevalence study and found a global rate of 24.2% with mental disorders in a rural setting. The proportion of psychotic patients was estimated to be 4.7%.

Involvement of the Cali Field Research Center in the WHO International Pilot Study of Schizophrenia (IPSS) since 1968 (WHO, 1973), and in the Determinants of Outcome of Severe Mental Disorders since 1976 (DOSMeD; Jablensky et al., 1992) provided unique clinical experiences and many opportunities for the refinement of concepts and techniques. These were a unique source of clinical experience and the development of teaching and research programs (León, 1986, 1992a; Von Zerssen et al., 1990).

THE CALI FIELD RESEARCH CENTER

In 1978, the Department of Psychiatry at the University of Valle, Division of Health Sciences, was designated as a WHO Collaborating Center for Research and Training in Mental Health. The center uses the facilities of the Mental Health Unit of the University Hospital (where the Department of Psychiatry is located). The center was conceived as a program rather than as an institution and thus has a semiautonomous structure, with strong ties to the University for teaching and research activities and with collaborations with other institutions in the health, education, and community development sectors. The center is represented in the Regional Council of Health and maintains close contact with the Municipal Secretary of Health in Cali. No specific funding, other than for salaries of the teaching staff of the Department of Psychiatry, is provided institutionally for the center, which finances its research activities through individual project grants. Other personnel involved in research studies are hired according to the type of project; funding is provided through several sources. Administrative support for accounting and promotional activities is given by Foundación para la Educación Superior (FES), a nonprofit local organization.

The Department of Psychiatry at the University of Valle has been vigorously involved in diverse research activities since its creation in the late 1950s. Participation in IPSS enhanced the research and training potentials of the Department of Psychiatry and widened its perspectives for dealing with mental health problems in developing countries. Since its designation, the center has participated in several major international WHO research projects such as DOSMeD, the Study on Dose Effects of Psychotropic Drugs in Different Populations, the Study on Strategies for Extending Mental Health Care, and the Study on Psychosomatic Sequela of Female Sterilization. It also collaborated with the Pan American Health Organization, the WHO Regional Office for the Americas (PAHO), in the design and testing of instruments for the Study of Dementia Disorders in Elderly People, and with the WHO Global Programme on AIDS in the testing of instruments for the study of knowledge, attitudes, and practices related to AIDS and to drug and alcohol abuse.

Under different auspices, members of the center have participated in the preparation of a manual of psychiatry for primary health workers, in designing curricular changes for medical and paramedical personnel for mental health activities in primary care, in research on the factors associated with drug abuse among the student population in Cali, and in the design of a prevention program. The center also participated in an international evaluation of a draft of ICD-10.

METHODS USED AT THE SITE

Defining the Long-Term Outcome Cohort

In Cali, a total of 127 probands were enlisted in the original study according to the IPSS protocol, of whom 101 were diagnosed as schizophrenic at the initial examination in 1968. The present follow-up study described in this chapter focused exclusively on this cohort of 101 ICD-8 "schizophrenic" students. In the aggregate ISoS tables, the total of 127 is used (see Table 9.1).

Case-Finding

Locating study subjects was an arduous and time-consuming process, not only because of the mobility of the cohort and the lack of appropriate communication services in many instances, but also because of fortuitous events (such as a change in street names in Cali) during the follow-up period. Case-finding procedures were designed on the basis of a directory of updated addresses, created for each case from psychiatric hospital records and from the list of addresses created for the 10-year follow-up in 1978. Each case history was reviewed in order to obtain the date of the patient's most recent hospital visit; however, this measure turned out to be insufficient since most of the subjects had not consulted with the facility in more than 10 years, and some subjects had never been back (26 years). A few addresses were obtained from the local phone book; in a very few cases, the subject was listed; in others, persons were located after finding a relative's listed phone number. After the directory was ready, two public health, auxiliary nurses familiar with the area were hired to search for the addresses (1 to 12 visits). If the subject or his or her family had moved from the given address, the auxiliaries discreetly questioned neighbors or acquaintances to obtain the most recent one. If the subject was found to be living outside the city, transportation

TABLE 9.1 Baseline and Short-Term Demographic and Clinical Description by Data Cohort

	Alive		*Dead*		*Lost to Follow-up*		*Total Schizophrenia*		*Non Schizophrenia*	
	N	%	N	%	N	%	N	%	N	%
Gender										
Male	37	51.4	9	75.0	7	41.2	53	52.5	3	11.5
Female	35	48.6	3	25.0	10	58.8	48	47.5	23	88.5
Birth Year										
Missing	0	0.0	0	0.0	1	5.9	1	1.0	0	0.0
1920–1929	2	2.8	1	8.3	2	11.8	5	5.0	3	11.5
1930–1939	16	22.2	6	50.0	4	23.5	26	25.7	12	46.2
1940–1949	41	56.9	5	41.7	9	52.9	55	54.5	8	30.8
1950–1959	13	18.1	0	0.0	1	5.9	14	13.9	3	11.5
Grouped Mode of Onset										
Sudden (IPSS Overnight)	9	12.5	0	0.0	2	11.8	11	10.9	1	3.8
Slow (IPSS > 24 Hours)	63	87.5	12	100.0	14	82.4	89	88.1	25	96.2
Other/Missing	0	0.0	0	0.0	1	5.9	1	1.0	0	0.0
Baseline Diagnosis Converted to ICD-10										
Paranoid Schizophrenia	10	13.9	5	41.7	5	29.4	20	19.8	0	0.0
Hebephrenic Schizophrenia	17	23.6	2	16.7	1	5.9	20	19.8	0	0.0
Catatonic Schizophrenia	11	15.3	0	0.0	2	11.8	13	12.9	0	0.0
Residual Schizophrenia	4	5.6	1	8.3	1	5.9	6	5.9	0	0.0
Other Schizophrenia	2	2.8	0	0.0	1	5.9	3	3.0	0	0.0
Schizoaffective	5	6.9	0	0.0	2	11.8	7	6.9	0	0.0
Acute Schizophrenia-like	20	27.8	4	33.3	5	29.4	29	28.7	0	0.0
Bipolar	0	0.0	0	0.0	0	0.0	0	0.0	3	11.5
Depression	0	0.0	0	0.0	0	0.0	0	0.0	9	34.6
Other Psychotic	0	0.0	0	0.0	0	0.0	0	0.0	2	7.7
Other Nonpsychotic	3	4.2	0	0.0	0	0.0	3	3.0	12	46.2
Grouped Baseline Diagnosis										
Schizophrenia	44	61.1	8	66.7	10	58.8	62	61.4	0	0.0
Nonschizophrenia/Missing	28	38.9	4	33.3	7	41.2	39	38.6	26	100.0
Grouped Short-Term Pattern of Course										
Complete Remission	21	29.2	2	16.7	2	11.8	25	24.8	9	34.6
Incomplete Remission	26	36.1	2	16.7	4	23.5	32	31.7	7	26.9
Continuously Psychotic	13	18.1	5	41.7	2	11.8	20	19.8	7	26.9
Other/Missing	12	16.7	3	25.0	9	52.9	24	23.8	3	11.5
Short-Term Follow-up Time										
0, Missing (Baseline)	0	0.0	1	8.3	5	29.4	6	5.9	1	3.8
18–30 Months (2 year)	2	2.8	0	0.0	0	0.0	2	2.0	0	0.0
5 Year	70	97.2	11	91.7	12	70.6	93	92.1	25	96.2
Total	72	100.0	12	100.0	17	100.0	101	100.0	26	100.0
Birth Year (19xx)										
N		72		12		16		100		26
MEAN		43.69		37.42		40.75		42.47		38.42
STD		6.27		6.96		7.42		6.82		7.76

was provided so the subjects could be interviewed in their homes. For deceased cases or for those living abroad, relatives who qualified as key informants were given a comprehensive interview. The locating and interviewing process, taking a total of 15 months (April 7, 1994, to July 5, 1995), was designed so that about six subjects per month could be studied.

Use of Study Instruments

At the Cali field center, most of the instruments used were the same as those employed by the 2-, 5-, and 10-year follow-ups. No translation and back-translation were required because almost all of the instruments had already been translated into Spanish for use either in the IPSS study or in other follow-up studies. One exception was the Life-Chart Schedule Scoresheet (LCS), which was filled in using the available information from other schedules designed to obtain psychosocial data. Also used in the Cali center were: Present State Examination (PSE); Broad Rating Schedule (BRS); Disability Assessment Schedule (DAS); Psychological Impairments Rating Schedule Scoresheet (PIRS—II); Substance Abuse Schedule (SAS); Basic Information on Study Subject (BIS); Basic Information on Informant(s) (BII); Scale for the Assessment of Negative Symptoms Scoresheet (SANS); Schedule for Deceased Patients (SDP); and Information on Refusers (IOR).

Three instruments designed for other studies or earlier follow-ups were also used. The Personal and Social History (HPS) based on the one used for IPSS, as modified during the 10-year follow-up (León, 1989, 1992a), includes data on the history, course, and symptoms of the disorder; hospitalizations; treatments received; personality characteristics; work; sexual adjustment; and interpersonal relationships. The Self Assessment Form and the Subjective Experiences Form were designed for the 5- and 10-year follow-up studies conducted in Cali and explore the subject's attitudes and notions regarding the disorder, its causes, and outcome, as well as their hope for the future.

The Physical and Neurological Examination instrument designed specifically for this follow-up was to be used by a general practitioner and follows uniform examination procedures applied for a general physical and neurological evaluation.

Information was also obtained from the subject's case histories and medical records. Case files were examined at the San Isidro Psychiatric Hospital, the Mental Health Unit of the University Hospital, and the Cali WHO Collaborating Center. In two cases, additional information was obtained from medical records of the social security clinic.

Data-Gathering Procedures

Once a case was located, an interview was scheduled with the subject or a key informant. All psychosocial information was obtained by two psychologists (project coordinator and research assistant) using the instruments designed for this purpose. If the subject was available, she or he was given a Rorschach test, interviewed by the psychiatrist to obtain an assessment of the present mental state, and then was given a complete physical and neurological examination by the general practitioner. The clinical interview and administration of the PIRS and SANS schedules were performed by the psychiatrist (C.A.L.) and, occasionally, by the psychologist (A.L.).

Reliability indexes were obtained using the Intra-Class Correlation Coefficient (ICC) (Bartko, Strauss, and Carpenter, 1980). In six exercises with the PSE, used by four raters, reliability coefficients between 0.75 and 0.92 for the scores in each section (mean=0.88) were obtained, as were coefficients between 0.84 and 0.99 for the general scores of psychoses, neuroses, and behavior (mean=0.86). Reliability levels between the two psychologists using the DAS and HPS in five different exercises showed a mean score of 0.90.

RESULTS

In spite of all the difficulties encountered, a total of 87 cases out of 101 were located. Sufficient information was obtained on 72 live subjects and on 10 deceased subjects to enable evaluation. No evaluation could be made on three live subjects who refused interviews or on two deceased subjects about whom insufficient information was available. Fourteen cases were lost to follow-up. All results presented in the following sections will refer to the 72 live subjects.

Baseline and Early Follow-Up

Gender and Age

Of the 101 subjects diagnosed as schizophrenic at initial examination, 53 were male and 48 female. The alive cohort evaluated at the 26-year follow-up is made up of 72 subjects; 37 men and 35 women (14 subjects were lost to follow-up, 3 refused to be evaluated, and 12 died during the follow-up period). The average age at initial examination was 24.9 for males and 26.3 for females, with an age range from 16 to 41. It is important to note that for close to 90% of the subjects the episode of inclusion was also the first episode of illness.

Mode of Onset and Diagnosis

The forms for recording the mode of onset at initial examination included only the categories "sudden" (overnight, or less than 24 hours) and "slow" (longer than 24 hours). Of the 72 cases, only nine (12.5%) had an onset shorter than 24 hours, while 63 (87.5%) were registered as having had a slow onset. Since the "sudden" category is too restrictive, in order to make our data more comparable to the standards used in the literature, we reviewed the psychiatric histories of all cases and reclassified the onset as: "acute" = a duration of up to 1 month, and "insidious" = lasting longer than 1 month. The number of cases in these revised categories is 37 (51.4%) and 35 (48.6%), respectively.

The use of a conversion table from the ICD-8 classification to the ICD-10 (WHO, 1994) allowed us to obtain a rough estimate of the number of cases that could be counted as schizophrenic according to the latter. In the cohort of 72 subjects, 44 (61%) were converted to an ICD-10 diagnosis of schizophrenia. This proportion is higher than those found in the other two IPSS centers. (Recall that Cali followed only subjects with a baseline diagnosis of ICD-8 schizophrenia.) No attempt was made to review the original psychiatric history or data from the initial examination in order to make an independent diagnosis using the ICD-10 criteria.

Because schizophrenia subtypes are notoriously unstable, the clinical picture was examined using longitudinal criteria which described the predominant clinical picture shown by each case throughout the whole period. The use of this approach revealed seven main categories: catatonic, paranoid, disorganized, mixed or changeable, affective, undifferentiated, and other (nonschizophrenic). Though these categories may not agree exactly with existing classification systems, they describe in the best possible way what was clinically observed over the follow-up period.

Table 9.2 presents a distribution of cases according to the initial ICD-8 diagnosis and the predominant clinical picture observed throughout the 26-year follow-up.

Pattern of Course at Early Follow-Up

About one-third of the cases were found to be in complete remission at the 2-year follow-up. For another 36%, the remission was incomplete, while 18% had remained continuously psychotic. The proportion of cases showing remission either complete or incomplete is similar to that of the Prague IPSS cohort, but it falls below that of Agra. For the full cohort of cases with a

TABLE 9.2 Initial (ICD-8) Diagnosis and Predominant Clinical Picture Observed Along the Follow-Up Period

Initial ICD-8 Diagnosis: Schizophrenia	*Predominant Clinical Picture*							
	Catatonic	*Paranoid*	*Disorganized*	*Mixed-Changeable*	*Affective*	*Undifferentiated*	*Other*	*Total*
Simple		1	1					2
Hebephrenic	1	5	2	8		1		17
Catatonic	2			3	3	3		11
Paranoid		9		1				10
Acute Undifferentiated	2	2	1	7	2	3	3	20
Latent		1			1		1	3
Chronic				2		1	1	4
Schizoaffective				1		2	2	5
Total	5	18	4	22	6	10	7	72
Percent	6.9	25.0	5.6	30.6	8.3	13.9	9.7	100

diagnosis of schizophrenia seen at the 22 to 27 months follow-up, the distribution of patterns of course was as follows: episode of inclusion followed by full remission, 19%; episode of inclusion followed by incomplete remission, 16%; several episodes followed by full remission, 13%; several episodes followed by incomplete remission, 26%; still in the episode of inclusion, 26% (WHO, 1973).

Alive Subjects

Symptomatology

The severity of psychotic symptomatology present during the last month of follow-up was rated with the use of a modified version of Manfred Bleuler's scale, derived from his criteria for end states (Bleuler, 1978, pp. 190–192). More than one-half of the live cohort (57%) was found to be recovered; 8% showed a mild condition; 24% a moderate condition; and 11% showed severe symptomatology. The difference in proportions of recovered cases in Agra (77%) and Cali is significant at the $p < .02$ level.

Evaluation of the symptoms present during the last month with the use of the Global Assessment of Functioning Scale (GAF-S) shows that about one-third of the cases (31%) are free of symptoms or show only a minimal number (GAF-S above 70); 20% show mild symptoms (61–70); 20% moderate symptoms (51–60); and 30% serious symptoms, reality impairment, and psychotic behavior (below 50). The differences in the proportions found in Agra (75% > 70) and Prague (74% > 70) are highly significant. For about two-thirds of the alive cohort, the observed trend for psychotic symptoms shows a concentration in the first 10 years of the follow-up period and a very low proportion of cases with symptoms spread throughout the period. It is also worth noting that 12.5% of the cohort did not show prominent psychotic symptoms in any of the three subperiods of the follow-up.

Course of the Illness

During the last 2 years of the follow-up period, more than one-third of subjects were regarded as being totally free of psychotic symptoms, whereas the rest showed varying degrees of pathology. The category listed as "continuous" does not necessarily imply that the person was overtly psychotic all the time; it rather describes a clinical condition where clinical symptoms of schizophrenia were present along the entire period. Hence, several cases with only a mild or moderate degree of disturbance could be included in this category. (This should caution against comparing Cali's "continuous" with those of other ISoS centers, for whom "continuous" meant continuously psychotic.) The distribution of cases according to the type of course observed during the last 10 years of the follow-up period is very similar to that of the last 2 years.

In order to register the course of the Cali cohort in a more objective way, we designed a matrix of coordinates in which the horizontal axis represented the time lapse and the vertical axis, the subject's clinical condition (León, 1989). This latter was classified in four categories operationally defined as normal, compensated, decompensated, and disintegrated. The course of the clinical condition through time was classified into three generic categories: episodic, mixed or intermediate, and continuous. Each one of these generic categories included three specific subtypes. Table 9.3 shows the distribution of cases according to the types of course observed for the full 26-year follow-up period. About one-half of the cases (48.6%) showed an episodic course; close to one-fifth (18.1%) a mixed or intermediate course; and one-third (33.3%) a continuous course.

TABLE 9.3 Distribution of Cases According to the Type of Clinical Course Observed During the 26-Year Follow-Up in Members of the Alive Cohort

Clinical Course			
Generic	*Specific*	N	Pct.
Episodic	Single Episode	3	4.2
	Occasional episodes	17	23.6
	Recurrent episodes	15	20.8
Intermediate or Mixed	Mixed with recovery	4	5.6
	Recurrent progressive	3	4.2
	Mixed without recovery	6	8.3
Continuous	Fluctuating	8	11.1
	Stationary	10	13.9
	Severe	6	8.3
	Total	72	100

For a full description of types and subtypes of course, see León (1989).

A definite overall trend toward improvement and attainment of full recovery was observed in 29% of the cases, and to this group should be added 7% with a tendency in this direction. The category "same" includes mostly cases who after coming out of the initial episode remained stable at a level of functioning below normal; this accounts for 37% of the cohort. (Other centers may refer to this overall trend as "somewhat better".) About one-fifth of cases remained continuously psychotic or became progressively worse. Some of these cases after initially attaining improvement, started on a downward course.

Our center constructed a variable, "global clinical outcome" (León, 1989), which operationalized the evolution of clinical status throughout the observation period. The categories were: excellent (full recovery), good (remission), mediocre (impairment), and poor (disability). Table 9.4 shows the distribution of global clinical outcome according to sex. More than one-half of the cohort (51.4%) had a satisfactory outcome (either excellent or good). For one-third of the subjects, the outcome was mediocre, and 15.3% had a poor outcome.

Reevaluation of Baseline Diagnosis

A reevaluation of the baseline diagnosis was not attempted in our center at the time of the 26-year follow-up because of the lack of means to engage independent evaluators with sufficient clinical experience to make reliable blind assessments. Instead, we made a special effort to document the predominant clinical picture shown by the subjects throughout the period (see Table 9.2).

TABLE 9.4 Global Clinical Outcome Observed at the 26-Year Follow-Up in Members of the Live Cohort According to Sex

Global Clinical Outcome	*Male*	*Female*	*N*	*Pct.*
Excellent	6	4	10	13.9
Good	13	14	27	37.5
Mediocre	14	10	24	33.3
Poor	4	7	11	15.3
Total	37	35	72	100

For a full description of the categories, see León (1989).

Living Arrangements

At the time of the 26-year follow-up evaluation, all cases were living in the community with the exception of one subject who was hospitalized temporarily because of a psychotic episode. Almost all (91.7%) lived in the company of relatives or friends, and only four (5.6%) lived alone. The same situation was observed for most cases during the last 2 years of follow-up; 69 (95.8%) lived independently for the entire 24 months, and the remaining three (4.2%) were living independently for a period between 13 and 23 months. The time spent in the hospital during those last 2 years was minimal. Most of the cases (97.2%) were never hospitalized during this period, and only two subjects (2.8%) were briefly hospitalized. No cases were reported as being homeless or vagrant during the past 2 years and none had been in prison during this period. For the last 10 years of the follow-up period, most of the cohort (97.2%) attained independent living for more than 95% of the period, with only two cases failing to do so.

Work

During the last 2 years of the follow-up period, more than two-thirds of the cohort (68%) were working at paid jobs and more than half of them (59%) had full-time employment for the entire 24 months. For 90% of subjects working for more than 12 months, the quality of work performance was rated as good or very good. Almost one-fifth of the cohort (18%) were engaged in full-time household work for the entire period, and the performance was rated as good or very good for close to 80% of those doing household work for more than 12 months.

Social Disability

On the evaluation with the Disability Assessment Schedule (DAS) for the last month, more than one-half of the cohort (52.3%) were rated as enjoying good or excellent social functioning, and only 9% were rated as poor. There was a single case rated as very poor and no one in the severe category. On the evaluation with the Global Assessment of Functioning-Disability (GAF-D), more than one-third of the cohort (36.6%) scored higher than 70, indicating good functioning, whereas about one-fifth (21.1%) had scores lower than

51, corresponding to serious impairment. For close to one-half of the cohort (43%), disabilities were prominent during the first third of the follow-up period only; one-fourth did not show disabilities at any time. In only two cases (2.8%) were disabilities prominent throughout the whole follow-up period.

Global social outcome was evaluated using data provided by the key informant and by other sources to estimate an average index of performance along the whole follow-up period in the following areas: family relationships, sexual or marital relations, work, social contacts, stigma and recreation. A composite score was obtained to indicate the level of social disability for each case.

As presented in Table 9.5, close to one-half of the members of the cohort (45.8%) did not show any disability or were affected to only a minimal degree. Cases with no disability or with only minimal or mild disturbances together amounted to three-fourths of the cohort while only two cases showed severe disability.

Violence and Suicide

No member of the cohort was involved in assaults or violent actions at any time during the last 2 years or 10 years of the follow-up period. One suicide attempt was registered during the last 2 years, and two subjects (one woman and one man) had each attempted suicide once within the last 10-year period.

Medications

Almost two-thirds of the cohort (64.8%) never received neuroleptics during the last 2 years of follow up, while about one-third of the subjects (31%) took them most of the time. For the last 10-year period, one-half of the cohort was never treated with neuroleptics, 20% were sometimes, and 27.1% most of the time. The situation for our center in this regard appears to be somewhat similar to that of Agra but very different from Prague. The time trend patterns over the last 10-year period show that the use of medications was predominant only during the first third of this part of the follow-up period for 41.7% of the subjects; whereas for one-quarter, medications were not predominant in any portion of the period. For more than one-half of the cohort (24 men, 14 women) (52.8%), treatment was received for 10% of the period or less, and only 10 subjects (five men, five women) (13.9%) remained under treatment for more than 75% of the follow-up period.

TABLE 9.5 Social Disability Observed at the 26-Year Follow-Up in Members of the Live Cohort According to Sex

Social Disability	*Male*	*Female*	*N*	*Pct.*
None or Minimal	18	15	33	45.8
Mild	12	8	20	27.8
Moderate	7	10	17	23.6
Severe	0	2	2	2.8
Total	37	35	72	100

Hospitalization

The time spent in the hospital by members of the live cohort during the last 2 years of follow-up was minimal. Only two subjects had been hospitalized, for a short time, during this period. Over the last 10 years, only about one-fifth of the cohort (20.8%) had spent some time in the hospital. The dominant trend observed was for hospitalizations to be prominent during the first third. In general, the number of hospitalizations was small and the duration was short: Eight subjects (11.1%) were never hospitalized, 60% of the cohort spent less than 1% of the follow-up time in the hospital, and less than one-tenth of the cohort was hospitalized for more than 2% of the follow-up time. The median number of days of hospitalization was 45.5 with a range of 0 to 366, the latter being an exceptional case, followed by the next highest with 262 days. Over 90% of the subjects spent a total period of less than six months hospitalized. The median number of hospitalizations was two, with a range of 0 to 11 for the entire period.

Deceased Subjects

A total of 12 subjects, nine men and three women, died during the 26-year follow-up period. A life table constructed for the cohort was compared with the survival rate observed for the population of Cali, with an average life expectancy at birth of 70 years, and no significant differences were detected. A woman, aged 37 years, committed suicide by hanging, and a man was killed by gunshot at the age of 21. For eight subjects, the cause of death was not established with certainty and so was registered as natural. For two others, there were discrepant versions among the informants and the true cause could not be determined. Mental condition at the time of death was reported to be good for six subjects; four were in the midst of a psychotic episode; and no information was available for the remaining two.

DISCUSSION

Assessing the Representativeness of the Alive Cohort

As mentioned previously, case-finding and retrieval were very difficult; thanks to the resourcefulness and stamina of two auxiliary nurses, the fieldwork turned out successfully. A comparison of the basic sociodemographic characteristics of the retrieved subjects with those lost to follow-up did not reveal any statistically significant differences between the two groups, although those lost to follow-up were older and more likely to be women—both of which are associated with better outcome in the literature.

Interestingly, an analysis of the changes in sociodemographic characteristics observed in the live cohort over the follow-up period showed favorable changes in marital status, educational level, and level of occupation. There was no evidence of deterioration in socioeconomic condition and positive characteristics were assessed in higher proportions than at the 10-year follow-up. The very low rate of persons refusing to be evaluated suggests the presence of a good working relationship between the subjects and the health personnel.

Interpreting the Status of Alive Subjects at Follow-Up

In the Cali cohort, the proportion of subjects who showed clinical and social recovery is similar to that mentioned in contemporary studies (McGlashan, 1988; Hegarty, Baldessarini, Tohen, Waternaux, and Oepen, 1994). A meta-analysis of more than 300 cohorts of patients diagnosed as schizophrenic found an average of about 40% "improvement" reported in follow-up studies of up to 10 years conducted during the present century (Hegarty et al., 1994). In our cohort, the worst clinical condition was observed around the 10th year of follow-up, and from then on a process of recovery was generally observed. This situation may correspond to the "positive turn observed to occur at advanced stages of the course of illness" (Huber, Gross, Schutler, and Linz, 1980).

There is a discrepancy between the finding that about one-third of the subjects were free from psychotic symptoms according to the GAF-S, whereas more than half of them (56.9%) were found to be "recovered" according to Bleuler's scale. The most plausible explanation may be that the Bleuler criteria for recovery are more permissive, allowing for inclusion in this category of probands in whom "a thorough medical examination uncovered some residues of delusional ideas [and] faulty perception relative to their former psychosis" (Bleuler, 1978). And a GAF-S cutoff of >60 (some mild symptoms) yields 50.7%, approximating the Bleuler rating.

Lack of correspondence between clinical and social evaluations of outcome is a frequent finding in long-term studies. The term *social recovery* is often used as a criterion for improvement in cases where no discernible changes in symptomatology could be observed. Most subjects in the Cali live cohort showed satisfactory levels of social functioning, even though some of them presented severe concomitant clinical symptoms. Identical findings were made at the 2-, 5-, and 10-year follow-up studies (WHO, 1979; León, 1989; Leff, Sartorius, and Jablensky, 1992). It is suggestive that a good outcome even in the presence of clinical disorder may be related to public attitudes toward mental patients, which in Cali appear to be more tolerant and benevolent than those observed in other cultures (Micklin and León, 1972). Possibly related, too, is the influence of a tolerant attitude on the part of relatives for accepting patients as bona fide members of the family who are entitled to share their living arrangements. This, in turn, may be reinforced by the traditional extended family pattern that still seems prevalent in our local culture.

The question of why schizophrenia shows significantly higher proportions of recovery in developing countries as compared with industrialized countries remains unresolved. The Cali cohort seemed to occupy an intermediate position between the two types of countries as observed in the 2- and 5-year follow-up of the IPSS.

For this present 26-year follow-up, there is no assurance that results may be comparable to those of Agra and Prague because of the differences in diagnostic composition and percentage successfully followed of the retrieved samples. For this reason, any attempt at comparison should be made with extreme caution.

CONCLUSIONS

On the basis of findings presented here, we draw the following interim conclusions: Among the most significant aspects of this follow-up is the fact that on four different occasions, we were able to interview and assess the subjects in the cohort. The proportion of cases assessed at the end of each follow-up period (85, 84, 84, and 82%, respectively) compares favorably to those of several other countries that participated in the IPSS 2- and 5-year follow-ups and in other long-term studies. In spite of the inherent difficulties in studies of this type, it has been demonstrated that a long-term follow-up study *can* be performed in a developing country with a high proportion of retrieved cases and full cooperation from subjects and their relatives. At the end of the 26-year period, one-half of the cohort showed a disappearance or substantial diminution of symptoms: At least half had a favorable clinical outcome; only 22% were found to be clinically disabled. Throughout the period, the stability of the clinical forms or subtypes of schizophrenia was very low: Only the paranoid type remained stable. Because of the lack of a classification system that can offer better longitudinal stability, it is more suitable to describe the predominant clinical picture observed throughout the follow-up period. Almost three-fourths of the cohort had a favorable social outcome, and only 8% were found to be severely disturbed. Close to two-thirds of the cohort were working full-time and in most cases the quality of their work was rated as good or very good. The proportion of cases with severe disorder did not increase after the first decade of the follow-up period. In most cases, the proportion of the follow-up period spent in overt psychosis or in the hospital is quite small. More than half of the cases did not require any psychiatric treatment during the second decade or the last 6 years of the observation period.

The results presented in this report point to a favorable evolution of the clinical and social conditions of people with a diagnosis of schizophrenia over a long period. The very low level of social disability is particularly noteworthy, as well as the short duration and the small number of hospitalizations as well as the sporadic use of treatment. Such evidence suggests the existence of a disease process less malignant than the one usually attributed to schizophrenia. Similar findings in several contemporary studies indicate the need for a change of paradigm—namely, the notion that schizophrenia inevitably evolves toward chronicity and deterioration should definitely be eradicated.

Acknowledgments Members of the 26-Year Follow-up Study on the Course and Outcome of Schizophrenia are: Professor Carlos A. León, M.D., M.S.—Director; Ms. Agatha León, M.P.H., Psychologist—Project Coordinator, Research Associate; Ms. Martha Maritza Salgado, Psychologist—Research Assistant; and Ms. Laura Abadía—Secretary. Other personnel, including physicians and auxiliary nurses, were hired on a contractual basis. The study was funded by two local agencies: the Margarita de Pacini—Fundación para la Educación Superior (FES) and Fondo Colombiano para la Investigación Científica (COLCIENCIAS).

References

Argandoña, M., & Kiev, A. (1972), *Mental Health in the Developing World: A Case Study in Latin America.* New York: Free Press.

Bartko, J. J., Strauss, J., & Carpenter, W. (1980), *Selecting Techniques for Evaluating the Reliability of Psychiatric Data, in Multivariate Statistic Methodologies Used in the I.P.S.S. Series GN: Methodology.* Rockville, MD: U.S. Department of Health and Human Services.

Bleuler, M. (1978), *The Schizophrenic Disorders—Long-Term Patient and Family Studies.* New Haven, CT: Yale University Press.

Climent, C., & de Arango, M. V. (1980), Strategies for extending mental health services to developing countries. I. Description of project. *Acta Psiquiát. Psicol. Amér. Lat.*, 26:48–53. (In Spanish)

——, ——Plutchik, R., & León, C. (1978), Development of an alternative, efficient, low-cost mental health delivery system in Cali, Colombia. Part I. The auxiliary nurse. *Soc. Psychiatry*, 13:29–35.

Departamento Administrativo Nacional de Estadística (1995), *Census of Population and Dwellings in Colombia 1993 (Preliminary Population Projections).* Bogotá: DANE. (In Spanish)

González Posso, C., Agudelo Calderón, C. A., Mendoza Villalobos, E., & Cuadros Ferré, M. I., (1991), *Health in Light of Mental Health: The National Plan.* Bogotá: División Comportamiento Humano, Ministerio de Salud. (In Spanish)

Guzmán Cuevas, M., Albarez Giraldo, E., Vesga Sánchez, A., & Ruíz Echeverry, P. (1995), *The New System of Social Security in Health.* Santiago de Cali, Colombia: Secretaría de Salud Pública Municipal. (In Spanish)

Harding, T. W., de Arango, M. V., Baltazar, J., Climent, C. E., Ibrahim, H. H. A., Ladrido-Ignacio, L., Srinivasa Murthy, R., & Wig, N. N. (1980), Mental disorders in primary health care: A study of their frequency and diagnosis in four developing countries. *Psycholog. Med.*, 10:231–241.

Hegarty, J. D., Baldessarini, R. J., Tohen, M., Waternaux, M., & Oepen, G. (1994), One hundred years of schizophrenia: A meta-analysis of the outcome literature. *Amer. J. Psychiatry*, 151:1409–1415.

Huber, G., Gross, G., Schutler, R., & Linz, M. (1980), Longitudinal studies of schizophrenic patients. *Schizophr. Bull.*, 8:591–605.

Jablensky, A., Sartorius, N., Ernberg, G., Anker, M., Korten, A., Cooper, J. E., Day, R., & Bertelsen, A. (1992), Schizophrenia: Manifestations, incidence and course in different cultures. A World Health Organization ten-country-study. *Psycholog. Med.*, 20(Monogr. Suppl.): 1–97.

Langner, T. S. (1962), A twenty-two item screening score of psychiatric impairment. *J. Health Soc. Behav.*, 3: 269–276.

Leff, J., Sartorius, N., & Jablensky, A. (1992), The international pilot study of schizophrenia: Five-year follow-up findings. *Psycholog. Med.*, 22:131–145.

León, C. A. (1967), Prevalence of mental disorders in an urban sector of Cali. *Rev. Colombiana de Psiquiatía*, 2:24–36. (In Spanish)

——(1970), The devil and the almanac (Changes in the content of psychopathological productions in relation to the passing of time). *Acta Psiquiát. Psicol. Amér. Lat.*, 16:105–116. (In Spanish)

——(1973), Social and community psychiatry. *Rev. deNeuropsiquiatría*, 36:81–91.

——(1977), Social psychiatry in Colombia. In: *Enciclopedia de Psiquiatría*, ed. R. J. Usandivaras, Buenos Aires: El Ateneo. (In Spanish)

——(1979), The evolution of the teaching of psychiatry in Cali. In: *Salud I: Reseña Histórica*. Cali, Colombia: División de Salud, Universidad del Valle, pp. 10–11. (In Spanish)

——(1981), "Barefoot" researchers: The potential role of rural students as mental health promoters performing prevalence surveys. *Bull. Pan Amer. Health Organ.*, 15: 362–369.

——(1986), Clinical course and evolution of schizophrenia in Cali, Colombia: A 10-year follow-up study. *Acta Psiquiát. Psicol. Amér. Lat.*, 32:95–136. (In Spanish)

——(1989), Clinical course and outcome of schizophrenia in Cali, Colombia. A 10-year follow-up study. *J. Nerv. & Ment. Dis.*, 177:593–606.

——(1992a), The schizophrenic and his (her) disorder: Subjective notions about the psychotic process. *Salud Mental*, 15:24–34. (In Spanish)

——(1992b), Drugs and violence in Colombia. In: *Social Psychiatry and World Accords*, ed. J. H. Masserman & C. McGuire-Masserman. Chicago: Masserman Foundation, pp. 77–83.

——Alvarez, O. (1972), Readmissions to the San Isidro Psychiatric Hospital: A 3-year follow-up study of patients hospitalized 1956–1964. *Rev. Colombiana de Psiquiatría*, 2:665–693. (In Spanish)

——Climent, C. E. (1968), An evaluation of instruments used to study the prevalence of mental disorders (Methodological trial in a semi-rural population). In: *Psiquiatría en la América Latina*. Bogotá: Editorial Tercer Mundo, pp. 208–237. (In Spanish)

——López, A. (1966), Follow-up of a sample of patients hospitalized at the San Isidro Psychiatric Hospital during the 10-year period 1956–1965. Unpublished.

——Micklin, M. (1971), Community opinions of mental illness and its treatment in Cali, Colombia. *Acta Psiquiát. Psicol. Amér. Lat.*, 17:385–394. (In Spanish)

López-Michelsen, A. (1987), *El Tiempo* (Bogotá), February 14. (In Spanish)

McGlashan, T. H. (1988), A selective review of recent North American long-term follow-up studies of schizophrenia. *Schizophr. Bull.*, 14:515–542.

Micklin, M., & León, C. A. (1972), Rejection of the mentally ill in a South American city: A comparative analysis. *Acta Psiquiát. Psicol. Amér. Lat.*, 18:321–329. (In Spanish)

——, ——(1978), Life change and psychiatric disturbance in a South American city: The effects of geographic and social mobility. *J. Health. Soc. Behav.*, 19:92–107.

Olivares-Mora, A. V. (1974), Schematic information on the outline of the mental health program in Colombia. Unpublished. (In Spanish)

Von Zerssen, D., León, C. A., Moller, H. J., Wittchen, H. U., Pfister, H., & Sartorius, N. (1990), Care strategies for schizophrenia patients in a transcultural comparison. *Compreh. Psychiatry*, 31:398–408.

World Health Organization (1973), *The International Pilot Study of Schizophrenia*. Geneva: World Health Organization.

——(1979), *Schizophrenia. An International Follow-Up Study*. New York: Wiley.

——(1994), *The ICD-10 Classification of Mental and Behavioral Disorders: Conversion Tables between ICD-8, ICD-9, and ICD-10*. Revision 1. (WHO/MNH/92.16.Rev.1). Geneva: World Health Organization.

Zambrano, E. (1967), Statistical analysis of the population of the San Isidro Psychiatric Hospital, *Rev. Colombiana de Psiquiatría*, 2:12–23.

Chapter 10

IPSS: Prague, Czech Republic

Ctirad Skoda, Pavel Baudis, and Eva Dragomirecká

CULTURAL CONTEXT

In the fifth and sixth centuries, the Slavs migrated into Prague, founding Prague Castle, which became a cultural and spiritual center. Prague was the capital of Bohemia from the ninth century on. In the 14th century under King Charles IV, it became the capital of the "Holy Empire of the German Nation," boasting the first university center in Europe (founded in 1348), and ranking as its third largest city after Constantinople and Rome. With the overthrow of the Austro-Hungarian Empire in 1918, Prague became the capital of Czechoslovakia. Since 1900, its population has increased fourfold. By 1967, the start of the IPSS, Prague had 1,102,060 inhabitants.

Prior to 1944, the German-speaking minority had great influence; however, following World War II, most returned to Germany, and the bilingual tradition was broken. Czech and Slovak, very similar at the dialect level, became the official languages. Members of both nationalities understand each other well, with the exception of some differences in technical or scientific vocabularies. In 1968, the armies of the Soviet Union and other Warsaw Pact countries invaded Czechoslovakia to counteract the Prague Spring Movement for freedom; the latter had been mounted to correct the totalitarian style of political and economic life imported from the U.S.S.R after the February 1948 coup by the Communist Party. Most people's memories of the communist period are dominated by images of waiting—to buy necessities and other goods, to get a phone, to get approval to buy a car, to get a child admitted to an institution of higher learning, to get bank approval to buy a small amount of foreign currency (which permitted one to apply, once in three years, for special permission, necessary even with a valid passport, to travel to a country west of the Iron Curtain).

Prague's participation in the IPSS began during the period of Soviet-induced "normalization" and participation in the DOSMeD started 10 years later (1978). Preparations for the ISoS were launched just after the November 1989 Velvet Revolution, when Soviet influence totally broke down and the 40-year dictatorship ended. Czechoslovakia then began the profound process of returning to the Western type of democracy that had been well established between the two world wars. Since 1989, the government has maintained a free market policy, a low unemployment rate, a relatively stable inflation rate (<10%), a balanced state budget, a growing gross national product, and rising reserves of foreign currency. The income range is far more differentiated when compared with the early 1980s. Economic activities, formerly totally run by the state, have steadily increased in the private sector, particularly in electrically powered machines (e.g., trams) and machine tool manufacturing, food processing, construction, and tourism. Commodities became available (no waiting for cars), as did foreign currency and visa-free travel to all European and most other countries. However, apartments are still scarce, and there are social changes brought about by previously unknown sources of stress and social pathology (unemployment, homelessness, and drugs).

In 1993, after 75 years of coexistence, Czechoslovakia became two independent states: in the west, the Czech Republic, comprising about two-thirds of its area and population, and in the east, the Slovak Republic. Prague remained the capital of the Czech Republic, and the Czech language became the only official language. The literacy level for the Czech Republic is 99%. Illiteracy, functional literacy, or language difficulties do appear among the Gypsy minority, which has problems with assimilation because of its cultural and linguistic differences and because some members live somewhat on the edges of society.

No Gypsies were included in ISoS. The reevaluations of both Prague ISoS subsamples (IPSS and DOSMeD) were conducted in the Czech language area in patients of Czech nationality. It is important to understand that the study took place during a period characterized by a return to Western-style democracy with freedom of speech based on a Bill of Human Rights; deep criticism of past deployment of national wealth, of past exploitation of national resources, and of pollution from power plants; a change from the social security model to individual responsibility for socioeconomic status; and negative attitudes toward involuntary inpatient treatment in mental hospitals nurtured by reports of the abuse of psychiatry in the former Soviet Union.

Migration

In 1989, the Czech Republic changed from a country from which people emigrated for political or economic reasons to a country traversed by people from the Balkans and other parts of Eastern Europe (Ukraine, Russia), China, Taiwan, and Vietnam on the way to the Federal Republic of Germany, mostly for economic reasons. Recently, there have been temporary residents from the United States and Canada (English language teachers, business people, journalists) and an annual return of about 35,000 former emigrants.

Employment

Prior to 1989, the right to work was secured by law, and it was not legally possible to be formally unemployed (except for women who were engaged in household activities). A large proportion of women worked in the health care, education, and business sectors. Restricted immigration to Prague, mostly because of the lack of housing, resulted in the lowest unemployment rate in the country (about 1% for both men and women). Since 1989, there has been a free employment market. The shadow economy disappeared as imported goods became available to all who could pay. Industrial, commercial, and administrative structures changed, and many people took new jobs. Job prerequisites no longer included political standing; for example, Communist Party membership, personal political views, or class of origin. Until 1990, time pressure on people was minimal, an attitude that is gradually changing, especially in those with private sector jobs. Unions have lost much of their former influence, and with the new *Code of Work* are unable to prevent employers from getting rid of ineffective employees.

Population

The population is largely homogeneous, with Czech nationality prevailing; however, there are small groups of Gypsies and foreigners whose stay is temporary. Leaders are usually drawn from the Czech nationality. People who profess no religious faith prevail, followed by Catholics and Protestants. About 30% of the population (mostly Catholics) believes in life after death. The population of Prague is older than the rest of the Czech Republic.

From 1995, the number of deaths exceeded the number of births. In the last 3 years, life expectation at birth reversed its long-term decline and increased. With forecasts of a steadily increasing proportion of retired persons, the Social Security Act is gradually raising the retirement age. In the last few years, previously high divorce and abortion rates have decreased. Criminality has increased. Average alcohol consumption has risen. The suicide death rates in the Czech Republic have slowly declined from a peak of 28.8 per 100,000 inhabitants in 1970 to 16.8 in 1995.

Prague has well-preserved historic districts, residential neighborhoods, and industrial districts. The typical household is two parents employed full-time and two children. Most families live on the outskirts in huge tenement house districts with minimal access to shopping, in apartments won after as many as 15 years on a waiting list. Adults commute to distant jobs by public transport (subway, bus, tram), leaving little time for children. The easiest way to spend free time is watching TV, as cultural opportunities are concentrated in the city center. Because of housing shortages, young people typically live longer with their parents than is usual in Western countries. On Fridays, families with a weekend or country house leave town.

Women's Role in Society

Legally, women are emancipated. No significant feminist movement existed in Czechoslovakia or exists in the Czech Republic. On average, however, working women hold inferior positions and earn less than men. Many must work because their husband's low income is insufficient to the family's needs. The study period was characterized by high employment rates for women and restricted availability of the newest medications, making long-term inpatient treatment of a mentally disturbed family member a necessity.

Attitude Toward Severe Psychiatric Disorder

From 1989, health care policy and the organization of services have been objects of stormy debates and often of political controversy. Most of the population views severe mental disorder as a result of external (psychogenous) factors, and as related to criminality, unpredictable behavior, violence, and aggression. The lay view is that schizophrenia is an incurable, progressive disease. In spite of open discussions, public interest, and education, public attitudes toward mentally ill persons are still conservative and negative. Recently, however, public pressure in favor of involuntary psychiatric treatment has lessened, and negative attitudes seem to be gradually changing. Patient advocacy organizations and societies providing social support to mentally ill and substance dependent persons have been established. In cases of severe mental disorder, relatives generally still ask for inpatient treatment, during which time they usually visit the patient. Some take care of their mentally ill relatives, but their motivation to do so weakens after 3 to 5 years of illness.

Impact of Mental Health Issues on Society

Daily average of sick leave (DASL) per insured population units, an indicator of the burden severe mental disorder imposes on society, is calculated on the basis of a random selection of 20% of all sick-leave forms completed by any physician in the country. (Physicians are required to certify short-term incapacity for work.) The time series for the Czech Republic (1968 to 1995) shows DASL rates in females to be twice those of males and to be classified mostly as neuroses. Between 1971 and 1989, DASL dropped from 1.8 to 1.1 per 1,000 insured females and increased in 1995 to 1.35. In males, a reduction in the DASL's classified with neuroses was compensated for by an increase in psychoactive substance abuse.

The role of the general practitioner was transformed from family doctor to an overworked dispatcher to various specialists; examinations averaged 5 minutes per patient contact. Hidden psychiatric morbidity in patients contacting general practitioners was noted (Skoda, 1978a, 1985). Surveys done in the United Kingdom (Shepherd, Cooper, Brown, and Kalton, 1966; Clare and Lader, 1982) were repeated in one region of Czechoslovakia of about 1 million inhabitants, and their results showed that about one-fourth of a general practitioner's clients have hidden psychiatric morbidity (Baudis, Mudra, Smutna, and Skoda, 1986).

THE MENTAL HEALTH SYSTEM

From 1950 to 1990, mental health care consisted chiefly of long-term inpatient treatment in large mental hospitals, fully state financed and managed. No private, self-help, or charitable organizations provided service. Beginning in 1992, officials sought to evolve from a paternalistic state administrative model to an efficient and economically feasible modern model with adequate state, private, and nonprofit voluntary and charity-based service providers. Legislative initiatives on health care included the creation of health insurance agencies, bills of rights for patients, limits on court-ordered "protective treatment," privatization of health care (especially outpatient services), and health care financing. With few exceptions, all health care including mental health services is still provided without direct payment by the patient. From 1988, the proportion of newly diagnosed cases with mental disturbance receiving benefits increased dramatically, and in 1994 reached 81 per 100,000 insured population.

Although most outpatient health care services financed by health insurance agencies were privatized, most inpatient care was not. Gradually, specialized departments of psychiatry in general hospitals began offering outpatient treatment. The number of psychiatrists rose from 0.87 per 100,000 population in 1960 to 4.29 per 100,000 by 1995. Nonstate institutions provide care for persons dependent on psychoactive substances, for persons severely mentally impaired, for mentally ill children, for the aged, and for the incurably ill (hospices). For long-term mentally ill patients, there are sheltered workplaces, sheltered living, clubs, and rehabilitation units. Complementary services include partial hospitalization, emergency and crisis intervention, child and adolescent services, matrimonial counseling, and substance abuse guidance/treatment. Some chronic mental disorders (mental retardation, brain disorders in old age, long-term psychotics) are the interest of social welfare and the newly organized voluntary and charitable organizations. The spectrum of care has widened to include psychological, social, and nonmedical alternatives; diagnostic and therapeutic quality has increased; and the patient-doctor relationship has improved. On the other hand, organizational control has decreased, several systems of preventive medicine (inoculation, active aftercare) are limited, and there has been a dramatic rise in health care expenditures from 4% of gross national product in 1970 to 7% at present. As of time of ISoS follow-up, there are 270 inhabitants per physician, about 1250 qualified psychiatrists, and a dearth of qualified nurses, especially in inpatient care.

In psychiatry, these changes were reflected in a lower average number of inpatients, in decreases in beds, bed utilization, and involuntary admissions, in a shortened average duration of stay, and in a reduction of involuntary alcoholic treatment. The period 1968 to 1993 showed a decrease in the proportion of the population staying in a psychiatric bed one year or longer, a lower proportion of cases of schizophrenia, and a higher proportion with brain disorder, mental retardation, and alcohol abuse. During the period covered by ISoS, the availability of psychiatric beds in Prague surpassed the average for the Czech Republic by about 45.1% in 1960 and by 27.5% in 1995; outpatient services in Prague, expressed by the rate of psychiatrists per 100,000 population, were two times higher in 1960 and 2.42 times higher in 1995.

Settings and Services Available in the Catchment Area

From 1968 to 1969 and 1978 to 1979, defined catchment areas were strictly adhered to, a restriction which ceased after November 1989. In general, psychiatric beds in general hospitals served only children and adolescents. For adults, only beds in teaching (university) hospitals were available, with access limited by teaching and research interests. Aging of the population contributed to the lack of beds for long-term treatment of brain disorders in the elderly. For discharged patients, owing in part to the severe housing shortage, alternatives other than their own or relatives' homes are still practically nonexistent (e.g., in the mid-1990s and only in the 7th and 8th Prague districts, only two apartments were adapted to posthospital residences for patients). Thanks to well-staffed departments of psychiatry that operate outpatient (polyclinical) health services, most of the supervision is provided by social workers, or home visits are made by general practitioners or psychiatrists. Data about the amount of such care are scarce.

Extramural (transition) services (such as day treatment) exist only sporadically, and mostly for those with neuroses and substance abuse problems. In the past, administrative or financial barriers made practically nonexistent or available only for a short duration such resources as emergency, crisis intervention, and walk-in services, substance abuse guidance and treatment, resocialization, vocational training or industrial rehabilitation units, or halfway houses. Only after 1989 were these barriers gradually removed; however, they still remain the preserve of individual specialists, partly supported by grants from local agencies and from abroad.

PSYCHIATRIC EPIDEMIOLOGY SINCE IPSS

At the founding of the Psychiatric Research Institute (PRI) in 1961, an Epidemiology Unit was headed by E. Ivanys. Together with J. Vana, he established and managed the Psychiatric Information System (PIS) covering all psychiatric beds in Czechoslovakia, and from 1963, the activities of outpatient departments of psychiatry. Data on every admission and discharge are collected and processed at the Institute of Health Information and Statistics (IHIS) in Prague, which publishes detailed analyses in a yearbook, *Psychiatric Care*. Among countries of the former Soviet bloc, the Czechoslovak PIS and its still complete yearbook series remain quite unique. From this database, epidemiological and service research studies covering a variety of topics were published—inpatient treatment incidence (Skoda, 1987a,b), sick-leave rates (Skoda, 1989), and general issues (Skoda, 1990a,b, 1995; Skoda et al., 1995). Patients not discharged within a fiscal year escaped the PIS but were captured by three censuses of the long-stay inpatient treated population in 1968 (Ivanys and Schwarzová, 1973), 1983, and 1993 (Skoda and Baudis, 1994). A substantial decrease in the long-stay population and changes in its diagnostic structure, treatment, and rehabilitation needs were observed over the past 25 years. A WHO-coordinated study of outpatient psychiatric morbidity pointed out problems in PIS methodology for outpatient services (Vana, 1979). Studies undertaken by the PRI Department of Social Psychiatry, established in December 1967 and headed by Dr. C. Skoda (1984, 1988), were presented at annual meetings of the Social Psychiatry Section of the Czechoslovak Psychiatric Association and published in Proceedings.

A time series of suicide rates for the Czech Republic since 1895, based on the register of births and deaths, has been continuously published, starting in 1967, by the IHIS in the yearbook *Suicides*; these were augmented by analyses of the circumstances of suicides and suicide attempts collected on special forms required by district departments of psychiatry.

The first survey of administrative psychiatric morbidity was done in the 8th Prague district. Based on an at-risk population of 80,000, estimates of average (1956–1960) treated prevalence rates per 1000 inhabitants were established (Ivanys, Drdková, and Vana, 1964): 38.03 for all mental disorders, 6.06 for all psychoses, 1.65 for schizophrenia, and 9.05 for alcohol abuse. The yearly incidence rates per 1000 inhabitants (Ivanys, Drdková, and Vana, 1965) were: 9.58 for all disorders, 1.34 for all psychoses (0.26 for schizophrenia and 0.16 for affective prognosis). The experiences were also analyzed from the methodological (Ivanys and Vana, 1965) and ecological points of view (Vana and Ivanys, 1969). The predictors of newly assigned rent subsidies awarded because of mental disorder were studied using a 33-month prospective follow-up of 381 patients (Baudis, Skoda, Vrbik, and Tomásek, 1981).

Using a procedure for estimating the size of a population from a single sample (Laska, Meisner, and Siegel, 1988), which was validated on a Czech population (Skoda, 1993), estimates of hidden psychiatric morbidity in several nonpsychiatric outpatient departments were calculated. Screening instruments that had previously been validated on teaching samples, for health, depression, schizophrenia, alcohol dependence, and neurosis were used (Skoda, 1992, 1994).

Three important contributions to service research were realized. First, periods of closed- and open-door policy in one mental hospital were compared and evaluated as to risks and advantages (Skoda, 1968). Second, neurotic patients were randomly assigned to three therapeutic programs (full inpatient treatment, day center, walk-in clinic) and followed up at 1, 2, and 11 years (Bouchal and Skoda, 1991; Skoda, Bouchal, Synkova, Baudis, and Tomásek, 1981). Third, a similar cohort was randomly assigned to short and long versions of the three treatment alternatives and followed up at 1 and 2 years (Skoda, Bouchal, Baudis et al., 1987).

Studies Based on the Prague Subsample of IPSS

Using IPSS samples, rates of inpatient treatment of mania (Matesová, Skoda, Kabesová, and Baudis, 1976; Baudis, Matesová, Skoda, Kabesová, and Skodová, 1977) and affective psychosis (Skoda, Baudis, Matesová, Kabesová, and Skodová, 1977; Skoda and Baudis, 1979) were compared in Prague, Aarhus, and London. Reliability substudies were broadened (Skoda and Husák, 1974; Skoda, Sartorius, Jablensky, and Husák, 1976) and the validity of K. Schneider's first-rank symptoms was evaluated (Skoda, 1978b,c). The diagnostic and prognostic value of PSE and BPRS classifications (both human and computer evaluations) was assessed (Skoda, Janouch, and Husák, 1980), and their differential diagnostic ability to detect microsyndromes was checked on the same sample (Skoda, Dostal, Kabesová, Syrová, and Skodová, 1976).

THE CENTER

Founded in 1961, the Psychiatric Research Institute (renamed the Prague Psychiatric Center [PPC] in 1991) has research, clinical, and informatics divisions. The Clinical Division is at the same time a pregraduate teaching program at Charles University's Third School of Medicine and, since 1991, a WHO Collaborating Center for Research and Training. The PPC Clinical Division has 50 beds and an EEG laboratory. PPC has no catchment area but rather admits patients that meet the criteria of current research designs. Most of its patients, however, are from the younger population of Prague, with few prior hospitalizations and a shorter duration of illness. The Research Division is comprised of Units of Psychometric Studies, Family Research, Biochemistry and Brain Pathophysiology, Clinical Psychopharmacology, Addiction Studies, and Psychiatric Demography. Collaboration in WHO-coordinated projects includes the IPSS, Utilization of Health and Social Services by the Mentally Ill, Cost Effectiveness of Treatment of Depression in Primary Care Settings, and DOSMeD. In 1976, the PPC also participated in biologically and diagnostically oriented WHO-coordinated studies as well as in WHO Training Programs in epidemiology and social psychiatry for developing countries.

The Psychiatric Demography Unit (PDU) consists of one senior scientist (C. Skoda), 0.5 research psychiatrist (P. Baudis), 0.75 research psychologist (E. Dragomirecká), and 1.5 technical assistants (M. Fricová and J. Ezrová). With a grant system, several other professional collaborators were hired and paid from grant budgets. The PDU directed ISoS, but actual data collection was completed by hired collaborators.

After 1989, the expenses of the Clinical Division were covered through Health Insurance Agencies, and research projects became subject to regular grant procedures. This change profoundly affected the usual work style of the PDU. For large-scale longitudinal studies, PDU designed the projects, developed the methodology, and went into the field to gain access to a representative population utilizing facility staff to collect the data. The field collaboration was easier during the period of state-managed health care. Under the new conditions, field collaborating physicians had to be motivated to cooperate by regular payment from the PDU. Lengthy and repetitive grant applications contributed to some timing problems. Delays eroded the willingness of some patients to cooperate, partly because their attitudes toward psychiatry and psychiatric research had changed.

METHODS USED IN THE SITE

Defining the ISoS Cohort

Between 1968 and 1969, the Prague Field Research Center (FRC), following the WHO inclusion and exclusion criteria, enrolled 125 patients from the mental hospital in the Prague-8 catchment area in the WHO International Pilot Study of Schizophrenia (IPSS). One hundred and eight patients were reexamined at 5-year follow-up and predictors of course and outcome of the disorder were analyzed (Skoda, Kabesová, and Tomásek, 1982, 1984).

From August 1978 to August 1980, 118 patients entered the study, and 107 were finally included into the WHO-coordinated study of Determinants of Outcome of Severe Mental Disorders (DOSMeD). As a treated incidence sample, however, the representativeness of the Prague cohort is questionable. First, a "leakage" study undertaken shortly after subject enlistment ended (Jablensky et al., 1992) determined that substantial numbers of first-onset psychosis (an estimated 257 possibly eligible cases) in the designated catchment area had been missed by the data collection methods used. Second, far from being assigned to "standard treatment," the greater part of the Prague DOSMeD cohort was followed by research clinicians at the PRI, which is a much better equipped facility than the average mental health care providers in the area.

In 1992, the last phase of preparations started for a WHO-coordinated international follow-up of both the IPSS, 25 years after inclusion, and DOSMeD, 15 years after inclusion. At the same time, the design and methodology of the unique, worldwide, long-term study of course and outcome of schizophrenia (ISoS) underwent final field testing (Sartorius, Gulbinat, Harrison, Laska, and Siegel, 1996).

Case-Finding

Present address and, if appropriate, year of death were retrieved from the Central Population Register (CPR) using the person's unique personal identification number. Most persons who were not found were later determined to have emigrated. An introductory letter was sent to all IPSS and DOSMeD subjects explaining the purpose of the follow-up and asking for cooperation. The psychiatrists and both social workers who participated in initial phases of the earlier studies were hired as external members of the research team in the hope that they had continued a therapeutic relationship with the subjects. Social workers, especially, were invaluable in enlisting the cooperation of the patients and their families and were instrumental in the collection of additional information from the very many sources available. Some of the subjects were still in Prague as psychiatric outpatients or in temporary inpatient care, which greatly enhanced the possibility of contact and cooperation. For many subjects, complete documentation of all hospitalizations was available either from the PPC (a computerized register of all 1961 to 1990 hospitalizations), from Prague-8 Mental Hospital, or from Department of Psychiatry archives.

Toward the end of 1994, we decided to pay the patients to participate. Despite the small amount of money offered and much to our surprise, they came. Even in the last weeks of data collection, subjects who had been considered "lost" appeared. The social worker was able to visit homes and this, too, brought other "lost" souls to be interviewed. The last minute receipt of additional funds enabled us to determine that a few subjects officially considered dead were in reality alive and could be reexamined.

Data-Gathering Procedures

An invitation letter suggesting a date and time for an interview (with instructions on how to change the appointment) was sent to each subject. By the time the subject arrived, all information available (previous contacts with the Center, PCP computerized case histories, IPSS, and DOSMeD rating sheets, and contacts with Mental Hospital Prague-8 or the University Department of Psychiatry) had been gathered by the social worker; then the subject was interviewed by the research psychiatrist. The already existing Czech version of the PSE 9th edition was complemented by Czech versions of all ISoS instruments, developed by Drs. Eva Dragomirecká and Ctirad Skoda. The resulting Czech coding sheets were then keyed by a technical assistant to the ISoS Epi Info database.

Tracing both Prague Subsamples

No problems were encountered in tracing the IPSS subsample that was on our computer. Our archives from the DOSMeD sub-study, however, were rather rudimentary and were only partly located. This research started with a full complement of 118 patients described in the Clinical Division archives, all of whom are included in the ISoS analysis (of these, six had not passed the original DOSMeD screening).

STUDY RESULTS

Baseline and Short-Term Follow-Up

Gender and Age Distribution

At inclusion, there was a preponderance of females in both Prague subsamples. Noted at the time of the short-term follow-up, these proportions were found to correspond to the population from which the subsamples were drawn. In this respect, the IPSS subsamples from Prague, Cali, Moscow, and Washington, DC, contrasted with those from Agra and London, where men prevailed. Male–female ratios in alive, dead, and lost were not significantly different from chance. Nonsignificantly, a higher proportion of women died than were traced alive or lost. With respect to age, the DOSMeD subsample is more skewed to younger subjects than the IPSS subsamples. This, together with the approximate 10 years difference between the starts of the substudies, explains many of the differences in mortality and somatic comorbidity in long-term follow-up to be commented upon later.

Compared with the rest of the IPSS sample (after subtracting the Prague frequencies from the total), Prague women are significantly overrepresented in original and dead subsamples but not in alive and lost subjects. Compared with the rest of the DOSMeD sample, Prague women are significantly overrepresented in all subgroups (alive, dead, and lost), a fact which may skew Prague in a more favorable direction compared with other ISoS centers.

Mode of Onset and Diagnosis

Fewer Prague IPSS subjects with sudden mode of onset were lost from long-term follow-up. Nonsignificant differences were also found in the Prague DOSMeD subsample, with a higher proportion of subjects with insidious onset in the lost than in the alive group. The Prague subsamples differ slightly from one another in their diagnostic profiles. Cases of mood disorder were included in the IPSS to widen its diagnostic profile; thus, 36 cases of affective psychosis complemented the 50 cases of schizophrenia, 20 cases of schizoaffective psychosis, four cases of acute schizophrenia-like disorder, eight cases of paranoid states, and five reactive psychosis cases. This was not the situation in the DOSMeD cohort, the diagnostic composition of which is more homogeneous and consistent with the final objectives of the ISoS.

Compared with the rest of IPSS, the Prague subsample of alive and dead subjects did not differ in the type of onset; lost subjects, however, are significantly more likely to have slow onset. The three center cohorts did differ at baseline: Agra had 50% slow onset, Cali had 90%, and Prague had 82%. The alive, dead, and lost subjects of the Prague DOSMeD cohort did not significantly differ from the DOSMeD sample on type of onset. Compared with the rest of the IPSS sample, there was a lower proportion of schizophrenic subjects in the original, alive, dead subjects of the Prague subsample. Only in the dead subjects of the Prague DOSMeD subsample was there a significantly lower proportion of schizophrenic subjects.

Pattern of Course at Early Follow-Up

There were no differences in short-term pattern of course in Prague IPSS and DOSMeD subsamples when comparing the alive versus the dead and lost combined. Prague is similar to the rest of the IPSS alive sample with respect to pattern of course. The DOSMeD alive subsample has a higher proportion of subjects with good outcome (complete remission).

Alive Subjects

In the analyses that follow, outcome in Prague is sometimes compared to other centers in IPSS and in DOSMeD. In these comparisons, figures in the ISoS tables have been adjusted to take this into account.

Symptomatology

Two simple observations—that the proportion of recovered is higher in Prague than in Cali and is similar to Agra, and that the proportion with severe psychopathology was higher in Prague than in the rest of the DOSMeD sample—describe differences that do not reach statistical significance and that cannot be understood without further inquiry into possible hidden factors. For both IPSS and DOSMeD, the proportions rated in Prague as mild or recovered versus severe or moderate on the Bleuler scale do not differ significantly from those seen in the remainder of the respective studies.

Global Assessment of Functioning-Symptoms GAF-S

After combining GAF-S scores 1 to 50 (because of low observed frequencies), we found no difference in distribution of Prague and other IPSS FRCs GAF-S scores, although Prague's proportions were lower. Compared with other DOSMeD centers, the Prague subsample had less severe psychopathology (GAF-S < 51), but more cases in the mid-range (GAF-S scores 51–70).

Living Arrangements

Compared with the totals of the remaining ISoS centers, both Prague subsamples show less favorable outcome where living arrangements are concerned. More IPSS subjects were ever in the hospital or in supervised residence during the last month, the last 2 years, or the entire long-term follow-up period. During the last month of the follow-up, fewer Prague subjects were living with family or friends and more were living alone. Fewer subjects were living independently during the last 2 years, as well as during the last 10 years rated in the IPSS. The Prague DOSMeD subsample distribution of last month's living arrangements did not differ from the rest of the sample combined. However, during the last 2 years a lower proportion of subjects was independent, and a higher proportion was in the hospital or in supervised residence. During the entire period, more subjects spent time in such institutions because of the high employment of women, preference for institutional treatment, and no services for social rehabilitation for most of the study period.

Work

Roughly a third of both DOSMeD and IPSS cohorts worked most of the last 2 years of follow-up, proportions which are slightly lower than their respective subsample totals. (Note that prior to the Velvet Revolution, "unemployment" did not exist in Czechoslovakia.) The distributions of work performance assessments in Prague IPSS and DOSMeD subjects employed full-time or part-time during the past 2 years, as well as subjects doing household work, did not differ significantly from those of the remaining centers in their respective subsamples.

Social Disability

The intensity of disability documented by all available information during the last month was rated using the GAF disability score (GAF-D). When compared with their respective subsamples, the distributions of the GAF-D score categories were in a more favorable (higher) direction for the IPSS sample but showed more psychopathology and disability in the DOSMeD subsample; however, neither difference reached statistical significance.

Assaults and Suicide

In the Prague, subsamples, assaults, and suicide attempts during the last 2 years and from first reexamination were similar to those seen in the total IPSS and DOSMeD samples.

Medications

In both Prague subsamples for both periods assessed (entire period and last 2 years), neuroleptics were used more frequently than in the other centers. This was especially the case in the IPSS subsample where the differences were highly significant.

Deceased Subjects

Losses by death and for other reasons were evidently lower for the DOSMeD group than for the IPSS group as would be expected from the time lag of 10 years between the two long-term follow-ups. The proportion of deaths caused by physical illness is much higher in the IPSS than in the DOSMeD study sample. Another contributing factor is the different diagnostic structure of the subsamples; the IPSS subsample included cases of affective disorders, which represented a high suicide risk—three times as high in the IPSS group as in the DOSMeD sample.

DISCUSSION

Most of the Prague ISoS data evaluation problems may be traced to the fact that the decision to complete a long-term course and follow-up study was made ex post facto. The original age range of both cohorts as set by inclusion criteria was adequate for the hypotheses tested at the time these studies were designed, but were not adequate for long-term observation, for which a larger and (with respect to age) more homogeneous cohort would have been more appropriate. In any event, we confront a troubled sea of descriptive data, predictably roiled by the aging of the sample—consider, for example, the complexity of aging as it influences marital status, living conditions, probability of retiring, impairment of physical health, and death. And our task is first to examine the trifling number of boats unaffected by such storms of time, and then, with deference to local sea traffic safety specificities of participating countries, to estimate international sailing risks.

A word should be said about some novel problems with subject cooperation encountered in the wake of fundamental socioeconomic changes introduced by the Velvet Revolution. During the preparatory phase of the study, a feasibility exercise was conducted, the results of which are available elsewhere (Sartorius et al., 1996). Actual data collection was then postponed several times, pending final development of study instruments, and finally occurred over a year ending March 31, 1995. Because the inclusion period for DOSMeD study had been expanded to 2 years, the Prague FRC had to start 1 year earlier. It was just at this time that the impact of a number of political and socioeconomic changes began to be felt. As described above, the last phase of the study was extremely demanding to the team; many things had changed. Besides the new freedoms the Velvet Revolution had won, strong criticism of the misuse of psychiatry in the former U.S.S.R. appeared in journals and TV, and radiated out to mental health care in general. This had a substantial effect on public opinion and on attitudes toward psychiatry. After a time of heavy discussions, it turned out that the abuses of Soviet psychiatry were not true of Czech psychiatry, but a heightened sensitivity remained in the population and had a visible impact on our ISoS efforts. In addition, the formerly complete police registration of the population lessened gradually, and tracking population movement became more difficult. As the start-up ISoS was delayed, the result of ever more refined versions of comprehensive data collection schedules, searches in the Central Population Register had to be repeated. There were few problems with subjects not yet recovered, as they were highly motivated to cooperate and their documentation (stored in the PCP PC database and readily available from archives) was at our disposal. But there were problems with the now fully recovered, "healthy" subjects, often living with a new partner and unwilling to be examined after many years without any contact with psychiatry. This seems to have caused losses from the more favorable outcome group within our samples.

Thus, a clear difference can be seen in the resistance of the ISoS subjects to participate compared with their former cooperative attitudes. Whereas nearly all IPSS and/or DOSMeD subjects responded positively to the invitation to be reexamined after the 2- and 5-year periods, *barely one-third* did so during the ISoS phase 15 to 26 years later. The remaining two-thirds refused the contact and were unwilling to present information about the further history of their illness, some despite the fact that participation in the 2- or 3-hour reexamination would be quite well paid. Lack of time and financial problems were the usual pretexts, but the real reasons were other: In the past they had been somewhat afraid of the possible consequences of refusing contact because they had to respect catchment area regulations in effect at the time. This was still true for those patients who remained in the care of PPC for a long period and showed good cooperation. Today, for those not in regular contact with the clinic, the old rules and their attendant fears no longer apply. For many of these, fortunately, we were able to include information about the course of illness by consulting records.

Some DOSMeD subjects who were mistakenly excluded many years ago or who did not participate in the 2- or 5-year follow-up (or, in one case, had been thought dead), were finally traced and invited to the reexamination. Interestingly, in several cases, the partner came instead of the subject, fully ready to give necessary information but choosing to protect the subject from a new contact with psychiatry.

Information about long-term course and outcome of the subjects in the study could hardly be wiped out of the minds of the ISoS psychiatrists who were asked to rediagnose the subjects on inclusion with the ICD-10 and DSM-III-R (APA, 1986) criteria. Methodological purists would have required that this be done before any contact with the patient at 15 or 25 years and that only the original documentation be used. These conditions could not be met, and so we must suspect that the rediagnoses have been contaminated by information about the long-term course. (The same information was, of course, used in determining the current ICD-10 and the overall ICD-10 diagnosis after thorough personal reexamination of the samples.)

We have earlier pointed to several drawbacks of a long-term course and outcome study that relies upon already existing samples, not originally designed for a longitudinal study. In a transcultural study investigating variation in socioeconomic policies and health care structures, many insurmountable problems arise owing simply to the age of subjects. In the event, an ambitious study winds up hostage to the ravages of time. We cannot escape the conclusion that less would have been more: About half of the time spent in reexamination could have been saved by omitting schedules that attempted to capture in minute detail what transpired in the 25 times 12 months of the follow-up period. The time saved could have been used to investigate the drop-outs in order to be better able to assess the potential biasing effects of the nonrandom selection processes that resulted in the alive traced sample. These issues have been especially sensitive in our center, burdened by a doubled load of ISoS samples, in a period of transition from the financing of research by the state to the "free market"-based sponsorship of a grant system with its merciless deadlines.

Acknowledgments The ISoS study undertaken by the Field Research Center of Prague was sponsored by grant No. Z-178 of the Ministry of Economic Policy and Development of the Czech Republic (later transferred to the Program for Health and Healthy Nourishment of the Population) and by grant No. 1809-1 of the Internal Grant Agency of the Ministry of Health of the Czech Republic. The last local grant expired at the end of 1994.

References

American Psychiatric Association (1986), *Diagnostic and Statistical Manual of Mental Disorders*, 3rd ed. rev. (DSM-III-R). Washington, DC: American Psychiatric Press.

Baudis, P., Matesová, A., Skoda, C., Kabesová, L., & Skodová, M. (1977), A comparison of first admission mania in Prague, Aarhus and London. A transcultural study linked with the WHO International Pilot Study of Schizophrenia. *Soc. Psychiatry*, 12:185–193.

——Mudra, M., Smutna, R., & Skoda, C. (1986), Psychiatric morbidity in the practice of general practitioners. *Zpravy VUPs*, No. 76. Prague. (In Czech)

——Skoda, C., Vrbik, J., Tomásek, L. (1981); Predictors of psychiatric invalidity. *Rep. Prague Res. Inst.*, 58. (In Czech)

Bouchal, M., & Skoda, C. (1991), Follow-up of neurosis randomly assigned to three alternatives of treatment programs 11 years later. *Psychiatry*, 87(5–6):230–241. (In Czech)

Clare, A. W. & Lader, M. eds. (1982), *Psychiatry and General Practice*. London: Academic Press

Ivanys, E., Drdková S., & Vana, J. (1964), Distribution of psychosis administratively evidenced from part of city population. I. Prevalence., *Csl. Psychiatry*, 60:152–160. (In Czech)

——, ——, ——(1965), Distribution of psychosis administratively evidenced from part of city population. II. Yearly incidence. *Csl. Psychiatry*, 61:47–57.

——Vana, J. (1965), Distribution of psychosis administratively evidenced from part of city population. III. Some methodological experience. *Csl. Psychiatry*, 61: 145–155.

——Schwarzová, H. (1973), Long-stay inpatients treated in psychiatric services in Czechoslovakia. (Final results and source tabulations of a census on June 30, 1968), *Rep. Prague Res. Inst.*, 24. (In Czech)

Jablensky, A., Sartorius, N., Ernberg, G., Anker, M., Korten, A., Cooper, J. E., Day, R., & Bertelsen, A. (1992), Schizophrenia: Manifestations, incidence and course in different cultures. A World Health Organization ten-country study. *Psycholog. Med.*, 20(Monogr. Suppl.): 1–97.

Laska, E. M., Meisner, M., & Siegel, C. (1988), Estimating the size of population from a single sample. *Biometrics*, 44:461–472.

Matesová, A., Skoda, C., Kabesová, M., & Baudis, P. (1976), Comparison of manic episodes incidence in Prague, Aarhus and London. Transcultural study joined to the WHO coordinated IPSS. *Csl. Psychiatry*, 72(3):164–169. (In Czech)

Sartorius, N., Gulbinat, W., Harrison, G., Laska, E., & Siegel, C. (1996), Long-term follow-up of schizophrenia

in 16 countries. *Soc. Psych. Psychiatr. Epidemiol.*, 31: 249–258.
Shepherd, M., Cooper, B., Brown, A. C., & Kalton, G. W. (1966), *Psychiatric Illness in General Practice*. Oxford: Oxford University Press.
Skoda, C. (1968), Statistical findings regarding the Open-Door-System problem. *Schw. Arch. Neurol. Psychiat.*, 102:223–234. (In German)
——(1978a), Differentially diagnostic value of K. Schneider's 1st rank order symptoms. Report from the WHO IPSS. In: *Psychiatry in 1978*, ed. E. Peterová, C. Skoda, & P. Baudis. *Rep. Prague Res. Inst.*, 49. (In Czech)
——(1978b), Psychiatric biometry. A contribution to standardization of documentation and of the diagnostic process in psychiatry. *Rep. Prague Res. Inst.*, 1:1–294. (In Czech)
——(1978c), Psychiatric biometry. A contribution to standardization of documentation and of the diagnostic process in psychiatry. II. *Rep. Prague Res. Inst.*, 2:295–439. (In Czech)
——(1984), Main results of epidemiological and social psychiatry research 1976–1982. XI. *Danube Symposium on Psychiatry, Sofia, October 8–10*, ed. T. Stankusev. Sofia, Bulgaria: Union wissenschaftlich-medizinischer Verbände, pp. 7–8.
——(1985), Psychiatric morbidity in general practitioners' practice. New knowledge. *Prakt. lékar*, 65:605–609.
——(1987a), Share of alcohol and other substance dependence in inpatient treatment incidence in CSR and SSR 1963 to 1985. *Protialkoholicky Obzor*, 22(5):257–264. (In Czech)
——(1987b), Inpatient treatment incidence of alcohol and other substances' dependence and abuse in CSR and SSR 1963 to 1985. *Protialkoholicky Obzor*, 22(4): 193–202. (In Czech)
——(1988), 20 years of social psychiatry in Czechoslovakia. *Csl. Psychiatry*, 84(65):412–419. (In Czech)
——(1989), Share of substance dependence in sick leave days' volume in Czechoslovakia 1960–1986. *Protialkoholicky Obzor*, 24(1):1–10. (In Czech)
——(1990a), Psychiatric assistance in Czechoslovakia. In: *The European Handbook of Psychiatry and Mental Health*, ed. A. Seva. Barcelona, Spain: Antropos, pp. 1911–1918.
——(1990b), Problems of mental health development in Czechoslovakia. In: *Psychiatrie in Wandel. Erfahrungen und Perspektiven in Ost und West*, ed. A. Thom & E. Wulff. Bonn, Germany: Psychiatric Verlag, pp. 430–439. (In German)
——(1992), Hidden psychiatric morbidity in a primary health care setting (GP, gynecology, orthopedic, surgery, internal medicine). In: *Aktuelle Aspekte der Psychiatrie*, ed. G. E. Khune. Jena, Czech Republic: University Verlag. (In German)
——(1993), Checking validity of "Estimating the size of a population from a single sample method." In: *WPA Symposium: Changing the Course and Outcome of Mental Disorders*. Groningen, September 1. *Abstr.*, Groningen, University Hospital.
——(1994), Screening to detect psychiatric morbidity in people with somatic complaints. A substudy of the WHO Project: Utilization of Health and Social Services by the Mentally Ill. In: *7th Symposium: Quality of Life and Disabilities in Mental Disorders. Abstr.*, Vienna: Association of European Psychiatrists.
——(1995), Culture, politics and mental illness in the Czech and Slovak Republics. In: *Handbook of Culture and Mental Illness: An International Perspective*, ed. A. Ihsan. Madison, CT: International Universities Press, pp. 249–268.
——Baudis, P. (1979), Inpatient treatment incidence of affective disorders in Prague, Czech and Slovak republics, and England. *Csl. Psychiatry* 75:346–355. (In Czech)
——, ——(1994), Long-stay inpatients treated in psychiatric facilities of the Czech Republic 1968, 1983, 1993. *Rep. Prague Res. Inst.*, 122:38. (In Czech)
——, ——Csémy, L., Dytrych, Z., Kubicka, L., & Libiger, J. (1995), Czech republic population mental health from the health care consumption point of view yesterday, today and tomorrow. Appendix of a closing report of task No. E. 2499-1 supported by Internal Grant Agency of Czech Ministry of Health. (In Czech)
——, ——Matesová, A., Kabesová, L., & Skodová, M. (1977), Inpatient treatment incidence of depressive episodes in affective psychosis in Prague (1963 to 1972). *Csl. Psychiatry*, 73(5): 321–328. (In Czech)
——Bouchal, M., Baudis, P., Boleloucky, Z., Hlavínová, J., Kulísková, O., Mudra, M., Placherová, A., Skalková, O., Sindelárová, & Tomásek, L. (1987), Effectiveness of short and long versions of three therapeutic programmes for neurotics. Results of three controlled studies. *Scripta Med.*, 60(2):91–96.
——, ——Synkova, J., Baudis, P., & Tomásek, L. (1981). Comparison of three therapeutic programmes. I. Project, method. *Csl. Psychiatry* 77:364–369. (In Czech)
——Dostal, T., Kabesová, L., Syrová, M., & Skodová, M. (1976), Differentially diagnostic ability of microsyndromes. Report from WHO International Pilot Study of Schizophrenia. *Csl. Psychiatry*, 72(2):88–97. (In Czech)
——Husák, T. (1974), Diagnostic agreement of groups of Czech and foreign psychiatrists who are being gradually exposed to an increased amount of information about patients. *Csl. Psychiatry*, 70(4):211–220.
——Janouch, J., & Husák, T. (1980), Prognostic informativeness of the PSE and BPRS: A comparison of their human and computer diagnostic assessments. In: *Multivariate Statistical Methodologies Used in the International Pilot Study of Schizophrenia*, ed. J. J. Bartko & W. Gulbinat. NIMH Series GN. No. 1. DHHS Publication No. (ADM) 80–630. Washington, DC: U.S. Government Printing Office.
——Kabesová, L., & Tomásek, L. (1982), Five-year follow-up of Prague sample of psychiatric patients, project, method. Report from International Pilot Study of Schizophrenia WHO. *Csl. Psychiatry*, 78(5):334–352. (In Czech)

——, ——, ——(1984), Five-year follow-up of Prague sample of psychiatric patients. Report from International Pilot Study of Schizophrenia. WHO. *Csl. Psychiatry*, 80(3): 155–164. (In Czech)

——Sartorius, N., Jablensky, A., & Husák, T. (1976), Diagnostic agreement of groups of Czechoslovak and international groups of psychiatrists presented with discrete sequences of information on patients. A report from the WHO IPSS. *Socijalna Psihijatrija*, 3(3):265–277. (In Czech)

Vana, J. (1979), Methods of epidemiology in psychiatric service research. *Rep. Prague Res. Inst.*, 53. (In Czech)

——Ivanys, E. (1969), Epidemiology of mental disorders in Prague-8. Paper presented at conference on the influence of the urban and working environment on the health and behavior of modern man. Prague, October 13–15.

Determinants of Outcome of Severe Mental Disorder (DOSMeD)

Vijoy K. Varma

The seminal contribution of the International Pilot Study of Schizophrenia (IPSS) was that schizophrenic patients in developing countries seemed to have less severe course and outcome than patients in developed countries with comparable initial clinical pictures. The next question was to test this finding in more epidemiologically robust samples of first episode cases presenting in defined populations. Accordingly, a subsequent study, the Determinants of Outcome of Severe Mental Disorder study (DOSMeD), was designed. Twelve centers in 10 countries participated, representing both the developing and developed world: Aarhus (Denmark), Dublin (Ireland), Honolulu and Rochester (U.S.A.), Moscow (Russia), Nagasaki (Japan), Nottingham (U.K.), Prague (Czech Republic), Agra and Chandigarh (India), Cali (Colombia), and Ibadan (Nigeria).

Over 2 years (1978–1980), all persons aged 15 to 54 from the catchment area (resident for at least 6 months), with symptoms suggestive of psychosis, were recruited on the basis of a first lifetime contact with a helping agency. Standardized instruments included the Present State Examination (PSE) and assessments of social and psychiatric history. Cases were followed up at 12 and 24 months. Although all centers contributed first episode case groups, only seven were able to identify all cases arising from defined populations which could be reliably estimated so as to generate robust Incidence rates.

Almost half of patients were in the age group 15 to 24, more so in developing countries. Eighty percent were assigned to the broad clinical diagnosis of schizophrenia and related disorders, and over half fulfilled the "restrictive" S+ diagnostic classification of the CATEGO program. The incidence of schizophrenia was found to be variable, though comparable, in different countries ranging between 1.6 and 4.2 (per 10,000) for a broad definition of schizophrenia and shrinking to 0.7 to 1.4 for the CATEGO S+ definition.

Following 2-year follow-up, patients were allocated to seven patterns of course type. Fifteen percent of subjects in developed countries had the best outcome as opposed to 37% in developing countries. Conversely, the worst outcome was recorded in 17.4% in developed, but in only 11.1% of subjects in developing countries. The study thus replicated the earlier finding of the IPSS. Surprisingly, even patients with a diagnosis of paranoid schizophrenia in developing countries showed a more favorable short-term pattern of course.

Of the original 12 field research centers, eight (Chandigarh rural and urban; Dublin, Honolulu, Moscow, Nagasaki, Nottingham, Prague, and Rochester) were able to participate in the ISoS and to carry out 15-year follow-up assessments of their cohorts.

Chapter 11

DOSMeD: Chandigarh, India

Vijoy K. Varma and Savita Malhotra

CULTURAL CONTEXT

Geographically, India consists of the great Himalayan range in the north, the Sutlej, Gangetic, and Brahmaputra plains in the middle, and the triangular Deccan plateau in the south. The Himalayas, barriers to climatic influences and to the movement of peoples, contain some of the highest peaks in the world and are the source of most rivers that flow through the vast Indo-Gangetic plains to the south.

Northern India, in which the Chandigarh center is located, has a rich cultural heritage tracing its roots to Indo-Aryan civilization. Aryans, who made a significant impact on Indian culture and beliefs, came to northern India between 2000 and 1500 B.C. The philosophy and belief system are largely dominated by religion. Hinduism is the dominant religion of India and of the part of North India that formed the catchment area of the present study. Certain religions, such as Buddhism, Jainism, and Sikhism, were offshoots of Hinduism, whereas Islam and Christianity came from outside, starting around the 12th and the 15th centuries A.D., respectively.

Fundamental to Hinduism are the beliefs that the individual human soul comes from the *Brahman* (world soul) and is destined to return to be absorbed by it, and that of the transmigration of souls, with which the ideas of *karma* and *sanskara* are closely bound. In actual practice, Hinduism is most aptly characterized as a "way of life" of wholesome and harmonious living. Hinduism has influenced the practice of the other religions in India. At the same time, India has historically been noted for religious tolerance; various religions existing side by side have exercised a mutually beneficial influence upon one another. The apparent strife between the religious groups that occurs from time to time in different geographical areas is mostly due to politics, not to intolerance.

A most striking feature of Hindu culture is the caste system. Although evidence of caste is to be found in many parts of the world, India originated the system and embodied it. The offshoots of Hinduism—Buddhism, Jainism, and Sikhism—do not have this system. Originally conceived of as a system of division of labor, in actual practice it led to a hierarchical stratification of the society. Until recently, society was rigidly divided into named castes, each with a well-developed life of its own. Distinct castes formed the scheme of social precedence; the status of a person depended on the traditional importance of the caste into which he was born. Thus, *Brahmins* stood at the apex of the social ladder, while ranked below were *Kshatriyas*, *Vaishyas*, and *Sudras*. In contrast to the high position enjoyed by *Brahmins*, the *Sudras* (untouchables) were subject to many restrictions—for example, not being allowed to use public roads or public wells, or to enter temples, and being forced to live on the outskirts of the city. Castes have been endogamous and continue to be largely so.

Since the 18th century, various reformist movements have affected the caste system. In the Constitution of India, which came into force in 1950, all citizens are guaranteed the right of equality. Not only was untouchability legally abolished with independence in 1947, but the Constitution also provides for the protection and social improvements of the "scheduled castes" (so called because these castes, primarily representing *Sudras* or untouchables, are enumerated in a special schedule of the Constitution). Though the formal authority of the caste system has diminished, its influence persists, and popular attitudes have changed relatively little.

The city of Chandigarh is located about 330 meters above sea level in the western foothills of the Shivalik mountain range, bound by two seasonal rivers, the Patiala Rao and Sukhna Choe in the northwest and southeast, respectively, and surrounded by the states of Punjab, Haryana, and Himachal Pradesh. It is a modern, fully planned city, built from scratch. The city was planned after the partition of India in 1947 as the new capital of the State of Punjab to replace the earlier capital, Lahore, which had been ceded to Pakistan. The first President of India, Dr. Rajendra Prasad, formally declared it open on October 7, 1953. On November 1, 1966, as a result of a reorganization of states, it became a federally administered Union Territory (UR) consisting of the city of Chandigarh, 57.6 sq km, and 22 rural villages; another 56.4 sq km of satellite towns, Panchkula and Mohali, have developed in the adjoining states of Haryana and Punjab, respectively. In addition to being a separate entity, Chandigarh is also the capital and seat of administration of the neighboring states of Punjab and Haryana. One elected member of the (Federal) Parliament represents this constituency.

Chandigarh, named after the local presiding deity, Chandi, the goddess of power, was designed by the French architect, Le Corbusier. It is noted for neat rows of houses, parks and gardens, and wide, tree-lined avenues in submountainous and undulating terrain. The city is modern; there are only a few small and medium industries, but it is a promising commercial center. It has electricity, road transport, sewerage, and a potable water supply.

In the decade 1981 to 1991, Chandigarh posted a growth rate of 42.16% as against 75.55% in 1971 to 1981. The literacy rate has increased to 77.81% from 74.81% in 1981. Sex ratio has improved from 769 to 790 females per 1000 males in 1991. The birth and death rates are very low. The majority of the population is Hindu (76.42%); Sikhs (19.78%), Muslims (2.57%), Christians (0.84%), Jains (0.26%), and Buddhists (0.11%) form the minority community. As compared to most states of India, the population of Chandigarh is characterized by lower representation of females, children, and the old. There is no significant ethnic population. The population of Chandigarh comprises the original residents who own the land, people who have immigrated from other areas, and people who have begun to migrate for employment and higher education. The phenomenon of immigration is an ongoing process, though it has slowed down.

Raipur Rani, the rural catchment area, is situated at the foothills of the Shivalik mountains about 50 km from Chandigarh in the adjoining state of Haryana, District Panchkula. The major source of livelihood is agriculture, and all trade and commerce revolve around it. All the villages have electricity, a potable water supply, asphalt roads, telephones, schools, post offices, telegraph offices, banks, and police. The population consists mainly of Hindus (80.1%), of which about 20% are members of the scheduled castes. The other minority communities are Muslims and Sikhs (20%). According to the 1991 census, there was decennial growth rate of 22.5%. The sex ratio was 844 females per 1000 males. The literacy rate in the rural area was 46%.

The social structure in the villages still reflects the caste system. The *Brahmins*, the *Kshatriyas*, and *Vaishyas* constitute the upper and dominant castes. Below them in the hierarchy are the lower castes consisting mainly of artisan groups. The scheduled castes stand at the bottom of the caste structure. The upper and dominant castes are usually the landholders. The scheduled castes labor in the fields and have little land of their own. The upper and dominant castes reside in the central part of the villages in permanent structures with relatively better sanitation, whereas scheduled caste people reside at the periphery of the villages in mainly thatched, semipermanent structures. Very often, caste considerations predominate in the constitution of village governing bodies. Migration is minimal in the rural areas.

The most commonly spoken language is Hindi. In Chandigarh, a majority of the people speak Hindi, Punjabi, and English, though a few also speak other languages, such as Kashmiri, Bengali, Marathi, Oriya, Kannada, Tamil, Telugu, and Malyalam. In Raipur Rani, the commonly spoken languages are Hindi and Haryanavi. A few also speak Punjabi and English. There are no problems in communication because a majority of the people speaking regional languages can also communicate in either Hindi or English. Because of linguistic homogeneity across all segments of society, the concepts, symptoms, and diagnosis of mental illness can be easily communicated.

IMPACT OF MENTAL HEALTH ISSUES ON SOCIETY

In India, psychiatric illnesses are being increasingly recognized, particularly in areas undergoing rapid social change and industrialization. People suffering from severe mental disorders become a burden for society and need constant care. By and large, the majority of the subjects in this region belong to close-knit families. Family ties are strong, and at times of crisis a satisfactory level of protection and social support is provided. Most subjects are accompanied by relatives when they visit the hospital for both inpatient and outpatient treatment, the cost of which is borne by the family. In most cases, the subjects engage in such light jobs as they can carry out. For those subjects who are unable to earn their own livelihood, economic support is provided by family members. Though mental illness is still considered taboo in society, widespread education has made it more acceptable to seek treatment.

Particularly in rural areas, significant stigma is attached to psychiatric disorders, popularly believed to be caused by evil spirits or ascribed to other magicoreligious forces. With increased education in the urban areas, a mixed belief system prevails regarding the causation of severe psychiatric disorder. External factors like food, climate, habits, environment, and also social factors are blamed. The medical disease model and genetic deficiency are less prevalent.

THE MENTAL HEALTH SYSTEM IN THE AREA

In India, health (including mental health) follows a three-sector model: government, private, and mixed. Each state is responsible for providing health services to everyone on a national health service model at little or no cost to the individual. The health services cater to the needs of the people through a network of government hospitals, primary health centers, subcenters, and government dispensaries. In addition to the government sector facilities, there are private sector facilities which include private nursing homes and private practitioners.

Organization and Policies

In India, by and large, the general health system is expected to also provide mental health service. Because of the paucity of qualified psychiatrists in the country (in total, fewer than 4000) and the absence of jobs for them at the primary care level, mental health is taken care of by general doctors or by the practitioners of other systems of medicine such as Ayurveda, homeopathy, or even magicoreligious healing. Mental health services by specialists are provided through mental hospitals, nursing homes, and psychiatric facilities in general hospitals located in big cities, generally utilized by a small proportion of the urban population. With the National Mental Health Program adopted in 1982, however, mental health care is envisaged as integrated with general health services, a concept that has yet to become an operational reality. The Mental Health Act of 1987 provided for all citizens to have the services of mental hospitals. People on their own or with the help of competent authorities, such as the police and even government organizations, can seek the help of a local government hospital psychiatrist for services or for suitable recommendation for help from other agencies.

Mental Health Facilities in the Catchment Areas at the Time of Follow-up

In Chandigarh, mental health services are provided by the Postgraduate Institute of Medical Education and Research (PGIMER), some privately operated psychiatric care agencies, a general hospital, and a medical college. The Department of Psychiatry of the PGIMER, provides a 24-bed general psychiatric inpatient unit and an active outpatient facility. It accepts all patients who come either directly or are referred by health agencies and practitioners in Chandigarh and in neighboring states. It also provides referral-consultation to other departments of the PGIMER. In addition, the department operates a separate 20-bed drug detoxification and treatment center with an outpatient facility. Mental health in- and outpatient facilities are also provided at a general hospital in Chandigarh, which has a variable number of beds available on a limited basis and a single qualified psychiatrist. Psychiatric services only became available at the Government Medical College, Chandigarh, a few years ago. At the time of follow-up, there was one private nursing home with four to six beds which provided inpatient facilities, and about 200 qualified doctors in Chandigarh.

In the rural catchment area of Raipur Rani, the state health services, the main vehicle for providing medical care to the catchment area, operates one primary health center with seven subcenters and 10 dispensaries, and one hospital that does not have any designated psychiatric beds. Severely ill subjects are referred to the district hospital at Ambala and to other psychiatric facilities outside the catchment area. Finally, in both catchment areas, there are traditional healers who provide treatment to mentally ill persons. Although there is no organized structure, most are known through personal contacts. Thus, their exact number could not be ascertained.

There is no formal system for coordinating care among different service providers. The care coordination between the mental health system and other health and social sectors is not very well organized and is primarily dependent upon the family.

Financial Support

Financial support for mental health services is similar to that of other medical services. For the population in general, the services are technically provided at little or no cost; however, the availability and quality of services in actual fact are rather limited. For civil servants, financial assistance is provided by their respective departments. For industrial or industry-related work, there are government dispensaries which provide medicines. Otherwise, for most cases, there is no financial help available for the treatment of the mentally ill. There have been no significant changes in the last 25 years (1970–1995).

PSYCHIATRIC EPIDEMIOLOGY

The earliest account of the rate of mental illness in India is given by Overbeck-Wright (1921) in his book, *Lunacy in India,* where he gave a figure of 0.26 per thousand on the census report in 1911. Although the need for assessing the prevalence of mental illness must have been felt by many, no mental morbidity surveys were undertaken in India until the 1960s. Dube (1970) refers to an effort by Govindaswamy in Bangalore, who conducted a survey through a questionnaire, but his results were inconclusive.

In the earliest reported field survey of mental morbidity in India, Surya, Dutta, Gopalkrishna, Sundaram, and Kutty (1964) surveyed a population of 2731 from 510 households in the Kurchikuppan locality of Pondicherry during June to September 1962, using a simple screening questionnaire with one informant per household. Informants were asked if they knew anybody with any of 25 listed symptoms. All the reported persons were identified, and clinical interviews were carried out by Surya himself. Twenty-six persons were found to be suffering from neuropsychiatric illness, making for a rate of 9.5 per 1000. Epilepsy accounted for 2.2, schizophrenia 1.5, alcoholism 3.6, and mental defect 0.7 per 1000, respectively. Depression was not represented, and no one appeared to be in need of institutional care.

Over the next 15 years, numerous studies were carried out in quick succession, and these were mainly on the general epidemiology (prevalence) of psychiatric morbidity in India. But there have been gross differences in such studies with regard to the methodology and the results. The size of the population varied from as low as 1060 (Nandi et al., 1975) to as high as 29,468 (Dube, 1970). The areas studied have been urban (Sethi, Gupta, and Rajkumar, 1967; Surya, Dutta, Gopalkrishna, Sundaram, and Kutty, 1964), semiurban (Verghese, Beig, Senseman, Sunder Rao, and Benjamin, 1973), and rural (Elnagar, Maitra, and Rao, 1971; Sethi, Gupta, Rajkumar, and Kumari, 1972). The interviews were generally conducted by clinical psychologists, physicians with psychiatric training, social workers, field workers, and psychiatrists. The methods used were screening questionnaire (Surya et al., 1964; Sethi et al., 1967; Sethi et al., 1972), interview method (Dube, 1970; Elnagar et al., 1971) and structured interview schedule (Kapur, Kapur, and Carstairs, 1974). Table 11.1 summarizes the major prevalence studies of mental illness in India (Varma and Das, 1995).

The prevalence rate for neuropsychiatric morbidity per thousand has varied from as low as 9.5 (Surya et al., 1964) to as high as 370.0 (Kapur, 1973). Data regarding certain disorders of the major morbidity groups have been lacking. The general findings of the studies indicate that the prevalence of "neuroses and miscellaneous disorders" was more than that of the psychoses, epilepsy, and mental retardation, except in some studies (e.g., Gopinath, 1968; Sethi et al., 1972, Nandi et al., 1975).

As regards the incidence of general psychiatric morbidity, such studies have been few. Nandi, Ajmany, Ganguli et al. (1976) carried out a longitudinal study of the epidemiology of mental disorders in a village near Calcutta over a one-year period and reported an incidence rate of 17.63 per 1000 per year for all psychiatric disorders (of 19 new cases, one had schizophrenia and one was mentally deficient). The latest study on prevalence of psychiatric morbidity in an urban population was carried out by Premarajan, Danabalan, Chandrasekar, and Srinivasa (1993) on a sample of 1115 which showed prevalence of 99.4 per 1000.

TABLE 11.1 Prevalence of Psychiatric Illnesses Reported by Various Authors

Author	*Year*	*Sample Size*	*Schizophrenia*	*Affective Psychosis*	*Organic, Epilepsy*	*MR*	*Neuroses and Misc.*	*Total*
Surya et al.	(1964)	2,731	1.5	—	2.2	0.7	5.7	9.5
Sethi et al.	(1967)	1,733	2.3	6.9	—	22.5	41.0	72.7
Gopinath	(1968)	423	—	7.0	2.4	4.7	2.4	16.5
Dube	(1970)	29,468	1.5	0.5	2.9	3.7	9.4	18.0
Elnagar et al.	(1971)	1,393	4.4	2.9	4.4	1.5	14.5	27.6
Sethi et al.	(1972)	2,691	1.1	1.5	—	25.3	11.5	39.4
Kapur	(1973)	1,233	—	8.1	—	5.7	253.0	370.0
Thacore	(1973)	—	1.9	1.5	2.7	3.7	71.4	81.6
Verghese et al.	(1973)	1,887	1.7	0.3	1.7	8.3	52.7	66.5
Nandi et al.	(1975)	1,060	2.8	37.7	10.4	2.8	49.0	102.8
Shah	(1980)	—	1.5	14.8	—	1.8	29.2	47.3
Nandi et al.	(1976)	1,862	5.3					
Isaac and Kapur	(1980)	4,209	0.9					
Bhide	(1982)	1,658	3.0					
ICMR	(1988)	146,380	2.2					
Padmavathi et al.	(1987)	101,229	2.5					
Nandi et al.	(1980)	4,053	2.2					
Nandi et al.	(1979)	1,622	4.3					
Premarajan et al.	(1993)	1,115	2.5					

Adapted from Varma and Das (1995)

The commonest disorders were neurosis (47%), alcohol dependence (30%), and psychosis (30%).

In the last three to four decades of the 20th century, schizophrenia formed an important focus of Indian research. Initial efforts were descriptive and cross-sectional, and in the latter part of the era have become more focused in nature. Prevalence has been studied in different parts of India and in different communities, and an average rate was determined to be 2 to 3 per 1000. Studies in the earlier phase were with smaller population groups of a few thousand. The more recent studies have covered up to 1 million people and have provided a more realistic base for the understanding of schizophrenia. Overall sample size has varied from 327 (Ganguli, 1968) to 146,380 (Indian Council of Medical Research, 1988), and calculated prevalence rates have ranged from 1.5 per 1000 (Surya et al., 1964) to 7.2 (Kapur, 1973). The differing rates reflect the differing methods used (e.g., of screening and case definition). Substantively, high rates of prevalence have been found to be associated with slums, low socioeconomic status, age 15 to 45 years, living alone, unemployment, and illiteracy.

As for the incidence rate of schizophrenia, sadly there is a dearth of studies. Barring the present DOSMeD cohort, only Nandi and Rajkumar and their colleagues have reported such research. Nandi, Ajmany, Ganguli et al. (1976) reported an incidence rate of 0.93 per 1000 in a rural sample whereas Rajkumar, Padmavathi, Thara, and Sarada Menon (1993) reported an incidence rate of 0.30 per 1000 in an urban area. An incidence rate of 0.35 per 1000 was found in slums of an urban area (Rajkumar et al., 1993).

THE CENTER

The Department of Psychiatry at the Postgraduate Institute of Medical Education and Research, Chandigarh, has been in existence since September 16, 1963, when Dr. N. N. Wig joined the Institute. An inpatient unit was established in 1964, and gradually, electroconvulsive therapy, occupational therapy, and other treatment modalities became available. During the first 5 years, because of staff limitations, efforts were concentrated on organizing essential psychiatric services for this general teaching hospital and on providing a training program for postgraduates in general medicine. The first major expansion took place in the years 1968 to 1970 when three more faculty members joined, and a postgraduate residency training program in psychiatry was introduced. The psychiatry ward was transferred to new specially designed premises in April 1971. A Ph.D. training program in clinical psychology was established in 1972.

The second major expansion took place in the years 1976 and 1977 when the department was designated a WHO Collaborating Center for Research and Training in Mental Health. A considerable expansion in research, training, and service activities followed, as well as augmentation of the staff. As a part of WHO-sponsored research projects, new commitments such as clinical services for alcohol and drug dependence and rural clinics for Raipur Rani were undertaken. In 1987, on expiration of the normal term of 10 years, official WHO collaborating center status ended; however, collaboration with the WHO on specific projects and programs has continued.

The third major expansion took place in 1988 and 1989 with the installation of a drug detoxification and treatment center. With this, the staff and bed strength almost doubled with 11 faculty members: one professor and head, two additional professors, two associate professors, and two assistant professors of psychiatry, and three additional professors and one assistant professor of clinical psychology. There are seven senior residents (qualified psychiatry specialists) and 11 junior residents (postgraduate students). Besides these, the other regular staff consists of one play therapist, four psychiatric social workers, one assistant clinical psychologist, and nursing staff. A number of research workers are also appointed from time to time.

METHODS USED AT THE SITE

The patient cohort was originally generated as a part of the WHO DOSMeD study. The methodology and many aspects of the results have been described in detail in a number of earlier publications (Varma, 1989; Jablensky et al., 1992; Wig, Varma, Mattoo et al., 1993; Collins et al., 1996; Varma, Brown, Wig et al., 1997; Varma, Wig, Phookun et al., 1997; Susser et al., 1998; Malhotra et al., 1998).

The Catchment Area

The Chandigarh Center in the present study consisted of two distinct catchment areas, the urban and the rural. The *urban catchment area*, spread over 58 square kilometers, was located in the Union Territory (UT) of Chandigarh in North India, about 250 km due north of New Delhi, the national capital. It consisted of the city of Chandigarh (45 sectors, excluding two sectors housing migratory defense personnel), its three labor colonies (temporary settlements for migrant workers), one periurban township, and three adjoining villages designated as urban agglomerations as per the Census of India (1971). The *rural catchment area* was centered about 50 km from Chandigarh in the Raipur Rani block of Narainpur Tehsil under the Ambala district of the state of Haryana. It is comprised of 145 villages located over an area of 455 sq km. At the midpoint of the intake period of the study, these areas were estimated to have a population of 348,609 and 103,865, respectively, with the populations in the 15 to 54 age group being 205,786 and 61,642, respectively.

Selection of Subjects

DOSMeD attempted to include all new cases from the defined catchment areas, by active recruitment, during the period of October 1, 1978, to September 30, 1980. As such, a list was made of all health facilities outside the area to which patients were likely to be referred, and active contact was maintained with these helping agencies to ensure that all cases from the catchment area with onset within the time period came to the attention of the study team. The recruitment process was supplemented by an analysis of the possible leakage of cases to confirm that all relevant cases were covered.

For the selection of the patients, the salient inclusion criteria were: age 15 to 54; residence for at least 6 months in the catchment area within the preceding year; and evidence, in the preceding 12 months, of at least one major psychotic symptom (i.e., hallucinations or delusions, qualitative thought or speech disorder, qualitative psychomotor disorder, or gross behavioral abnormalities), failing which at least two of a list of six lesser disturbances were required. Those with a history of admission, diagnosis, and/or treatment for a psychotic disorder at any time before the past 3 months preceding the screening were excluded. The idea was to select patients with first onset of schizophrenia or certain other related psychotic conditions. Cases with clinically manifest organic cerebral disorder, severe or moderate mental retardation, or organic CNS damage due to alcohol or drug dependence were also excluded.

The objective of DOSMeD was to study the incidence, natural history, and factors affecting the outcome of severe mental disorders. With the help of various case-finding agencies and methods of case identification, 268 patients of first onset severe mental disorder were identified in the defined rural and urban catchment areas over a 2-year period. These subjects, after initial assessment, were followed up regularly and evaluated using standardized schedules at 1 and 2 years from the date of inclusion.

Defining the ISoS Cohort

The ISoS cohort was taken from the DOSMeD study. Table 11.2 summarizes the process of screening of the population for the selection of the study cohort. The ISoS cohort was selected on the basis of the broad diagnosis of schizophrenia assigned to these subjects by WHO on ICD-9 or as CATEGO class S+ or SPO. The final schizophrenic cohort comprised 210 cases which included 155 urban and 55 (including one missed as a "leakage" case in the original DOSMeD Study) rural cases. Before working on the present study, a feasibility study was carried out. Centers were asked to locate subjects randomly selected by WHO. More than 75% of these subjects in both urban and rural areas were traced, qualifying the center for participation in ISoS.

Case-Finding

Fixing prior appointments or checking the availability of the study subject or informant in advance was not possible. In the urban catchment area, a home visit was initially made to locate and contact subjects and/or informants. Once the subject was contacted, a subsequent appointment was fixed for interviews with the subject and informants. On average, it took around half an hour to reach the home or workplace and 30 to 40 minutes to locate the subject and to fix the appointment. In certain cases, the study subject and the informants were not available at the same place and time; so each was interviewed separately. Repeat visits were also necessary for those who were not available at home during the first visit. A number of cases had changed their place of residence within the catchment area; special efforts were made to obtain their new addresses and to locate them. A number of cases had left the catchment area for various reasons such as job transfer or subjects marrying outside the catchment area; an effort was made to trace relatives and to contact the study subject through them. In a few cases, it was possible to call the subject to Chandigarh for an interview. Many subjects were available only on Sundays and holidays; they were contacted accordingly. All this required a great deal of effort over a 6-month period, and the relatives had to be visited again and again during this period.

Some study subjects and their informants refused to be interviewed for various reasons. An attempt was

TABLE 11.2 Summary of Screening Process for the Selection of the Study Cohort

	Urban	*Rural*	*Total*
Total Population	348,609	103,865	452,474
Population 15–54 years	205,786	61,642	267,428
Cases Screened	2338	317	2655
Cases Identified	199	69	268
Evaluation Not Possible	32	4	36
Evaluation Completed	167	65	232
Excluded, Diagnostic Reason	12	11	23
Final Size of DOSMeD			
Cohort (M/F)	155 (91 M, 64 F)	54 (27 M, 27 F)	209 (118 M, 91 F)
Died (M/F)	14 (8 M, 6 F)	10 (7 M, 3 F)	24 (15 M, 9 F)
Lost to Follow-Up (M/F)	61 (40 M, 21 F)	7 (4 M, 3 F)	68 (44 M, 24 F)
ISoS Alive Cohort (M/F)	80 (43 M, 37 F)	38 (16 M, 22 F)	118 (59 M, 59 F)

made to convince them of the necessity of the study, and in a few cases the time-consuming effort was successful. In the case of female subjects who had gotten married since inclusion in the study cohorts, we had to wait for their visits to their parents' homes on occasions of festivals or family functions (as is customary) in order to interview for ISoS. Much discretion needed to be exercised in this regard.

Almost all cases in the rural catchment area were contacted by making home visits. It took about two hours to reach the particular village and 30 to 40 minutes to locate the subject. All efforts were made to conduct as much of the interview on that same day (with either the study subject or the informant) and to schedule the rest of the interview. At times, the subjects, with the help of distant relatives or neighbors, were away at their farms or workplaces. In cases where it was not possible logistically to call informants or subjects within the stipulated time, a date was fixed for a revisit, and subjects and relatives were requested to remain at home at that agreed upon time.

A strategy similar to that used with urban subjects was employed in cases where the subject had left the catchment area. In the rural catchment area, however, the recontact visits were fewer than in the urban catchment area. Special efforts were required to visit or locate many rural cases not only because of the logistics involved, but also because a poor communication network, extreme weather, and inhospitable geographical conditions combined to make some villages inaccessible for weeks or months.

Use of Study Instruments

The Life Chart Schedule, Disability Assessment Scale, and Family Interview Schedule were translated into Hindi by a psychologist. In the first draft, an attempt was made to include colloquial terms to make it easy for the local population to understand. This first draft was discussed with one social worker and two psychiatrists, and necessary changes were incorporated to make the final Hindi version. Though most of the interviews were conducted using these translated versions, there was no difficulty in switching to other locally spoken languages when required.

Prior to the actual study, a preliminary study was carried out to establish reliability. The instruments were administered to 10 subjects each and were rated by a number of investigators. The data were analyzed at the WHO Center at the Nathan Kline Institute, Orangeburg, NY. After data analysis, the results were discussed at this center with an expert from WHO.

Data-Gathering Procedures

With most of the study subjects and their informants, the interview was conducted in Hindi. BIS, BII, FIS, DAS, LCS (partly), and IOR were filled out by the psychologists and took about 2 hours/subject to complete. PSE, LCS (partly), SANS, PIRS, SAS, SDP were filled out by the psychiatrist, and it took around 1 ½ to 2 hours to complete these schedules. No fixed pattern of interview was adopted. The entire interview was very time-consuming, and, in most cases, had to be completed in two sittings. Most of the time, the subjects and the informants were interviewed together as is the usual practice in India. Confidentiality is not an issue between the subject and the primary caregiver; rather, subjects feel more secure and comfortable with the relative's presence during interview. In case of disparity between the study subjects' and informants' version of information, the interviewer's own judgment was used. The order of administration of scales varied from case to case according to the comfort of subjects. After completing the interview, the interviewer reviewed the subject's records for filling out the LCS, DSS, and BRS. The information provided by subject and informant(s) was also cross-checked against the intake data and follow-up information.

RESULTS

The DOSMeD sample consisted of 155 subjects in the urban and 54 in the rural cohort. The ISoS cohort consisted of one extra subject in the rural cohort, identified on the basis of the "leakage" study (Table 11.2).

In the urban area, 61 subjects were lost to follow-up, and 14 had died, whereas in the rural area only seven subjects were lost to follow-up and 10 had died. This suggests that "lost to follow-up" rate is higher in urban areas as compared to rural areas; more males than females were lost to follow-up; and mortality was much higher among rural males. Regarding age distribution, the mean year of birth for the dead was very much earlier (1938) in the rural sample than in the urban group (1952). There was no difference in the mean ages of the "alive" and the "lost to follow-up" cohorts. Birth year distribution at follow-up was similar to that at entry, while there was a higher proportion of females alive for both cohorts.

Mode of Onset and Diagnosis

The distribution according to the mode of onset in the alive cohort was similar to that of the original DOSMeD study. A majority of the subjects in the alive cohort had acute onset, in both urban and rural cohorts. More subjects in the urban alive cohort had insidious onset than in the rural alive cohort. In the urban area, only 34% of the alive cohort of 80 received a baseline diagnosis of schizophrenia (using ICD-9 to ICD-10 conversion), which is similar to that seen in the original study cohort. In the rural alive cohort, only 26% had a baseline diagnosis of schizophrenia. In the urban area, the mortality rate was much higher among schizophrenics, whereas in the rural area mortality was higher among nonschizophrenics. The largest diagnostic category for the alive group was acute schizophrenia-like disorder (urban, 35%; rural, 47%), quite similar to the original cohort.

Pattern of Course at Early Follow-up

Forty-six of the 80 subjects (57%) in the urban alive cohort had a favorable, short-term (two-year) pattern of course (episodic with full remissions between episodes). In the rural cohort, 28 of the 38 subjects (74%) had a favorable short-term pattern of course. This is very similar to the original study cohort. Death rate was higher among subjects who had been continuously psychotic or who had incomplete remission.

ALIVE SUBJECTS

Symptomatology

Classified according to the Bleuler severity scale, 66% of the 80 persons in the alive urban cohort had recovered; 18% had mild and 11% had moderate symptomatology, and only 5% suffered severe symptoms. In the rural cohort 61% of the 38 persons had recovered, 16 and 24% had moderate and mild symptoms, respectively, and no person suffered severely. A similar impression of current symptoms was gained from the results of the Global Assessment of Functioning Scale for Symptomatology (GAF-S). Seventy-five percent of the urban cohort and 81% of the rural cohort showed "no significant" or only mild symptoms (GAF-S above 60). The relative prominence of psychotic symptoms over time tends to conform to this pattern. Only 3% of the combined Chandigarh cohorts were found to have had prominent psychotic symptoms throughout their illness period, which is considerably less than the other DOSMeD centers (11.3%). Such symptoms were never prominent in 26 and 29% of subjects in the urban and rural cohorts respectively, whereas in other DOSMeD centers, only 3% of subjects never had prominent symptoms.

Course of Illness

Of the 80 urban alive subjects, 64% had no psychotic episodes over the immediately preceding two years, 19% had been continuously psychotic, and 9% were classified as episodic. In the rural cohort of 38 subjects, 71% had no psychotic episodes over the past 2 years; 8% were continuously psychotic; and another 8% were classified as episodic. This pattern was significantly different from the total of other DOSMeD centers (47% had no psychotic symptoms, 30% continuously psychotic, and 20% had episodic illness). As expected, the course of illness over the entire period showed a different pattern. Seventy-five percent of subjects in the urban cohort had episodic illness, and 15% were continuously psychotic; the corresponding figures in the rural cohort were 79 and 10%, respectively. A majority of the subjects (51.2% of the urban and 63.1% of the rural) had either recovered or had shown improvement. In the urban group, the illness had worsened in 4% of subjects, which is similar to other DOSMeD centers. But as compared to other centers, the outcome of this center was better. (In the "Overall Time Trends" for Chandigarh, the "other" category refers to subjects who were fully recovered.)

Living Arrangements

At the follow-up assessment, most subjects were living in the community: 91% of the 80 urban subjects and 97% of the 38 rural subjects were living with their families. Figures for independent living were similar to the other DOSMeD centers as a whole, although the subjects from Honolulu and Nagasaki showed a smaller tendency to be living with family and were more often living either in a hospital or a supervised residence. More subjects in Moscow, Nottingham, and Rochester were found to be living alone as compared to other centers. For the most part, this situation was stable for the 2 years preceding the assessment. More than 90% in both the urban and rural cohorts spent all of the immediately preceding 2 years in an independent residence. Only 5% of urban subjects spent time in hospitals; there were no hospitalizations in the rural cohort. As compared to other DOSMeD centers, more subjects from the Chandigarh center were living independently. Honolulu and Nagasaki centers had many more subjects who had never lived independently during the last 2 years of follow-up. Over the course of the entire follow-up period, each subject had lived independently in the community for some time. Ninety-eight percent of subjects in the urban cohort had stayed independently for more than 90% of the time, whereas in the rural cohort, all the subjects had managed to live independently for more than 95% of the time. This figure was far better than most of the other DOSMeD centers. At the time of follow-up, 99% of urban subjects and 95% of rural subjects had never been homeless or vagrant in the preceding 2 years, which was similar to the findings in other centers. None of the subjects had been in jail during the last 2 years. Over the course of the entire follow-up period, only 9% of urban and 10% of rural subjects were found to be homeless or vagrant and that, too, for less than 5% of the time. Three subjects in the urban cohort but none from the rural cohort spent time in jail. This picture is similar to almost all other DOSMeD centers. Low rates of homelessness and jail were common throughout the ISoS centers. Only Honolulu had substantially higher rates on these measures.

Work

Sixty-four percent of urban and 45% of rural subjects had worked at paid jobs at some point in the last 2 years of follow-up; most of the subjects (54% urban and 37% rural) had worked for the entire 24 months. For those working most of the time, performance was judged as good in 89% of urban and 67% of rural subjects. In addition, 28% of urban and 58% of rural subjects were engaged in fulltime household work, and their performance was also generally rated as "good" to "very good." Only two urban subjects had retired and no one was classified as a student. Global work performance (looking only at those subjects ever employed and those ever engaged in household work) was rated as poor in only 11% amongst both urban and rural subjects.

Social Disability

With respect to overall functioning in the last month, only 10% of subjects both in the urban and rural cohorts were rated "poor" to "severe" on the Disability Assessment Scale (DAS). On the Global Assessment of Functioning Scale for Disability (GAF-D), 14% of urban and 5% of rural subjects had scores lower than 51 indicating serious impairment. On the other hand, 63% of urban and 71% of rural subjects were rated good to excellent on the DAS, and 59% of urban and 68% of rural subjects scored higher than 70 on the GAF-D, indicating good functioning. For 7.5% of the alive urban cohort, disabilities were prominent throughout the follow-up period; for 5% they were more prominent during the last third of the period, while for 57.5% disability was a prominent feature of only the first third. Twenty-two out of 80 (27.5%) experienced no prominent disabilities at any time. For 57.9% of the rural alive cohort, disability was a prominent feature of only the first third; 31.6% experienced no prominent disabilities at any time; and none suffered prominent disabilities throughout the follow-up period.

Violence and Attempted Suicide

Eight subjects (10%) of the 80 alive urban cohort and three subjects (8%) of the 38 alive rural cohort had been involved in assaults on other people in the last 2 years of follow-up. None resulted in serious injury. Over the entire course, 19 urban subjects (24%) and eight rural subjects (21%) had been involved in assaults on other people. Assault rates are higher in Honolulu and Nagasaki, but much lower in Dublin (9%). Only three subjects (4%) in the urban cohort attempted suicide in the last 2 years. During the entire follow-up period 15 urban subjects (19%) and four rural subjects (11%) deliberately harmed themselves at some point. For the total DOSMeD sample, rates of self harm are 4% in the last 2 years and 20% for the entire period.

Medications

In the immediately preceding 2 years, 11 (14%) of urban subjects had been prescribed neuroleptics at least once, and 26 (32.5%) had taken them for most of the time. Thus, 43 subjects (54%) had not been prescribed neuroleptics at all during the last 2 years of follow-up. All cohort subjects had been on medication at sometime during the follow-up period; 27 subjects (34%) had taken neuroleptics for most of the entire period.

In the rural cohort during the preceding 2 years, five subjects (13%) had been prescribed neuroleptics at least once, and 3 (8%) had taken them for most of the time. Thirty subjects (79%) had not been prescribed neuroleptics at all during the last 2 years. Thirty-four subjects (90%) had been on medication at some time during the follow-up period; only two subjects (5%) had taken neuroleptics most of the entire period, and two subjects had never taken neuroleptics. An examination of time trends over the entire period reveals that for 38 urban subjects (48%) and 21 rural subjects (57%), medication use was prominent only in the first third of the follow-up period; for two urban and two rural subjects (2.5%) and (5.4%) respectively, it was prominent only in the latter period. In the case of 32% of urban and 35% of rural subjects, medication was never prominent.

Hospitalization

Four subjects of the urban cohort (5%) had spent some time in the hospital in the 2 years prior to the follow-up. Seventy-six subjects (95%) had never been hospitalized. In the rural area, no one was hospitalized in the last 2 years. As compared to the DOSMeD centers, the rate of hospitalization of Chandigarh center was quite low. Twenty-eight subjects (35%) in the urban cohort were admitted to a hospital at least once during the entire follow-up period whereas in the rural cohort only five subjects (13%) had been thus admitted. The other DOSMeD centers had higher rates of hospitalization. For more than half of the urban subjects ever hospitalized (57%), hospitalization was prominent in the first third of the entire period only; for only one subject was it a consistently prominent feature. For nine subjects (30%), hospitalization was never prominent. In the rural cohort, for only one subject was hospitalization prominent in the first third of the entire period, and for one it was prominent in the recent period.

DECEASED SUBJECTS

At the time of this follow-up, 14 subjects in the urban cohort were deceased. Four (31%) had committed suicide, four subjects had died of natural causes, and one had died in an accident. Cause of death for five subjects could not be determined. Four subjects (36%) were known to be in an episode of illness at the time of death, one was in partial remission, and six were well at the time of death. In the rural cohort, 10 subjects were deceased (7 men and 3 women). One had committed suicide, six had died of natural causes, and three had died for other or unknown reasons. Only one subject was in an episode of illness at the time of death, three were in partial remission and six were well at that time.

DISCUSSION

The field research center at Chandigarh had the unique distinction of following two cohorts, urban and rural, in order to capture the influence of such sociocultural factors that are specific to each setting. There are vast differences between urban and rural living in India. Another unique feature of the Chandigarh cohorts was that after recruitment and 2-year follow-up as a part of the DOSMeD study, both were systematically and extensively followed up 5, 7, and 12 years after intake using local funding. Thus, subjects were in contact with the center and were very closely monitored. Details of their course of illness, clinical status, and other life circumstances (such as migration, physical illness, and death) commonly were known. Most subjects remained on active follow-up and treatment. One social worker, who has been a member of the research team from intake through all the follow-ups including ISoS, knows each individual case. His contribution to locating and contacting subjects, getting their cooperation, and collecting information about lost-to-follow-up, deceased, and refuser cases has been most valuable. Moreover, the extensive records of the 5-, 7-, and 12-year follow-ups were available to the ISoS research team.

A small proportion of subjects who remained in active contact with the psychiatric outpatient department at the Postgraduate Institute of Medical Education and Research, Chandigarh, were assessed at the clinic. For all other subjects, field visits were made by the research team to their homes or workplaces.

The strategies for follow-up assessment of the ISoS cohort were carried out in tandem with DOSMeD strategies because the cohort was the same, and the subjects had been in contact with the research team until the 12-year follow-up. In fact, the ISoS investigation team was equipped with almost up-to-date information about the subjects which made the planning and execution of ISoS follow-up strategy relatively easy. The success rate in follow-up (counting alive and dead) of the urban and rural cohorts was 61 and 87%, respectively; the urban rate was lower because migration was more common there. Chandigarh, a new city coming into existence only after India became independent, has virtually no native population. As most of the people in the Chandigarh urban center belong to the service class, they are likely to move out of the catchment area to return to their native communities either because of job transfers or after retirement.

The death rate among males in the urban cohort was high, and four subjects (31%) had committed suicide. On the other hand, in the rural cohort, deaths were more often due to natural causes and had no relation to their mental illness.

In our center, on the whole, there were very few refusers or uncooperative subjects. There was no selection bias in the sample followed for the ISoS study. There were no significant differences in our "alive," "dead," and "lost to follow-up" cohorts with regard to gender, age, mode of onset and diagnosis, and pattern of course at early follow-up. With respect to symptoms and functioning, there were no substantial discrepancies among the scores of the Bleuler Severity Scale, Global Assessment of Functioning (Symptoms), and Global Assessment of Functioning (Disability).

As in other centers, the vast majority of the subjects spent most of their time in "independent" living arrangements. "Living with the family" is the core of the Indian social system rather than an indication of special need. Interdependent living rather than independent living is the sociocultural ideal. No other alternative arrangements of living prevail; in India there are no supervised homes, and there is no disability pension for mental illness. But the number of subjects requiring constant care and support in the Chandigarh cohorts was very low, not exceeding four or five subjects.

The rate of hospitalization was also very low in the Chandigarh Center as compared to other ISoS centers. The cohort was in continuous contact and had regular follow-up by psychiatrists who assessed the need for hospitalization. Facilities for hospitalization in Chandigarh indicated lesser need for hospitalization and, hence, better outcome, rather than reflecting an absence of services.

In the Chandigarh center, most of the subjects were either successfully employed or were engaged in commensurate occupations. These rates are not unusually high because in Indian society there is a natural tendency for the social support system to mobilize in favor of a person who has serious illness. By and large, people are sympathetic, have lower expectations, and exhibit greater tolerance. Generally, job situations for persons with severe mental illness are not very demanding. Those in rural areas are accepted as handicapped on account of illness and are assigned work that they can easily perform. In the urban setting, they are usually switched to lighter jobs. Generally, work output of these persons is adequate at the lower level of functioning, because of less strenuous, less stress provoking, nondemanding work environments and relationships with colleagues and superiors.

Subjects were rediagnosed basically using the WHO Conversion tables of ICD-9 to ICD-10. Records of symptoms and history at intake were consulted for clarification on the subtype of the broad diagnosis. In this exercise, the case narratives were found to be more useful than the structured schedules. The rater for the ISoS schedules was not blind to the original intake diagnosis; however, retrospective rediagnosis of the cohort on ICD-10 was done by a team of researchers who were not involved in the intake diagnostic process. Nevertheless, the team had access to the entire case record including course and outcome; however, this was deliberately not consulted for diagnosis. On the whole, confidence in the reliability of rediagnosis is high.

In India, mental illness is accepted by the subject and the family members as an affliction beyond the control of the afflicted person. On account of the attribution of mental illness to an external locus of control and, to some extent, a fatalistic attitude, the personal responsibility of the subject to account for the illness was minimized. The family members minimized their demands on and expectations of the patient to the extent of not burdening him or her with responsibilities. In addition, they were less critical and more tolerant of behavioral deviations and deficiencies. Even friends and colleagues pitched in. Many who showed good recovery and adjustment had a limited social network and did not have to deal with many people. Limited but positive interactions helped in recovery. On the other hand, in families where illness was highly stigmatized and considered as an aberration, where the subject was criticized for his or her deficiencies and where expectations were high, the outcome was poor.

Our impression is that it was the positive emotional relationship with supportive and accepting family members that worked as the driving force to recovery from illness. On many occasions, subjects expressed a desire to get well for the sake of family members who depended on them. In India, these conditions in fact are not purposefully created but are natural social institutional forces that help create a more dependent, accepting, tolerant relationship between persons with severe mental illness and their social environment. Thus, it is the interdependent family system in the sociocultural set-up that appeared to be the key factor in recovery—the antithesis of the independent "autonomous" man, a Western value.

Acknowledgments The ISoS was carried out under the guidance of Professor V. K. Varma, Principal Investigator, and Dr. Savita Malhotra, Co-Principal Investigator. Dr. P. J. Santosh and Dr. M. Balaji, psychiatrists, and Dr. Manju Mohanty and Ms. Rajvans Sandhu, psychologists, helped in gathering the data. Dr. A. K. Misra, the senior social worker who had participated in the initial DOSMeD study, helped in planning strategy for the present follow-up.

At this center, ISoS is a follow-up to the previous WHO study, Determinants of Outcome of Severe Mental Disorder (DOSMeD), which generated the intake cohort over a 24-month period, October 1978 to September 1980, and carried out a 2-year follow-up completed in 1982. Professor N. N. Wig (1977–1980) and Professor V. K. Varma (1980–onwards) were the Principal Investigators of DOSMeD. Other research workers included Drs. D. K. Menon, A. K. Misra, P. B. Behere, C. B. Khare, and H. R. Phookun, Ms. Harminder Bedi, and Ms. Mala Khare.

References

Bhide, A. (1982), *Prevalence of Psychiatric Morbidity in a Closed Community in South India.* M.D. Thesis, Bangalore University.

Collins, P., Wig, N. N., Day, R., Varma, V. K., Malhotra, S., Misra, A. K., Schanzer, B., & Susser, E. (1996), Psychosocial and biological aspects of acute brief psychoses in three developing country sites. *Psychiatric Quart.*, 67:177–193.

Dube, K. C. (1970), A study of prevalence and bio-social variables in mental illness in a rural and urban community in Uttar Pradesh, India. *Acta Psychiatr. Scand.*, 46:327.

Elnagar, M. M., Maitra, P., & Rao, M. M. (1971), Mental health in an Indian rural community. *Brit. J. Psychiatry*, 118:499–503.

Ganguli, H. C. (1968a), Prevalence of psychological disorders in an Indian industrial population. Part I. *Ind. J. Med. Res.*, 58:754–760.

——(1968b), Prevalence of psychological disorders in an Indian industrial population. Part II. *J. Med. Res.*, 58: 761–766.

——(1968c), Prevalence of psychological disorders in an Indian industrial population. Part III. *J. Med. Res.*, 58: 767–776.

Gopinath, P. S. (1968), Epidemiology of mental illness of an Indian village. *Trans. All India Inst. Ment. Health*, 8:68.

Indian Council of Medical Research (1988), *Multicentered Collaborative Study of Factors Affecting Course and Outcome of Schizophrenia.* New Delhi: Indian Council of Medical Research.

Isaac, M., & Kapur, R. L. (1980), A cost effectiveness analysis of three different methods of psychiatric case finding in the general population. *Brit. J. Psychiatry*, 137: 540–546.

Jablensky, A., Sartorius, N., Ernberg, G., Anker, M., Korten, A., Cooper, J., Day, R., & Bertelsen, A. (1992), Schizophrenia: Manifestations, incidence and course in different cultures. A World Health Organization ten-country study. *Psycholog. Med.*, 20(suppl.):1–97.

Kapur, R. L. (1973), An illustrative presentation of a population survey on mental disorders—A cross-cultural study in an Indian setting. WHO Seminars on Organization of Mental Health Services. Addis Ababa, EM/SEM DRG MH.

——Kapur, M., & Carstairs, G. M. (1974), Indian psychiatric survey schedule (IPSS). *Soc. Psychiatry*, 9:71–76.

Malhotra, S., Varma, V. K., Misra, A. K., Das, S., Wig, N. N., & Santosh, P. J. (1998), Onset of acute psychotic states in India: A study of sociodemographic, seasonal and biological factors. *Acta Psychiatr. Scand.*, 97:125–131.

Nandi, D. N., Ajmany, S., Ganguli, H., Banerjee, G., Boral, G. C., Ghosh, A., & Sarkar, S. (1975), Psychiatric disorders in a rural community in West Bengal—an epidemiological study. *Ind. J. Psychiatry*, 17:87–89.

——, ——, ——, ——, ——, ——, ——(1976), A clinical evaluation of depressives found in a rural survey in India. *Brit. J. Psychiatry*, 128:523–527.

——Das, N. N., Chaudhari, A., Banerjee, G., Dutta, P., Ghosh, A., & Boral, G. C. (1980), Mental morbidity and urban life. An epidemiological study. *Ind. J. Psychiatry*, 22:324–330.

——Banerjee, G., Boral, G. C., Ganguli, H., Ajmany (Sachdev), S., Ghosh, A., & Sarkar, S. (1979), Socioeconomic status and prevalence of mental disorders in certain rural communities in India. *Acta Psychiatr. Scand.*, 59:267–293.

Overbeck-Wright, A. W. (1921), *Lunacy in India.* London: Baillière, Tindall & Cox.

Padmavathi, R., Rajkumar, S., Kumar, N., Manohanan, A., & Kamath, S. (1987), Prevalence of schizophrenia in an urban community in Madras. *Ind. J. Psychiatry*, 31(3):233–239.

Premarajan, K. C., Danabalan, M., Chandrasekar, R., & Srinivasa, D. K. (1993), Prevalence of psychiatry morbidity in an urban community of Pondicherry. *Ind. J. Psychiatry*, 35(2):99–102.

Rajkumar, S., Padmavathi, R., Thara, R., & Sarada Menon, M. (1993), Incidence of schizophrenia in an urban community in Madras. *Ind. J. Psychiatry*, 35(1):18–21.

Sethi, B. B., Gupta, S. C., & Rajkumar, R. (1967), 300 urban families—A psychiatric study. *Ind. J. Psychiatry*, 9: 280–284.

——, ——Rajkumar, R., & Kumari, P. (1972), A psychiatric survey of 500 rural families. *Ind. J. Psychiatry*, 14:183–196.

Surya, N. C., Dutta, S. P., Gopalkrishna, R., Sundaram, D., & Kutty, J. (1964), Mental morbidity in Pondicherry. *Trans. All Ind. Instit. Ment. Health* (Bangalore), 5:50–61.

Susser, E., Varma, V. K., Mattoo, S. K., Finnerty, M., Mojtabai, R., Tripathi, B. M., Misra, A. K., & Wig, N. N. (1998), Long-term course of acute brief psychosis in a developing country setting. *Brit. J. Psychiatry*, 173: 226–230.

Thacore, V. R. (1973), *Mental Illness in an Urban Community*. Allahabad: Allahabad Publishers.

Varma, V. K. (1989), *Final Report of Severe Mental Disorders. A Prospective Five-year Follow-up Study*. New Delhi: Indian Council of Medical Research.

——Das, M. K. (1995), Mental illness in India: Epidemiology, manifestations and outcome. *Ind. J. Soc. Psychiatry*, 11(1):16–25.

——Brown, A. S., Wig, N. N., Tripathi, B. M., Misra, A. K., Khare, C. B., Phookun, H. R., Menon, D. K., & Susser, E. S. (1997), Effects of level of socio-economic development on course of non-affective psychosis. *Brit. J. Psychiatry*, 171:256–259.

——Wig, N. N., Phookun, H. R., Misra, A. K., Khare, C. B., Tripathi, B. M., Behere, P. B., Yoo, E. S., & Susser, E. S. (1997), First-onset schizophrenia in the community: Relationship of urbanization with onset, early manifestations and typology. *Acta Psychiatr. Scand.*, 96:431–438.

Verghese, A., Beig, A., Senseman, L. A., Sunder Rao, P. S. S., & Benjamin, V. (1973), A social and psychiatric study of representative group of families in Vellore Town. *Ind. J. Med. Res.*, 61:618–620.

Wig, N. N., Varma, V. K., Mattoo, S. K., Behere, P. B., Phookun, H. R., Misra, A. K., Srinivasa Murthy, R., Tripathi, B. M., Menon, D. K., Khandelwal, S. K., & Bedi, H. (1993), An incidence study of schizophrenia in India. *Ind. J. Psychiatry*, 35:11–17.

World Health Organization (1994), *The ICD-10 Classification of Mental and Behavioral Disorders: Conversion Tables between ICD-8, ICD-9, and ICD-10*. Revision 1. (WHO/MNH/92–16. Rev. 1). Geneva, Switzerland: World Health Organization.

Chapter 12

DOSMeD: Dublin, Ireland

Aine Finnerty, Fiona Keogh, Anne O'Grady Walshe, and Dermot Walsh

CULTURAL CONTEXT

Since the late 19th century, there has been preoccupation with major functional psychotic illness in the Irish because of high hospitalization rates for mental illness and because of reportedly similar high rates among the emigrant Irish, particularly in North America. Speculation has centered on whether incidence is higher among the Irish than in other populations and, if so, whether this is due to a high incidence rate and/ or to an abnormally poor outcome. In the 1960s, these concerns led to considerable research through both fieldwork and improved mental health information systems in Ireland. To begin with, critical examination of hospitalization figures revealed artifactual difficulties indicating that hospital-derived data were unreliable; for example, the term *first admission* was not rigorously defined, so that there was a substantial overreporting of first admissions. Thus, as an incidence indicator, first admission was invalid perhaps to a greater degree than in other jurisdictions. Second, traditions and practices established in the 19th century and continued into the 20th ensured that Irish mental hospitals became an indiscriminate repository for social problems. Thus, elderly, mentally handicapped, and destitute people flooded into institutions, mirroring the impoverishment caused by the great Irish famines of the 19th century. The catch-all nature of institutions continued until comparatively recently; in 1963, no less than 16% of psychiatric hospital inpatients were mentally handicapped, not mentally ill. Third, only during the past two decades has accurate diagnostic information (ICD diagnoses) on inpatients become available.

It is not suggested that what is described here is unique to Ireland, but that these factors contributed to hospitalization prevalence rates twice those of its European neighbors. However, when reexamination of inpatient populations was carried out using more rigid diagnostic practices, first admission incidence of schizophrenia, for example, declined substantially. Thus, the explanation for high hospitalization rates in Ireland is largely a structural one: The overgenerous 19th-century supply of asylum places became a vacuum in the face of a population which had declined from approximately 8 million at the time the mental hospital construction program began in the 1830s, to 3 million in the 1960s—and society (no less than nature) abhors a vacuum.

The incidence of schizophrenia in Ireland on a community basis (as distinct from an institutional one) was established in a study based on the Irish Psychiatric Case Registers. Cohorts showed that schizophrenia incidence figures were no greater than those reported elsewhere (Ni Nullain, O'Hare, and Walsh, 1987). Participation in the WHO-coordinated Determinants of Outcome of Severe Mental Disorder Study (DOSMeD) was a logical development of Irish concerns. Follow-up of the incidence cohort from DOSMeD assembled some 15 years ago from two catchment area services, St. Loman's in Dublin and a midland rural Irish county, forms the basis of this report.

Social and Demographic Characteristics

In 1922, the country of Ireland was established by the secession from the United Kingdom of 26 of the 32 counties of the island of Ireland. Six northern counties remained within the United Kingdom. Politically autonomous, the two geopolitical entities share a common border but have no political boundary with any other nation. Ireland geographically consists of one large urban conurbation, Dublin, with a population of 1.2 million, and aside from Cork, Limerick, and Galway, each having populations of under a quarter of a million, there is no other urban setting of more than 100,000 persons. Although Ireland remains a strongly agricultural country, as with most other Western European nations, the agricultural population has been declining, the urban population growing, and industrialization increasing—often through the attraction of foreign multinationals to the country by reason of an extensive and educated workforce and, in the European context at least, low production costs. Much recent industrial investment has been in small specialized sectors such as the computer industry; coincidentally, there has also been growth in employment in the financial services sector.

Although still among the poorer Western European countries, Ireland's economy has performed very well in recent years with low interest rates, a stable economy, and, even though governments have changed, a relatively stable political system—mainly of the center right. Despite relative affluence, unemployment remains a problem, running at approximately 15% in recent years. The nation's population has tended to be generally youthful, with 45% currently under age 25 and with 12.5% aged 65 or over, a relatively low proportion of elderly. Indications are that during the 21st century, the number of elderly will increase substantially. High fertility, that had been an average of four children per dyadic pair, has recently started to decline. The Irish population is ethnically and religiously homogeneous, with 95% of the population at least nominally Roman Catholic. Until recently, the majority of Roman Catholics were practicing, but there has been some decline in churchgoing (particularly among young people).

Ireland has long been a conservative country in terms of substance abuse, recourse to suicide, and sexual behavior. With increasing "Europeanization" or "internationalization" over the past two decades, much of this has changed. Although the Irish had generally been perceived as a hard drinking nation, this impression was fallacious at least within Ireland, where consumption of alcohol was among the lowest in Europe. From the early 1960s to the early 1990s, however, per capita consumption of alcohol in the population aged over 15 years more than doubled, from just over 5 liters per person in 1961 to just over 11 liters in 1994, moving Ireland into 11th place in mean alcohol consumption in Europe and equaling that of neighboring countries, the United Kingdom and Denmark. Suicide rates in Ireland had been traditionally low, and although underreporting had been substantial, this wasn't simply an artifact of the recording system. Official statistics on mortality rates from suicide—which in the 1950s had been reported as 2.5 deaths per 100,000 population—are now approximately 10 per 100,000 population. Underreporting has been eliminated, and the real rate of suicide has approximately doubled. To a substantial degree, this increase has been among young men, a trend which is not uncommon among other European countries, and Irish suicide rates are now very similar to those in the United Kingdom. Likewise, young Irish people have traditionally been conservative in their sexual behavior, and pregnancy termination in Ireland remains illegal. However, evidence suggests that sexual mores have liberalized, and the pregnancy termination rate among Irish women (who obtain their abortions legally in the United Kingdom) is now not much lower than that of the indigenous British.

There are two official languages in Ireland: Irish and English. Although Irish is spoken as the everyday language in some isolated Western rural localities, English is, for practical purposes, the ordinary working language.

The Catchment Areas

The St. Loman's catchment area is a predominantly working class, almost exclusively urban area of 250,000 in West Dublin. Much of the catchment area consists of new, almost all publicly funded housing estates that have replaced green fields and are occupied by newly married or cohabiting couples with a very high index of unemployment—as high as 50%. There is a great deal of social chaos, petty criminality, and social deprivation. The older and more settled parts of the catchment area with elder folk, for example, and where privately owned units prevail, are much less deprived and much more socially cohesive with fewer overt social problems. Many housing areas have a sense of community in that they focus centrally around a church or parish, shopping areas, complexes, or schools. Educational opportunities in the catchment area (as well as in the nation) have improved considerably since the mid-1970s. Formerly, very few people would have completed a primary education (terminating at age 15); now, however, the majority have completed secondary education (up to age 18), and many have gone on to the third level, enrolling in university or technical courses.

County Westmeath, the second catchment area in this study, is a rural midland Irish county of approximately 62,000 persons. Two towns, each with approximately 8000 persons, account for 16,000 of the total urban population of 28,000. The remainder of the community is made up of rural dwellers who are engaged in farming activities of one kind or another.

MENTAL HEALTH CARE IN IRELAND

The district lunatic asylums, built in the mid-19th century, served catchment areas largely identical to those today; however, through a national policy of sectorization, a pivotal element in mental health care delivery, catchment areas of approximately 100,000 people have been subdivided into smaller geographic sectors, each staffed by its own multidisciplinary team (at least multidisciplinary in aspiration, if not always in achievement). The principle of providing mental health care near to a patient's residence has been achieved by the setting up in each geographic area of mental health centers and sector headquarters, which usually incorporate a day hospital and where mental health workers are based. Since 1970, successive policy documents have urged integration of specialist mental health services with primary care services and have recommended that inpatient care be delivered from small psychiatric units in general hospitals. Currently, following the sale, closure, or partial closure of the parent mental hospitals, over half the catchment inpatient services are located in general hospitals. It is estimated that early in the 21st century all inpatient mental health care will be so delivered, and all of the 19th-century mental hospitals will have been closed.

Concurrent has been the growth of community alternatives to hospitalization. Day places (a combination of day hospital and day center places) and community-based residences for mentally ill persons are each provided at an average rate close to 1 per 1000 of population. The intent is to increase this ratio to 1.5 places per 1000. Also being developed are specialized services including child psychiatry, adolescent psychiatry, psychiatry of later life, forensic psychiatry, rehabilitation psychiatry, substance abuse psychiatry, and liaison psychiatry within general hospitals; however, specialization does not override the primary commitment to the geographic delivery of care.

Health services in Ireland, including the voluntary sector, are financed by a central agency, the Department of Health, that distributes funds to eight health boards which have the responsibility of running local services, including psychiatry. The mental health services are comprehensive in that the full range of mental health services, institutional and community, are provided by the same administration—a seamless service unlike many other European mental health administrations where there is a dichotomy between the institutional and the community services—that greatly facilitates the movement of patients and staff, as well as finances, among the various service elements.

Private psychiatric services, which largely consist of two Dublin-based traditional psychiatric hospitals of approximately 200 beds each with little by way of community facilities, are funded in the main by state-run voluntary health insurance which pays for hospital maintenance and for medical and drug treatments. Recent European Union regulations have opened up the health insurance market to outsiders who compete with the national voluntary health insurance scheme.

The Westmeath Psychiatric Service

Westmeath is one of two counties comprising the Westmeath/Longford mental health service in the Irish midlands. The catchment area comprises three sectors, two of which are in and serve County Westmeath; each contains a mental health center and sector headquarters out of which the mental health teams operate. The inpatient component operates from a typical Victorian psychiatric hospital of some architectural elegance, the patient capacity of which has been much reduced. Plans include the provision of inpatient service in the local general hospital, at which point the psychiatric hospital will close.

The St. Loman's Psychiatric Service

The St. Loman's service had its origin in the late 1960s with the sectorization of psychiatric services in the Dublin area catering to approximately 250,000 of the population of Dublin city and county. St. Loman's Hospital, the inpatient base of the service, a former tuberculosis sanitarium built in the 1950s, became a 200-bed inpatient psychiatric unit in the 1960s. Reduced to approximately 95 beds, St. Loman's was finally closed in 1999; inpatient accommodation for this catchment area will be transferred to a 50-bed psychiatric unit in a newly built general hospital.

The catchment area is subdivided into a number of sectors, each sector served by a consultant-led, multidisciplinary team. The service provides post-graduate training in psychiatry for medical graduates, nurses, and other staff, which includes social work, psychology, and occupational therapy. There is a close relationship between the specialist psychiatric service and primary medical care teams. General practitioners are encouraged to make referrals and to consult. A number of community and voluntary organizations such as the Mental Health Association and the Schizophrenia Association of Ireland operate in the catchment area.

PSYCHIATRIC EPIDEMIOLOGY IN IRELAND

Psychiatric epidemiology in Ireland can be said to have had its beginnings in 1967 with the establishment of the Medico-Social Research Board (renamed the Health Research Board), a government funded, statutory body which investigates medicosocial problems to help in the development of social-health policy. The Mental Health Section of the Board develops psychiatric epidemiology. As a first step, a psychiatric recording and reporting system was established and since the 1960s, has recorded every admission to and discharge from (or death in) every psychiatric inpatient facility, public and private, within the country. Each entry is accompanied by substantial demographic and clinical data. From these data, the Health Research Board publishes annual reports on the activities of Irish psychiatric hospitals.

The Health Research Board has established two psychiatric case registers covering all phases of psychiatric care (outpatient, day hospital, day center, and community residential accommodation): one for a three-county area in the east, middle, and west of Ireland and the second for the St. Loman's catchment area. Together they cover approximately one-tenth of the national population and have been the basis of considerable epidemiological research: the intercounty variation in Irish psychiatric hospitalization rates (Walsh and Walsh, 1968), the impact of season of birth on the incidence of schizophrenia (O'Hare, Walsh, and Torrey, 1980), and the prevalence and incidence of schizophrenia (Ni Nuallain, O'Hare, and Walsh, 1987, 1990). The last study did not sustain the previously held belief, based on first admissions, of a raised incidence of schizophrenia in Ireland. A study of prevalence produced the important finding that over half the patients identified from case register and other inpatient sources did not meet the cut-off point for caseness, suggesting that the continued hospitalization of symptomatically recovered cases has given rise to the mistaken impression that the prevalence of schizophrenia is unduly high. Substantial differences between cases ascertained by hospital admission data and those arrived at by standardized diagnostic interview techniques have been pointed out. Register studies of incidence and prevalence were supplemented by key informant community studies (Buckley, Ni Nuallain, O'Hare, and Walsh, 1989) that did not find significant numbers of incidence or prevalence cases missed by the case register. A 2-year outcome follow-up study of schizophrenia, based on a cohort of first contact schizophrenic patients identified by the Three County Case Register in the mid-1970s, was conducted to assess symptomatic and social outcome. Only 14% of the cohort enjoyed full remission at the 2-year follow-up period; 19% experienced partial remission; over one-third had at least one subsequent episode; and another third were still in the episode of inclusion (Walsh, O'Hare, Ni Nuallain, O'Connor, and McHugh, 1991).

During the 1980s, Irish/United States collaboration and United States funding made it possible to extend epidemiological studies in schizophrenia through extensive proband recruitment from the Three County Case Register. Because one of the case register counties, County Roscommon, contributed a substantial number of schizophrenic probands and a number of affective patients, this study became known as the Roscommon Family Study. Control probands from the general population in the same county were randomly selected, and first degree relatives were identified. Both proband and relative groups living in Ireland and in the United Kingdom were then clinically examined in standardized fashion by trained field research workers. The study examined many parameters of the familial distribution of schizophrenia and like conditions, with particular emphasis on Schizophrenia Spectrum Disorder (Kendler, McGuire, Gruenberg, and Walsh, 1994). The Roscommon Family Study led naturally to studies of the genetic epidemiology of schizophrenia based on families multiply affected by schizophrenia throughout Ireland. Early results have already been published (Straub et al., 1995), and work is continuing on genetic analysis.

The research team here has participated in a number of WHO mental health projects since the 1960s including the Mental Health Services in Pilot Study

Areas project, and a member has acted as a consultant to the European Regional Office for many years. The research team for ISoS consists of the project director, a field psychiatrist researcher, and a field social researcher with administrative and data processing participation from the Health Research Board.

METHODS USED IN THE DUBLIN STUDY

Defining the ISoS Cohort

In 1978, the first subjects were selected and assessed following the DOSMeD protocol. The cohort was drawn from those in contact with the psychiatric hospital, mental health centers, outpatient service, and psychiatric social workers from a catchment area incorporating the St. Loman's and the Westmeath mental health services. Eighty-three subjects passed the initial DOSMeD screening and 67 were included in the original incidence study. Three subjects were excluded from the ISoS followup.

Case-Finding

The St. Loman's Hospital Case Register records all contacts with St. Loman's psychiatric service, both at inpatient and outpatient levels. The social researcher involved in the study (AF) initially consulted the St. Loman's Case Register to establish the last known address of each subject. In the case of the subjects from the rural area, the medical records department of the local psychiatric hospital was consulted. Following this, AF made contact with all community psychiatric nurses in the relevant catchment area. Where the subject was still in contact with the service, AF made contact by telephone or house call. Following an explanation of the study, an interview was scheduled with those subjects who agreed to participate.

In the case of those subjects no longer in contact with the service, the social researcher attempted to contact the subjects at their last known address. Of the 65 subjects, only 23 still resided at the original address. A variety of means was used to trace those who had changed residence including consulting the local telephone directory, checking all case records, post office records, and local authority housing lists; interviewing outpatient secretarial staff; and in several cases visiting the subject's last known address and asking if the present occupant had any knowledge of the whereabouts of the previous occupant.

Despite these efforts, 12 subjects were untraceable; 8 subjects had died; and 33 were found to be living at different addresses. The effort required to locate cases ranged from minimal, in the case of subjects still in contact with the psychiatric service and known to all key personnel, to very difficult, requiring painstaking and repeated contacts (see Table 12.1).

The following illustrate some of the difficulties encountered in finding cases:

1. A number of subjects had moved several times within the Dublin area. Efforts to trace one such subject involved unsuccessful attempts at contact by letter and telephone, inspection of the local authority housing lists, and contact with the post office.
2. One subject had not been in contact with the local psychiatric service since 1978. He lived at the outer extremities of the catchment area in an isolated cottage in the Dublin mountains. The social researcher and psychiatrist spent a half day driving along an unmarked track, eventually locating the subject in a barely habitable barn-type dwelling where conditions were extremely primitive. The subject, unkempt and disheveled, had a hostile demeanor. Although no longer in contact with the psychiatric service, he appeared to be quite unwell. He was unwilling to consider participating in the study. As the

TABLE 12.1 Dublin Center Subjects. Number of Contacts

	Interviewed	*Deceased*	*Refused*	*Untraceable*	*Total*
Subjects	37	8	8	12	65
No. of Phone Calls	22	0	8	10	40
No. of House Calls	105	9	13	25	152
Letters/Staff	62	18	16	24	120
Total No. of Contacts	189	27	37	59	312

whereabouts of his next of kin were also unknown, regrettably no further information was available on this subject.

3. The most unusual example of case-finding was that of a subject who had moved from the catchment area to another part of Dublin some years prior to follow-up. All attempts to contact him at his last known address were unsuccessful. While interviewing another subject for the study, the psychiatrist noticed a painting of the untraceable subject. Through this contact, the subject was eventually traced but unfortunately refused to participate in the study.

Data-Gathering Procedures

All patient assessments were carried out by the same psychiatrist (AO'GW). All family interviews were conducted by the social researcher (AF). The Diagnostic Schedule Scoresheet was completed by a senior investigator (DW) and the psychiatrist (AO'GW) who conducted the subject assessments. The interviews were carried out in a variety of settings, as follows: subject's own house, 21; hospital, 3; day hospital/health center, 9; and telephone, 1. Nineteen informants were interviewed. Thirteen subjects refused to allow access to informants. In some cases, this was because their next of kin were unaware of their psychiatric history. A further three informants were unwilling to participate, and in seven cases, no relative or other informant was available. Time taken for interviews with the subject ranged from 1½ to 4 hours. Interviews with relatives-informants took ½ to 3½ hours.

All death certificates for the entire country are located in the Office of Births, Deaths and Marriages in Dublin city. By contacting this register, death certificates for all eight deceased subjects were obtained and the cause of death recorded. Where possible, the relatives of deceased subjects were interviewed, and case notes were consulted for additional information. Finally, the two psychiatrists met to assign a current, lifetime, and original rediagnosis to each subject, including deceased subjects and untraceable subjects.

RESULTS

Baseline and Early Follow-Up

Of the 67 subjects from the original sample selected in 1978, 37 (55%) were successfully followed up, 8 subjects had died (12%), and 22 (33%) were lost to follow-up. Of the 22 patients who were lost to follow-up, 12 had moved away and could not be traced, 8 refused to be interviewed, and 2 had had some contact prior to entry and were excluded from follow-up.

Gender and Age

There were slightly more males than females in the Dublin cohort at the beginning of the study (54% versus 46%). Similar numbers of males and females were either successfully followed up or lost to follow-up; fewer females died. Most of the sample was born in the two decades 1940 to 1949 and 1950 to 1959.

Mode of Onset and Diagnosis

In the baseline cohort, 52% of subjects had an onset of greater than one month, with 33% having a more acute onset of 1 week up to 1 month; 15% were missing onset. There was a larger proportion of subjects in the greater than 1 month mode of onset group in Dublin (60%) at follow-up, compared to 44% or less in most of the other centers. This difference in mode of onset between the Dublin and other DOSMeD followed-up cohorts may be important as mode of onset has been shown to be related to outcome (Jablensky et al., 1992). In the ISoS study, for the entire DOSMeD cohort, 57% of those with onset <1 month had never been psychotic in the last 2 years; for those with onset >1 month, the figure was 47%.

Four diagnostic categories accounted for 90% of the baseline cohort: schizoaffective disorder 25%, paranoid schizophrenia 24%, hebephrenic schizophrenia 21%, and acute schizophrenia-like disorder 19%. Most of those with hebephrenic schizophrenia were followed up, as were two-thirds of the schizoaffective group; but fewer than half of those with paranoid and acute schizophrenia-like illness were available at follow-up.

The group of subjects who were followed up is somewhat different from the other centers on diagnostic composition. The Dublin cohort had a substantially higher proportion of subjects with a schizoaffective diagnosis (30%) compared to less than 10% in most other centers; more subjects with a diagnosis of hebephrenic schizophrenia than all centers except for Nagasaki; and fewer subjects with a diagnosis of paranoid schizophrenia than over half of the centers. It was specified in the inclusion criteria that a schizoaffective diagnosis should be included in the selected cohort, but it remains unclear why the proportion in Dublin was higher than in other centers at the point of inclusion. The center closest to Dublin both culturally and in terms of service provision and operation is Nottingham, yet these two alive cohorts differ substantially, with two-thirds of the Nottingham subjects being male (compared to 49% in Dublin), and 4% having a diagnosis of schizoaffective disorder (compared to 30% in Dublin). Unfortunately, this precludes any in-depth comparisons between the two centers as both diagnosis and gender are related to outcome.

Pattern of Course at Early Follow-Up

The analysis of the short-term pattern of course shows that the largest single group was made up of subjects with an incomplete remission, comprising almost one-half of the cohort (42%). Almost one-third of subjects had a complete remission and a further 12% were continuously psychotic; in 13% information was missing. A similar distribution is seen in the alive subjects who were followed up in the study. The pattern of course at early follow-up for the Dublin cohort lies somewhere in the middle of the other centers, with some having a poorer short-term outcome (for example, Moscow, Honolulu, and Nagasaki) and the rest showing a somewhat better short-term outcome.

ALIVE SUBJECTS

Symptomatology

A little over one-third (37%) of subjects were in the recovered group as classified by the Bleuler Severity of Symptoms Scale, with a further 31% reporting mild symptoms. However, one-fifth of subjects reported moderate and 11% reported severe symptoms at follow-up. The Dublin center had one of the lowest proportions of recovered subjects (only Nagasaki was lower) but had the largest proportion in the mild symptom group. Thus, for Dublin subjects, it seems that while relatively few made a complete recovery, many have only mild symptoms at follow-up.

An examination of the Global Assessment of Functioning Scale for Symptomatology (GAF-S) mean score shows that the Dublin cohort (60.0) is quite similar to three other DOSMeD centers; three are much higher and one is slightly higher. A slightly different picture is seen on examining the distribution of GAF-S scores. Twenty-nine percent of the Dublin cohort suffered from serious symptoms (GAF-S scores <51), with a further 29% having no significant symptoms (GAF-S scores >70). Thus, the largest group in the Dublin cohort had symptoms in the moderate range (43%). The pattern was very different across DOSMeD centers: Four had proportionally fewer subjects in the serious symptom range; three had proportionally more.

A different gender breakdown was also seen on GAF-S scores for the Dublin cohort compared to the DOSMeD cohort. The mean score for females was lower than males in Dublin (58 versus 62), and there were more females in the serious symptoms category (32% versus 25%), both indicating more serious symptomatology for female Dublin subjects. A contrasting picture was observed in the DOSMeD cohort where the mean score was lower for males (64 versus 67), and more males were in the serious symptoms category (24% versus 22%), denoting serious symptomatology for males overall, although the gender difference in the entire cohort is not very pronounced. The trend of psychotic symptoms over the entire study period showed that, in common with most other centers, symptoms for the majority of Dublin subjects (54%) were prominent in the first third of the study period only.

Course of the Illness

In the 2 years prior to the follow-up interview almost one-third of the subjects (31%) had no psychotic episodes, 44% were continuously psychotic, and 19% were classified as episodic. The Dublin cohort had one of the highest proportions of continuously psychotic subjects in this 2-year period compared to the other DOSMeD centers (only Nagasaki was higher and Honolulu similar), and one of the lowest proportions of subjects with no psychotic episodes. Considerably more females than males were not psychotic in this period (37% versus 24%) while even proportions of males and females were in the not psychotic group in the DOSMeD cohort (53 and 50%, respectively). The pattern of course since the first interview for Dublin subjects shows the same proportion in the continuously psychotic and episodic categories (46%), a pattern not seen in the other centers (except Nagasaki and Honolulu), where many more subjects were classified as episodic. In spite of this relatively poor course of illness, the overall time trend for Dublin subjects shows 74% in the much better or somewhat better categories, one of the highest proportions in any center, with only 9% scoring as somewhat worse. A gender difference was also observed in this outcome with more females having a much better or somewhat better time trend than males (79 and 69%), while no females had a somewhat worse rating compared to 19% of males. Overall, for Dublin subjects in terms of symptomatology, females either do very well or very poorly, while males are represented at all points on the spectrum.

Reevaluation of Baseline Diagnosis

At the completion of the follow-up interviews, the two psychiatrists on the research team (DW and AO'GW) met to reevaluate the baseline diagnosis. Using only the information available at the first interview, all subjects were rediagnosed. There was no identifiable source of bias in this rediagnosis process as similar baseline information was available for all alive subjects. Of the 20 subjects with schizophrenia, 60% were reclassified as schizophrenia, with four diagnosed as other psychotic, two as bipolar/depression, and two as schizoaffective disorder. Of the 11 subjects with a diagnosis of schizoaffective disorder at baseline, only one received a reclassification of schizoaffective disorder, with five rediagnosed as schizophrenia, three as bipolar/depression, one as other psychotic, and one as acute schizophrenia-like disorder. Thus, the diagnostic difference evident between the Dublin cohort and others at baseline with respect to schizoaffective disorder may be somewhat spurious as most of those so diagnosed received a different diagnosis following the reevaluation exercise. Of the five subjects with a diagnosis of acute schizophrenia-like disorder at baseline, three were reclassified as schizophrenia, one as schizoaffective disorder, and one as bipolar/depression. Thus, the largest group following the reevaluation of the baseline diagnosis was schizophrenia (54%), followed by bipolar/depression (19%), other psychotic (14%), schizoaffective disorder (11%), and acute schizophrenia-like disorder (3%).

Living Arrangements

At the follow-up interview, most of the Dublin cohort were living with family or friends in the community (81%), and a further 11% were living alone. Almost half were in marital relationships (49% married or cohabiting), with 35% never married. Thus, for many of the subjects living with family it was their own family and not their parents they were living with. The Dublin cohort was exceeded only by the Chandigarh cohorts in respect to the numbers living with family or friends, perhaps reflecting the extended family or informal support structures which exist in the two countries. Four of the centers had no subjects living in supervised accommodation, compared to 8% of Dublin subjects. This may be more indicative of the availability of such accommodation in each country than of differences in subjects. This pattern of living arrangements for Dublin subjects was reflected in the 2 years prior to the follow-up interview, with most (72%) living independently throughout, and only 6% having no independent living in this time period, and also for the entire study period with 89% of the cohort in independent living for over 90% of the time.

Three subjects (8%) spent some time in the previous 2 years either homeless or vagrant. In total, four subjects spent less than 5% of the entire study period homeless—three males and one female. One subject spent some time in prison in the 2 years prior to the follow-up interview, with a further three subjects (all male) spending short periods of time in prison over the entire 15-year study period. These low rates of homelessness and time in prison are seen in all the DOSMeD centers, with the exception of Honolulu.

Work

Most of the Dublin subjects were unemployed in the 2 years prior to the follow-up interview (65%), with only 35% being employed at best part-time for this period, evenly split between males and females. This was the lowest rate of employment in the DOSMeD centers. For most of the subjects who had been employed full time for more than 12 months, their work performance was judged good to very good. Nine subjects (24%, all female) had been engaged in full-time household work in the 2-year period and the performance of most was reported as good to very good. The majority of Dublin subjects (51%) received a disability pension for the entire 2 years prior to follow-up. With the exception of Prague, this was the highest proportion in all the DOSMeD centers.

Social Disability

Overall social functioning in the month prior to follow-up was assessed on the Global Assessment of Functioning Scale for disability (GAF-D). The mean GAF-D score was 61.3, similar to three other DOSMeD centers with means around 61, with the two Chandigarh cohorts, and Moscow reporting higher means (denoting better functioning), and Nagasaki and Rochester showing lower means. The mean GAF-D score was lower for males compared to females (58 vs. 65) in Dublin and in all the DOSMeD centers (62 vs. 66), reflecting poorer social functioning in males.

On the Disability Assessment Schedule (DAS), overall social functioning was rated poor to severe for 43% of subjects, one of the higher proportions in all the DOSMeD centers. This evaluation is somewhat skewed in that it was not reported for a significant number of subjects in some centers, and so it is difficult to interpret this finding. Because there were few interviews with relatives, 43% of DAS ratings for Dublin subjects were missing. The trend of disability over the 15-year study period showed that for one-third of Dublin subjects (34%) disability was most prominent for the first 5 years of the study only. This was slightly lower than most of the other centers, excepting Moscow (much lower at 17%), and both Chandigarh cohorts (which was much higher at 58%). Twenty-nine percent of subjects had prominent disability for the entire study period, a slightly higher rate than Nagasaki, Nottingham, and Rochester, and much higher than the remainder of the DOSMeD cohorts.

Violence and Suicide

Only one subject (male) attempted suicide in the 2 years prior to interview, and there was no record of any assaults. In the entire study period, five subjects attempted suicide, and three subjects were recorded as having committed an assault. The Dublin cohort had the lowest rate of assaults compared to all other DOSMeD centers and one of the lowest attempted suicide rates.

Medications

In the 2 years prior to the follow-up, three-quarters of the subjects had been on neuroleptic medication for most of the time; only 11% were never on neuroleptics during that time. This pattern is similar only to Nagasaki (84 and 7%, respectively) and presents an atypical pattern in comparison with the remainder of the DOSMeD centers. This pattern is repeated in an examination of neuroleptic medication over the entire study period, with most Dublin subjects being on this medication for most of the time (78%) and the remainder being prescribed neuroleptics for some of the time. Again, this pattern is seen in Nagasaki but not elsewhere.

Hospitalization

Most of the subjects had not been in the hospital in the 2 years prior to follow-up (72%). Two subjects spent those 2 years in the hospital, and the remaining eight (22%) were in the hospital for fewer than 12 months. This represents a low rate of hospitalization in common with most other DOSMeD centers. (The exceptions were Honolulu and Nagasaki, where over 20% of subjects were hospitalized for the entire 2-year period.) An examination of time spent in the hospital or in a supervised residence over the entire study period shows that the majority of Dublin subjects spent less than 5% of this period (42%) or were never (17%) institutionalized for the 15-year study period. No subjects spent more than 50% of the time in the hospital, and only one spent 26 to 50% of the time in the hospital. These low rates of hospitalization were seen in some, though not all, DOSMeD centers. Again, the exceptions were Honolulu and Nagasaki, with 28 and 39% of their subjects, respectively, hospitalized for more than 25% of the entire period. Hospitalization for Dublin subjects was most prominent in the first 5 years of the study period only (46%), a pattern with at least this high a percentage also seen in most other centers.

DECEASED SUBJECTS

Eight subjects from the original Dublin ISoS cohort died before completion of the study, accounting for 12% of the cohort. Six males and two females died, the mean age at death was 35.9 years. The Dublin subjects showed a significantly increased death rate in comparison to the rest of the population with a standardized mortality ratio (SMR) of 4.10. Males accounted for this significant difference with an SMR of 5.14 compared to the female SMR of 2.55, which did not differ significantly from the general population. Of the eight deaths, five were suicides and three were of natural causes—myocardial infarction, subarachnoid hemorrhage, and septicemia.

DISCUSSION

To some extent, the results of the follow-up were disappointing in that only 37 subjects (55% of the original in take) were successfully followed up and evaluated

15 years later. Of those unavailable at the expiration of the follow-up period, 8 were deceased, 8 were traced but refused to cooperate, 12 were untraceable, and 2 were excluded. However, it was possible to obtain information, clinical and social, from case notes and other documentary evidence, from relatives, and from professional careers. The mean follow-up time for each of the first three groups was as follows: deceased, 3.9 years (range 0–7); refusals, 6.3 years (range 0–16); untraced, 3.5 years (range 0–12). In the case of the deceased subjects, the death certificate relating to each of them was obtained from the General Registrar's Office so it was possible to determine the mode of death. In relation to those untraced, it is possible that some may have died, but since we were unable to ascertain whether this was the case, it was not possible to determine the cause of death. Because of the availability of data on the deceased, the refusals, and the untraced, it was possible to supply information for most of the variables studied on short-term follow-up for the entire group. Obviously, such data were not available for the entire period of follow-up.

For 12 of the subjects, a current correct address could not be identified, possibly reflecting the social characteristics of the catchment area with a highly mobile population living in rented accommodation—the mobility being within Dublin city, within Ireland, and between Ireland and the United Kingdom and continental Europe. The high refusal rate was surprising when compared with the much more compliant behavior of rural Irish subjects as evidenced from the Roscommon Family Study (Kendler et al., 1994). Lower cooperation rates may be more characteristic of the Dublin area, or it may be that the very long follow-up period created difficulties. Many subjects had not been in contact with the psychiatric services for some time, and, for purposes of the follow-up interview, were approached by people with whom they had never been in contact. It is also noteworthy that some of the refusers were obviously not well and that their refusal might have been a consequence of their disturbed mental state.

The loss of over 40% of the intake cohort raises serious difficulties in interpretation. Can it be that those who were lost to follow-up have had a more favorable outcome than those traced? Is it likely that more of the socially upwardly mobile patients have left the catchment area than remain in it, or does outward migration simply reflect migration to other impoverished center city areas or local authority housing estates? Greater proportions of the lost to follow-up or untraced group had acute onsets, and it may be hypothesized that such individuals had better prognosis and were therefore more likely to move away from the catchment area than those with insidious onsets and poorer outcomes. Likewise, some of those with acute onsets and good outcomes may have figured among the refusals who, because of their recovery, were not anxious to be reminded that they had been ill. An additional important finding in terms of representativeness is that there are no gender differences either in the total sample or in those followed up—surprising, in view of the preponderance of males with schizophrenia in Ireland and elsewhere—and so, once again, the question of the representativeness of the Dublin sample is raised.

Of the 67 subjects comprising the original cohort, all but 4 qualified for an ICD-9 schizophrenic diagnosis (including 17 given a schizoaffective diagnosis and 13 given an acute schizophrenia-like diagnosis). At rediagnosis on the successfully traced 37 patients, there were now 13 subjects with a nonschizophrenia diagnosis (included 6 classified as other psychotic and 7 as bipolar/depression); of the original 24 with a schizophrenia diagnosis, 4 were now schizoaffective, 1 was acute schizophrenia-like, and the remainder were schizophrenia. The reason for the conversion may well reside in the inclusion criteria which allowed in psychotic, but not necessarily schizophrenically psychotic, subjects. Comparison of rediagnosis with the DOSMeD cohort as a whole showed the Dublin cohort to have fewer acute schizophrenia-like cases (2.7% compared with 16.2%). The Irish cohort, on the other hand, had a slightly higher proportion of affective disorder cases (19 vs. 15%) on rediagnosis. Both for the entire period and the last 2 years, the Irish sample outcome was significantly worse in relation to the proportions continuously ill (with nearly twice as many in this category for both time periods), and, for the last 2 years, the proportion of individuals psychotic. In addition, the Dublin subjects had lower mean global functioning than the DOSMeD subjects as a whole, although this difference was not as great as the illness differences.

There was a greater tendency for Dublin subjects to improve symptomatically over the follow-up period compared with DOSMeD, with only 9% being worse at the end of the assessment period than at the beginning. Outcome by rediagnosis was as expected for Dublin subjects: with a smaller proportion of schizophrenic subjects never psychotic in the last 2 years than was true of bipolar/depression subjects; none of those with schizoaffective disorder met this criterion. However, it must be remembered that the numbers in the schizoaffective and bipolar categories are very small. Still, these findings are substantiated by outcomes in the Roscommon Family Study, where schizophrenic probands had far worse outcomes than did bipolar and unipolar depression cases. It must be noted that this latter study did, however, differentiate between good and poor outcome in schizoaffective disorder, and it may be that the four subjects in this category were, by chance, poor outcome cases.

As regards disability in the past month, because there were no available informants for almost half of the Dublin subjects, information is missing. Of those for whom information is available, none was regarded as having an excellent outcome on global evaluation. Forty-three percent of Dublin subjects were evaluated as having poor, very poor, or severe outcomes compared with 32% of DOSMeD subjects. On employment, Dublin subjects compared unfavorably with DOSMeD as a whole with only slightly more than one-third being employed at some point in the past 2 years compared with over half of DOSMeD subjects; however, this may reflect the high unemployment situation in the catchment area rather than any difference in social outcome.

Two important differences in living arrangements were observed for the Dublin cohort compared to most of the other centers. The Dublin cohort had one of the highest proportions of subjects living with family or friends (81%). The concern has been expressed that this does not represent independent living as such, but rather some form of sheltered accommodation. As this aspect of the living arrangements was not assessed, this concern remains speculative. It is more likely to be true, perhaps, in the situation where an individual is living with parents; however, half the Dublin subjects who lived with family, lived in their own marital family, which suggests a high degree of independent living. A further 8% of the Dublin cohort lived in supervised accommodation, again higher than most other centers. It is likely, however, that this represents the availability or lack of such accommodation in the centers as much as the functioning of the individuals concerned. The use of these measures—living arrangements and independent living—as outcome measures is open to question as they reflect so many other factors within the service and culture of a particular country that they do not necessarily denote good or poor outcome.

Dublin subjects had the lowest assault rate and one of the lowest suicide rates compared to other DOSMeD centers. In relation to medication, most of the Dublin subjects were taking neuroleptic medication for most of the study period, a pattern seen only in one other center. However, Dublin subjects had a fairly low rate of hospitalization over the study period, which may in some part be due to the medication.

An examination of deceased subjects as an independent group has not been particularly fruitful given that only eight of the Dublin cohort figured in this category. Nevertheless, they did comprise 12% of the cohort, and of the eight, five died from suicide, comprising almost 7% of the entire cohort. It must be remembered, however, that there is no indication of how many of the untraced subjects may have died. The proportion of suicides among traced Irish subjects was higher by one-half than that seen across all DOSMeD subjects.

One of the difficulties in using occupational–employment status as an outcome measure is exemplified by the Dublin Center. In the area from which subjects were drawn, unemployment was rife, and in some parts of the catchment area (particularly for males) was as high as 50%. In such a competitive job environment, people with disabilities are less likely to be able to secure a job. A combination of high unemployment and the ready availability of disability benefits seems to result in poor outcomes for the Dublin cohort compared to some other areas, when in fact they rather represent the context—the socioeconomic condition—of the study in Dublin.

The movement of some previously schizophrenic subjects to the affective category may simply reflect the broad nature of the inclusion criteria of DOSMeD, which admitted a substantial number of affective psychotic subjects. However, a greater proportion of Dublin subjects (approximately half of those alive, deceased, or lost to follow-up) had an insidious onset and an illness history of greater than 1 month. On short-term follow-up, only a minority proved to have had one episode with a complete remission. On the other hand, a higher proportion of short-term follow-up patients had a poorer outcome with upwards of two-thirds of alive patients having continuous illness or episodic illness with incomplete remission since onset. This also held true for the deceased and lost to follow-up categories. But it is interesting that the overall symptomatological time trend for Dublin patients is toward improvement, contrasting with discrepant findings for DOSMeD as a whole on this particular parameter.

Comparing the mode of onset of the Dublin cohort with the DOSMeD group as a whole shows a clear preponderance of insidious onsets in the Dublin group, and this must go some way to accounting for its relatively poor outcome. A more recent analysis of the DOSMeD data (Craig, Siegel, Hopper, Lin, and Sartorius, 1997) disaggregates developed and developing countries and shows that the developed centers can themselves be divided into good and poor outcome groups. With this reexamination Dublin falls into the poor outcome group of the developed centers, with only 38% having a good outcome as measured by pattern of course compared to 60% in Nottingham, the center socioculturally closest to Dublin.

The overall outcome for Dublin subjects was quite good with only a substantial proportion (44%) being continuously psychotic over the last 2 years of follow-up, and the remainder having partial or complete remissions. Similarly in terms of symptomatology, one-third were scored as recovered with another third having mild symptoms. While these outcomes are among the worst in the DOSMeD centers, as were the disability scores, which were quite poor for the Dublin subjects, on other outcome measures (time spent homeless, assaults by subjects, and suicide rate) they were better than most other centers. It may be that the loss of many Dublin subjects and the composition of the follow-up group, particularly in terms of type of onset and diagnosis, had an important influence on the type of outcome evidenced by the remaining group.

References

Buckley, H., Ni Nuallain, M., O'Hare, A., & Walsh, D. (1989), Community studies in psychiatry. *Irish J. Psychiatry*, 2:11–15.

Craig, T. J., Siegel, C., Hopper, K., Lin, S., & Sartorius, N. (1997), Outcome in schizophrenia and related disorders compared between developing and developed countries. *Brit. J. Psychiatry*, 170:229–233.

Jablensky, A., Sartorius, N., Ernberg, G., Anker, M., Korten, A., Cooper, J. E., Day, R., & Bertelsen, A. (1992), Schizophrenia: Manifestations, incidence and course in different cultures: A World Health Organization ten-country study. *Psycholog. Med.*, 20(Monogr. Suppl.): 1–97.

Kendler, K. S., McGuire, M., Gruenberg, A., & Walsh, D. (1994), Outcome and family study of the subtypes of schizophrenia in the west of Ireland. *Amer. J. Psychiatry*, 151(6):849–856.

Ni Nuallain, M., O'Hare, A., & Walsh, D. (1987), Incidence of schizophrenia in Ireland. *Psychol. Med.*, 17:943–948.

——, ——, ——(1990), The prevalence of schizophrenia in three counties in Ireland. *Acta Psychiatr. Scand.*, 82:136–140.

O'Hare, A., Walsh, D., & Torrey, F. (1980), Seasonality of schizophrenic births in Ireland. *Brit. J. Psychiatry*, 137: 74–77.

Straub, B., Mac Lean, C., O'Neill, A., Burke, J., Murphy, B., Duke, F., Shinkwin, R., Webb, B., Zhang, J., Walsh, D., & Kendler, J. (1995), A potential vulnerability locus for schizophrenia on chromosome p24–22: Evidence for genetic heterogeneity. *Nature Gen.*, 11:287–293.

Walsh, D., & Walsh, B. (1968), Some influences on the intercounty variation in Irish psychiatric hospitalization rates. *Brit. J. Psychiatry*, 114:15–20.

——O'Hare, A., Ni Nuallain, M., O'Connor, A., & McHugh, B. (1991), Outcome of schizophrenia in Ireland—A two-year follow-up study. *Irish J. Psychiatry*, 2:6–13.

Chapter 13

DOSMeD: Honolulu, Hawai'i

Anthony J. Marsella, Edward Suarez, Thomas Leland, Heather Morse, Barbara Digman, Alice Scheuer, and Martin M. Katz

CULTURAL CONTEXT

Geography

Hawai'i consists of eight major volcanic islands and more than 200 small islets totaling 6450 square miles in the middle of the Pacific Ocean, approximately 2100 miles southwest of San Francisco, California. Volcanic activity continues to add landmass from eruptions that flow from the Kilauea Crater to the ocean. The Hawaiian Islands are a lush tropical paradise of flora and fauna that thrived because of their isolation from other lands and people (Nordyke, 1989).

Population

According to the 1990 census, Hawai'i has more than 1,150,000 people with ethnocultural minorities making up more than 75% of the population; there are Caucasians, Japanese, Filipinos, Chinese, African-Americans, Koreans, pure and part-Hawaiians, Samoans, Hispanic/Latinos, and other mixed races. More than 98 different foreign languages are spoken in Hawai'i, most frequently, Japanese, Tagalog, Ilocano, Chinese, Korean, Spanish, Samoan, Hawaiian, and Vietnamese. In 1990, about 23% of the population aged 5 or older spoke a non-English language at home. Though Christians, led by Roman Catholics, predominate in numbers, there are also substantial numbers of Buddhists, especially among Japanese, Chinese, and other southeast Asians. There is a small but growing population of believers in Islam and in new-age religions.

Early History

The Hawaiian Islands were first inhabited around 100 A.D. by settlers from the Polynesian Islands of the Marquesas and Tahiti. In 1778, British Captain James Cook arrived with two ships, the first contact of the native peoples with Europeans. Within a short period of time, sizable numbers of Western whalers, businessmen, and missionaries came to the Islands. The precontact population of Hawai'i has been the topic of considerable debate, estimated between 200,000 and 875,000 people. Postcontact, the population declined sharply because of imported communicable diseases against which they had no immunity, infertility, high infant mortality, outmigration, war, intermarriage, the adoption of tobacco and alcohol, and, some say, despair. More than 15,000 Native Hawaiian people died in a single smallpox epidemic in 1853. Some native Hawaiian people speak of their history as genocide (Nordyke, 1989; Stannard, 1992).

Missionaries and Businessmen

In 1820, the first New England missionaries arrived destroying much of the ancient Hawaiian culture and purchasing much of the land that is still held by their descendants today. By the 1850s, American businessmen had begun to import large numbers of Chinese and Japanese contract workers for the sugar plantations. In the 1890s, they were joined by Filipino and Puerto Rican workers. In 1893, the Hawaiian monarchy (*Onipaa*) was overthrown, and the land was annexed as an American territory. In 1959, Hawai'i became a state.

Contemporary Mental Health Issues

Today, three major mental health issues have important implications for Hawai'i: (I) the Felix-Waihee Consent Decree, in which the courts ruled that the state is obligated to provide mental health services to youth, has increased public expenditures and concerns for cost; (2) deinstitutionalization has expanded the need for community-based services and has resulted in the release of numerous mentally ill persons from the State Hospital without adequate provision of care; and (3) issues of cultural insensitivity have arisen as a result of Caucasian dominance of the mental health professions.

THE MENTAL HEALTH SYSTEM

The state operates child and adult mental health services employing not only practitioners of Western medicine but also indigenous healers from various ethnocultural groups (e.g., Hawaiian kahunas, Filipino hilots and herbolarios, Japanese shiatsu massage and religious healers). As of July 1993, the state's community mental health centers were authorized to provide care to severely mentally ill persons only. Today, public financial support for mental health services has diminished, and private health insurance pays for mental health services provided by private practitioners. At the same time, there has been an increase in profit-making medical insurance corporations and a decrease in the numbers of patients being seen in the public sector services. Hawai'i has more than 150 private and charitable social service agencies that offer different kinds of mental health services (e.g., Salvation Army, Catholic Social Services). New approaches to managing the mental health care system have also emerged: case management, managed care, capitated financing, wraparound services, assertive community care, interdisciplinary teams, supported full and partial employment, and biopsychosocial rehabilitation. These are aimed at reducing institutionalization, hospital admissions, length of hospital stay and costs, and at improving patients' quality of life through better community and social functioning.

RECENT PSYCHIATRIC RESEARCH ON HAWAI'I

Given the multiple national lineages of the Hawaiian people, it is not surprising that inquiries in psychiatric epidemiology have focused on ethnic diversity.

Research by Kinzie and Tseng (1978) showed that Caucasians were overrepresented in the utilization of mental health and adolescent services, a finding they attributed not to heightened levels of psychopathology, but to an inclination among Caucasians to resort to professional services rather to rely on family and other social networks (that may, in any event, not be present) (Choy, 1981). Caucasian clients sought mental health services for depression (33%), anxiety (25%), interpersonal difficulty (15%), and schizophrenia (12%). Japanese and Chinese clients were more likely to seek help for more severe disorders. The former sought help for schizophrenia (23%), self-destructive acts (19%), depression (19%), and anxiety (14%); the latter, for schizophrenia (29%), interpersonal difficulties (29%), anxiety (21%), and depression (21%). Different rates of help-seeking do not simply mirror rates of disorder; they also reflect such factors as willingness to seek treatment or to tolerate disruptive family members.

In a study of admission rates to Hawai'i State Hospital, Kalal (1982) found that although Japanese have the lowest proportional admission rates compared to Caucasian, Chinese, Filipino, and Hawaiian populations, they had a higher rate of functional psychotic first admissions. Again, this suggests that though Japanese may be hesitant to use mental health services, they do seek professional care when problems are severe. Leong (1989) studied the treated prevalence rates and symptomatology of Caucasian, Chinese, Filipino, and Japanese schizophrenic patients admitted to Hawai'i mental health centers. He also found that Japanese and Chinese had significantly higher rates of treated schizophrenia than Caucasians or Filipinos, a finding consistent with Sue's (1977) comparison of Asian Americans and other minority groups in Seattle, Washington.

A study among the four major ethnic groups showed that Caucasians constituted 41.2% of first admissions from 1980 to 1981 to inpatient services and 41.6% of admissions to outpatient services, resulting in a service estimate (an index derived by dividing population by service utilization) of 162%. Comparable estimates were 101% for Hawaiians, 99% for Filipinos, 46% for Japanese, and 39% for Chinese (Ostrowski, 1982). During this period at least, Caucasians disproportionately used the state public mental health services. Conversely, in 1995, Japanese cases formed the leading ethnic group in admissions to Hawai'i State Hospital, followed by Caucasians and Hawaiians. Japanese are disproportionately higher than their estimated population on Oahu (approximately 20%), while Caucasians are disproportionately smaller than their estimated population on Oahu (22%). This may be a function of the increased service needs of the Japanese population who have higher proportions of elderly in comparison to the other groups (Nathan, 1995; Peel and Wylie, 1996).

With respect to ethnic differences in symptomatology, Katz, Sanborn, Lowery, and Ching (1978) compared psychotic behaviors of different ethnic groups in Hawai'i using a "normal" baseline. Japanese patients were found to be more "suspicious, negative, anxious, and bizarre" when compared to a normal community sample of Japanese, a result clearly different from the clinical picture in their previous study which reported Japanese patients to be "withdrawn" and "apathetic" (Katz, Sanborn, and Gudeman, 1969; Katz, Gudeman, and Sanborn, 1969). Such results suggest that Japanese psychotic behavior becomes problematic when it violates local standards of Japanese acceptable normality, not when it conforms to the clinical standards of "acceptance," "passivity," and "withdrawal."

Takemoto-Chock (1985) compared the symptomatology of 104 first episode psychotic patients from the WHO DOSMeD study and found that psychotic Japanese had much higher levels of anxiety, depression, and muscular tension than psychotic Hawaiians who had higher levels of lack of insight. The Japanese had higher levels of delusions of misinterpretation, assistance, catastrophe, and appearance, while Caucasians had higher levels of religious delusions, and Hawaiians had higher levels of pseudo/true and visual hallucinations. Takemoto-Chock's interpretation again honed in on the tendency of Japanese to come to treatment later in the trajectory of their disorders, only after their behavior has become severe, antagonistic, or dangerous. In the hospital, they tend to withdraw and to respond to medications with passivity and submission (cf. Sartorius, Jablensky, and Shapiro, 1978).

Leong (1989) found ethnocultural variations in 11 of 23 symptoms associated with schizophrenia. Still, the four groups (Japanese, Chinese, Filipinos, and Caucasians) did not differ significantly in the presentation of suspicions, delusions, social withdrawal, and depressed mood—the core symptoms of the disorder. Other, more distal symptoms showed ethnocultural nuances. In a later study of clinical symptomatology among 82 first episode psychotic patients who participated in the WHO DOSMeD study, Marsella, Suarez, Morse, and Scheuer (1997) reported that schizophrenic patients had higher frequencies of Schneiderian signs than nonschizophrenic psychotic patients (affective psychoses and brief psychotic reactions). The fact that the differences across diagnostic groups were not statistically significant suggests that such signs are sensitive to psychosis but not specific to particular psychotic diagnoses. Japanese and Hawaiians had much higher frequencies of Schneiderian signs at admission than Caucasians, suggesting that the former groups may present with more severe symptomatology.

THE HAWAI'I CENTER

In 1978 with funding from WHO and the U.S. National Institute of Mental Health (NIMH), the WHO/NIMH Hawai'i Psychiatric Research Center was established at the Queen's Medical Center, the largest private medical center in Hawai'i. The Hawai'i Center was invited to participate in the Determinants of Outcome of Severe Mental Disorders (DOSMeD) study. In 1993, the Center was asked to participate in ISoS, to follow up subjects from DOSMeD.

DOSMeD

Oahu was chosen as the catchment area site for the DOSMeD study. Although it occupies only 10% of the state's total land mass and ranks third in size among the islands, Oahu contains approximately 80% of the population and is the commercial and governmental center. Every resident of the catchment area, aged 15 to 54, who at any time in the previous 6 months had made a first contact with any helping agency because of problems suggesting the presence of a psychotic illness was identified. Subjects selected to be followed had to be in the early stages of their illness; be evaluated as closely as possible to the point of their first contact with a helping agency; and be reassessed over a defined period of time. Subjects were excluded if they had organic damage, a chronic or recent history of severe alcohol/substance abuse, and/or any previous history of severe mental disorder. The two major psychiatric hospitals and 30 other potential sources of inpatient and outpatient cases were contacted, and 15 psychiatrists and psychologists in private practice were used as contact points. Less than 1% (0.43%) of total cases screened between December 1978 and the end of 1983 were ultimately included in the sample.

ISoS

Case-finding in Honolulu included two phases. Phase I consisted of 68 cases who were interviewed from 1979 to 1981 and were included in the DOSMeD Incidence study. Although case-finding continued until the end of 1983 (phase II), these additional cases are not included in ISoS. The ISoS cohort consists of the

68 cases from phase I plus an additional three cases who had passed the initial screening for phase I but had not been included in the final cohort. Twenty-four of the 68 cases had only marginal baseline evaluations and no follow-up at all; these cases account for much of the missing data at baseline and short-term follow-up. The remaining 44 cases were the major focus for the ISoS case finding. With respect to ethnicity, the follow-up cases were equally represented by Caucasian and Japanese and slightly less by part-Hawaiians.

The Hawai'i Center used a variety of methods for locating cases: trying telephone numbers in the DOSMeD case records; accessing electronic national telephone directories and checking local directories; checking mental health system and Hawai'i State Hospital records; checking death records; calling psychiatrists, mental health professionals, and other service providers who had previously treated the subject; requesting the postal service to send mail to a forwarding address; and checking criminal records at the State Attorney General's Office.

Center staff contacted subjects by telephone, reminded them of their previous participation, and invited them to join the study. The purpose of the study was explained, and they were offered $30.00 for being interviewed. Where telephones were not available, a letter was sent to the subject's address asking him or her to contact the Center.

All subjects were interviewed at either the centrally located Kalihi-Palama Mental Health Center, at the University of Hawai'i WHO Center; at the Department of Psychiatry at the Queen's Medical Center; or at the Hawai'i State Hospital. Approximately 10 cases had to be transported to and from an interview site. In general, the subjects were first administered the PSE, DAS, and PIRS by Drs. Leland or Marsella and then the other instruments by the staff. Subjects were thanked and told that the study team would be in contact to monitor their progress.

RESULTS

Baseline and Short-Term Follow-Up

Gender and Age

At entry into the index study period (1979–1981), the Honolulu cohort (N=71) consisted of 41 (57.7%) males and 30 (42.3%) females. Twenty-six cases, 14 (53.8%) males and 12 (46.2%) females, were located by the end of 1996. Forty-one cases had not been located and were deemed lost to follow-up; four cases, all males, had died.

The average mean birth year of the cases located at the 15-year follow-up was 1955. The average birth year for the entire DOSMeD subsample was 1951; thus, the Hawai'i alive cohort was 4 years younger on average. Birth-year distribution of the follow-up cohort was similar to that of the original cohort, with the modal birth decade of those followed up being 1950 to 1959. This finding also held true for those who had died during the follow-up period; three of the deceased cases were born in the 1950 to 1959 period, and one in the 1920 to 1929 period. Thus, relative to the alive cases, age did not appear to be a factor in those who died during the follow-up period.

Mode of Onset

Of Hawai'i's 26 alive cases, the majority (42%) had insidious onset (>1 month). Other onset patterns included precipitous (<1 week) (19%), acute (up to 1 month) (19%), and other/missing (19%). The distribution of modes of onset in the original study cohort included other/missing (44%), insidious (28%), precipitous (10%), and acute (18%). In comparison to the other DOSMeD centers, Hawai'i ranked approximately in the middle for insidious mode of onset. The mode of onset distribution for the deceased and lost-to-follow-up cases was similar to that of the alive cases, except that none of the four deceased had an acute mode of onset, and 61% of the lost-to-follow-up cases were categorized as other/missing onset pattern.

Diagnosis

Paranoid schizophrenia is the most common baseline diagnosis in both the original and the 15-year follow-up cohorts when using the converted ICD-9 to ICD-10 diagnostic criteria. Thirty-nine percent of the alive cases and 29% of the lost-to-follow-up cases were diagnosed with paranoid schizophrenia, similar to the rate of 32% in the original study cohort. Compared to the other DOSMeD centers, Hawai'i's baseline rate was moderate; results from the entire DOSMeD cohort revealed that rates for paranoid schizophrenia ranged from 63.5% in Moscow to 5.3% in the rural areas of Chandigarh.

Additionally, at follow-up as well as at baseline, the grouped baseline diagnosis was evenly distributed between schizophrenia (50%) and nonschizophrenia (46%). Other diagnostic subgroups of note in the alive cohort included acute schizophrenia-like psychoses (19%) and bipolar/depression (15%). Schizophrenia was an equally common diagnosis in the lost-to-follow-up group (51%), followed by schizoaffective (15%), acute schizophrenia-like psychoses (12%), other psychoses (10%), and bipolar/depression (7%). A comparison of the baseline diagnostic distribution across the various DOSMeD centers revealed that Hawai'i's rate of 50% for schizophrenia cases ranked it approximately in the middle of all centers. Reported DOSMeD results for the schizophrenia diagnosis ranged from 91.2% for Nagasaki to 21.2% for Rochester.

Reevaluation of Baseline Diagnosis

Of the 13 cases in the alive cohort with schizophrenia diagnoses at baseline, 9 cases (69%) received the same diagnosis at long-term follow-up reevaluation of baseline diagnosis (i.e., given in 1995 to 1996, but using only clinical material available at the time of study entry). The others were rediagnosed as schizoaffective (8%), schizophreniform (8%), nonpsychotic (8%), and missing/unknown (8%). Of the five cases diagnosed with acute schizophrenia-like (schizophreniform) psychoses at baseline, three (60%) cases received the same diagnosis at reevaluation, while the rest were rediagnosed with schizophrenia (20%) and bipolar/depression (20%). In contrast, 100% of the four cases diagnosed with bipolar depression at index/baseline (1979–1981) received the same diagnosis at long-term follow-up reevaluation.

The net change in diagnostic categories from initial/baseline to reevaluation baseline was an 8% decrease in schizophrenia, a 20% decrease in schizophreniform, a 25% increase in bipolar/depression, and a 50% increase in unknown/missing (a function of the small number of cases in the category). Subsequent analyses here make use of the reevaluated baseline diagnoses.

Pattern of Course at Early Follow-Up

For the alive cases with a specified early course (1979–1981), the modal pattern was incomplete remission (30.8%); this was also true for all cases (i.e., alive, dead, and lost to follow-up). The largest change over time was the percentage decrease between the cases with an unspecified/missing pattern of course for those alive at 15-year follow-up (27%) and the total cases at the time of study origin (59%). This may reflect the relationship between quality of information at index interview, and the subsequent availability/participation of subjects in the 15-year follow-up. Complete remissions were much less common in the Honolulu follow-up cohort (23%) when compared to the entire DOSMeD subsample (47%). This maybe an artifact of the greater number of more severe cases in the Honolulu follow-up cohort.

ALIVE CASES

Symptomatology

According to the Bleuler Severity Scale, only 42% of the alive cases had recovered by the 15-year follow-up; however, the majority of cases (54%) had mild to moderate psychotic symptoms, while only one case (4%) was classified as severe. For the DOSMeD centers, the majority (56%) of cases had recovered while 38% were in the mild to moderate range. The Honolulu cohort appeared to be worse symptomatically than the total DOSMeD subsample, perhaps as a result of a selection bias in the 26-member Honolulu sample (i.e., 73% had been part of the 2-year follow-up cohort, and chronic cases may have been easier to locate because of their continued presence in the state registries).

The results of the Global Assessment of Functioning Scale for symptomatology (GAF-S) (i.e., index of symptom severity during past month) indicate that 27% showed no significant (or only mild) symptoms (i.e., GAF-S scores greater than 70), while 42% of the cases presented serious symptoms (i.e., GAF-S scores below 51). When mean GAF-S scores were compared across the international centers, the Honolulu cohort (m=58.2, sd=21.0) was among the most severely symptomatic. Only the Rochester (m=55.8, sd=21.6) DOSMeD center had a lower mean GAF-S score. The overall DOSMeD center average for the GAF-S was 65.2 (sd=20.5).

Although numbers are small, analysis by diagnostic category suggests that the most severe current symptomatology occurred in those cases with schizophrenia rediagnoses (m=45.0, sd=17.5), compared to the acute schizophrenia-like (m=69.8, sd=16.4) and bipolar/ depression (m=84.0, sd=2.7) rediagnoses. Based on the GAF-S distribution of scores, 58% of the schizophrenia cases presented serious symptoms (scores of less than 51), but none (0%) of the schizophrenia cases showed "absence of" or "only mild" symptoms (scores greater than 70). By contrast, 50% of acute schizophrenia-like cases, and 100% of bipolar/depression cases showed "absence of" or "only mild" symptoms.

The results also revealed an interesting relationship between mode of onset and symptomatic outcome. Among the 10 cases with sudden or acute onset of illness (<1 month), the mean GAF-S score was 64.2, whereas among the 11 cases who had an insidious onset (>1 month), the score was 56.5, suggesting that mode of onset may predict symptom severity at 15-year follow-up.

Analysis by gender showed a greater percentage (50%) of the 14 male cases were rated as having "serious" symptoms compared to 33% of the 12 female cases. In addition, 33% of the female cases versus 21% of the male cases were rated as having "mild" to "no significant" symptomatology (i.e., GAF-S scores greater than 70).

Course of Illness

In the last 2 years of the 15-year follow-up period, half (50%) the cases were never psychotic, whereas the remainder were either continuously (42%) or episodically (8%) psychotic. Most (67%) of the cases rediagnosed as schizophrenic had a continuous course of illness; 33% of the subjects in that group were never psychotic. In contrast among those rediagnosed as schizophrenia-like psychosis, 25% were continuous, and 50% were never psychotic, while in the bipolar/depression group, none was ever psychotic.

Course of illness for the total DOSMeD subsample was 52% never psychotic, 26% continuous, and 17% episodic. Thus, by comparison, the Honolulu cohort tended to have a more continuous and a less episodic course of illness. Only Dublin (44%) and Nagasaki (55%) had higher rates of continuous illness than Honolulu, while the other centers had higher rates of episodic courses during the same period. Throughout the last 15 years, 32% of the cases were never psychotic again, while the majority (68%) relapsed. Among those cases who relapsed, 44% were continuously psychotic, and 24% were episodically psychotic.

For 77% of the cases, the overall trend was improvement over time (with 42% much better and 35% somewhat better), while for 15% of the cases, the overall trend was worsening. While seemingly contradictory to the high percentage of schizophrenia in the Honolulu sample, this finding can be explained by noting that improvement was rated relative to the individual. Thus, a case could show improvement despite continuous symptomatology given his or her baseline.

Analysis by rediagnosis category showed that only 25% of the schizophrenia cases were getting much better versus 100% of the bipolar/depression cases and 50% of the acute schizophrenia-like cases. However, 42% of the schizophrenia cases were getting at least somewhat better, and only three schizophrenia cases (25%) were getting somewhat worse during the entire follow-up period.

Using baseline rediagnoses to look at the course-type over the first 2 years of follow-up indicated that only for schizophrenia cases was early short-term pattern of course (1979–1981) superior to most recent pattern of course (1994–1996). Among the schizophrenia cases, the early short-term course distribution showed that 25% were continuously psychotic, 42% were incomplete remission, and 8% were complete remission. For the most recent 2 years, 67% were continuously psychotic, 0% were episodically psychotic, and 33% were never psychotic. The most recent pattern of course for the acute schizophrenia-like cases was 25% continuously psychotic, 25% episodically psychotic, and 50% never psychotic, while for the bipolar/depression cases, 100% were never psychotic. Unlike the schizophrenia cases, a higher percentage of the latter two disorders had a superior recent course versus early short-term course. The early short-term course for the acute schizophrenia-like cases was 25% continuously psychotic, 0% incomplete remission, and 25% complete remission. For the bipolar/depression cases, 0% were continuously psychotic, 40% incomplete remission, 40% complete remission. (The percentages do not add up to 100% because of missing or other cases.) These variations in course may be expected because of the differences in the nature of these disorders. At the same time, because reevaluation diagnoses may not be blind to subsequent course and outcome, some rater bias may have crept in.

Living Arrangements

At the time of long-term follow-up, most cases (69%) were living in the community with family/friends (54%) or were living alone (15%). Twelve percent of the cases were in a psychiatric hospital, and 19% of the cases were in supervised residences for mentally ill persons. There was a greater tendency for subjects in Honolulu to be placed in the hospital or in supervised settings away from family and friends, probably reflecting the relatively greater availability of residential alternatives as well as the relatively greater overall symptom severity of the sample.

For the 2-year period prior to follow-up interviews, almost one-third (31%) never achieved independent living status, while the remainder of the cases spent at least half the period in independent living. These findings were similar to those of Nagasaki; however, they stand in contrast to the entire DOSMeD sample, in which 93% of the cases maintained independent living for most of those previous 2 years, and only 6% of the cases were never in independent living situations. Over the course of the entire follow-up period, 28% had spent a substantial portion (greater than 25%) of this time "hospitalized" or in "supervised settings," including three cases (12%) who never attained independent status at all. Nonetheless, 72% of the cases did manage to live independently for over half of the period, while over half of the cases (52%) did so for more than 90% of the time. Analysis by gender revealed that females spent a greater percentage of their time in independent living than males (90 vs. 76%).

Two (8%) subjects had been homeless during the 2 years preceding assessment, and two (8%) of the cases had spent time in jail. In comparison, the total DOSMeD subsample had lower rates of homelessness (2%) and imprisonment (1%) in the preceding 2 years. Over the course of the entire follow-up period, homelessness and imprisonment were more common in Honolulu than in any other DOSMeD center; 36% spent some time homeless and 20% spent some time in jail. In comparison, the percentage of all DOSMeD cases spending some time homeless was 6%, while 4% spent some time in jail. These results may be attributed to environmental and sociologic variations. Homelessness constitutes a more readily available option in Honolulu because of the tropical climate and the ease of outdoor living. Before homelessness was considered a major societal problem, it was not uncommon for people in Hawai'i to live outdoors.

Work

Fifty-four percent of subjects worked at paid jobs (including part-time employment) for some time during the last 2 years of follow-up. For the 23% who worked full-time for at least 12 months, performance at work was reported to be good to very good. A substantially larger percentage of DOSMeD cases (37%) were employed (full- or part-time) for most (>12 months) of the preceding 2 years, compared to just 23% of the Honolulu cases. This difference in employment rates probably reflects the comprehensiveness of the disability coverage in Honolulu, where 54% of cases received some form of disability income in the previous 2 years. Disability recipients in Honolulu realize that taking paid employment puts them at risk of losing their financial assistance. Five cases (19%) engaged in full-time household work; four of them for most of the 2-year period. Of these cases, half (50%) were rated as poor to very poor in their performance and half as good to very good. Only one case was classified as a student at any time in the past 2 years of follow-up, and no one had retired.

Social Disability

Regarding overall functioning in the most recent month, 19% were rated poor to severe on the Disability Assessment Scale (DAS), and 23% were rated lower than 51 (seriously impaired) on the Global Assessment of Functioning Scale for Disability (GAF-D). Meanwhile, 35% of the cases were rated fair, and 46% of the cases were rated good to very good in terms of overall functioning on the DAS. In addition, 42% of the cases scored between 51 and 70 on the GAF-D, indicating fair to moderate functioning, while 35% of the cases scored higher than 70 on the GAF-D, indicating good functioning. The ratings of current social functioning are higher than would be expected given the high level of current symptomatology among the cases, most pronounced when comparing GAF-S scores to DAS scores: 73% of the cases were judged to have moderate to severe symptomatology, whereas 81% (77% according to GAF-D) were considered to be functioning (in social/occupational spheres) moderately to very well. It appears that these general dimensions of recovery (i.e., disability and symptomatology) may vary independently. There is a general agreement between the two disability indices (DAS and GAF-D) across the recovered, mild/moderate, and severe outcome indices; however, the Bleuler and the GAF-S indices differ strongly, especially for the severe category (Bleuler = 4% and GAF-S = 42%). This may be a function of the finer distinctions in the GAF-S scale (0–100) versus the Bleuler (1 to 4 scale).

A baseline reevaluation diagnosis of schizophrenia was more often associated with poorer functioning when compared to the group of other psychoses; 50% of schizophrenic cases rated below 51 (serious symptoms) on the GAF compared to none of the other psychoses cases. Average GAF-D scores were as follows: schizophrenia (m=52.6; sd=13.1; acute schizophrenia-like psychosis (m=73.0; sd=9.6); and bipolar/depression (m=83.2; sd=3.5). Similarly, good to excellent global evaluations on the DAS were given to only 17% with a reevaluation diagnosis of schizophrenia compared to 100% with bipolar/depression and 75% with schizophreniform diagnoses.

Violence

Only one person (5%) assaulted others in the last 2 years of follow-up. Over the entire course, eight cases (36%) were involved in assaults on other people. Assault rates for the total DOSMeD sample were higher for the most recent 2-year period (11%), but lower for the entire follow-up period (24%). Compared to Honolulu, Nagasaki (41%) was the only center with a higher assault rate for the entire course. The Hong Kong (34%) and Beijing (33%) centers followed close behind Honolulu.

Suicide

One case (4%) attempted suicide in the last 2 years of follow-up, while seven cases (28%) had attempted suicide during the entire follow-up period. For the total DOSMeD sample, rates of self-harm were 4% in the last 2 years, and 20% for the entire period.

Medication

In the last 2 years of follow-up, the majority of the cases (52%) had been on neuroleptics most of the time, while an additional 8% of cases had been on neuroleptics some of the time, leaving 10 cases (40%) who were never on neuroleptic medication. Percentages of cases never on neuroleptic medication ranged across centers from 1% in Hong Kong to 79% in Chandigarh rural.

Over the entire course of follow-up, 83% of the 23 cases for whom information was supplied had been on neuroleptics at least some of the time (including 52.2% on neuroleptics most of the time and 30.4% some of the time). Neuroleptic figures for the entire DOSMeD cohort tended to be only slightly higher. Honolulu was moderate in this regard, relative to the practices of the developing (i.e., typically less medication-oriented) and the developed (i.e., typically more medication-oriented) centers.

Examination of time trends over the entire period shows that for the largest number of subjects (8; 31%) medications were most prominent only in the first third of the period, while for the next largest group (6; 23%) medications were most prominent only in the last third. For an additional 19%, medications were equally prominent in the last two-thirds. This trend toward medication prominence later in treatment may reflect a trend toward improvement in medication compliance over time, which in turn may reflect improved insight of patients regarding their psychotic conditions as well as major improvements in the quality of neuroleptic medications over the past decade. For the total DOSMeD cohort, neuroleptic medications tended to be more prominent initially (39%) and continuously (32%). Nearly 92% of those who had a reevaluation diagnosis of schizophrenia were on neuroleptic medication during the last 2 years of follow-up, whereas only one-third of those rediagnosed with acute schizophrenia-like psychoses and none of the bipolar/depression or other psychotic disorder rediagnosis groups were on neuroleptic medication at all during this time.

Hospitalization

Ten subjects (38%) had spent some time in a hospital or in a supervised residence in the last 2 years of follow-up, compared to 23% of the entire DOSMeD cohort. Nineteen subjects (76%) did so at least once during the entire follow-up period, including four subjects (16%) who spent the majority of the follow-up period in such a setting. Similarly, three-quarters of the entire DOSMeD cohort spent some time in supervised residence during this period. For half of the subjects, hospitalization was most prominent only in the first third of the follow-up period, while for 19%, it was most prominent only in the most recent third.

DECEASED SUBJECTS

Fifteen years after study entry, four male subjects were deceased. Three of these were classified as unnatural deaths; one (age 59) was murdered and two (ages 28 and 33) were suicides (one by hanging and one by jumping from a high building). The fourth subject (age 44) died of complications of tuberculosis. Comparison to the general population of Honolulu shows an increased death rate for this cohort. The standard mortality ratio (SMR) for males of 4.22 was significantly different from 1 at the 5% significance level. It is unknown but suspected that the individuals who died of unnatural causes were in episodes of mental illness at the time of death.

DISCUSSION

Disability and Symptomatology

Whereas the majority of the Honolulu cases were judged to have moderate to severe symptomatology, they were also considered to be functioning moderately to very well in terms of social and occupational adjustment; thus, the indices of disability and symptomatology seem to be somewhat independent depending on the scale used (e.g., Bleuler scale scores tend to yield fewer severe outcomes than GAF-S scores). The differences may be a function of the brevity and lack of specificity of the Bleuler scale when compared to the more refined distinctions provided by the GAF-S.

Work

The differences in the employment rates between Honolulu and the other DOSMeD centers may be a function of the many resources (including comprehensive psychiatric disability coverage, unemployment compensation, food stamps, aid to dependent children, and job training) available in Hawai'i to persons with mental disorders. Thus, the mental health and social welfare systems may foster dependency by providing a wide spectrum of human services. Then, too, the subjects' self-reports of performance could be influenced by a variety of personal biases.

Potential Bias in the Reevaluation Diagnosis

The Honolulu staff had been concerned that the follow-up procedure would be biased by the relatively greater ease of locating the episodically or continuously ill versus the recovered. Based on updated information, however, there does not appear to be evidence of systematic bias, in terms of symptoms, disability, or demographic status, in locating subjects. The staff that made the original diagnoses and the staff that made the rediagnoses 15 years later were different. Still, the current staff could not completely ignore the interim data on the cases. This may constitute a mild bias since the cases were supposed to be rediagnosed solely on the basis of index information.

Other Cultural Influences on the Course of Recovery

Family seemed to be an important source of social support in nearly every case in which the participant was locally born and raised, except when their tendencies toward crime or living on the streets created excessive stress/burden. In a few case, hallucinated behaviors (such as communicating with deceased ancestors) could be viewed as culturally normative by the individual and his or her ethnic group and not necessarily indicative of impaired psychiatric functioning.

SUMMARY

The original cohort of 71 individuals was assembled between 1979 and 1981 on the Island of Oahu, a geographically diverse island of approximately 1 million people with no dominant ethnic or racial majority (75% of the Island population is non-white). Of the cases identified as having a first-episode psychosis, there was an overrepresentation of males (58%). This distribution dissipated somewhat by the time of the 15-year follow-up because of the greater likelihood for males to be lost to follow-up. Males and females were nearly equally represented among the 26 alive cases in the 15-year follow-up cohort. There were four deaths, three of which were classified as unnatural causes (i.e., two suicides, one homicide).

At follow-up using only information available at baseline, 12 cases (50%) of those not missing received an ICD-10 rediagnosis of schizophrenia, five (21%) bipolar/depression, four (17%) acute schizophrenia-like disorder, and one case (4%) each of the following: schizoaffective, other psychotic, and other nonpsychotic. Nine of the 13 cases (69%) receiving a baseline diagnosis of schizophrenia retained that diagnosis in the reevaluation. Two of the five cases given baseline diagnoses of acute schizophrenia-like psychoses were rediagnosed differently: one with schizophrenia (20%) and one with bipolar/depression (20%).

Forty percent of subjects had never been on neuroleptics at any time in the most recent 2-year follow-up period. Approximately two-thirds lived independently. A substantial proportion of cases (36%) had been homeless for some time during the entire follow-up period. In addition, one-fifth of the cohort had been jailed during the follow-up period. Over half (54%) of the cases had been employed during the 2 years preceding follow-up, and an additional five cases (19%) had been involved in full-time household work though their self-rated performance was often poor. Disability income was received by the majority of subjects for some part of the last 2 years and continuously by 42% of them. The availability of disability income may have diminished the need/motivation for employment within the Honolulu sample.

Forty-two percent of the alive cases were judged to have recovered while 54% were experiencing mild or moderate psychotic symptoms. Overall, the course trend was improving for 77% of the cohort and worsening for 15%. Social and occupational disability was good to excellent for nearly half the cases and poor for 19%. Those with baseline reevaluation rediagnoses of schizophrenia were much more impaired socially and symptomatically.

Half of those so diagnosed, for example, had serious to persistently dangerous symptoms, whereas none of the nonschizophrenic groups had cases rated this low. Similarly, only 17% with baseline reevaluation diagnoses of schizophrenia were considered to be well-adjusted socially, compared to 100% of bipolar/depression subjects, and 75% of schizophreniform subjects.

Diagnostic differences appeared to be the most potent predictor of treatment, course, and outcome in this cohort. For example, while short-term course of schizophrenia was most likely to be characterized by incomplete remission (42%) during early (2-year) course, in the most recent 2-year period, course was either continuous (67%) or never psychotic (33%). Conversely, early course in bipolar/depression was typically full (40%) or partial (40%) remission, compared to 100% never psychotic from 1994 to 1996.

The Honolulu data revealed that mode of onset appeared to be associated differentially with symptomatology at follow-up. Those cases with insidious onset appeared to be more symptomatic and more disabled than those cases with precipitous, acute, and sudden onset. This result is consistent with well-documented findings regarding the relationship between poor premorbid personality and chronic course and outcome.

Gender also appeared to be an influential factor in course and outcome, with the majority of females experiencing only mild to moderate symptoms, and the majority of males experiencing moderate to severe symptoms. Greater equivalence between genders on social-occupational disability levels, however, indicated less influence of gender for this outcome domain.

Acknowledgments The staff gratefully acknowledges the support of the Department of Psychiatry, University of Hawai'i, Honolulu, Hawai'i; Mental Health Services, Queen's Medical Center, Honolulu, Hawai'i; Adult Mental Health Division, Department of Health, State of Hawai'i. The staff also extends deep appreciation to the subjects and their families and their gratitude to the former members of the project who conducted the early phases.

References

Choy, S. (1981), Adolescent psychiatric hospitalization and ethnic origin. Hawaii, 1979. *Hawaii Med. J.*, 40:320–322.

Ikeda, K., Ball, H., & Yamamura, D. (1964), Ethnocultural factors in schizophrenia: The Japanese in Hawaii. *Amer. J. Sociol.*, 68:242–248.

Kalal, B. (1982), *Changes in Psychiatric Admissions at Hawaii State Hospital: 1940–1979.* Unpublished Master's Thesis, Department of Psychology, University of Hawai'i, Honolulu, Hawai'i.

——(1989), *Clinical, Social, and Demographic Predictors of First Incidence Psychosis in Hawaii.* Unpublished Doctoral Dissertation, Department of Psychology, University of Hawai'i, Honolulu, Hawai'i.

Katz, M., Gudeman, H., & Sanborn, K. (1969), Characterizing differences in psychopathology among ethnic groups in Hawaii. A preliminary report on Hawaii-Japanese and mainland American schizophrenics. In: *Mental Health Research in Asia the Pacific*, ed. W. Caudill & T. Lin. Honolulu, Hawai'i: East-West Center Press.

——Sanborn, K., & Gudeman, H. (1969), Characterizing differences in psychopathology among ethnic groups in Hawai'i. In: *Social Psychiatry*, ed. F. Redlich. Baltimore: Williams & Wilkins.

——,——Lowery, A., & Ching, J. (1978), Ethnic studies in Hawaii. On psychopathology and social deviance. In: *The Nature of Schizophrenia: New Approaches to Research and Treatment*, ed. L. Wynne, R. Cromwell, & S. Matthysee. New York: J. Wiley, pp. 572–585.

Kinzie, D., & Tseng, W. (1978), Cultural aspects of psychiatric clinic utilization: A cross-cultural study in Hawaii. *Internat. J. Soc. Psychiatry*, 24:177–188.

Leong, F. (1989), Cultural variations in the treated prevalence rate and symptomatology among Chinese, Japanese, Filipino, and Caucasian schizophrenic patients in Hawai'i. In: *Schizophrenia: Scientific Progress*, ed. C. Schultz & C. Tamminga. New York: Oxford University Press.

Marsella, A. J., Suarez, E., Morse, H., & Scheuer, A. (1997), Results from the WHO determinants of outcome study in Hawai'i. Paper presented at American

Psychological Association Annual Convention, Chicago, August 15–19.

Nathan, J. (1995), *Prevalence Estimates of Mental Disorders in the State of Hawai'i.* Unpublished technical report, Honolulu, Hawai'i: Adult Mental Health Division, Department of Health, State of Hawai'i.

Nordyke, E. (1989), *The Peopling of Hawai'i.* Honolulu: University Press of Hawai'i.

Ostrowski, B. (1982), *Selected Ethnicity Data (1979–1980): State of Hawai'i Mental Health Division.* Unpublished technical report, Honolulu, Hawai'i.

Peel, J., & Wylie, M. (1996), Psychiatric diagnoses of consumers at Hawai'i's community mental health centers by ethnic background. Paper presented at Hawai'i Psychological Association Annual Convention, October, Honolulu, Hawai'i.

Sartorius, N., Jablensky, A., & Shapiro, R. (1978), Cross-cultural differences in the short-term prognosis of schizophrenic psychoses. *Schizophr. Bull.*, 4:102–113.

Sue, S. (1977), Community mental health services to minority groups: Some optimism, some pessimism. *Amer. Psychologist* 32:616–624.

Stannard, D. (1992), *American Holocaust: The Conquest of the New World.* New York: Oxford University Press.

Takemoto-Chock, N. (1985), *Ethnocultural Variation in Psychiatric Symptomatology in Hawaii.* Unpublished Doctoral Dissertation, Department of Psychology, University of Hawai'i, Honolulu, Hawai'i.

Chapter 14

DOSMeD: Moscow, Russia

Sergey Tsirkin

CULTURAL CONTEXT

In the late 1970s, an administrative district of Moscow was chosen to participate in the Determinants of Outcome of Severe Mental Disorders study (DOSMeD), a WHO-coordinated epidemiological study of new cases of schizophrenia. The population of this district was then approximately 400,000, of whom about 230,000 were aged 18 to 54, the age of inclusion in the study. (The population of the City of Moscow, now about 9 million, was then about 8 million.) The selected catchment area does not include historic central Moscow, but is a relatively new area that has more factories and fewer offices, theaters, and museums. The population, having migrated to the catchment area during the last decades to improve their living conditions, is accordingly more numerous and younger. Most of the houses, erected in the sixties, are much larger than those in other parts of the city. Several hostels house relatively young workers from the provinces who came with the obligation of taking menial jobs in specific factories with manpower shortages.

The early 1990s witnessed great economic and political change, the impoverishment of the population in particular (acknowledged by the authorities). Some people, especially the elderly, tried speculation as an additional source of income. Many younger people were eager to work in private businesses, even to establish their own firms; however, many of these mostly trading or service companies thrived during their initial years only to collapse. Migration to Moscow from provincial areas became attractive to businessmen, because it became possible to get residence permits and to buy flats, and to refugees fleeing tense social situations (e.g., Russians who, since the dissolution of the U.S.S.R., were no longer welcome in many former Soviet republics). The local population and administrative bodies are reluctant to accept these migrants because they need apartments, money, and jobs; if they have no relatives in Moscow, they face a very hard time.

In the 1990s, a greater variety of goods has begun to appear in the shops eliminating the need to spend hours waiting in line to make purchases. The majority of people are distressed, however, because they cannot afford to buy much. People are no longer sure whether they will receive their salaries and pensions on time or whether they will be able to keep their jobs. Wealthy people are statistically insignificant; social experts assert that there is now actually no middle class in Russia. The majority of the population is affiliated with the Russian Orthodox church, although other religions (e.g., Islam) are also practiced. Recently, many religious sects have become active in Moscow, finding adherents largely among the young (and not infrequently among mentally ill persons) and causing parents alarmed concern.

That mental disorders are a consequence of stressful experiences is a popular idea; so, too, is the notion that hereditary factors influence their development. Despite recent popularization, Freud's theories are still not really accepted by ordinary people. Belief in witchcraft is more widespread, especially as such ideas have circulated more freely as part of the "democratization" process. Belief in extrasensory influences also excite much curiosity in the population.

Linguistic Characteristics

The majority of the population is Slavic; except for Tartars and Jews, other nationalities are relatively rarer in Moscow. There is only one spoken language (Russian), though in some non-Russian families, people also speak their own languages. Compared with

English, Russian has more words, many of which, though borrowed from foreign languages, are used with very narrow and specific meanings. During recent decades, only a small number of people have been able to use the Russian language skillfully and perfectly. Differences in linguistic competence are substantial but not striking; those with technical educations are intermediate between teachers and workers in competence.

Impact of Mental Health Issues on Society

Acccording to some estimates (Shevchenko, 1993), the total national expenditure related to mental diseases corresponds to 0.4% of the gross domestic product. This includes treatment and rehabilitation, pensions in cases of disability, boarding houses for those who are mentally disabled, cash compensation in cases of temporary loss of working capacity, education of psychiatric staff, and construction of mental hospitals, but does not include costs associated with alcoholism and drug addiction. Among direct expenditures, one-third is spent on compensation for temporary and persistent loss of working capacity (Shevchenko and Solokhina, 1995). Indirect expenditures include losses in national income because of the lack of productivity of mentally disordered or disabled persons—1% per year (Shevchenko, 1993). Indirect expenditures are 50% greater than direct ones (Shevchenko and Solokhina, 1995).

Previously, acute cases of mental disorders resulted in stigmatization of patients and their families. Ordinary people tend to regard mentally ill persons with pity, mixed with fear of aggression. They are usually of the opinion that mentally disordered persons (even during long and seemingly full remissions) are irresponsible with respect to delinquent or criminal behavior and that they are free to do whatever they want without fear of the consequences.

Even without enabling legislation, it is now easier for an employer to fire a mentally ill person, especially in private firms. Monetary support (pensions) and other benefits (such as free medication, preferential consideration in housing, etc.) do not totally cover the losses families suffer from unemployment in cases of chronic disorder. Treatment of acute disorders recently became a larger financial burden when some hospitals ran out of funds, and relatives of patients were asked to pay for their food and medicines. Vocational rehabilitation formerly allowed patients to earn money in many large hospitals, outpatient clinics, and factories; economic difficulties and the cessation of state support for these programs have made them unprofitable. Unless supported by wealthy relatives, mentally disabled persons have very low economic status; those who have retired can choose which pension, old age or disability, is most advantageous.

MENTAL HEALTH SYSTEM

There are several mental health systems in Russia. To the territorial system of psychiatric service belong institutions affiliated with the Ministry of Health. Patients are referred to outpatient clinics, to day clinics affiliated with outpatient clinics, and to hospitals, depending on place of permanent residence. Each catchment area contains a local mental hospital where beds for area patients are readily available, and it is also the most likely place for a patient from the catchment area to be admitted in case of psychotic relapse. Pyschotropic drugs are still available there free of charge. The local mental hospital for subjects of the DOSMeD cohort is the largest one in Moscow, admitting patients from several administrative districts; the outpatient clinic serving subjects included in the DOSMeD study is actually situated on the territory of the neighboring district and provides psychiatric help free of charge. In cases of emergency admission outside their catchment area, patients are sooner or later transferred to their local hospitals. Special institutions for children and adolescents (to age 18) are also territorially organized.

A second source of psychiatric services is some general/somatic hospitals and polyclinics (general/somatic outpatient clinics), where there are special wards (for patients both somatically and mentally ill) and psychiatrists who counsel patients referred by general practitioners (mostly with somatoform disorders, mild depressions, anxiety, and phobic disorders). Patients with special disorders may also be referred by their local psychiatric services to research institutions that belong either to the Ministry of Health or to the Academy of Medical Sciences. Admission to these clinics, however, is limited. Yet another health system is organized for professionals by their corresponding ministries. Persons employed by the Ministry of Defense can be (and usually are) referred to special polyclinics and hospitals, railway people are referred to special institutions of their own, and some large factories provide psychiatric services in their general outpatient clinic. The Ministry of Welfare operates special boarding houses for chronically disabled persons who are not dangerous but who are in need of constant help. Finally, a private health system has recently taken shape, where psychiatrists (but not psychotherapists) are officially forbidden to work since their services should be free of charge. In actuality, many psychiatrists work there disguised as psychotherapists. Nowadays, many patients seek help from "magicians" and "extrasensory" healers.

District outpatient clinics for mentally ill persons (affiliated with the Ministry of Health), which are independent from hospitals, are responsible for maintaining a case register. The hospitals in the district are responsible for sending information on admitted patients to the District outpatient clinic. Previously, there was only one undifferentiated type of psychiatric registration which imposed social limitations on all mentally ill persons. Since the adoption of a new psychiatric law several years ago, only severely ill mental patients are officially registered by the outpatient clinics. Others are registered unofficially: Case notes on mildly disordered persons are kept confidential, so that when such people apply for driver's licenses, for example, their documents do not indicate that they are registered as psychiatric patients. Formerly psychotic patients who have not been referred to psychiatric services for at least 5 years are removed from the official case register. Another major impact of the new psychiatric law is a substantial decrease in admission rates. Psychiatrists are reluctant to admit a patient involuntarily for fear they would not be able to prove (to officials of the health system who receive complaints from patients and their relatives) that the patient posed a potential physical threat to himself or to others. Another reason for the decrease in admission rates is the antipsychiatry campaign led by a mass media that for decades kept silent about political and mostly nonpolitical abuse in psychiatry and now is making up for lost time.

In cases of nonpsychotic episodes, people can choose among a greater variety of services in Moscow, but much depends on their own or their relatives' ability to pay. Mental health is not a matter of insurance in Russia. Money for medical (among them psychiatric) services is supposed to come from a special tax (5.8% of personal income).

PSYCHIATRIC EPIDEMIOLOGY

Epidemiologic studies of schizophrenia in Moscow have used a broad traditional concept of this disease that corresponds to schizophrenia plus paranoid psychoses in ICD-9. There are two inclusion criteria for schizophrenia, either of them sufficient for diagnosis: psychotic symptoms (such as catatonia, mood incongruent delusions and hallucinations) and peculiar personality deficits (negative symptoms such as social withdrawal and emotional blunting). The exclusion criteria are psychogenic or organic origin of these symptoms.

According to data from the Research Center for Mental Health of the Academy of Medical Sciences, the great majority of persons with schizophrenia are treated mostly as outpatients. Only patients with a malignant form of schizophrenia (about 3% of all schizophrenics) are treated chiefly in hospitals; all other schizophrenic patients spend only 7% of time after the onset of their disorder in hospitals. Because they kept the case registers, outpatient clinics were chosen for a prevalence study of schizophrenia in Moscow. In four district outpatient clinics, about 7000 persons with schizophrenia were examined personally by officers of the center from 1965 to 1990. The total prevalence rate for schizophrenia was found to be 10.22 per 1000. In the age range 7 to 19, prevalence was low (0.48); in the age range 20 to 29, it was higher (7.10). The age groups 30 to 39 and 40 to 49 had the highest prevalence rates (15.27 and 16.82, respectively). The slight decrease in prevalence rates of schizophrenia in the population over 50 suggests that a certain proportion of affected persons at this age are no longer being referred to psychiatric institutions (or have already died).

Among different forms of schizophrenia, the highest prevalence rate was for the psychotic form with episodic course: 5.66 per 1000 of general population, or 55% of all cases of schizophrenia. The malignant form of schizophrenia was the rarest: prevalence 0.33. Paranoid schizophrenia with continuous course had a prevalence of 1.30. The remaining patients (nearly one-third of all schizophrenics) had a sluggish (latent or pseudoneurotic) form of schizophrenia with a relatively favorable outcome. Schizophrenia was nearly equally distributed among males and females, though its prevalence in males was a little bit higher: 10.66 versus 9.91. Differences between males and females were more prominent by form of schizophrenia: Malignant schizophrenia was slightly more than two times more frequent in males; recurrent schizophrenia (schizoaffective psychoses) was two times more frequent in females; and sluggish schizophrenia was 1.5 times more frequent in males.

Schizophrenia of all types, not only in those with acute psychotic onset, most frequently began in adolescence. Frequency of onset gradually declined in subsequent age groups. Rarely did schizophrenia begin after 55: less than 1% of all cases. When only overt psychotic symptoms of schizophrenia onset were taken into account, differences in disease manifestation became less prominent. An early onset of schizophrenia (in adolescence) was more probable for males. On the other hand, in females there was a noticeable increase of cases with onset between ages 40 to 44 that could not be detected in males.

A first incidence study of schizophrenia was conducted in Moscow in the 1970s using the same broad national concept of the disease (Liberman, 1974). The age of onset was assessed retrospectively by the first (usually nonpsychotic) signs of the disease. The total incidence rate was 1.91 per 10,000 per year (1.98 for males and 1.65 for females).

In the late 1970s to early 1980s, another incidence study of schizophrenia in which both broad and narrow concepts of schizophrenia were used was undertaken as a part of the DOSMeD. Some subjects from that study were followed up in ISoS. Under the broadest concept, all schizophrenic patients were included (even if their ICD-9 diagnoses were paranoid states, acute paranoid reaction, alcoholic hallucinosis, schizoid personality disorder, and some others). The Moscow incidence rates were 2.5 for males and 3.1 for females (total rate, 2.8 per 10,000 per year for population aged 18–54). Using the narrowest concept, only cases diagnosed as CATEGO class S+ (schizophrenic psychoses) were included. With this approach, incidence rates were 1.0 for males and 1.4 for females. These findings contradict previous epidemiological data from Moscow that showed males are affected with schizophrenia more frequently than females. Differences between males and females were most prominent (though still not reaching the level of statistical significance) for paranoid schizophrenia with episodic course and schizoaffective syndromes. As compared with those at other WHO centers, incidence rates in Moscow were particularly high in females in the age group 50 to 54 (3.85–1.71, depending on the concept of schizophrenia used). These rates were actually 1½ times higher than those for younger females from Moscow.

The most thorough study of long-term course and outcome of schizophrenia in Moscow was done in the 1970s at the Institute for Psychiatry of the Academy of Medical Sciences (Shternberg et al., 1981). The authors examined more than 1000 patients with a 20-year duration of disease. Because of numerous methodological incompatibilities, direct comparisons of data from that study with ISoS cannot be made. The study was retrospective and included only old persons registered in local outpatient clinics; this meant, in particular, that cases of "recovery" were not captured. The most important findings are the following: Although types of course of schizophrenia are rather stable for decades, three main phases of the evolution of the disease are discernible—an active phase in which its manifestations (symptoms) are more intense and phases of stabilization with reduction of psychotic symptoms; long-term course (taking into account both clinical and social criteria) is not invariably poor but shows prospects for some improvement when compared to the early years; there is a trend toward simplification of the clinical picture of schizophrenia in old age; negative symptoms usually do not become more severe after the first several psychotic episodes; and duration of episodes is relatively stable, but they become less frequent from age 40 to 49 and more frequent in those age 50+.

THE CENTER

The Research Center for Mental Health (now Institute for Clinical Psychiatry) of the Academy of Medical Sciences was established in the early 1980s, an outgrowth of the Institute for Psychiatry founded by the Academy of Medical Sciences in 1944. The Institute for Clinical Psychiatry has about 350 beds for psychiatric inpatients; its research has focused on schizophrenia and the development of a course type classification scheme now widely used in Russia. The Institute has participated in such WHO projects as the International Pilot Study of Schizophrenia (IPSS), DOSMeD, and studies in biological psychiatry. Also organized was the Institute for Preventive Psychiatry whose clinicians work in general hospitals and polyclinics with general practitioners. In this institute, somatoform, neurotic, mild affective, and stress-related disorders are studied; a new concept of psychiatric pathology has been elaborated (the concept of psychopathological diathesis). Both institutes participated in the field trials of ICD-10.

METHODS

From 1978 to 1982, 228 subjects were recruited for the DOSMeD study in Moscow. During most of the first year, new cases of schizophrenia were sought only in the district psychiatric outpatient clinic because it was assumed, wrongly, that all new cases of mental diseases would be registered there. In fact, the majority of new cases of schizophrenia were admitted to mental hospitals without first having been referred to the local outpatient clinic and without proper registration there, as outpatient doctors preferred to wait for diagnostic assessment to be made at the hospital. Excerpts from hospital case notes were received in local outpatient clinics only after discharge and often with some delay. Such cases could not be included in the study because the protocol called for subjects to have been referred to psychiatric services no more than 3 months before inclusion in the study. As a result of appropriate changes in the case-finding method at the end of the first year of the study, it became possible to include about five to six subjects every month instead of one to two cases as in the beginning of the study. Under such circumstances, data from subjects entered in the first year of the DOSMeD (30 cases) were considered invalid epidemiologically for a treated incidence study, and they were not followed up. (This material was also clinically biased as it excluded cases with the most acute type of onset, emergency admissions to the hospital who were not registered in local outpatient clinics.) Since it was impossible to follow up all subjects from years 2 to 4 included in the DOSMeD study, and since the longest possible follow-up period for ISoS was preferable, only subjects from the second year of the DOSMeD study were traced.

The author of this chapter examined nearly all Moscow subjects in the DOSMeD study, an investigation coordinated by Professor R. A. Adzharov. In the ISoS study, subjects were examined at follow-up by the same psychiatrist. A nurse who participated in the DOSMeD study and was known to many subjects continued to schedule appointments with the subjects and to collect information on them mostly from case notes in the district outpatient clinic. Tracing of the 72 subjects began several years before actual follow-up examination, including obtaining information from mental health services that might have seen the subject and then contacting subjects. The nurse phoned subjects using numbers dating from the DOSMeD study. Inquiries were also made at the local outpatient clinic. If a subject had been admitted to a district facility, outpatient case notes usually mentioned this, and excerpts from hospital case notes were then ordered. If subjects still could not be traced, information from the address bureau was sought.

At contact, subjects were reminded that more than 10 years ago they had been included in a psychiatric study (and had come to no harm) and told that in the near future, they would be asked for another interview. Many subjects remembered the initial examination and interviewer and consented, some eagerly. Others were rather reluctant, but if contacted frequently, they could finally be persuaded to participate. Since over the intervening years, there had been many opportunities for contact, the subjects were prepared for the request; only one subject refused to be interviewed. (She was not only reluctant but lived several hours away from Moscow.) The total interview did not usually exceed 1.5 hours, in part because in the majority of cases it was possible to review accumulated medical information before the interview. Initially, interviews of family members were to be undertaken by the nurse, but as the follow-up examinations were delayed (while awaiting the beginning of the formal study) and time pressures increased, it was not possible for her to put aside her routine work. (There was only one exception: when a subject came to the interview with her mother.) The PIRS was excluded as no one in Moscow was properly trained in its use. Study instruments were not translated into Russian; instead, the single interviewer used the English version but put the questions to the subjects in Russian, as had been done in the DOSMeD study.

STUDY RESULTS

The ISoS sample is the 72 subjects initially included in the second year of the DOSMeD study, November 1979 to October 1980. The follow-up period was 15 years. Twenty subjects could not be examined at follow-up: 10 had died, seven could not be traced, two moved far away, and one refused.

The 10 deceased subjects included one certain case of suicide, three possible cases of suicide (drowned or poisoned), and two cases of death from somatic diseases (heart failure and brain infarction). For the other four cases, it was impossible to get any information of value from neighbors. In Moscow, there was a clear-cut decrease in death rates during the follow-up period, tentatively explained by the effect of suicide on the statistics: All four cases occurred during the first several years of the follow-up period. Mean age of female deceased subjects was the same as in the total DOSMeD sample (41.8 vs. 42.3), but that for deceased male subjects (57.5) was higher than Moscow female subjects and DOSMeD male subjects (38.0). The mean age of death for mentally ill males is actually a bit lower than for the general Russian male population.

Although sex distribution was nearly equal in the total DOSMeD sample, in Moscow because of their superior numbers in the general population, there were more females in the total cohort (59.7%), as well as in the alive (63.5%) and deceased (60.0%) groups. Incidence rates for females in Moscow were somewhat higher than for males; only among the lost-to-follow-up subjects were the rates higher for males (60.0%). When these cases were examined, they were found to have been mostly young and living in hostels, having been recruited from the provinces by the large factories. Young men are best suited for such work and living conditions. Should they marry, they usually live in their spouses' flats; but if unmarried and affected by a severe mental disorder, they tend to return (often after first discharge from the hospital) to their places of birth, there to live with and receive support from their parents. We hypothesize that it is for this reason that 90% of the lost-to-follow-up subjects in Moscow had short-term follow-up time, not exceeding 17 months. In the total DOSMeD sample, such cases made up less than 55%. To corroborate this explanation, data on birth year of subjects were examined. The majority of lost to follow-up subjects (70%) were born in the 1950s or later, an age-group that made up one-third of the Moscow sample. On the other hand, most of the deceased subjects in Moscow (90%) were born before the 1950s. Overall, subjects in Moscow were 8.5 years older than DOSMeD subjects.

Examination of type of onset in the Moscow sample showed a larger portion with insidious onset as compared with the total DOSMeD cohort (47.2% vs. 32.3%, respectively). Adjusting percentages to take account of missing data, however, significantly narrows the gap, raising the DOSMeD figure to 41.3%.

When baseline diagnoses converted to ICD-10 are compared between Moscow and all centers, a number of discrepancies appear. First, it should be noted that these differences could reflect the distinctive way in which the original ICD-9 classification was applied in Moscow (Jablensky et al., 1992, pp. 28, 78), as well as the preference at that time in Russian psychiatry for the schizophrenic diagnosis. If clinical rediagnoses, as opposed to converted diagnoses conversion are studied, differences between the two cohorts became less prominent: Schizophrenia accounted for 71.2 and 53.3% of Moscow subjects' total DOSMeD alive cohorts, respectively, when converted diagnoses were used, but for only 55.8 and 48.1%, respectively, when clinical rediagnosis was the method. Not surprisingly, changes in diagnostic distribution were more prominent in Moscow; schizophrenic subjects were rediagnosed as nonschizophrenic (usually "other psychotic disorder") in nearly one half of cases, whereas in the total DOSMeD sample this occurred far less frequently (in about a quarter of cases).

To explore further whether real differences in psychopathology exist between the Moscow and the total DOSMeD cohorts, we compared frequencies of nonaffective psychotic disorders (all disorders except "bipolar disorders/depression" and "other nonpsychotic disorders"). In Moscow and in all centers, such disorders made up from 81 to 87% of the samples. Thus the results of the present study indirectly confirm the higher reliability of ICD-10 as compared with ICD-9, although some doubts about diagnostic discrepancies with ICD-10 remain, especially when algorithmically converted diagnoses are used.

Returning to converted baseline diagnoses, it is interesting to note some differences in type of schizophrenia diagnosed. On the one hand, 65.3% of subjects in the Moscow sample were diagnosed as paranoid schizophrenics, whereas in the total DOSMeD sample the portion of paranoid schizophrenia was less than half as much (about 30%). On the other hand, hebephrenic schizophrenia in Moscow was not so frequent as in the total DOSMeD cohort (4.2% vs. 10.7%) and catatonic schizophrenia was not diagnosed here at all (2.7% in the total DOSMeD sample). Putting aside the "nosological status" of mental disorders, the different diagnoses in which delusional symptoms usually predominate (such as paranoid schizophrenia, other psychotic disorders, acute schizophrenia-like disorders) are more frequent in the Moscow cohort than in the total DOSMeD cohort (79.2% vs. 55.7%) One explanation might be that delusional symptoms were not more frequent among Moscow subjects but were more frequently dominant in the clinical picture of their mental disorders. Acute schizophrenia-like disorders were next in frequency in the Moscow cohort (13.9%), nearly as frequent as in the total DOSMeD sample (18.9%), the majority of which were rediagnosed as schizophrenic. Equally frequent in Moscow, though much rarer in DOSMeD total (13.9% vs. 4.6%), were "other nonpsychotic disorders."

When patterns of short-term course are compared, the results in Moscow and in all DOSMeD centers look roughly alike: The percentages of course with single psychotic episodes, two or more psychotic episodes, and continuous psychotic illness are nearly the same. The most striking difference appears when assessment of the types of remission is made: In Moscow, remissions were assessed as incomplete much more frequently (62.5%) than as complete (16.7%), while in the total DOSMeD sample complete remissions were more common than incomplete (38.4 vs. 29.4%). In Moscow, the usual reasons for assessing a remission as incomplete include the presence of some signs of personality change, such as emotional bluntness and/or narrowing of interests. Nonpsychotic episodes after single psychotic episodes were found nearly two times more frequently in Moscow than in the total DOSMeD sample. About one-third of subjects in both samples had courses limited to a single psychotic episode without nonpsychotic episodes. This percentage is somewhat higher than in previous studies in Moscow; in the latest (Seyku and Morozova, 1989), it was about one-quarter (26.2%), a fact probably accounted for by the longer follow-up period (usually at least 15 years) in those studies. (It is worth noting that in the study cited above, only 0.9% of cases had complete remission.)

Assessment of the severity of psychotic symptoms with the modified Bleuler scale showed that in Moscow, about 92% of alive subjects were rated mild or "recovered" (no psychotic symptoms; only residual signs). Severe or moderate levels were found in about 18% of alive subjects. In the total DOSMeD sample, these figures were 75 and 25%, respectively.

The dead and lost-to-follow-up groups frequently revealed much more severe or moderate levels of psychotic symptoms in all centers and in Moscow. In the latter case, they were found in 30% of dead and in 60% of lost-to-follow-up subjects (compared with 8% of alive subjects). In part, this difference may be explained by different periods of assessment. Remissions last much longer than psychotic episodes in a great majority of cases of episodic course (and continuous course was observed in only 5.8% of subjects). So, if the period of assessing psychotic symptoms is only 1 month, as for alive subjects, it is more probable that they were in remission. If most of the relatively short follow-up period is assessed, as for deceased and lost-to-follow-up subjects, the probability of including a psychotic episode increases. As noted earlier, lost-to-follow-up subjects usually left Moscow for home in the provinces soon after discharge from a psychiatric hospital; for such subjects, rating severity of symptoms meant taking into account psychotic episodes lasting the greater part of the follow-up period with only short intervals of remission. We simply don't know how their clinical picture evolved in the ensuing months. At odds with this methodological explanation for the discrepancy, however, are real differences in severity of symptoms: Suicidal subjects among the dead group and seriously socially maladjusted subjects among the lost-to-follow-up group are more likely to have clinically unfavorable outcomes.

ALIVE SUBJECTS

In Moscow, alive subjects during the last 2 years of follow-up were usually not psychotic (67.3%), while in all DOSMeD centers over one-half (51.8%) were not psychotic. Episodic course during this period was registered far less frequently (26.9%) but more frequently than in the total DOSMeD sample (17.0%). The most clear-cut difference between the Moscow and the total DOSMeD cohort was in the proportions of subjects with continuous course (5.8% vs. 26.4%). When type of course since first episode is assessed, the same trends in differences between the Moscow and the total DOSMeD sample may be seen. For example, episodic course was registered in 78.8% of subjects in Moscow and in 63.4% of subjects in the total DOSMeD sample.

Ratings made on the Global Assessment of Functioning Scale for Symptomatology (GAF-S) showed that severe symptoms (< 51) during the past month are rarer in Moscow (9.5% of cases) than in the total DOSMeD sample (23.0%). Absent or minimal symptom levels (81–90) were observed more frequently in all centers (31.8%), especially in Moscow (51.9%). Time trends of psychotic symptoms during the entire follow-up period were similar to those of all DOSMeD centers. Most frequently, symptoms were prominent during the first third of this period only: 55.8% of subjects in Moscow and 61.8% in all centers. Consistently low levels of symptom severity were registered in 15.4% of cases in Moscow and 8.9% of the whole DOSMeD sample, and consistently high levels of symptom severity were 13.5 and 9.1%, respectively. Other types of time trends were rare. A general trend of improvement over time was registered in 57.6% of subjects in Moscow and in 50.2% of the total DOSMeD sample. No changes were observed in 38.5% of subjects in Moscow and in 26.2% of cases in all centers. Subjects rarely got somewhat worse (3.8% in Moscow and

12.2% in all centers). The most unfavorable outcome (getting much worse) wasn't registered in Moscow at all, and in the total DOSMeD sample was true for only 17 subjects (3.5%).

Only a relatively small percentage of subjects was hospitalized during the past 2 years in Moscow (17.3%; all of them for a period of less than 12 months), and in the total DOSMeD sample (20.8%; nearly three-quarters of whom spent less than 12 months in hospitals). Mean duration of hospitalization in Moscow was much less than in all centers (2.2 months vs. 8.6 months), a difference that can be attributed to the general rule in Russia that an admission to an ordinary mental hospital should not exceed 3 months. Otherwise, it is recommended, though not strictly obligatory, that patients be sent to special hospitals or boarding houses for chronic psychiatric patients. Usually patients and their relatives are reluctant (because conditions there are worse than in hospitals) and prefer discharge, to be followed later, if necessary, by a new admission.

Subjects at the time of follow-up examination were usually living with families or friends: in Moscow (71.2%) and in the whole DOSMeD cohort (74.0%). Less frequently, subjects lived alone, 26.9% in Moscow, and 15.6% of the whole sample. During the greater part of the last 2 years of follow-up, all Moscow subjects had independent living arrangements, as did the vast majority of subjects in all other centers. In general, living arrangements during the entire follow-up period were not much different from those that were found during the recent 2 years. No subjects in Moscow were homeless or vagrant during those past 2 years, and there were only 11 (2.3%) such subjects in the total DOSMeD sample. During this period of time, in the whole cohort only five (1.0%) were imprisoned, none in Moscow.

Global evaluation of disability during the last month of follow-up showed the rarity of extreme ratings in the Moscow sample. A similar trend is observed also in the total DOSMeD sample, though not so prominently. Fair and higher levels of adjustment were achieved in 63.4% of cases in Moscow and in 68.2% of cases in the total sample. Another rating of disability during the past month was made with the Global Assessment of Functioning Scale (GAF-D). Severe levels of disability (<51) were rare in Moscow (17.3%), less so in all centers (30.1%). Mean values on this scale were 69.1 for the Moscow sample and 64.4 for the total DOSMeD sample. With respect to time trends of disability over the entire period, for the majority of cases in Moscow (61.5%) disability was not prominent during the whole period of follow-up, while in the total DOSMeD sample, disability most frequently (41.9%) was prominent in the first third only.

During the last 2 years of follow-up, 36.5% of subjects in Moscow and 49% of subjects in all DOSMeD centers were never employed. For the majority of subjects who were, the duration of employment exceeded 12 months in 93.8% of Moscow subjects and 75.3% of DOSMeD subjects. Work performance was good or very good in 93.3% of cases of full-time employment in Moscow and in 89.1% of such cases in the total DOSMeD cohort. Mean values of duration of full-time employment over those last 2 years were 23.2 months in Moscow and 21.6 months in all DOSMeD centers. Only two Moscow subjects worked part-time (averaging 22 months) and only two female subjects were engaged full-time in household activities. Part-time employment and full-time household activities are gradually becoming a more frequent kind of social engagement, but they are still not very usual in Moscow.

During those most recent 2 years, there was a significantly larger proportion of retired persons in Moscow (36.5%, nearly all of them women), than in all DOSMeD centers (5.8%), meaning that the majority of retired subjects in the total DOSMeD sample were from Moscow. This may be explained, first, by the early retirement age in Russia (55 for women, 60 for men), and second, by the average 8.5 years higher age of alive cohort subjects in Moscow where females prevailed in the older groups. Only two Moscow subjects (12 in all centers) received pensions for medical (somatic) conditions during those last 2 years. Disability pensions for mental conditions were received by 15.4% of subjects in Moscow and by nearly twice that proportion in the total DOSMeD cohort (29.3%). In Moscow, such pensions were always (and in all centers, nearly always) received for more than half of the last 2 years. None of the Moscow subjects were students during this period, versus four in all other centers.

Assaults during the last 2 years were rather infrequent both in the Moscow (11.5%) and in the total DOSMeD (10.8%) samples. During this period, there were no suicide attempts among alive Moscow subjects, and only 20 subjects (4.3%) from other centers made attempts. When the entire follow-up period is examined, assaults are more common, occurring in 19.2% of Moscow cases and 24.2% in all centers. The difference in the frequency of suicide attempts between the

Moscow and the total DOSMeD samples was much greater (1.9% vs. 20.3%).

During those most recent 2 years, nearly one-half of Moscow subjects took no neuroleptics, but for the entire follow-up period, all but one were on neuroleptics, the majority taking them sometimes. In most other (7 of 8) DOSMeD centers, neuroleptics were taken more frequently (most of the time). Many patients dislike taking psychotropic drugs, neuroleptics especially, because of side effects, and there is a serious problem with compliance. Many Russians believe that "chemical compounds" can be harmful. Less frequent neuroleptic treatment also correlates with lower levels of psychotic symptoms and with relative rarity of continuous course. Females were more often on neuroleptic treatment most of the time during the past 2 years (36.4%) than males (15.8%). This may be explained, first, by a greater frequency of cases with psychotic episodes or with continuous course during those past 2 years in female subjects as compared to male subjects (42.4 vs. 15.8%); and second, by lower compliance in males. Trends in taking medications during the entire period of follow-up were similar for the Moscow cohort and for all centers: Medications were prominent during the first third of the follow-up period for 46.2 and 39.0% of subjects, respectively. One-third of subjects were rather intensively medicated during the entire period. About one-tenth of subjects did not use much medication (if any) at any time. During the past 2 years, diagnostically different groups of subjects were equally often treated with neuroleptics (except for nonpsychotic subjects).

Nearly two-thirds of subjects in both the Moscow and the total DOSMeD samples were hospitalized during the first third of the follow-up period only. Other trends in hospitalization were relatively infrequent.

Mode of onset proved a poor predictor of outcome in Moscow: Contrary to expectation, those with acute or sudden onset proved no less likely than those with insidious onset to have had psychotic episodes in the last 2 years of follow-up (35 vs. 31%, respectively). On closer examination, however, the lack of difference is probably an artifact of the disproportionate number of subjects with (converted) schizophrenia diagnoses in the noninsidious groups. Fully 77% of those with onset of less than a month (vs. 65% of those with onset greater than 1 month), received a converted diagnosis of schizophrenia. Thus, whatever favorable prognostic tendency acute mode of onset confers may have been counteracted by the less favorable tendencies of the schizophrenic diagnosis.

In Moscow as elsewhere in DOSMeD, in cases where the early course of episodic illness was characterized by complete remissions, mean values of scores on the GAF-S scale were higher than in cases of incomplete remissions or continuous illness. Cases showing complete remissions early on also have much better overall time trend. Global evaluation of adjustment also correlated with complete remission (60% of whom had good or excellent adjustment) whereas 90% of those with early incomplete remission or continuous illness had fair, poor, or very poor adjustment. A similar distribution occurred in the total DOSMeD sample. Subjects with complete remissions were also assessed as having higher scores on the GAF-D scale, as compared to their counterparts (a difference in mean value of about 11 points).

Subjects clinically rediagnosed as having schizophrenia on first contact were less frequently not psychotic during the last 2 years of follow-up, as compared to other diagnostic categories. This prognostic difference for diagnosis holds for the total DOSMeD sample as well. Compared to subjects with other psychoses, those with schizophrenia less frequently improved over the follow-up period, instead remaining the same or even becoming worse, in both Moscow and the total DOSMeD samples. Differences between subjects with schizophrenia and those with other psychoses were not seen, however, in global evaluations of disability.

DISCUSSION

The substantial time devoted to persuading subjects to be interviewed allowed assessment of all but one found case in Moscow. Many other lost-to-follow-up subjects are believed to have migrated from Moscow, mostly back to their places of birth, because of illness and social maladjustment. Having come to take jobs unpopular among Muscovites, they wound up losing both employment and their rooms in hostels owing to disruptive manifestations of the disorder. If one assumes that their subsequent clinical course remained unfavorable, this would mean that the alive Moscow ISoS cohort would be biased in the direction of better outcome.

In Moscow, many patients with psychotic disorders are still obliged to register at local outpatient clinics. Referring to this fact sometimes helped to get a subject's consent for an interview. Other subjects, however, had negative attitudes toward outpatient clinics, and investigators learned to avoid such references. Information about cause of death was difficult to come by in Moscow, not because of reluctance on the part of relatives or neighbors, but because they had little interest in the subjects and little motivation to recall information once known.

Comparison of clinical data on the Moscow and the total DOSMeD samples showed that in the former cohort there were substantially fewer cases of continuous course type (5.8 vs. 26.4%). Accordingly, the percentage of cases with absent or minimal symptom levels (during the past month) on the GAF-S scale was higher in Moscow than in other centers, though differences in the mean values of symptoms between the two cohorts were not substantial (73.5 vs. 65.3%, respectively). The same trend can be seen when Bleuler severity scores are analyzed. The discrepancy between subjects in Moscow and those in other DOSMeD centers might be attributed partly to the early loss (hypothesized above) of subjects likely to have less favorable outcome. This does not explain, however, the small number of cases of continuous illness in the alive Moscow sample (only two such subjects were lost to follow-up).

With respect to early (2-year) course of illness, remissions among Moscow subjects, in contrast to the total DOSMeD sample, were usually assessed as incomplete (mostly because of emotional bluntness and insufficient insight into illness). The Russian concept of schizophrenia viewed such symptoms as the result of a psychotic episode (so-called deficit symptoms); recently, it has become apparent that such signs may be to a large extent inborn peculiarities. There was also a larger proportion of subjects with nonpsychotic episodes after a single initial psychotic episode in Moscow that can be attributed to the method of collecting information (i.e., nonpsychotic episodes were well documented in case notes made by local outpatient clinics).

Ratings of disability on the GAF scale in Moscow ran parallel to those of symptom severity; extreme levels of disability were rare here. Global evaluation of disability showed less difference between the Moscow and the total DOSMeD samples, though extreme ratings (excellent adjustment as well as very poor adjustment or severe maladjustment) were less common in Moscow. Disability tended not to be prominent during any particular interval of the follow-up period in Moscow, while being more prominent in the first third for the total DOSMeD cohort. This time trend in disability in the whole sample accords with trends in symptomatology. During first psychotic episodes subjects were hospitalized in Moscow. In assessing disability trends, these hospitalization periods weren't taken into consideration in Moscow, not only because their duration made up only a small part of the first third of the follow-up period, but also because it was difficult in a general rating to combine properly periods of good adjustment in society during remissions and periods of treatment in hospitals.

Unemployment rates for Moscow subjects were lower than for the whole DOSMeD sample, and employment lasted longer in Moscow. Unemployment in Russia became a real social problem only in the 1990s, but as compared to other regions, Moscow is an exception with negligible levels of unemployment (especially until 1995). It is rather easy for a person, even with some degree of disability, to keep a job, especially in a state-run enterprise, because of regulatory protections. Salaries in state-run enterprises are rather low, and in the 1990s many people quit their jobs there to get jobs in private business. But as such change of employment is risky, subjects with episodes of mental disorder usually preferred not to run the risk.

There was a substantial difference in frequencies of suicide attempts, which were very low in Moscow. This may be because attempts are underreported in Moscow; if the three possible cases are added to the one confirmed case of suicide the rate would be comparable to that of the total DOSMeD sample. Besides, it is well known in Moscow that suicide attempts are grounds for involuntary admission, so patients are reluctant to disclose them.

As compared to the total DOSMeD sample, neuroleptics were taken less frequently in Moscow. The most obvious explanation for this discrepancy is its correlation with the relative rarity of continuous course of psychotic disorders and lower levels of psychotic symptoms in Moscow, although such medications are often prescribed preventively. In addition, the general population harbors ideas about the "harmfulness" of psychotropic drugs which often manifests itself in noncompliance on the part of patients, with the tacit complicity of doctors. A shortage of neuroleptics in the early 1990s could have led to interrupted schedules of medication, but in nearly half the cases during the last 2 years of follow-up, they were not taken at all.

Conversion tables between ICD-9 and ICD-10 (WHO, 1994) are useful for statistical purposes, particularly when large groups of subjects need to be diagnosed anew. But because the diagnostic principles underlying these two classifications are different, the translations cannot be precise. Rediagnosis is more accurate; but when done retrospectively, the process may be contaminated by additional diagnostically significant information that might not have been available at the time of the original diagnosis. In Moscow, there was practically no additional information about the clinical picture of first contact psychotic episodes, except for its duration. Other potential sources of bias are clinical course of the disease and overall trend for better or worse. To study the possibility of bias, cases of schizophrenia according to converted diagnosis were compared with clinical rediagnoses. Rediagnosed schizophrenia cases showed less favorable course and outcome than cases with converted schizophrenia diagnoses. There was practically no difference in the frequencies of continuous course during the last 2 years of follow-up: 6.9% in rediagnosed schizophrenia and 8.1% in converted schizophrenia. Nevertheless, more subjects with converted schizophrenia were nonpsychotic during the past 2 years as compared to rediagnosed schizophrenics (67.6 vs. 55.2%). Overall time trends were also more favorable in converted schizophrenia subjects; changes for the better were noted in 56.7%, whereas in cases of schizophrenia rediagnoses were noted in only 44.8%. So, in the rediagnosis process some prognostically more favorable cases theoretically could be excluded, though in the Russian concept of schizophrenia as well as in ICD-10, type of course is not supposed to be taken into account.

The main result of ISoS is that long-term course and outcome of schizophrenia and related psychotic disorders is somewhat better in Moscow as compared to all other DOSMeD centers. This cannot be attributed to selection into the original Moscow cohort of more prognostically favorable cases. Moscow had relatively more cases of schizophrenia (both rediagnosed and, especially, converted) and cases with insidious mode of onset of the disorder, parameters that tend to be associated with less favorable course and outcome. Moreover, short-term course and outcome of schizophrenia and related psychotic disorders were no better in Moscow as compared to all centers; according to the DOSMeD study, they were actually the same as in the majority of developed countries and worse than in developing countries. Speculations about what factors cause such a difference yield only two that have changed in Russia during recent years: level of well-being and instability. If instability is not a characteristic of developing countries, then only one explanation is left.

SUMMARY

A long-term follow-up study proved to be feasible in Moscow as 52 (72.2%) of 72 subjects initially included in the second year of the DOSMeD study were successfully traced and examined. Ten subjects (13.9%) had died and 10 subjects (13.9%) were otherwise lost to follow-up. In the majority of cases of schizophrenia (and related psychotic disorders), long-term outcome is relatively favorable; as compared with the early years of the disorder, subjects improved substantially as indicated by ratings on general trend over the 15-year time period as "change for the better" (57.6%), by the absence of psychotic symptoms during the last 2 years of follow-up (67.3%), and by their prominence in the first third only (55.9%). At the time of follow-up examination and during the last 2 years, disability was not a serious problem for a majority of subjects: During the last month, 63.4% of cases showed fair and higher levels of adjustment, and global assessment of functioning (GAF) revealed lower levels of disability (51–90) in 82.7% of subjects. The majority of Moscow subjects were employed during the greater part of the past 2-year period, and their work performance was good or very good.

There were a number of differences between the Moscow and the total DOSMeD cohorts. The baseline examination revealed higher rates of paranoid schizophrenia over catatonic and hebephrenic forms in Moscow. As schizophrenia (especially its paranoid form) and other psychotic disorders (in which delusions and hallucinations are essential symptoms) were more frequent in Moscow than in other centers, it is possible to conclude that delusional (and/or hallucinatory) symptoms dominated the clinical picture more frequently in Moscow. When compared with all DOSMeD centers, long-term outcome of schizophrenia was in some respects better in Moscow. Moscow subjects were more often nonpsychotic during the last 2 years of follow-up. If psychotic, the course of the disorder was more often episodic and less frequently continuous. Severity of symptoms in the Moscow subjects was also lower, and the greater percentage of incomplete remissions and twice greater number of cases with nonpsychotic episodes could be explained by detection of minor negative symptoms in the detailed clinical data available from case notes in outpatient clinics. Assessment of disability on global evaluation did not reveal substantial differences between subjects in Moscow and those in all centers, but severe levels of disability on the GAF scale were rare in Moscow. Hospitalization and neuroleptic treatment during the last 2 years were also rare among Moscow subjects. This can be explained by the relative infrequency of continuous course of the disease, by lower levels of psychotic symptoms, by regulations in the local mental health system, and by attitudes toward medication. There was one confirmed and three cases of suspected suicide; but such attempts are likely underreported, possibly because subjects fear rehospitalization. Compared with other diagnostic groups, subjects with schizophrenia had less favorable outcome, as assessed by overall time trend. They had lower levels of adjustment than subjects with nonpsychotic disorders, bipolar affective disorders and depressions; but not than subjects with "other psychotic disorders."

References

Jablensky, A., Sartorius, N., Ernberg, G., Anker, M., Korten, A., Cooper, J. E., Day, R., & Bertelsen, A. (1992), Schizophrenia: Manifestations, incidence and course in different cultures: A World Health Organization ten-country study. *Psycholog. Med.*, 20 (Monogr. Suppl.): 1–97.

Liberman, Yu. K. (1974), The problem of schizophrenia incidence. *Zhurnal Nevropatologii i Psikhiatrii*, 74(8): 1224–1233. (In Russian)

Seyku, Yu. V., & Morozova, V. (1989), Prevalence of single episode schizophrenia in an epidemiological study. *Zhurnal Nevropatologii i Psikhiatrii*, 89(10):81–86. (In Russian)

Shevchenko, L. (1993), Russia and the commonwealth of independent states. In: *International Handbook on Mental Health Policy*, ed. D. R. Kempe. Westport, CT: Greenwood Press, pp. 346–347.

——(1995), Evaluation of social detriment from mental diseases. In: *Fifth Congress of the World Association for Psychosocial Rehabilitation, Abstr.*, Vol. 1. Rotterdam, The Netherlands.

——Solokhina, T. (1995), Economic aspects of functioning of mental health services. *Zhurnal Nevropatologii i Psikhiatrii*, 95(1):81–85. (In Russian)

Shternberg, E., Gavrilova, S., Druzhinina, T., Kontsevoy, V., Medvedev, A., Modchanova, E. (1981), *Evolution and Outcome of Schizophrenia*, Moscow: Meditsina. (In Russian)

World Health Organization (1994), *The ICD-10 Classification of Mental and Behavioral Disorders: Conversion Tables between ICD-8, ICD-9, and ICD-10*. Revision 1. (WHO/MNH/92.16. Rev.1). Geneva, Switzerland: World Health Organization.

Chapter 15

DOSMeD: Nagasaki, Japan

Yoshibumi Nakane, Koichi Takada, Kazuyasu Yoshitake, and Keiko Hatada

CULTURAL CONTEXT

Located in the western part of Kyushu Island of the Isles of Japan and in the southern part of Nagasaki Prefecture, Nagasaki City is home of the prefectural government of Nagasaki and a center of economic activity: industry, business, and trade. It extends 25 km from east to west and 25.9 km from north to south, for a total area of 240.43 sq km. According to the October 1995 census (Statistical Bureau, Prime Minister's Office), the population of Nagasaki City is 438,724 (204,252 men and 234,472 women), and the population of Nagasaki prefecture is about 1,545,000.

In the 17th century, an isolationist policy closed Japan to the outside world. Only the Dutch and the Chinese were allowed to carry on very restricted trade with Japan and only through Nagasaki harbor. Thus, for nearly 250 years, Nagasaki was Japan's only window to foreign culture. Even after the opening of Japan in the mid-19th century, Nagasaki remained an important entry point for foreign culture and technology. Among its innovations were a training school for sailors and the first steel ingot factory, which marked the beginning of modern technological industry in Japan and set the stage for the development of Japan's major industries.

In the past 60 years, Nagasaki has suffered several disasters, the best known of which was the atomic bomb dropped in August 1945. Many survivors still receive medical support from the government. In the 1980s and early 1990s, Nagasaki suffered a disastrous flood and was ravaged by a giant typhoon, each of which did substantial damage to people, property, and industry. Unemployment has increased slightly of late because the main industry of the city, shipbuilding, has shifted from a high- to a low-growth economy. As orders for ships decreased, shipbuilding and related companies have laid off employees.

Most people in Nagasaki are Buddhists, and there are a small number of Christians. Religion seldom influences lifestyle or medical treatment. Japanese is spoken by everyone regardless of class, age, gender, or educational background. Very few speak other languages.

Impact of Mental Health Issues on Society

Many schizophrenic and alcoholic patients languish in the wards of psychiatric hospitals in every city and prefecture in Japan. The number of psychiatric beds is over 50 per 10,000 population in Nagasaki prefecture, the second highest in Japan. The mean length of stay per admission is over 700 days, and 30% of the psychiatric inpatients remain in the hospital for more than 10 years because old persons cannot be discharged. Stigma is slowly lessening, however, and length of stay for newly admitted patients is decreasing. The shortage of a community-based support system, a major reason for the long stay of inpatients, is a problem which the government is tackling at long last.

Generally, understanding of psychiatric disorders has been improving, but prejudice against such patients is still strong. Many people still believe that severe psychiatric disorders cannot be cured or that psychiatric disorders are indications of inherited genetic deficiency. In the 1980s and 1990s, however, the number and utilization of day care and outpatient clinics has grown, and the number of former schizophrenic patients working after discharge has increased, although anyone who suspends work activity is not thought well of and is taboo.

THE MENTAL HEALTH SYSTEM

Responsibility for regulating mental health services lies locally with the Department of Hygiene and Welfare of the Nagasaki Prefectural Office and nationally with the Ministry of Health and Welfare. Operating under the national Mental Health Act, the system basically has not changed in the years surrounding ISoS.

Structure of the Mental Health Services System

In 1900, the Mental Health Act established a mental health system for the first time in Japan. The act was revised in 1950, and again in 1988 to protect the human rights of psychiatric patients and to provide for their social rehabilitation. As a general rule, the act recommends that admission to psychiatric hospitals be voluntary. Persons who need treatment but who refuse admission to a psychiatric hospital or mentally ill persons who have committed a crime must be examined by two psychiatrists qualified by the Ministry of Public Health before commitment. In 1995, the act was revised again to improve psychiatric and medical treatment and psychiatric rehabilitation and to ensure coordination among the mental health system and other health, social service, and administrative sectors. For example, psychiatrists are available at the family court and at the juvenile classification home which makes psychological reports and recommendations to family court. The Public Health Center provides day service (once or twice per month). The mental health system and the welfare system jointly coordinate services for the more than 30% of psychiatric patients on public support. Mental health facilities that treat alcoholic patients are connected with Alcoholics Anonymous and other self-help groups. In the mid-1990s in Nagasaki City, the connections among the public hospitals, private hospitals, private clinics, Department of Hygiene and Welfare, health centers, welfare offices, children's welfare clinics, and other mental health systems have been moving closer to providing for the social rehabilitation of psychiatric patients.

At present, all public and private psychiatric hospitals have outpatient clinics, and independent outpatient clinics are affiliated with psychiatric hospitals. In addition, there are special hospitals that care for alcoholic and adolescent patients. When psychiatric patients have serious physical complications, they are sent to those general hospitals that have departments of psychiatry.

Financial Support

Medical care is provided by the National Health Service which is funded through general taxation and from monthly fees based on grade of employment and family size. Currently, the National Health Service is underfunded, so fees may be increased shortly. Most Japanese also buy private health insurance. Hence, a patient usually pays 10 to 30% of the cost of medical treatment but no more than approximately $600 per month per household.

More than 80% of inpatient care for persons with severe mental illness is provided by private hospitals, the rest by public hospitals. Before June 1995, for psychiatric outpatients who applied to the public system for official support for outpatient treatment, 50% of the cost was paid by the prefecture and the nation, 35 to 50% was paid by the patient's insurance, and patients paid 0 to 15%. In July 1995, the system changed, so that outpatients with official support pay at most 5% of the cost. Outpatients who do not apply for official support pay 10 to 30% of the cost of medical treatment. For atomic bomb survivors, treatment for any disease is rendered without charge.

PSYCHIATRIC EPIDEMIOLOGY

Clinical Characteristics of Patients with Mental Illness on an Isolated Island in Nagasaki Prefecture

A study of schizophrenic patients who visited Goto Central Hospital for the first time between 1961 and 1972 (Ohta, Nagaoka et al., 1976; Nagaoka and Ohta, 1978; Ohta, Nakane et al., 1985) demonstrated the sociocultural factors affecting schizophrenia. It was found that schizophrenic patients who had their first breakdown in the Goto Islands (a rural region) showed the delusion of being observed more frequently than patients having onset elsewhere. On the other hand, among schizophrenic patients who had onset outside of the Goto Islands (in an urban area), the delusion of being followed was observed significantly more than in other schizophrenic groups. Further investigation showed that significantly more schizophrenics with first breaks in the Goto Islands had an abulia-autistic state. Conversely, those with onsets occurring away from their native islands showed more florid symptoms (namely, a hallucinatory-delusional state). Schizophrenic patients in the Catholic, Buddhist, and Kakure-Christian (hidden-Christian) village communities were investigated to determine the relationship among the subtypes of schizophrenia, the initial clinical features, and the cultural backgrounds of the three religions' social psychologies. Differences in the subtypes of schizophrenia and in the clinical features at onset were observed only between the Catholic group and the Kakure-Christian group.

Seasonal Distribution of Births of Schizophrenics

A study of seasonal distribution of birth in 3094 patients diagnosed as schizophrenic from 1950 to 1978 (Ohta, Ishizawa et al., 1979) showed that more schizophrenic patients were born in winter or early spring than in other seasons. Furthermore, as part of the DOSMeD, and with the cooperation of all the mental health facilities in Nagasaki City, birth dates of 107 first break schizophrenic patients during 2 years starting January 1979 were also analyzed. The birth rate of persons with paranoid type schizophrenia was higher in winter with marginal significance; that of patients with hebephrenia was significantly higher in summer.

Epidemiological Studies of Schizophrenia in Japan

As part of DOSMeD, collaborating researchers interviewed all new patients, who met specified inclusion criteria, visiting any of the 30 institutions in Nagasaki. There were 107 subjects (61 males; 46 females) (Nakane, Ohta, and Radford, 1992).

1. The Administrative Incidence Rate (Nakane, Takahashi, Tominaga et al., 1985) and Morbidity Risk (Nakane, Takahashi, and Ohta, 1986) of Schizophrenia

The incidence rate for schizophrenia in Nagasaki City was 2.0 per 10,000 (male, 2.4; female, 1.6). The peak incidence of schizophrenia in Nagasaki was in the age group 24 years and below. For males, the peak incidence occurred in the 15 to 19 age group, although it was still relatively high in both the 20 to 24 and the 25 to 29 age groups. For females, the peak occurred in the 20 to 24 age group. The total incidence rate for males was higher than that for females. The morbidity risk rate for males was 0.90 and for females 0.62. Both incidence rates and estimated morbidity risk for Nagasaki are somewhere in the middle of the eight other centers in the DOSMeD study. In general, although some differences in schizophrenia subtypes have been found, prevalence and incidence rates of schizophrenia in Japan are not significantly different from those reported in other countries.

2. First Rank Symptoms of Schizophrenia (Araki et al., 1984)

Ninety-three subjects had thorough PSE interviews. The frequency of (Schneiderian) first rank symptoms for all the subjects was 57%, for cases of hebephrenic type, 50%, and for cases of paranoid type, 67%. Lower relative frequencies suggest that the hebephrenic type is becoming less symptomatic.

3. Study of Life Events of Schizophrenia (Ishizawa, 1980)

A substudy of the life events of schizophrenia was carried out on 80 cases. Sixty-three cases (78.8%) experienced at least one life event of some kind during the 3 months preceding onset. Fifty-five percent of subjects experienced at least one independent life event (not caused by the onset of the illness) during the last 4 weeks before onset. Patients with acute-subacute onset had significantly more independent life events than patients with chronic onset during the 3 months prior to onset, particularly during the 4 weeks immediately prior, suggesting that the more acute the onset of schizophrenia, the greater the triggering effect of life events. The number of patients who had at least one event during the 3 months prior to onset was a little larger among paranoid cases than among hebephrenic cases, and it was significant during 9 to 12 weeks before onset—45.8% in paranoid cases versus 16.7% in hebephrenic cases. In paranoid cases, the number increased gradually until the last 4 weeks before onset, suggesting that life events affect paranoid cases and hebephrenic cases in different ways.

4. Epidemiological Study of the Association between Schizophrenia and Malignant Neoplasms (Ohta, Nakane, and Takahashi, 1981; Ohta, 1982)

In a DOSMeD substudy, 3107 schizophrenic patients who resided in Nagasaki City from 1960 to 1978 were examined for malignant neoplasms. The incidence rates for all patients (and females especially) were statistically higher than those of the general and female population (no difference was found for male schizophrenics). A significantly higher incidence of malignant neoplasms was observed in younger schizophrenic patients born after 1925, as compared with the incidence of malignant neoplasms in their counterparts in the general population. Among the malignant neoplasms by site, only breast cancer showed a significantly higher rate for female schizophrenic patients, especially in younger females born after 1925, than in the corresponding general female population.

5. Epidemiological Study of Physical Morbidity in Schizophrenics (Ohta, Nakane, Mine et al., 1988)

The incidence of tuberculosis among 3251 patients diagnosed as schizophrenic residing in Nagasaki City between 1960 and 1978 was significantly higher for both males and females than that of the general population. Similarly, the incidence rates of tuberculosis among schizophrenic patients born before 1925 and those born after were significantly higher than those of the corresponding age groups in the general population.

6. Features of Patients with Schizophrenia and Depression as Observed by Family Members (Ohta and Nakane, 1989)

A comparative study of two groups of patients, one with schizophrenia and one with depression, looked at symptoms and social behaviors, the performance level of socially expected activities and of free-time activities, and the family members' levels of expectations with respect to activities as measured by the Katz Adjustment Scale (KAS; Katz and Lyerly, 1963). The evaluation of symptoms and social behaviors by family members clearly reflected the clinical features of schizophrenia and depression. Depressive patients were evaluated by their families at significantly higher performance levels of socially expected activities than were schizophrenic patients. As for free-time activities, there were no differences between the two groups in levels of performance, but the family members of the depressive group expected a significantly higher level of free-time activities than was achieved, while the significant discrepancy between expectation and performance was not observed for the schizophrenic group.

7. An Epidemiological Study of Mortality in Persons with Schizophrenia with Exposure to Radiation Caused by the Atomic Bomb in Nagasaki City (Ohta, Ueki, Mine et al., 1991)

A comparison of cause of death of schizophrenic persons who were exposed to radiation from the atomic bomb with that of all atomic bomb survivors in Nagasaki City showed significantly higher rates of heart disease, pneumonia, cerebral vascular disease, and suicide in survivors with schizophrenia.

8. Ecological Structure and Incidence Rates of Schizophrenia in Nagasaki City (Ohta, Nakane, Nishihara, and Takemoto, 1992; Ohta and Nakane, 1993)

The relationship between incidence and residential situation was analyzed using the results of the 1980 national census and data on new schizophrenic patients collected in 1979 and 1980. The incidence rate was relatively high in males in central commercial areas of the city, areas of less education, and lower occupational status, as well as in areas with long-term residents. Contrary to the findings of many other studies conducted in Western cities, no statistically significant differences were observed, although it seemed that incidence rates were comparatively higher in the lower social classes. These results possibly reflect differences in cultural and social values and structures.

THE NAGASAKI CENTER

In 1907, the Department of Neuropsychiatry of Nagasaki University School of Medicine was established, and in 1913, clinical work was begun in Nagasaki University Hospital, a hospital near the middle of the city that serves the southern part. The department also receives emergency patients from outside as well as from the other departments in the hospital. As of the time of follow-up, there are 56 psychiatrists in the department. Nagasaki University Hospital has 829 regular beds. Of these, 48 beds (including two in isolation rooms and two in intensive care units) belong to the Department of Neuropsychiatry. Built in 1912 and renovated in 1977, the primary ward is not yet a completely open-door system. Inpatient staff is 12 psychiatrists and 16 nursing staff. The chief treatment is medication and individual psychotherapy, while recreation therapy is also used. There is some integration with outpatient and day-care treatment. Outpatients total some 400 to 500 per year.

The Nagasaki Center conducts its own clinical work, research, and education. There are four main research groups: biochemistry, genetics, psychopathology, and social psychiatry. The center has pursued not only problems of general psychiatric importance but also has intensively researched some issues arising from the uniqueness of Nagasaki. The social psychiatry group is conducting studies on schizophrenia, expressed emotion of family members, affective disorders, mental health of the aged, psychiatric disorders in childhood and adolescence, and the epidemiology of mental disorders among the Nagasaki atomic bomb survivors.

Participation in WHO Studies

Since 1972, the Nagasaki Center has participated in the mental health program of WHO as one of the regional research centers. On August 31, 1979, the Department was officially designated a WHO Collaborating Center for Research in Functional Psychoses and, in 1989, was redesignated a WHO Collaborating Center for Research and Training in Mental Health. The projects carried out at the center include: Study on Depressive Disorders; Collaborative Study on the Determinants of the Outcome of Severe Mental Disorders (DOSMeD); Field Trials of the Diagnostic Criteria for Research (DCR) of ICD-10; Field Trials of the ICD-10 Multiaxial Presentation; Collaborative Project on Psychological Problems in General Health Care (PPGHC); Study on Long-Term Course and Outcome of Schizophrenia (ISoS); and Study on Quality of Life (QOL) of Patients with Malignant Tumors.

The ISoS study team has changed during the 15 years of the study. The team currently numbers 12, all of whom are psychiatrists with at least 6 years of experience in clinical work.

METHODS

Defining the ISoS Cohort

The original members of the study cohort were selected according to the protocol of the DOSMeD study. However, for subjects who moved out of Nagasaki Prefecture and whose whereabouts were unknown at the time of 5- and 10-year follow-up studies, no further searches were made for the following reasons: (1) In order to find the new addresses, legal procedures would have been needed to gain access to resident registry cards. (2) Most of the subjects had moved within 2 years after the start of the DOSMeD study, meaning that they had not been followed up for more than 10 years. The possibility of getting the subjects' or their families' consent was considered low. (3) Psychiatrists from clinics and hospitals in the catchment area understood the purpose of the study and were cooperative enough to talk to subjects and their families to encourage their participation in the study, while psychiatrists outside Nagasaki might not have been so cooperative. (4) Considering the low probability of success, the time and the expense involved in locating the subjects and in traveling for an interview were too great.

Case-Finding and Data Collection

In 1984 to 1985 and 1990 to 1991, Nagasaki Center carried out 5-year and 10-year follow-up studies on the course and the outcome of the subjects in DOSMeD. The results of these studies and various information collected at that time (e.g., subjects' residences, hospitals/clinics, etc.) were useful in tracing them for this study.

Subjects in Treatment

The subjects for whom follow-up data are available were easily found for ISoS because most such subjects had not changed psychiatrists; several cases have been continuously treated by psychiatrists in the Nagasaki Center. Cases who had changed hospitals/clinics within Nagasaki Prefecture were also easy to find. Collaborating researchers explained to the treating psychiatrists the purpose, method, and importance of ISoS and asked them to assess if interviewing a subject directly would have an adverse effect on the subject's condition or on the relationship between the subject and his or her psychiatrist. The researchers asked for information about the subjects. Where no information was available from subjects' families, their psychiatrists were their key informants. For a few subjects, very little useful information was available. If a psychiatrist agreed to contact the subject, he or she was requested also to obtain consent and to ask the subject's family to participate in the study. There were a few cases where the subject refused to allow contact with the family. In cooperative cases, the researchers made direct contact with the subject/family as suggested by the psychiatrist. With their consent, interviews were conducted at the outpatient clinic of the center, at the psychiatric institutions where the patients were hospitalized or visiting, or at their houses.

Subjects Not in Need of Treatment, Who Had Discontinued Treatment or Whose Whereabouts Were Unknown

Maps and public telephone books were searched for clues to the location of missing subjects. After reviewing records of the psychiatric institutions which subjects had last visited and obtaining the consent of psychiatrists in charge, researchers, in order to protect privacy, directly telephoned only those family members who would have known about the subjects' prior receipt of psychiatric services. The researcher first confirmed that the person who answered the phone knew that the subject had received psychiatric services and asked about the subject's current situation. Then the purpose, methods, and importance of ISoS were explained. The families were asked to assess the effect of an interview on the subject and then to give consent. Sometimes, while the researcher was on the phone, the family explained the study to the subject, and the subject himself agreed to an interview; in other cases, the family refused to allow contact with the subject. For those consenting, face-to-face interviews were then scheduled.

Use of Study Instruments

A Japanese version of each instrument was prepared. For those instruments used in the DOSMeD study, translations had already been prepared. The others were translated by collaborating researchers, not professional translators, and mistranslations were corrected by conducting back-translation. For difficult terms, a note in English was included. The interviews were conducted by psychiatrists who had done the reliability exercises for ISoS.

STUDY RESULTS: PATTERNS AND VARIATIONS

Baseline and Short-Term Follow-Up

Study Population

There were 107 (61 males and 46 females) subjects in DOSMeD that the Nagasaki Center defines as its ISoS cohort. Table 15.1 (and the baseline tables in the Appendix) show a total of 115 subjects, the cohort used for baseline comparisons by other centers. The original Nagasaki cohort was modified after the DOSMeD incidence cohort was selected: Eight cases of questionable schizophrenia were removed (and are excluded from this chapter's analysis) and seven originally screened and excluded were added—five picked up as part of a leakage study (Jablensky et al., 1992) and two who had been outside the case-finding period. In the ISoS study, 7 subjects (four males and three females) died, 43 subjects (28 males and 15 females) were lost to follow-up, and 57 (29 males and 28 females) were successfully traced (see Table 15.1).

Gender and Age

There were more males than females in the original DOSMeD subjects (the ratio of male to female was 1.33), and in the total DOSMeD slightly more males than females (1.09). Among the cases lost to follow-up in Nagasaki Center, the difference was greater and the male to female ratio was 1.87; while in the alive cohort, the ratio was 1.04. The percentage of subjects who were lost to follow-up was 33% for females and 46% for males. The age of the subjects at study intake was 25.8±8.2 years (males 24.8±7.5, females: 27. 0±8.9) on average; with a median of 23 years (both genders). Sixty-eight percent of the subjects whose birth years were between 1940 to 1949 were lost to follow-up. The age distribution of those lost to follow-up was slightly older than those of the successfully traced subjects, but not significantly so.

Mode of Onset and First Contact Rediagnosis

Among the original DOSMeD subjects, the number of subjects with insidious mode of onset (> 1 month) was large, as was true in most other developed countries. Of 34 subjects with insidious onset, 25 subjects were successfully traced for the ISoS (74%). Of 19 subjects with acute onset (< 1 month), 12 subjects were traced (63%). Of 27 subjects with sudden or precipitous onset (< 1 week), 16 subjects were traced (59%). Subjects with more acute onset seemed to be more difficult to follow.

Thirty-nine of the alive cohort of 57 (68%) received a first-contact rediagnosis of schizophrenia, and 28% were classified as "other psychotic disorders." This distribution is similar to that seen in both the original study cohort and those lost to follow-up.

TABLE 15.1 Baseline and Short-Term Demographic and Clinical Description by Data Cohort

	Alive		*Dead*		*Lost to Follow-up*		*Nagasaki Defined Total*		*Excluded from Cohort*	
Nagasaki	N	%	N	%	N	%	N	%	N	%
Gender										
Male	29	50.9	4	57.1	28	65.1	61	57.0	1	12.5
Female	28	49.1	3	42.9	15	34.9	46	43.0	7	87.5
Birth Year										
1920–1929	1	1.8	0	0.0	0	0.0	1	0.9	0	0.0
1930–1939	5	8.8	1	14.3	1	2.3	7	6.5	0	0.0
1940–1949	5	8.8	1	14.3	13	30.2	19	17.8	1	12.5
1950–1959	29	50.9	2	28.6	18	41.9	49	45.8	4	50.0
1960–1969	17	29.8	3	42.9	11	25.6	31	29.0	3	37.5
Grouped Mode of Onset										
Up to 1 Week	16	28.1	3	42.9	8	18.6	27	25.2	1	12.5
Up to 1 Month	12	21.1	0	0.0	7	16.3	19	17.8	2	25.0
Greater than 1 Month	25	43.9	1	14.3	8	18.6	34	31.8	0	0.0
Other/Missing	4	7.0	3	42.9	20	46.5	27	25.2	5	62.5
Baseline Diagnosis Converted to ICD-10										
Paranoid Schizophrenia	14	24.6	0	0.0	17	39.5	31	29.0	0	0.0
Hebephrenic Schizophrenia	33	57.9	4	57.1	16	37.2	53	49.5	1	12.5
Catatonic Schizophrenia	1	1.8	0	0.0	1	2.3	2	1.9	0	0.0
Residual Schizophrenia	0	0.0	1	14.3	0	0.0	1	0.9	0	0.0
Other Schizophrenia	4	7.0	1	14.3	5	11.6	10	9.3	0	0.0
Schizoaffective	1	1.8	0	0.0	0	0.0	1	0.9	0	0.0
Acute Schizo-like	3	5.3	1	14.3	1	2.3	5	4.7	0	0.0
Depression	0	0.0	0	0.0	0	0.0	0	0.0	1	12.5
Other Psychotic	0	0.0	0	0.0	0	0.0	0	0.0	6	75.0
Other Nonpsychotic	1	1.8	0	0.0	3	7.0	4	3.7	0	0.0
Grouped Baseline Diagnosis										
Schizophrenia	52	91.2	6	85.7	39	90.7	97	90.7	1	12.5
Nonschizophrenia/Missing	5	8.8	1	14.3	4	9.3	10	9.3	7	87.5
Grouped Short-Term Pattern of Course										
Complete Remission	16	28.1	0	0.0	6	14.0	22	20.6	2	25.0
Incomplete Remission	20	35.1	2	28.6	10	23.3	32	29.9	1	12.5
Continuously Psychotic	19	33.3	3	42.9	9	20.9	31	29.0	0	0.0
Other/Missing	2	3.5	2	28.6	18	41.9	22	20.6	5	62.5

Nagasaki	Alive		Dead		Lost to Follow-up		Nagasaki Defined Total		Excluded from Cohort	
	N	%	N	%	N	%	N	%	N	%
Short-Term Follow-up Time										
0, Missing (Baseline)	1	1.8	2	28.6	16	37.2	19	17.8	5	62.5
1–17 Months (1 year)	6	10.5	2	28.6	8	18.6	16	15.0	1	12.5
18–30 Months (2 year)	50	87.7	3	42.9	19	44.2	72	67.3	2	25.0
TOTAL	57	100.0	7	100.0	43	100.0	107	100.0	8	100.0
Birth Year (19xx)										
N	57		7		43		107		8	
MEAN	54.47		54.71		53.53		54.11		56.25	
STD	8.83		11.07		7.36		8.35		7.09	

Baseline Diagnosis Converted to ICD-10

It was remarkable that Nagasaki Center had a much higher rate of hebephrenic schizophrenia (57.9%) than the other DOSMeD centers when baseline diagnosis was converted to ICD-10. However, it is possible that the subtyping of the schizophrenia by using ICD-9's descriptive diagnostic classification was greatly influenced by the conventional Japanese concept of schizophrenia subtypes prevailing at the time the study began, especially since hebephrenia was the most common subtype in Japan (Inoue, 1993). Among the 53 subjects originally diagnosed as hebephrenic type (295.1) using ICD-9 in DOSMeD, only 15 subjects were diagnosed with hebephrenic schizophrenia (F20.1) in the ICD-10 rediagnosis. The main changes were: 14 (26%) paranoid schizophrenia, nine (17%) undifferentiated schizophrenia, seven (13%) acute schizophrenia-like, and five (9%) other nonpsychotic.

Pattern of Course at Early Follow-Up

Subjects with continuous psychotic course during the early 2-year follow-up were observed more in the Nagasaki Center than in the total DOSMeD sample. If one excludes subjects with missing data or inadequate information, no significant differences are seen between the Nagasaki subsamples (alive vs. lost to follow-up) (Takada, Yoshitake et al., 1997).

Because of the difference in the duration of symptom evaluation period, we cannot simply compare severity of symptoms among different cohorts (deceased, lost to follow-up, and alive), but it is notable that there are no subjects with severe symptoms in the lost-to-follow-up group. In the alive group, severity of symptoms ranged widely from severe symptoms to recovered, while in the deceased group, 86% were moderate or severe.

Alive Subjects

Symptomatology

A rather different impression of current symptoms is gained from the results of the Global Assessment of Functioning Scale for symptomatology (GAF-S). The percentage of subjects with lower than 51 points on the GAF-S indicating severe symptoms was 28%, while the percentage of subjects with severe symptoms on the Bleuler scale was 12%. Among those scoring less than 51 on the GAF-S, females were predominant (46% of the alive female subjects); only 10% of the alive male subjects scored in this range. Almost the same rate of subjects (30%) showed no significant or only mild symptoms (GAF-S scores >70) as were rated as recovered (28%) on the Bleuler scale. These latter rates were similar to Dublin and at the low end among DOSMeD centers. If one looks at symptom trend over the entire period, the percentage of subjects with symptoms predominant only in the early one-third of the entire period was about 50%, which was similar to that in the total DOSMeD sample (62%). The percentage of subjects with symptoms predominant only in the last one-third of the entire period was 12%, or much higher than those of other DOSMeD centers (0–5%), except Honolulu (12%) and Prague (8%).

TABLE 15.2 Severity of Symptoms (Bleuler Scale)[a]

	Alive		*Lost to Follow-Up*		*Deceased*	
	N	%	N	%	N	%
Nagasaki						
Severe	7	12.3	0	0.0	3	42.9
Moderate	19	33.3	19	44.2	3	42.9
Mild	15	26.3	10	23.2	1	14.3
Recovered	16	28.1	14	32.6	0	0.0
Total	57	100.0	43	100.0	7	100.0

[a] Duration for symptoms is "most of the period" for the deceased and lost-to-follow-up groups but only "the past month" for the alive cohort.

Course of the Illness

One-fourth of the 57 subjects had no psychotic episodes over the last 2 years of follow-up, 16% were episodic, and about half were continuously psychotic (55%). This high rate of continuous course was double that of the total DOSMeD sample (26%). Through the entire period, 45% of subjects had continuous course, much like the course in the last 2 years. This high rate of continuous course is similar to Dublin (46%) and to Honolulu (44%), but again quite a bit higher than those of the rest of the DOSMeD centers (6–27%) or the total DOSMeD sample (23%). With respect to relapses, the subjects who had only one psychotic episode with incomplete remission in short-term course had at least one more relapse without exception during the entire period (Takada and Nakane, 1996). The overall time trend was evenly divided into thirds: for subjects getting better, staying the same, and getting worse. This distribution was less favorable than the overall time trends in the other DOSMeD centers or in the total ISoS sample.

Reevaluation of Baseline Diagnosis

In Nagasaki, ICD-10 clinical rediagnosis was done by at least two investigators utilizing only information available at first contact and blind to subsequent course of the illness (see Table 15.1). For the alive cohort, all 57 subjects were reevaluated using ICD-10 criteria. Of the 52 subjects diagnosed with schizophrenia (using the baseline diagnosis converted to ICD-10), 38 (73%) were reevaluated with a diagnosis of schizophrenia, eight (15%) acute schizophrenia-like, four (8%) other psychotic, and two (4%) nonpsychotic. Of the five remaining cases: One was diagnosed as schizoaffective by both methods as were three classified as acute schizophrenia-like; the last case was reevaluated as schizophrenia from a converted diagnosis of nonpsychotic.

Living Arrangements

Currently, subjects are either in a hospital (33.3%) or living with their families (61.4%); none was in a supervised residence or nursing home. The one-third of successfully traced subjects still in the hospital was far higher than in other DOSMeD centers (0–11.5%) and in all ISoS subsamples (1.1–7.5%). During the last 2 years of follow-up, 41 of 57 subjects (72%) have been living independently most of the time. Fourteen subjects (25%) have not lived independently in this period, and were in the hospital. No differences were seen in duration of independent living by sex and age.

About half of the subjects (47%) had been in the hospital for some period during those past 2 years, and about half of those subjects (26%) had been in the hospital for more than 1 year. This high rate of long stay at hospital/supervised residence was similar to Honolulu (DOSMeD) and Groningen and Mannheim (Disability), but was far higher than that of all subsamples (DOSMeD, 6.6%; IPSS, 2.2%; Disability, 17.8%; Invited, 7.9%). No subjects were homeless in the past 2 years, and one was detained at a police station for 1 day for violence.

Over the entire period, nearly all (98%) of the subjects had experienced independent living for some time, but 23% of them have lived independently less than half of the entire period, which was far higher than the average of the DOSMeD centers (5.5%) and other subsamples (3.4–13.7%). Likewise, the percentage of subjects who lived independently more than 95% of the entire period was only about 30%, or about half of the average of the DOSMeD centers (61%). Fifty-one of 57 (90%) subjects experienced hospitalization, again higher than the total DOSMeD centers (75%). About a fourth (22.8%) were in the hospital for more than half of the entire period, a rate five times higher than that of the total DOSMeD sample (4.7%).

No subject was homeless through the entire period, although one subject left home for a few days without telling her family. Two cases were detained at a police station, one of whom was committed involuntarily to a hospital. The other case was detained for a few days at a police station under suspicion of indecent behavior forced on a child but was released because it was concluded that the conduct was due to psychiatric symptoms. No subject was arrested or on trial.

Work

Forty percent of the subjects worked at paid jobs at some point in the last 2 years of follow-up; most of them (65%) did so for at least 12 months. For those working most of the time, performance was mostly (77%) judged as good to very good. Although somewhat lower, these rates were not so different from those of the total DOSMeD sample. Thirteen of the 28 successfully traced female subjects (46%) engaged in household work (although six also were employed outside the home). Another three worked full-time, and one part-time. In total, 17 of the female subjects (67%) engaged in some kind of work, while this was true for only 13 of the 29 successfully traced male subjects (45%). Of the subjects doing household work more than one year, however, 44% of them were evaluated as poor or very poor. With respect to the global performance of the 30 subjects doing work outside the home and/or household work in the last 2 years, this was rated as good in almost half the cases, comparable to the total DOSMeD sample. In the same 2 years, there were no retired or student subjects in the Nagasaki Center. About one-fifth (21%) of the subjects were on a pension for mental disabilities; none received a pension for physical disabilities.

Social Disability

With respect to overall functioning in the last month, 59% were rated poor to severe on the DAS, while 49% had scores on the GAF-D lower than 51, indicating serious impairment. At the same time, 25% were rated good to excellent on the DAS and 32% scored higher than 70 on the GAF-D, indicating good functioning. Nagasaki and Rochester had lower mean GAF scores than the other DOSMeD centers. As for the time trend of disability, the percentage for whom disability was predominant only in the first one-third of the period was 39%, similar to that of most of the DOSMeD centers except Chandigarh (both urban and rural) and Moscow. However, 21% of the subjects had disability throughout the entire period, which was similar to Dublin, Nottingham, and Rochester (24–29%).

Violence and Suicide

Assaults were seen in 12 of the 57 subjects with available data (21%) in the last 2 years of follow-up, all but one of which were mild (and that was only slightly more severe). In the entire period, 23 of the 56 subjects (41%) committed assaults at least once, but all except the one mentioned were mild. These rates were about twice as high as those of the total DOSMeD sample (past 2 years: 11%; entire period: 24%), but the apparent difference may be attributable to differences in the definition of assault; in the Nagasaki Center, a slap is considered an assault.

There was only one mild suicide attempt in the most recent 2 years. Throughout the entire period, 12 of the 56 subjects (21%) experienced at least one suicide attempt: 8 mild, 3 moderate, and one severe. This rate (21%) of suicide attempts was the same as that seen in the total DOSMeD (20%), but an additional four subjects who succeeded in their suicides are not included.

Medications

In the last 2 years of follow-up, 52 (93%) of the 57 subjects received neuroleptics; only four subjects (7%) received no medication. Information is missing on one subject. In the entire period, all subjects received neuroleptics for some or all of the period. When the percentage of subjects on neuroleptics most of the time is examined, the rates are much higher in Nagasaki than for the total DOSMeD sample, for both the past 2 years (84 vs. 48%) and the entire period (86 vs. 47%). In Nagasaki, few patients were under treatment by nonpsychiatrists; almost all of those who needed medication consulted psychiatrists. If one examines time trends over the entire period, it is clear that most subjects (61%) received some kind of medication throughout the entire period. Only Nagasaki and Dublin (80%) had far higher rates than those of the other DOSMeD centers (0–38%).

Hospitalization

As mentioned earlier, 27 subjects (47%) had spent some time in the hospital during the last 2 years of follow-up. Fifty-one (90%) did so at least once during the entire follow-up period. In 38% of the subjects, hospitalization was predominant only in the first third of the period; for 20%, it was prominent only in the last third of the period, a figure three times higher than that of the total DOSMeD sample (6%).

Deceased Subjects

At the time of this follow-up (15 years after study entry), seven subjects were confirmed dead. Comparison to the general population of Nagasaki Center shows an increased death rate (SMR=5.71). Four had committed suicide: two by drowning (a man, aged 30, and a woman, aged 27 at time of death); one with a sharp object (a woman aged 45); and one by jumping from a high place (a man, aged 28). In addition, there was one suspicious suicide case (a man, aged 31), who drowned in a bathtub after taking an excessive amount of medication; however, suicidal intent was not clear. Two deaths were from natural causes (a man, aged 26, from heart failure; a woman, aged 48, from renal disease). One suicide was committed in partial remission, and the mental status of one suicide is unknown. The remaining subjects who had died were determined to be in a psychotic episode at the time. Suicide rates in Japan were between 16 and 20 per 100,000 from 1980 to 1990. The rates in people aged 20 to 59 were between 15.7 and 27.3 per 100,000 (1982). Compared to those in the general population, the suicide rate among the subjects—4 or 5 of the original 107 cases—is extremely high.

DISCUSSION

The alive cohort in the Nagasaki Center had some distinctive features: a higher rate of schizophrenia, more severe social disability, and more continuous course type than those for the other DOSMeD centers. One probable reason is that at study entry, Nagasaki Center excluded as "false positives" those subjects who received a rediagnosis of nonschizophrenia. Longer stay in the hospital may be a reflection of limited community-based living arrangements (hostels, nursing homes, supervised residences, group homes, etc.) and lack of a social support system. Wide utilization of neuroleptics may reflect the clinicians' tendency to give neuroleptics as maintenance therapy that is relatively inexpensive for patients, especially when compared to medications prescribed for physical illness.

The representativeness of the alive cohort is somewhat problematic because of the substantially high rate of the subjects lost to follow-up and the differences between alive and lost to follow-up in the mode of onset, male-female ratio, and severity of symptoms. In tracking, the main difficulties arose because the reason for "early dropouts" had not been determined. However, the rates for those whose vital status was known has been approximately 60% at the 2-year, 5-year, 10-year, and 15-year follow-ups. Mobility may potentially be the main reason. Locating patients was mainly based on information from psychiatrists in original case-finding network, so the likelihood of locating and assessing subjects with less favorable outcomes may have been higher.

Fewer symptoms and better social ability were commonly seen among the subjects with better outcome, while half of 28 subjects with severe social disability (GAF-D<51) showed only moderate to mild severity of symptoms (GAF-S>50). This discrepancy meant that social disability was not parallel to the symptomatology. The disability scores could have been suppressed by under-participation in work.

The term *independent living arrangement* was difficult to interpret in Japanese settings. Some subjects lived with their families, as is the convention for people not suffering from illness, and so lived their lives literally "independently"; there were, however, a small number of subjects who received continuous informal support from the families with whom they lived. Therefore, "independent living" is not a reliable indicator of independence in Japan.

High rate of hospitalization is also a poor indicator of outcome and need. Historically, easy accessibility of hospitalization, long-standing segregated care (now changing), lack of community-based care resources, financial difficulties of the family, and prejudice by the subject's family or community have contributed to high rates.

Unusually high rates of unemployment among the subjects was seen compared to remarkably low unemployment rates (less than 3%) in the general population in Japan. One probable reason is lack of promotion of the idea of employing mentally disabled people by governmental bodies and corporations.

As discussed earlier, reevaluation ICD-10 diagnoses did not conform very much to the baseline diagnoses converted to ICD-10, especially in subtyping of schizophrenia. However, a large percentage (73%) of the subjects diagnosed as schizophrenic at baseline received the same diagnosis at reevaluation.

CONCLUSIONS

The original cohort was assembled during 1979 and 1980 in Nagasaki City, Japan, and consisted of 107 subjects. There were more male (male to female ratio was 1.33) with an age at study intake of 25 years (on average) or 23 years (median). Fifteen years later, the present follow-up effort relocated 53% of the original subjects; the alive 57 analyzed here showed no apparent bias with respect to age, baseline diagnosis, or short-term pattern of course, but did show differences to some extent with respect to gender, mode of onset, and severity of symptoms.

At follow-up, 39 subjects (68% of those alive and evaluated) received an ICD-10 rediagnosis of schizophrenia; 11 (19%) a diagnosis of acute schizophrenia-like disorder; one (2%) a diagnosis of schizoaffective; and four (7%) a diagnosis of other psychotic disorder. Only two subjects (4%) were rediagnosed as "other nonpsychotic" disorder. It was noteworthy that Nagasaki Center had a small number of nonschizophrenia (ICD-9) (9%), and few rediagnoses of nonpsychiatric disorder (4%). Thirty-eight (74%) of the 52 subjects receiving a baseline diagnosis of schizophrenia retained that diagnosis in the reevaluation; eight (15%) were rediagnosed as acute-schizophrenia-like; four (8%) were rediagnosed as other psychotic disorder; and two (4%) received a rediagnosis of nonpsychotic.

Nearly one-third of the alive subjects were judged to have recovered, although the same percentage still showed evidence of some symptomatology and about half had suffered continuously from psychotic symptoms during the last 2 years of follow-up. Over half of the subjects showed evidence, too, of substantial impairment in social and occupational functioning, while about 30% were rated as good or excellent in their social functioning. Over 80% of the subjects were currently prescribed neuroleptic medications. The majority of subjects were living independently, though in a certain number of cases, this term masks the significant support received from family; 26% were on a long stay ward and none lived in any kind of sheltered accommodation outside the hospital. Almost 40% had experienced paid work during the past 2 years, and another 12% were engaged in full-time household activities only. Overall, the trend of the course of the illness was rated as improving in a third of the alive subjects; another third were worsening.

The characteristics of the results in Nagasaki Center compared to other centers were generally summarized as the following: (1) lower follow-up rate; (2) higher content of schizophrenia in study population; (3) higher rate of continuous course type; (4) more severe social disability; (5) longer stay in hospital; and (6) wider utilization of neuroleptics.

Acknowledgments The authors thank collaborative investigators: Drs. T. Douma, S. Kawaguchi, J. Kim, H. Sugasaki, M. Tsukasaki, J. Uchino, K. Ueki, H. Utsunomiya (ISoS group); Drs. K. Araki, M. Ishizawa, S. Michitsuji, I. Nakama, Y. Ohta, R. Takahashi, Y. Tominaga (DOSMeD group). The authors also thank the psychiatrists of the case-finding network in Nagasaki for allowing their patients to be included in this study. This study was supported in part by a Grant-in-Aid for Scientific Research (C) No. 06670966 from the Ministry of Education, Science and Culture, Japan.

References

Araki, K., Ohta, Y., Nakane, Y., & Takahashi, R. (1984), First-rank symptoms (Schneider, K.) in schizophrenics. *Clin. Psychiatry [Seishin Igaku]*, 26:59–67. (In Japanese).

Inoue, S. (1993), Hebephrenia as the most prevalent subtype of schizophrenia in Japan. *Japan. J. Psychiatry & Neurol.*, 47:505–514.

Ishizawa, M. (1980), Study on life events in schizophrenia: I. Relationship of life events to onset of illness. *Nakasaki Med. J.*, 58:117–140. (In Japanese)

Jablensky, A., Sartorius, N., Ernberg, G., Anker, M., Korten, A., Cooper, J. E., Day, R., & Bertelsen, A. (1992), Schizophrenia: Manifestation, incidence and course in different cultures: A World Health Organization ten-country study. *Psychol. Med.* 20(Monogr. Suppl.): 1–97.

Katz, M. M., & Lyerly, S. B. (1963), Methods for measuring adjustment and social behavior in the community: I. Rationale, description, discriminative validity and scale development. *Psycholog. Rep.*, 13:503–535.

Nagaoka, K., & Ohta, Y. (1978), Psychopathology of persecution and place. In: *Culture and Psychopathology*, ed. K. Ogino. Tokyo: Kobundo. (In Japanese)

Nakane, Y., Ohta, Y., & Radford, M. H. B. (1992), Epidemiological studies of schizophrenia in Japan. *Schizophr. Bull.*, 18:75–84.

——Takahashi, R., & Ohta, Y. (1986), Morbid risk of schizophrenia in Japan. *Clin. Psychiatry [Seishin Igaku]*, 26: 421–426. (In Japanese)

——,——Tominaga, Y., Ohta, Y., Ishizawa, M., Nakama, I., Michitsuji, S., & Araki, K. (1985), The incidence rate study of schizophrenia in Nagasaki City. *Clin. Psychiatry [Seishin Igaku]*, 27:771–781. (In Japanese)

Ohta, Y. (1982), The epidemiological study on the association between schizophrenics and incidence of malignant neoplasms. *Kyushu Neuropsychiatry*, 28:221–242. (In Japanese with English abstract)

——Ishizawa, M., Nakama, I., Michitsuji, S., Araki, K., & Nakane, Y. (1979), Seasonal distribution of births of schizophrenics. *Bull. Neuroinform. Lab., Nagasaki University*, 6:39–46. (In Japanese)

——Nagaoka, K., Matsunaga, F., Kawazoe, M., Masui, K., Moriyama, K., & Ogino, K. (1976), Transcultural psychiatric research in the Shimo-Goto Islands, Nagasaki

Prefecture. *Clin. Psychiatry [Seishin Igaku]*, 18:1271–1278. (In Japanese)

——Nakane, Y. (1989), Features of schizophrenic patients and patients with depression as observed by family members: Symptoms, social activities and social performance. *Japan. J. Psychiatry & Neurol.*, 43:29–36.

——, ——(1993), Urban ecology and incidence rate of schizophrenia results from a study in Nagasaki City. *Japan. Bull. Soc. Psychiatry*, 1:31–52. (In Japanese with English abstract)

——, ——Matsunaga, F., & Nagaoka, K. (1985), Study of the association between schizophrenia and culture defined by religion in Shimo-Goto, Nagasaki Prefecture. *Bull. Neuroinform. Lab., Nagasaki University*, 12:1–16.

——, ——Mine, M., Nakama, I., Michitsuji, S., Araki, K., Tominaga, Y., & Uchino, J. (1988), The epidemiological study of physical morbidity in schizophrenics: 2. Association between schizophrenia and incidence of tuberculosis. *Japan. J. Psychiatry & Neurol.*, 42:41–47.

——, ——Nishihara, J., & Takemoto, T. (1992), Ecological structure and incidence rates of schizophrenia in Nagasaki City. *Acta Psychiatr. Scand.*, 86:113–120.

——, ——Takahashi, R. (1981), Physical morbidity pattern of schizophrenic patients. 1. Association between schizophrenia and incidence of malignant neoplasms: A report from the WHO project on determinant of outcome of severe mental disorder—First report. *Clin. Psychiatry [Seishin Igaku]*, 23:875–884. (In Japanese)

——Ueki, K., Mine, M., Otsuka, T., Sugasaki, H., Tsukasaki, M., Yoshitake, K., Uchino, J., Araki, K., Michitsuji, S., & Nakane, Y. (1991), An epidemiological study of mortality in schizophrenics with exposure to radiation caused by the atomic bomb in Nagasaki City. *Clin. Psychiatry [Seishin Igaku]*, 33:165–173. (In Japanese)

Takada, K., & Nakane, Y. (1996), Relapses of schizophrenia: The results from a 15-year follow-up study of an incident cohort of schizophrenia patients. *J. Japan. Assn. Psychiatric Hosp.*, 15:637–643. (In Japanese)

——Yoshitake, K., Otsuka, T., Sakyo, T., Hatada, K., Sata, M., Imamura, Y., & Nakane, Y. (1997), Nagasaki schizophrenia study: Outcome of a 15-year follow-up of an incident cohort. *Acta Med. Nagasakiensia*, 42: 39–44.

Chapter 16

DOSMeD: Nottingham, U.K.

Glynn Harrison and Peter Mason

CULTURAL CONTEXT

For centuries, England and Scotland have been ruled by a centralized monarchy. England achieved the transition to parliamentary democracy in the 17th century with only one major civil war. Surrounded by its ocean "moat," Shakespeare's "sceptered isle" resisted invasion by Spain and France and, in this century, by Germany. Some believe this has nurtured a sense of insularity and even unhealthy jingoism; others argue that it has generated a distinctive independence of thought and social cohesion. Seafaring trade and conquest built a global British empire, which led to the widespread diffusion of English language and culture. Following the transition to a self governing Commonwealth of nations, the United Kingdom (England, Scotland, Wales, and Northern Ireland) resumed its status as a relatively small island off the coast of Europe and joined the European Union in 1971.

Since the early 19th century, the population has grown steadily from about 12 million to nearly 60 million, owing to a broadly positive balance between birth and death rates and between inward and outward migration. Following the Second World War, there was a sizable influx of refugees, especially from Eastern Europe, who formed small but distinctive communities, usually located in large urban areas. After 1957, immigration from the Commonwealth and from the Caribbean, India, and Pakistan gained momentum because of skill and labor shortages. Second- and even third-generation offspring often preserve distinctive ethnic and cultural identities, especially among Asian groups. Inevitably, though, intergenerational cultural conflict can occur and the threat of cultural assimilation has led some ethnic minority leaders to call for segregated schooling to preserve distinctive cultural and religious values.

Although all of the indigenous inhabitants of the United Kingdom speak and understand English, strong regional dialects and accents persist. Some members of ethnic minorities know little English and continue to speak their original languages within tightly knit communities. Most people in the United Kingdom profess some form of religious belief, but less than 10% of the population attends a place of worship on a regular basis. The traditional "established" religion is Protestant Christian. Following the break with Rome during the reign of Henry VIII in the 16th century, the national church of England became Protestant, although now it encompasses diverse evangelical and Anglo-Catholic traditions. Scotland is predominantly Presbyterian, the Welsh tend to follow a strong tradition of Methodism, and Northern Ireland has strong Protestant and Catholic communities. In present-day multicultural Britain, there are growing numbers of mosques and temples alongside traditional churches. Even as strong regional identities and local cultures endure, inward migration has resulted in a pluralist, multicultural society, although many of the traditional divisions of class and status persist, as do significant social class gradients in mortality and morbidity. Over 40% of schoolchildren progress to some form of higher education, and the number of working mothers has risen steadily. Over one-third of marriages end in divorce, one of the higher rates in Western Europe. After a sharp rise in the early 1980s, unemployment in the late 1990s stands at around 4.8%—well below the European average.

The Area of Nottingham

Nottingham is an urban area of 600,000 located in the Midlands region of England. Although there have been huge improvements in the health of the population of Nottingham over the past decades (Wilson, 1995), there remain pockets of high deprivation. Unemployment stands at over 30% in some areas, remaining stubbornly high despite employment initiatives. The main employment opportunities are in service industries and in light engineering, tobacco, and knitwear. The employment profile of Nottingham and its surrounding districts has been affected by a severe reduction in deep mining for coal, although this has been compensated for, to some degree, by the arrival of overseas car makers and the movement of government departments into the area. Nearly 70% of households in Nottingham live in owner occupied accommodation with less than 1% of households lacking the use of either a bath/shower or an inside bathroom facility. Over 65% of households have cars and just over 1% live at a density of more than one person per room; 13% have at least one child under age 5. Around 5% of households have three or more children under age 16, and 25% were one person living alone (OPCS, 1992). The largest ethnic minority group in Nottingham is black Caribbean forming 3.2% of the population; South Asians constitute about 3% of the population.

The National Health Service

The health services of the United Kingdom are financed largely through central government taxation. The National Health Service was established in 1948 as a comprehensive service providing most treatment "free at the point of need." Ninety-eight percent of primary care physicians work in the National Health Service, and the vast majority of hospitals in the United Kingdom also provide treatment within the National Health system. There is a growing private sector, however, whose expansion was until recently encouraged by government policy. Mental health services have a significant proportion of the National Health budget, accounting for 9% of the £30.7 billion expenditure in 1993 and 1994 (Department of Health, 1994). Sixty-four percent of the mental health budget was spent on inpatient services, 10% used for day and outpatients, and 9% went to community mental health services. Patients with schizophrenia and related psychotic disorders account for the majority of general adult inpatient costs for long-term care. Davies and Drummond (1994) estimate that schizophrenia patients consume direct health service costs of £397 million (1.6% of the entire health care budget) and indirect annual costs of lost production of £1.7 billion. The most severely disabled 10% of patients (requiring long-term inpatient care or intensive community facilities) consume 79% of total direct treatment costs for schizophrenia. Although few in number, these most disabled patients make the heaviest demands upon resources.

The Mental Health System in Nottingham

The policy of community care for mentally ill people and the process of deinstitutionalization effectively began in the mid-1950s. The second half of the 19th century had seen a rapid expansion of county and city asylums, with bed numbers reaching a peak of 148,100 in 1954. Thereafter, the number of beds began to fall quite steeply, and the official policy of closing the old-style institutions (made explicit in 1962) built upon a process already under way. Both patients and professionals perceived the old county asylums as remote and intimidating; studies described the phenomenon of "institutionalization," whereby custodial care was found to accentuate the negative symptoms of schizophrenia. The average number of psychiatric beds in institutions fell steadily between 1960 and 1990, with the total number of beds in 1985 in England and Wales falling to 64,800. In England, it now stands at 47,296 (Audit Commission, 1995). Beds in the old institutions have been replaced with acute units in general hospitals, smaller community psychiatric units, and home care programs.

In addition to community care reforms, other reforms to the National Health Service in the late 1980s had a profound impact on psychiatry. These reforms introduced a distinction between those charged with the responsibility for "purchasing" health services (Purchasers) and those able to "provide" them (Providers), although so far the fundamental commitment to treatment "free at the point of need" has been maintained. Previously, those *providing* health care were also responsible for the *allocation* and *distribution* of resources. Now, Providers compete for the attention of Purchasers charged with allocating resources on the basis of evidence of clinical effectiveness and efficiency. Primary care doctors were also encouraged to become Purchasers (called fund-holders), managing their own budgets and purchasing care on the basis of *their* prioritization of the needs of their patients. The Labor government elected in May 1997 reversed some of these changes in an attempt to reduce competitiveness between Providers, and fund-holding for general practitioners was abolished. The Purchaser/Provider contractual basis was swept away and new service standards (the "National Service Framework") were introduced, which were to be achieved by strong performance management.

Following accelerated deinstitutionalization of the mentally ill in the 1980s, there developed a massive increase in residential care facilities, since these were funded by the central government rather than by social services controlled by local authorities. In response to this disincentive to more innovative models of community care, the government transferred funding for residential care from central to local government. Social service departments were charged with carrying out comprehensive assessments and with allocating their resources according to need, whilst health authorities remained responsible for the psychiatric and medical care of the mentally ill. These structural reforms radically altered the organization and financing of the mental health system, provoking concern that the fragmentation between Purchasers and Providers, and between health and social services, would lead to the most vulnerable patients "falling through the net." In Nottingham, this risk was attenuated by retaining most psychiatric nurses on community mental health teams, by making those with more severe disorders a priority, and by a local policy of joint strategic planning between health and social services.

Structure of the Local Services

The post-World War II policy of deinstitutionalization was accelerated in Nottingham. The process of "sectorization" began in 1973 and mental health services are now provided by one single Provider—Nottingham NHS Healthcare Trust. Acute psychiatric services are organized into six multidisciplinary mental health teams, each serving a population of about 100,000. These teams interface with a single citywide rehabilitation service for continuing care, currently maintaining over 500 patients with severe mental disorders in community and residential settings. The community mental health teams each have a community base close to their target population and comprise a range of health care professionals, working closely with physicians in primary care and managing their own inpatient facilities. The six acute inpatient wards are located in three units: One is in a local general hospital, another on the old Mapperley Hospital site, and the third in refurbished accommodation on another small former hospital site.

Brewin et al. (1997) report that about 90 first episode cases of schizophrenia and related psychotic disorders present to the Nottingham psychiatric services each year. A typical pathway of care begins with the patient's general practitioner, who is usually called in to see a patient with developing symptoms by family members or concerned friends. Over 20% of first episode cases are judged to be at risk and require a compulsory admission to the hospital under the 1983 Mental Health Act; half have informal hospital admissions, and about 30% of patients are not admitted at all during their first episode. In the acute phases of the illness, patients are cared for by the sector team. Almost all receive some form of neuroleptic medication, with depot preparations commonly used. Those who achieve remission may continue to be cared for in the acute general psychiatry services, while those with chronic symptoms or complex needs will be transferred to the rehabilitation services.

PSYCHIATRIC EPIDEMIOLOGY

The task of measuring psychiatric morbidity and describing patterns of resource utilization in Nottingham began with creation of the Nottingham psychiatric case register in 1958. With the establishment of the academic psychiatric unit of the new medical school in 1972, the Nottingham psychiatric case register was computerized and used to track records of patient stay. Since then, it has continued to produce data confirming the position of Nottingham as a leader in the reconfiguration of psychiatric services. A census of psychiatric inpatients in Nottingham in 1960 showed that the inpatient prevalence rate was already lower than that found either nationally or in other local studies (Howat, 1979). This appeared to be due almost entirely to the reduced number of long-stay patients, with the most striking difference for those admitted between 1945 and 1958, reflecting the success of the policy of preventing prolonged admissions. A follow-up study showed accelerated attrition of that cohort compared with levels found elsewhere, which was attributed to the increased rate of discharge from the hospital into the community. A subsequent follow-up of discharged long-stay patients reported a pattern of high rates of readmission, frequent redischarges, and a final low overall level of dependence on inpatient services (Howat and Kontny, 1982).

Professor J. E. Cooper took forward the cause of psychiatric case registers and argued cogently for their place in providing service planners and administrators with accurate information (1989; 1990). Work by the register team with other U.K. case registers revealed striking differences in psychiatric treatment received by patients in different age groups in Nottingham, Salford, and Southampton. In 1981, the register provided data used to reorganize the psychiatric sectors and to determine workloads in a comprehensive community psychiatric service (Kontny, Jones, and Cooper, 1986). Data from the register showed that from 1980 to 1985, the number of psychiatric admissions fell significantly (4.5% a year) compared with national figures (0.46% a year). Admissions were reduced mostly for affective psychosis, neuroses, and personality disorders. The average duration of admission fell by 3.6% a year and use of inpatient beds was reduced by 37.5% (Tyrer, Turner, and Johnston, 1989). The case register was used as a sampling frame for several other epidemiologically based studies in the Nottingham area. Using spatial analysis techniques, Giggs (1972) and Giggs and Cooper (1987) explored the geographic distribution of selected populations of schizophrenic and other psychoses and found a consistent pattern of concentration in the inner residential areas of the city. Exploratory multivariate analyses further revealed that incidence rates of schizophrenia were closely correlated with a specific set of unfavorable life circumstances—notably, low social class, high unemployment, and low social cohesion. Dauncey, Giggs, Baker, and Harrison (1993) later mapped the lifetime geographic mobility of 67 patients with an ICD-9 diagnosis of schizophrenia in an attempt to investigate the processes leading to a threefold rate of schizophrenia in the most socioeconomically deprived area of the city. Although numbers were small, the spatial distribution of birthplaces of incidence cases of schizophrenia suggested that their skewed distribution toward deprived inner city areas begins early in their lives and is well established at least 5 years before initial contact with the psychiatric services.

Some observers have recently proposed that schizophrenia may be dying out (Eagles and Whalley, 1985; Der, Gupta, and Murray, 1990; Harrison, 1993), a hypothesis based upon data showing a decline in hospital admissions in Scotland and England over the last three decades and falls in first episode cases of diagnosed schizophrenia among all service contacts in some parts of the United Kingdom. Harrison, Cooper, and Glancarczyk (1991) analyzed data from the case register to show that in Nottingham rates for first onset schizophrenia remained stable between 1975 and 1987 with no evidence of decline. The proportion of patients *admitted* within 3 months of first contact had fallen steadily over this period, but when all service contacts were included, there was no evidence of an overall decline. Similarly, Brewin et al. (1997) carried out a 2-year prospective study of first episode cases in the same area and found that over the period 1992 to 1994, rates for broadly defined schizophrenia based upon ICD-10 DCR operational criteria were very close to those reported in the original DOSMeD in 1978 to 1980. Although there were some differences in diagnostic grouping at onset, with a decline in F20 schizophrenia and an increase in acute and transient (F23) psychoses, this was eliminated when diagnoses were reviewed at 3-year follow-up (Amin et al., 1998; Brewin et al., 1997). Although these two "snapshot" reports of incidence rates cannot be relied upon for trend, they are consistent with the case register data reported above.

The above trend is probably explained, at least in part, by an increase in the denominator of the proportion of "second generation" migrants in Nottingham entering the age risk period for schizophrenia. Researchers in Nottingham produced widely cited data demonstrating an increase in the incidence of schizophrenia and related psychoses among second generation migrants from the Caribbean. In the early 1970s, Giggs (1973) analyzed case register data and reported high rates of schizophrenia among first generation immigrants. Although consistent with other findings for psychoses among migrant groups, such results were criticized because they relied upon retrospectively determined case note diagnoses and imprecise estimates of the population at risk. Harrison, Owens, Holton, Neilson, and Boot (1988) and Harrison, Holton et al. (1989) used a prospective methodology in a defined population and found high rates of schizophrenia in second generation migrants to the United Kingdom from the Caribbean. They also found a greater proportion of this group of high-risk patients had symptoms for 6 months or more prior to psychiatric contact and experienced greater delays in their pathway to care, with higher rates of compulsory admissions, findings later confirmed by Owens, Harrison, and Boot (1991). These findings of elevated rates of schizophrenia among second generation migrants provoked considerable interest because it had been believed that rates in the second generation would converge toward those of the "host" population. Here, rates in British-born offspring appeared to be even higher. In addition, the data had considerable face validity in terms of the perceptions of mental health workers in many parts of the country, especially those working in inner city populations. These findings have been replicated in a series of studies using a range of different methodologies (Wessley, Castle, Der, and Murray, 1991; Thomas, Stone, Osborn, Thomas, and Fisher, 1993; van Os, Castle, Takei, Der, and Murray, 1996; King, Coker, Levey, Hoare, and Johnson-Sabine, 1994; Harrison et al., 1997) in different parts of the United Kingdom. The evidence for an excess of psychotic disorders associated with this group has been considered sufficiently well established to justify a major multicenter U.K. study (Nottingham, Bristol, and London), funded by the Medical Research Council, investigating potential etiologic factors.

THE NOTTINGHAM ISoS CENTER[1]

Methods Used in the Site

Defining the ISoS Cohort

Selection of subjects into the Nottingham cohort followed the protocol of the DOSMeD study. In brief, the cohort consisted of patients (ages 15–54) with psychotic symptoms making their first ever contact with psychiatric services including inpatient admissions in Nottingham (population 390,000; ages 16–64) between the dates August 1, 1978, and July 31, 1980. The screening schedule used was deliberately overinclusive and was based on symptoms rather than on diagnosis. Patients with a clear organic cause for their symptoms and those with severe mental retardation were not included in the cohort. Ninety-nine subjects were identified by the screening schedule and subjected to a battery of interview schedules at entry to the study. In the current 13-year follow-up, an attempt was made to trace all 99 of these subjects (Harrison, Mason, Glazebrook et al., 1994; Mason, Harrison, Glazebrook et al., 1995). A previous publication (Jablensky et al., 1992) reported a sample size of 92 for Nottingham. This difference arose when investigators decided to exclude two subjects who had a previous psychiatric contact (although never psychotic) and five others who had mania (although with symptoms of psychosis at entry). In ISoS we decided to follow up all 99 subjects to ensure a complete sample of all first episode psychoses from this catchment area.

Case-Finding and Data Collection

Most of the cases were traced using the Nottingham Case Register and the Medical Records Department at Mapperley Hospital, Nottingham. Others were found using the electoral register and the registrar for births, deaths, and marriages. A few had left the Nottingham area and were traced using the National Health Service Central Register and various Family Health Service Authorities throughout the United Kingdom. The study instruments took up to 2 hours to complete, and up to 1 hour was spent with relatives and/or informants. In two cases, English was not spoken, and family members acted as translators. Subjects who were still in contact with the psychiatric services were approached for interview by their psychiatrist or their care coordinator. For those patients out of contact, approaches for an assessment were made through their general practitioner. Most of the interviews were conducted in the subjects' homes. Where subjects refused to give their consent to interview, consent was sought to speak with their relatives, doctors, or other health care professionals. General practice and hospital case records were also scrutinized for information on symptoms, treatment and hospitalization, employment, and residence. Cleaning, entering, and analyzing the data were undertaken by S. Docherty, C. Glazebrook, and T. Croudace. I. Medley assisted with the reliability exercises.

Study Results: Patterns and Variations

Baseline and Short-Term Follow-Up

Of the 99 subjects who entered the study, 95 were traced to residence or death. Four subjects were lost to follow-up; three were lost in the first year of follow-up,

1. The University Department of Psychiatry was established following the creation of the Medical School in 1971. Professor John Cooper took the foundation chair. Professor Cooper directed the original DOSMeD research group involving academic and National Health Service colleagues and directed research programs in social psychiatry and epidemiology. In 1994, Professor Glynn Harrison was appointed to the foundation chair of Community Mental Health and built upon earlier collaboration with Professor Cooper and colleagues to establish a research team to carry out the ISoS study. In 1997, he left to take up the Chair of Mental Health at the University of Bristol.

and the other was lost in the seventh year. Information was available on this subject up to year 7 in the hospital case records. Nine of the cohort were dead, and 15 subjects refused to be interviewed. Information on those subjects refusing an interview was available from informants and from general practice and hospital case records. We obtained face-to-face interviews with 69 subjects. An additional two subjects refused face-to-face interviews but agreed to telephone interviews. For these, the data set was complete, apart from the PIRS and SANS which require face-to-face interviews.

Gender and Age

At entry to the DOSMeD study, the cohort comprised 65 men and 34 women and of these, 57 men and 29 women completed the 13-year follow-up. There were almost twice as many men as women, in contrast to the distribution in other DOSMeD centers. This excess was most apparent in the younger age groups (Cooper et al., 1987; Jablensky et al., 1992). Fifty-seven of the 99 subjects entering the study were born between the years 1950 and 1969; their mean age was 29.6 (standard deviation = 10.1). The age distribution of those subjects completing the follow-up was similar to that at entry.

Mode of Onset and Diagnosis and Pattern of Follow-Up

The distribution of mode of onset of the alive cohort is very similar to that in the original study total. Fifty-four (63%) of the 86 alive subjects received a baseline diagnosis of schizophrenia, using the ICD-9 to ICD-10 crosswalk tables, which is similar to that of the original study cohort. The proportion of subjects with this diagnosis in the DOSMeD study as a whole is smaller (53%), but there is a relative excess of subjects in DOSMeD with acute schizophrenia-like psychotic disorder compared to the Nottingham cases (19 and 4% respectively). Fifty (58%) of the 86 alive subjects had a favorable short-term (2-year) pattern of course (episodic with full remissions between episodes). This is very similar to the pattern of course determined for the alive cases at 2-year follow-up and a more favorable short-term outcome compared with the DOSMeD centers as a whole (47%). Overall, comparing those subjects dead or lost to follow-up and those completing the 13-year follow-up, there were no statistically significant differences with respect to gender, birth year, type of onset, diagnosis, and short-term pattern of course.

Alive Subjects

Symptomatology

Classified according to the Bleuler Severity Scale, 61% of the 85 subjects for whom information was available had no symptoms in the last month of follow-up. This is a markedly different finding to those of Bleuler (1978) and Ciompi (1980) who found that only 30% of their samples had recovered. It is also noteworthy how few (5%) of our sample were rated as exhibiting *severe* symptoms: 15% of Bleuler's sample and 20% of Ciompi's sample were left with severe symptoms at long-term outcome, although biases because of follow-up attrition are partly responsible for this difference. The findings of the Nottingham sample are remarkably similar to those of the DOSMeD sample as a whole, with almost three-quarters of both samples achieving a mild/recovered outcome. Symptomatology over the last month, as measured by the GAF-S scale, showed similar mean scores for Nottingham and for the total DOSMeD cohort (mean scores 61 and 65, respectively). Scores of 61 and above on the GAF-S scale are generally recognized to represent a favorable outcome; 53% of the Nottingham cohort had a score of 61 or above, compared to 63% of the remaining DOSMeD cases. Using the cut-off of 61, further univariate analyses were performed to explore differences in GAF scores for the Nottingham center predicted by gender, types of onset, short-term (first 2 years) pattern of course, and diagnosis. The only significant finding was for short-term pattern of course: 33 (66%) of the 50 subjects who had a short-term episodic course with complete remissions between episodes scored 61 or above on the GAF-S scale (mean score = 65.76), compared to 11 (34%) of the 32 subjects with a continuous course or episodic course with incomplete remissions between episodes (mean score = 53.63) (chi-square = 6.63, $p < .02$).

Course of the Illness

Over the 13 years of follow-up, 24% (21 out of 86) of the sample experienced continuous psychotic symptoms. The majority of the sample (69%) had an episodic course with only 7% having a course not typified by either continuous or episodic symptoms. These findings are similar to the proportions in each course type for the DOSMeD sample as a whole but differ from the findings of Ciompi's long-term follow-up of 289 patients in Lausanne (Ciompi, 1980). He found 52.2% of subjects had an episodic course, with 47.8% having a simple (continuous) course. These differences may reflect variation in definition of course type and the extent of completeness of follow-up of the respective samples (Ciompi followed up 18% of a cohort of 1642 consecutive admissions to the hospital between 1960 and 1962). Over the last 2 years of follow-up, 50 (59%) of the 85 subjects on whom there was sufficient information had not experienced any psychotic symptoms: Nine (11%) had an episodic course, and 23 (27%) had continuous psychotic symptoms. There were no significant differences comparing Nottingham data and those from the pooled DOSMeD cohorts, with respect to the proportions of subjects experiencing psychotic symptoms over the last 2 years (Nottingham=41%, DOSMeD, excluding Nottingham=50%), and the proportions of subjects experiencing continuous psychotic symptoms (Nottingham=27%, other DOSMeD=26%). In univariate analyses, only a diagnosis of schizophrenia (and not gender, nonacute onset, poor short-term course of illness) predicted global values for symptomatic outcome over the last 2 years of follow-up. Of subjects with a diagnosis of schizophrenia, 35.8% had a continuous course in the last 2 years compared to only 13.8% of subjects with a nonschizophrenia psychotic diagnosis (chi-square=4.39, $p<.04$). However, no correction factors were applied for multiple testing. In separate multiple linear analyses reported elsewhere (Harrison, Croudace et al., 1996) a model which included age, gender, marital status, speed of onset, and early (2-year) course type showed significant prognostic ability, enabling the prediction of over 30% of the variance of global ratings of symptoms and disability at 13-year follow-up. The extended analysis held for both the original ICD-9 project classifications and the reclassification to ICD-10 (see below).

The trend of psychotic symptoms as recorded in the Life Chart reveals a similar pattern to the course type over the entire 13 years. Nineteen (22%) of 86 cases experienced psychotic symptoms of much the same severity in each third of the follow-up period, and 59 (69%) experienced most prominent psychotic symptoms in the first third of the follow-up. The overall time trends revealed that only 5 (6%) of the 86 subjects completing the follow-up in Nottingham were somewhat worse at 13 years than they had been at onset. This is considerably less than the 18% with a worse outcome found for the pooled data from the other DOSMeD centers. Fifty-six percent of the Nottingham cases had a better overall time trend, which was similar to the 49% in other DOSMeD centers. Thirty-eight percent had an overall time trend rated as unchanging, considerably more than the 24% for the other DOSMeD centers.

Reevaluation of Baseline Diagnosis

The conversion tables used to convert ICD-9 to ICD-10 diagnoses yielded 61 subjects with schizophrenia at entry to the study. Of the 86 subjects completing the follow-up, 54 met ICD-10 criteria for schizophrenia determined by this method. ICD-10 diagnoses were also made independently by the investigators at the Nottingham Field Center (Mason et al., 1997). This rediagnosis exercise was conducted at 13-year follow-up. All the original project assessments for each subject together with case narratives were reviewed, blind to outcome, by GH who assigned a diagnosis according to ICD-10 Research Diagnostic Criteria (WHO, 1993). This method relied upon a Diagnostic Schedule (a diagnostic decision tree which systematically guides the researcher through the criteria for all psychotic disorders in ICD-10). The rediagnosis exercise was possible given the extensive baseline clinical data collected at entry to the study. A reliability exercise was carried out. Pairwise agreement for both 2- and 3-digit ICD-10 codes was 90%, with kappas of 0.79 ($z=7.1$) and 0.88 ($z=10.1$) respectively. Forty-eight of the 86 subjects available for 13-year follow-up were assigned a diagnosis of schizophrenia at this rediagnosis exercise. All 48 of these were also classified as schizophrenia by the ICD-9 to ICD-10 conversion tables. The additional six subjects given a diagnosis of schizophrenia using the conversion tables included two assigned to acute schizophrenia-like psychotic disorder, two with a delusional disorder, and two with affective psychoses. It is likely that the greater detail regarding duration criteria and differences in "weight" accorded to symptoms in the Nottingham rediagnosis exercise accounted for these differences. For the purposes of this report, the diagnoses derived from the conversion tables based upon the original ICD-9 diagnoses are used for consistency with the other centers.

Living Arrangements

Eighty-two (95%) of the entire alive sample were in independent community living during the last month of the 13-year follow-up. Two subjects were on psychiatric wards, one subject was on a medical ward, and one was living in a supervised residence. The remaining pooled DOSMeD data show that overall 11% spent the last month of the follow-up in either the hospital or in supervised residences. These findings underline the fact that our data represent *treated* and *administrative* outcomes: Differences with other centers are likely to reflect the comprehensive nature of community psychiatric services in Nottingham and local social conditions. Over the last 2 years of follow-up, only two subjects had not spent any time in independent community living.

Sixteen (19%) of the 86 subjects had been admitted to the hospital in the last 2 years for psychiatric reasons but only one of these spent more than 12 months in the hospital. More men (23%) had spent time in the hospital or in supervised residences than women (14%). The mean length of stay for men was considerably longer than for women, although this result is skewed by one male subject who had spent all of the last 2 years in supervised residences and another who had spent more than twelve months on an acute psychiatric ward. Only one member of the Nottingham cohort had spent any of the last 2 years homeless—the only person to have spent any time in prison over the last 2 years of follow-up. Over the entire follow-up period, all 86 subjects had spent some time in independent living. Indeed, only one subject spent less than 50% of the time in independent living; this was a male subject who had spent all but 2 years in either a psychiatric hospital or a supervised residence. The percentage of people spending 96 to 100% of the time in independent living at follow-up is similar for Nottingham and the total DOSMeD cohort (63 and 60% respectively). Women spent more time in independent living.

Eighty-one subjects had spent some of the follow-up period as psychiatric inpatients; of these subjects, seven also spent some time in supervised residences (six in supervised residences for people with mental health problems, and one in a probation hostel). Five subjects (6%) were never admitted to a psychiatric hospital over the entire course of their illness, including the first episode. The percentage of time spent in the hospital or in supervised residences was greater for men than for women; the percentage of time spent in the hospital was considerably less in Nottingham than for the rest of the DOSMeD centers. The mean period of time spent in the hospital and in supervised residences in Nottingham was 6% compared to 11% for the whole DOSMeD cohort. Two males (2%) of the Nottingham cohort had spent some of the entire follow-up period homeless, but neither had spent more than 10% of the time homeless. The proportion of the subjects spending some time homeless or in prison is similar for the DOSMeD cohort as a whole. The number of subjects spending time in prison was similar for the Nottingham cohort and the DOSMeD cohort as a whole, with only three (4%) of the Nottingham sample spending any time in prison.

Work

During the last 2 years of the follow-up, 39 (45%) of the 86 subjects had been employed at some point. Twenty-nine of these had full-time employment for more than 12 months, and for 27 of these subjects on whom information was available, their work performance was described as good or very good. Three subjects did full-time work for less than 12 months and the other seven subjects did part-time work only. Eighteen subjects undertook full-time household activities at some point during the last 2 years, and of these, 16 were in full-time household work for more than 12 months. Of the two subjects not doing full-time household work for more than 12 months, one obtained part-time employment, and the other became the main household worker when a relative with whom he was living became ill. For the 16 subjects who had been in full-time household work for more than 12 months, performance was described as good or very good. Twenty-four of the subjects employed full-time were men compared to only eight women. For part-time work there were seven women and only one man, and for full-time household work there were 16 women and two men. Two subjects had been retired for the last 2 years, both men. Thirty-six subjects were in receipt of disability living allowance, of whom 32 were receiving it for their mental condition.

Social Disability

Fifty-five (64%) of the 86 subjects completing the follow-up in the Nottingham sample achieved a fair to excellent outcome with respect to disability in the past month as measured by the DAS global ratings. This is slightly less than the 68% of the total DOSMeD cohort achieving fair to excellent social adjustment at 13 years. Simple univariate analyses of gender, type of onset, short-term pattern of course, and diagnosis were unable to predict social adjustment at 13 years. Mean GAF-D scores for disability were 63.3 for the Nottingham cohort and 64.4 for the entire DOSMeD cohort. Using the cut-off of 61 and above to represent favorable outcome, 55% of the Nottingham and 56% of the total DOSMeD cohorts achieved a favorable outcome. Male gender and a diagnosis of schizophrenia corresponded with unfavorable outcome on the GAF-D scale (chi-square=4.54, $p<.05$, and chi-square=4.26, $p<.05$, respectively). Fifty-four percent of the male subjects had an unfavorable GAF-D score compared to only 28% of the female subjects, and for those subjects with schizophrenia, 52.8% had an unfavorable GAF-D score compared to 37.5% with a nonschizophrenia diagnosis. The remaining candidate variables examined with univariate analyses (type of onset and short-term pattern of course) were unable to predict outcome on the GAF-D scale. The most common time trend was for greater disability in the first third of follow-up, accounting for 40% of subjects. The next most common trend was no prominent disability throughout the follow-up, describing 24% of subjects. The time trends for the Nottingham cohort are broadly similar to those for the DOSMeD cohort as a whole. As for symptoms, there was no evidence of a "late recovery" effect in this period of follow-up.

Violence and Suicide

Six subjects had been involved in assaults on other people in the last 2 years of follow-up. Five of these subjects were men, and all six had an ICD-10 diagnosis of schizophrenia. All of these assaults involved either kicking or punching close acquaintances or relatives, and no injuries were sustained of greater severity than bruising. Over the entire course, an additional 10 subjects had been involved in assaults against other people. In total, 14 of the male subjects and two of the female subjects had been involved in assaults. The most serious assault was a nonfatal stabbing which resulted in the subject's compulsory detention in a psychiatric hospital. One of the other subjects received a 6-month prison sentence for grievous bodily harm (aggravated assault). The rates of assaultive behavior in the Nottingham cohort are slightly less than in the total DOSMeD sample. Eight subjects had deliberately harmed themselves in the last 2 years of follow-up, all of whom were male. This proportion of subjects harming themselves is higher than that found in the total DOSMeD cohort. The rate of deliberate self-harm over the entire follow-up period is considerably higher in the Nottingham cohort than in the remaining DOSMeD cohorts (41 and 16%, respectively). This difference is statistically significant (chi-square=23.34, $p<.001$). A diagnosis of schizophrenia did not alter the risk compared to the group of psychoses as a whole.

Medication

Over the last 2 years of follow-up, 49 (58%) of the 85 subjects for whom information was available had been prescribed neuroleptics at some point. Of these, 43 subjects had taken neuroleptics for most of the last 2 years, and there were 36 subjects who had taken neuroleptics for most of the entire follow-up period. Only six subjects had never taken neuroleptics, and over the last 2 years, there were 36 subjects who had not been prescribed neuroleptics. Gender, type of onset, and short-term pattern of course did not predict which subjects were more likely to be taking neuroleptics in the last 2 years of follow-up. Interestingly, the proportions prescribed neuroleptics were similar for both schizophrenia and for the group of psychoses as a whole.

Hospitalization

As we have noted above, 16 subjects had spent some time in the hospital for treatment of their mental condition in the last 2 years of follow-up. Time trends for hospitalization showed the majority of subjects of the Nottingham cohort (80%) had most of their hospitalizations in the first third of the follow-up. This was the same pattern for the total DOSMeD cohort, although the percentage was slightly lower at 63%. We have shown elsewhere (Mason et al., 1995) that, relying upon the original ICD-9 classification of schizophrenia, the median survival time to readmission was 1.75 years, and to relapse was 1.4 years. For those patients who had a second hospitalization, the risk of readmission was almost completely consumed by 4 years after the first episode.

Deceased Subjects

At the time of the 13-year follow-up, nine of the subjects were deceased. Four had committed suicide, two by self-poisoning (a man and a woman, ages 47 and 42 at the time, respectively), one by drowning (a man, age 31 at time of death), and the other by jumping (a woman, age 49 at the time). All of these subjects were in an episode of illness at the time of their deaths. Three of the subjects were found dead at home (all men, ages 28, 44, and 48). In two of these cases, the bodies were in an advanced stage of decomposition, and the cause of death could not be ascertained; in the remaining case, the cause of death was found to be bronchopneumonia. These three subjects were living alone at the time of their deaths: Two were thought to be in partial remission, and in the third case, the state of mental health could not be determined. The remaining two subjects were both female and died of natural causes.

DISCUSSION

The completeness of follow-up of the Nottingham case group, with high-quality data available on most of those who refused face-to-face interviews, suggests that selection biases have not seriously compromised the representativeness of the data. The gender distribution was uneven compared to other cohorts in the present series of studies, with more than twice as many men as women. This appears to be a stable epidemiological feature of the Nottingham area; we recently reported a similar finding (Brewin et al., 1997) in an inception cohort identified between 1992 and 1994, using almost identical methodology.

The long-term outcome data reported here illustrate the need to consider the dimensional nature of outcome across the domains of symptoms, social disability, and service use. The most simple cross-sectional clinical measure was perhaps the Bleuler Severity Scale, with 61% of the entire sample showing no psychotic symptoms in the last month of follow-up. Another common historic measure of outcome (whether the subject is hospitalized) shows an even more remarkable level of "recovery" with less than 2% in the hospital at the point of follow-up. These crude measures, however, obscure the diversity and range of disabilities across the longitudinal course. Disability measures showed significant continuing social impairment in nearly half of the surviving case group; this must also be considered alongside the attrition which had already taken place on account of suicide and premature deaths. Although there was a strong association between symptoms and disability (Mason et al., 1995), the potential independence of these dimensions is apparent from our review of the individual narrative summaries. For example, one man had had continuous auditory hallucinations throughout the entire follow-up period and yet was able to work full-time in professional employment. Another subject who suffered continuous auditory hallucinations and persecutory delusions was successfully caring for her son who was severely disabled by his schizophrenia.

Although the residential data showed that nearly two-thirds of cases were living either alone or with family, it was not possible to undertake objective measures of family burden or to carry out a systematic needs assessment. We judged, however, that for those subjects still living with families, 10% imposed such a severe burden of care that they would be incapable of independent living when their caretakers eventually died or became unable to continue this level of care. These included one person disabled by a cerebrovascular accident, another with severe and florid delusions of persecution demanding continuous vigilance from his caretakers, and four patients with severe and enduring deficit symptoms. This identifies a significant pool of pent-up demand for residential mental health services, linked with the mortality of informal caretakers. Our findings for full-time employment rates are similar to other studies: Leary, Johnstone, and Owens (1991) reported 22.5% of their sample in full-time employment at 3- to 13-year follow-up, and Carone, Harrow, and Westermeyer (1991) reported that 33% of their sample were employed at 5-year follow-up. Although recent (1996–1998) strong improvements in the U.K. employment market offer new opportunities, prospects for those with psychiatric disabilities continue to be bleak as employers seek applicants with higher levels of skills and teamwork competencies.

Although only a small proportion of patients was hospitalized in the last few years of follow-up, 58% of the entire case group had been prescribed neuroleptic medication in the last 2 years and 53% were using specialist mental health services at follow-up. Only 34% were no longer in contact with specialist services and taking no psychotropic medication. This moderates the overall findings of "good" outcome and "recovered or mild" ratings in symptoms and social disability. Several patients were functioning well but should be considered as being "in treated remission" rather than having achieved a complete recovery. Compared with the other DOSMeD groups, and the invited centers, outcome data for the Nottingham case group are generally close to aggregated follow-up data from all the DOSMeD cohorts. Regrettably, because of the relatively small numbers in some of the DOSMeD center case groups, and the different follow-up biases operating across centers, comparisons between centers should be treated with caution. The sample sizes especially do not allow sufficient power to determine whether or not there are meaningful differences in course and outcome between centers, across a range of outcome variables examined. Broadly, however, when the Nottingham data are compared with other centers there are trends for less assaultive but more self-harming behavior, comparable levels of psychosis and disability, and less good work performance.

These findings emphasize the heterogeneity of schizophrenia and related psychotic disorders. They underline the need for concepts of administrative outcome based upon representative samples with complete follow-up data. Although a first episode of psychotic illness (and especially syndromal presentation with schizophrenia) has serious repercussions for the long-term health and social competency of the sufferer and his or her family, these data show that many subjects achieve remarkably good outcomes. This is important for health professionals as well as for patients. When reviewing the predictors of long-term outcome elsewhere (Harrison, Croudace et al., 1996) we emphasized the predictive strength of duration of untreated psychosis (DUP) and early 2-year course type. This offers the prospect that earlier intervention at onset, and assertive treatment in the early course, may have important implications for the long-term outcome of the disorder. Evidence would need to be provided in controlled trials, but the notion that early intervention may have effects enduring for decades afterward is intuitively appealing. Besides mitigating social losses, the potential biological and psychological effects of reducing the time in active psychosis may be considerable. These follow-up data therefore have twofold importance: They emphasize heterogeneity of outcome in psychosis and warn against the overly pessimistic prognostications of the past. And they hold out the prospect that earlier intervention aimed at reducing time in psychosis and mitigating the adverse social effects of the illness can produce enduring benefits lasting over 10 to 20 years. Mental health professionals must plan and work for long-term, as well as the short-term, recovery of their patients.

References

Amin, S., Brewin, J., Singh, S. P., Harrison, G. L., Medley, I., & Kwiencinski, R. (1998), Diagnostic stability of first onset psychoses: Implications for epidemiology. *Schizophr. Res.*, 29:1–2, 9.

Audit Commission (1995), *Review of Adult Mental Health Services. Nottingham Healthcare NHS Trust.* London: Audit Commission.

Bleuler, M. (1978), *The Schizophrenia Disorders: Long-Term Patient and Family Studies*, tr. S. M. Clemens. New Haven, CT: Yale University Press.

Brewin, J., Glazebrook, C., Cantwell, R., Dalkin, T., Fox, R., Kwiecinski, R., & Harrison, G. (1997), The incidence of schizophrenia: Two Nottingham cohorts. *Brit. J. Psychiatry*, 171:140–144.

Carone, G. J., Harrow, M., & Westermeyer, J. F. (1991), Posthospital course and outcome in schizophrenia. *Arch. Gen. Psychiatry*, 48:247–253.

Ciompi, L. (1980), Catamnestic long-term study on the course of life and aging of schizophrenics. *Schizophr. Bull.*, 6:606–618.

Cooper, J. E. (1989), Information for planning: Case registers and Korner. In: *Health Services Planning and Research: Contributions from Psychiatric Case Registers*, ed. J. K. Wing. Gaskell: Royal College of Psychiatrists.

——(1990), Some aspects of psychiatric case registers in the United States and in Europe. *Aging* (Milano) 2(1):88–93.

——Goodhead, D., Craig, T., Harris, M., Howat, J., & Korer, J. (1987), The incidence of schizophrenia in Nottingham. *Brit. J. Psychiatry*, 151:619–626.

Dauncey, K., Giggs, J., Baker, K., & Harrison, G. (1993), Schizophrenia in Nottingham: Lifelong residential mobility of a cohort. *Brit. J. Psychiatry*, 163:613–619.

Davies, L., & Drummond, M. (1994), Economics and schizophrenia: The real cost. *Brit. J. Psychiatry*, 165 (Suppl. 25):18–21.

Department of Health (1994), *Department Report, Department of Health and Office of Population Censuses and Surveys*. London: Her Majesty's Stationery Office.

Der, G., Gupta, S., & Murray, R. (1990), Is schizophrenia disappearing? *Lancet*, 335:513–516.

Eagles, J. M., & Whalley, L. J. (1985), Decline in the diagnosis of schizophrenia among first admissions to Scottish mental hospitals from 1969–1978. *Brit. J. Psychiatry*, 146:151–154.

Giggs, J. A. (1972), The distribution of schizophrenics in Nottingham. *Trans. Inst. Brit. Geographers*, 59: 55–76.

——(1973), High rates of schizophrenia among immigrants in Nottingham. *Nurs. Times*, 69:1210–1212.

——Cooper, J. A. (1987), Ecological structure and the distribution of schizophrenia and affective psychoses in Nottingham. *Brit. J. Psychiatry*, 151:627–633.

Harrison, G. (1993), Disappearing schizophrenia? *Schizophr. Monitor*, October:1–3.

——Cooper, J. E., & Glancarczyk, R. (1991), Changes in the administrative incidence of schizophrenia. *Brit. J. Psychiatry*, 159:811–816.

——Croudace, T., Mason, P., Glazebrook, C., Docherty, S., & Medley, I. (1996), Predicting the long-term outcome of schizophrenia. *Psycholog. Med.*, 26:697–705.

——Glazebrook, C. Brewin, J., Cantwell, R., Dalkin, T., Fox, R., Jones, P., & Medley, I. (1997), Increased incidence of psychotic disorders in African Caribbean migrants to the U.K. *Psycholog. Med.*, 27:799–806.

——Holton, A., Neilson, D., Owens, D., Boot, D., & Cooper, J. (1989), Severe mental disorder in Afro-Caribbean patients, some sociodemographic and service factors. *Psycholog. Med.*, 19:683–696.

——Mason, P., Glazebrook, C., Medley, I., Docherty, S., & Croudace, T. (1994), Residence of incident cohort of psychotic patients after 13 years of follow-up. *Brit. Med. J.*, 308:813–816.

——Owens, D., Holton, A., Neilson, D., & Boot, D. (1988), A prospective study of severe mental disorder in Afro-Caribbean patients. *Psycholog. Med.*, 18:643–657.

Hegarty, J. D., Baldessarni, R. J., Tohen, M., Waternaux, C., & Oepen, G. (1994), One hundred years of schizophrenia: A meta-analysis of the outcome literature. *Amer. J. Psychiatry*, 151:1409–1416.

Her Majesty's Stationery Office (1971), *The Nottingham Psychiatric Case Register. Findings 1962–1969.* Statistical Report Series no. 13. London: Her Majesty's Stationery Office.

Howat, J. G. M. (1979), Nottingham and the hospital plan: A follow-up study of long stay in-patients. *Brit. J. Psychiatry*, 135:42–51.

——Kontny, E. I. (1982), The outcome for discharged Nottingham long stay in-patients. *Brit. J. Psychiatry*, 141:590–594.

Jablensky, A., Sartorius, N., Ernberg, G., Anker, M., Korten, A., Cooper, J. E., Day, R., & Bertelsen, A. (1992), Schizophrenia: Manifestations, incidence and course in different cultures. A World Health Organization ten-country study. *Psycholog. Med.*, 20(Suppl):1–97.

King, M., Coker, E., Levey, G., Hoare, A., & Johnson-Sabine, E. (1994), Incidence of psychotic illness in London: A comparison of ethnic groups. *Brit. Med. J.*, 309:1115–1119.

Kontny, D. E. L., Jones, S., & Cooper, J. E. (1986), An example from the Nottingham case register: The design of a zoning system. In: *Psychiatric Case Registers in Public Health: A Worldwide Inventory 1960–1985*, ed. G. H. M. M. ten Horn, R. Giel, W. H. Gulbinat, & J. H. Henderson. New York: Oxford.

Leary, J., Johnstone, E. C., & Owens, D. G. C. (1991), Disabilities and circumstances of schizophrenic patients—a follow-up study. II. Social outcome. *Brit. J. Psychiatry*, 159(Suppl. 13):13–20.

Mason, P., Harrison, G., Glazebrook, C., Hedley, I., Docherty, S., Dalkin, T., & Croudace, T. (1995), Characteristics of outcome in schizophrenia at 13 years. *Brit. J. Psychiatry*, 167:596–603.

——, ——Croudace, T., Glazebrook, C., & Medley, I. (1997), The predictive validity of competing diagnostic systems. *Brit. J. Psychiatry*, 170:321–327.

OPCS (1992), *1991 Census, County Report.* London: Her Majesty's Stationery Office.

Owens, D., Harrison, G., & Boot, D. (1991), Ethnic factors in voluntary and compulsory admissions. *Psycholog. Med.*, 21:185–196.

Thomas, C. S., Stone, K., Osborn, C., Thomas, P. F., & Fisher, M. (1993), Psychiatric morbidity and compulsory admission among UK-born Europeans, Afro-Caribbeans and Asians in central Manchester. *Brit. J. Psychiatry*, 163:91–99.

Tyrer, P., Turner, R., & Johnston, A. L. (1989), Integrated hospital and community psychiatric services and use of in-patient beds. *Brit. Med. J.*, 299:298–300.

van Os, J., Castle, D. J., Takei, N., Der, G., & Murray, R. M. (1996), Schizophrenia in ethnic minorities. Clarification of the 1991 Census. *Psycholog. Med.*, 26:203–208.

Wessley, S., Castle, D., Der, G., & Murray, R. M. (1991), Schizophrenia and Afro-Caribbeans: A case control study. *Brit. J. Psychiatry*, 159:795–801.

Wilson, S. (1995), Aiming for health in the year 2000. *Annual Report of the Director of Public Health 1995.* Nottingham Health District.

World Health Organization (1992), *The ICD-10 Classification of Mental and Behavioral Disorders.* Geneva: World Health Organization.

——(1993), *The ICD-10 Classification of Mental and Behavioral Disorders, Diagnostic Criteria for Research.* Geneva: World Health Organization.

CHAPTER 17

DOSMeD: Rochester, New York

Lyman C. Wynne and Sharon Holmberg

CULTURAL CONTEXT

Metropolitan Rochester, New York, is located at about the midpoint of the southern shore of Lake Ontario, 550 km northwest of New York City. Rochester is the core city for an area about 110 km from east to west and about 80 km north to south. Monroe County, which runs some 60 km from east to west, is the jurisdiction within this metropolitan area in which most of the mental health services are provided. While surrounding counties have some of their own services, persons with severe problems, such as psychosis, come into the city medical facilities. Rochester's strategic location has meant that there is very little duplication of resources within the area. From the epidemiological standpoint, this has two consequences: (1) At the time of primary data collection, there was no significant "leakage" from the area of persons with acute psychoses; all were screened through the Emergency Department of Strong Memorial Hospital, the site of the Rochester WHO Center. (2) Mobility is primarily from one neighborhood to another (e.g., from the inner city to the suburbs). People tend to stay within Monroe County and continue to receive public health care services within the same jurisdiction.

Population

For several decades, Monroe County as a whole has had a relatively stable population, estimated at 714,000; however, for at least 30 years, population has shifted steadily from the city of Rochester primarily into the surrounding suburbs of Monroe County. Since 1970, the population within the Rochester city limits has shrunk by about 100,000 to about 230,000. From the standpoint of schools and many public services, the inner city has undergone moderate deterioration. Although not so severely as in many other American cities during this time period, Rochester has unmistakably failed to thrive when compared to its much more affluent suburbs; despite repeated efforts at rejuvenation, major retail stores have steadily moved to suburban shopping malls. The county includes a full range of residence types—from deteriorated "tenements" in part of the crowded, relatively impoverished, racially mixed inner city, to the more culturally homogeneous, white, and affluent suburbs, and to a rural periphery of farms and small villages. The major hospitals and health care services have remained in the city, though not at its core.

Racial and Ethnic Characteristics

Epidemiologically, Rochester has a racial and ethnic mix that is remarkably similar to that of the United States as a whole, a mixture not found in the rural South and Midwest or in such cities as Boston, New York, Philadelphia, Washington, Atlanta, Houston, Los Angeles, or San Francisco. In its racial distribution, a critical issue in the United States, it includes about 14% blacks and a substantial Hispanic population, mostly from Puerto Rico and Cuba, sufficient in size to necessitate Spanish-speaking staff in major clinics. Ethnically, the largest immigrant groups are German and Italian, scattered throughout the suburbs, and Ukrainian, mostly in one neighborhood. There is also a small Native American (Seneca tribe) population within the city; others live nearby. After the Vietnam War, there was a noteworthy influx of Laotian, Cambodian, and Vietnamese refugees. Although the parents in these families have had difficulty finding work and have continuing language problems, their children usually assimilate more easily into

American culture. There is also a rapidly growing minority of nonrefugee, well-educated Japanese, Chinese, and Pakistanis who are English proficient and often have obtained medical, scientific, or academic employment.

Religious, Gender, and Political Affiliations

The religious distribution follows expected patterns given the ethnic and racial mix. The majority of the population is Roman Catholic and traditional Protestant, but Greek Orthodox, Jewish, Muslim, and evangelistic Christian sects are also represented. Rochester is said to have been the first American city to have elected an openly homosexual man to the city council and has controversially taken national leadership in accepting homosexual clergy. Politically, as in most American cities, the inner city is now predominantly Democratic and the suburbs are predominantly Republican, with an uneasy and only sporadically effective collaboration between city and county governments.

Employment Patterns

Socioeconomically, because of the technological nature of the major local industries, the area is somewhat atypical in that a higher than usual proportion of the work force is employed in white-collar positions. Ordinarily, the unemployment rate in Monroe County is 1 to 2% lower than in most of the rest of New York state. Kodak, which had 48,000 employees in Rochester in 1970 and at the time of this follow-up study has about 30,000 employees, provides jobs at varying salaries for a wide racial mix and subsidizes a great many of the cultural activities in the city; Xerox, the second largest employer, has a reputation for having an unusually high proportion of black executives. During the past 25 years, considerable numbers of small electronics and computer companies have located in the suburban periphery of Rochester.

Impact of Mental Health Issues on Society

Over the past 25 years, the mental health policy of deinstitutionalization of state hospital inpatients and drastically shortened length of stay for all psychiatric inpatients has had a major impact on service delivery. The availability of psychotropic medications and the belief that smaller, locally managed treatment settings could provide better care for persons with persistent mental illnesses led to the development of federally funded (for a delimited time) community mental health centers (CMHCs). Funding for community care, however, has not increased in proportion to need.

The patient census of Rochester Psychiatric Center (RPC), the regional New York State-operated psychiatric hospital, dropped from about 3000 in 1970, to 1,400 in 1977, and to 175 in 1996. After federal funding expired, CMHCs, which were underfunded by the state, tried to cope with increasing numbers of outpatients. Alternative facilities—especially boarding houses, partial hospitalization (day hospital) facilities, and community-based social clubs for mentally ill persons—began to emerge, at times to the distress of host communities. In recent years, these facilities have become linked to management of persons with dual diagnoses, especially mental illness plus alcoholism or street-drug abuse.

THE MENTAL HEALTH SYSTEM

In 1891, the Monroe County Insane Asylum, which had been established in 1864, was converted to a hospital run by the New York State Department of Mental Hygiene. Originally, this institution was physically south of the populated area, but as the city grew around it, the asylum became relatively centrally located. In 1927, outpatient care began, and a 16-bed inpatient unit was established within the new Strong Memorial Hospital, the primary facility in the University of Rochester Medical Center. In 1946, the Department of Psychiatry was founded in the Medical School, and a series of new inpatient facilities in Strong Memorial Hospital soon followed.

On January 1, 1960, monitoring of all psychiatric services in the county began with the establishment of the Monroe County Psychiatric Case Register (Miles and Gardner, 1966). On that date, all patients under psychiatric care were registered, and all subsequent psychiatric contacts were reported to the Register from the University inpatient, outpatient, and emergency services, from all the state hospital (now called Rochester Psychiatric Center) facilities, the county children's services, the court clinic, and 56 of 60 psychiatrists in private practice (Liptzin and Babigian, 1972). For the next 30 years, the Register was what the epidemiology chief at the National Institute of Mental Health called "the only viable data collection operation of its kind and scope in the US" (Kramer, 1978).

In 1968, community mental health clinics were opened, and the number of inpatient beds in the state hospital decreased. So that better services could be provided by the new CMHCs and that more detailed data could be obtained for the Case Register, the county was divided into four mental health catchment areas, delineated in "pie-like" fashion and extending in quadrants from the center of the city to the periphery. Area A in the southwest sector, the location of the University of Rochester Medical Center and WHO Center headquarters, and from which the original sample for ISoS was obtained, has a total population of 132,719, of whom 18.6% are black.

Current Structure

During the 1970s and 1980s, overall increase in the use of mental health facilities was due largely to an increase in ambulatory care. Changing state regulations made it difficult to admit elderly patients to RPC. Socially disadvantaged groups greatly increased their utilization of CMHC services. Studies using Case Register data showed that distance from available services was highly significant in determining utilization rates (Babigian, 1977). When partial hospitalization programs were opened in various sectors of the community, patients became more compliant with care after inpatient stays. However, with inpatient stays becoming steadily shorter—now less than 2 weeks, even for grossly psychotic patients—the frequency of relapse appears to have increased, but the relationship between length of inpatient stay, type of ambulatory care, and relapse of psychotic symptoms has not yet been adequately studied.

Financial Support

The shift from long-term state hospital care for psychotic patients to outpatient CMHCs was succeeded in the 1980s and 1990s by care at agencies paid for at levels often considered to be below what is optimally needed, by private insurance plans in combination with Medicare (for those over 65) and Medicaid (for the disabled and indigent). In the mid-1980s, a capitation payment system, Integrated Mental Health (IMH), was experimentally introduced. This "voluntarily formed, not-for-profit corporation" included a Contract Revenues System in which all public funding and matching local funding were rolled into performance-based contracts, paid for by stabilized, prospective, predictable quarterly payments. Eligibility was based on treatment history at RPC, with different levels of payment specified for patients needing chronic inpatient care, intermittent care, and outpatient treatment. In addition, 300 patients with no qualifying history of care at RPC were enrolled. Staff, patients, and families were strongly motivated to obtain the most satisfactory and cost-effective care within the limits set by the capitation system. While highly successful in some respects, the capitation system could not be integrated administratively with new forms of private insurance coverage and managed care that have become important in the 1990s.

PSYCHIATRIC EPIDEMIOLOGY

Using the data from the Monroe County Psychiatric Register, Lehman, Babigian, and Reed (1984) estimated the annual treated incidence and prevalence of chronic and nonchronic mental disorders. Based upon the definition of a chronic illness as one requiring at least three inpatient hospitalizations or at least 365 inpatient days during a 5-year follow-up period, the annual treated incidence of chronic mental disorders did not change significantly between 1964 and 1965 (0.47/1000) and 1969 and 1970 (0.41/1000). The annual treated prevalence of chronic disorders also remained unchanged at 0.6% between 1965 and 1970; nonchronic disorders rose by 43%, from 1.4% in 1965 to 1.9% in 1970, coinciding with the development of the CMHCs.

THE CENTER

The Rochester WHO Center was organized in 1978 as a function of the University Department of Psychiatry. Data collection took place in two phases: first, in "WHO-1," from August 1978 to July 1980 (58 patients), and second, after an interruption of funding, in "WHO-2," from July 1981 to January 1983 (87 patients). The subjects for the present follow-up come from the first cohort.

METHODS

Defining the ISoS Cohort

The enrollment of subjects in the initial study precisely followed the DOSMeD protocol. Between August 1,

1978, and July 31, 1980, all patients who came through the Emergency Department of Strong Memorial Hospital were screened to determine eligibility for the study. The screening schedule was completed on all potential subjects and reviewed by one of the primary investigators within 24 hours of the patient's admission. Since all patients were required to have a preadmission screening evaluation in the Emergency Department, there was essentially no "leakage" of patients from this catchment who met study criteria.

Case-Finding at Follow-Up

Case-finding was complicated by the substantial requirements imposed by local Institutional Review Boards to protect the privacy and human rights of research subjects. In the intervening 16 years, the Monroe County Psychiatric Case Register was discontinued, and data from the register could not be used to obtain information about individuals. The further division of the mental health catchment areas and the growth of independent mental health services providers further increased the complexity of follow-up. Before a subject could be contacted through an agency, the research proposal had to be reviewed by the agency to ensure clear and accurate procedures for informed consent. Because there was no initial follow-up information about where, or if, subjects were currently receiving treatment, and because each individual agency review potentially required several months, it was impractical to obtain primary information from individual agencies. Therefore, preliminary approval of the protocol at Strong Memorial Hospital (SMH), where all subjects were initially registered, and at the Rochester Psychiatric Center (RPC) was obtained, and then Institutional Review Board (IRB) responsibility was transferred to the Nathan S. Kline Institute for Psychiatric Research. Once the subjects had agreed to participate, they were asked to sign a release for their medical records so that information about current treatment could be requested from the agencies.

Within the approved framework, several procedures for finding subjects were used. Researchers had personal knowledge of, or relatively recent contact with, about 10% of the original cohort. A brief letter from one of the original investigators (LCW) was sent to the last known address of each subject, reminding him or her of previous participation, providing information about the planned follow-up, and then requesting the individual's participation. A few subjects called the research office, but most did not respond. Many letters to subjects who had relocated since their last treatment contact were returned.

Other efforts at case-finding involved cycles of reviewing patient records, telephone directories, and other public documents for the subject or relatives and then following up leads via telephone. One difficulty encountered was the frequency with which telephones were answered by machine, requesting the caller to leave a message, and saying that the call would be returned. When left, messages were carefully worded to protect the confidentiality of the subject. Many calls were not returned, leaving the researchers uncertain whether or not the correct person had been reached or whether a family member might have ignored the necessarily nonspecific message, perhaps believing that this was a disguised merchandising call, and failed to pass it on to the subject. Telephone contact was established with a number of persons who were uncertain about their willingness to participate, especially in a face-to-face interview. Some eventually agreed, others agreed to an extended telephone interview to discuss their life situations and illness, while a third group ultimately refused to participate. Making contact with the WHO Center was entirely the recipient's decision; it was impossible to ascertain whether the subject had been located and, if so, chose not to respond. In several cases, we were quite certain that we had located a subject, but direct communication could not be established because there was no personal response to letters or telephone calls. At least two additional letters were sent to these persons as well as to all remaining unlocated persons in the initial cohort, explaining the importance of their participation in the study. In the first letter, we enclosed a checklist and a return envelope. The checklist requested the recipient to check one of the following: "I am not the person you are seeking; I am the person you are seeking and do not wish to participate; I am the person you are seeking and am willing to participate in the follow-up study." In this way, a few more subjects were identified. A final mailing was sent to nonresponders near the close of the study. This letter was a personal appeal, explaining in very practical, specific, and direct language, the importance of each individual's contribution to this long-term study; subjects were told that even our simply knowing that they had been located was a relevant contribution. Once again, few responses, but these were sometimes useful in obtaining data on the status of the subjects, especially on their reasons for not wanting to participate. A final attempt to contact several subjects for whom we believed we had a correct address was through home visits which, although they did not net interviews, did confirm the location of three subjects.

The State Department of Motor Vehicles will, for a relatively small fee, provide the most recent address of persons with a state driver's license. This source proved relatively fruitless since apparently persons with continuing psychiatric symptoms are unlikely to have a driver's license. Other sources (e.g., Social Security Administration) were willing to forward a message, but would neither provide a current address nor assure researchers that a message was received.

Use of Study Instruments

Most of the subjects were native speakers of English. During and after World War II, there had been a large influx of people from central Europe, but the ISoS cohort included their offspring, many of whom were at least partially bilingual, with English as their dominant language. One subject's elderly parents were the informants but spoke Italian as their first and dominant language. With the subject's sibling acting as translator, they eventually agreed to an interview, enabling us to understand the current status and functioning of the subject. This sibling asked many questions about mental illness during the interview and openly expressed appreciation for the explanations provided. He explained that his parents' earlier evasiveness and their continuing refusal to allow direct contact with the son was based upon their firm conviction that exposing him to the mental health system would somehow "bring back" the illness. While face-to-face contact with this subject was never achieved, the family provided abundant evidence of their son's economic achievements and involvement with his children and church.

Data-Gathering Procedures

Most subjects and informants (52.6%) were interviewed in the research office; 13.2% were interviewed in their homes; and 29.0% by telephone at their request. One subject was interviewed in a psychiatric hospital. One informant very much wished to participate but was only willing to meet at her job site (a shopping mall), so the interview took place early in the morning before stores opened. The majority of interviews were conducted by one of the primary investigators (SKH); for several, both were present. Diagnoses were reviewed and discussed, with the senior investigator (LCW) making final diagnosis decisions.

Interviews were usually completed in one or two sessions over 2 to 4 hours. The initial phase explained reasons for the interview, covered the anticipated content of discussion, and solicited informed consent. Next, the subject was asked for a life review, using the Life Chart, beginning with the events that led up to the first hospitalization and continuing to the present. As the respondent talked, specific details about employment, residence, symptoms, and treatment were explored. At appropriate points, specific instruments, such as the Present State Examination or the Substance Abuse Schedule, were completed. Most observational schedules, such as the Scale for the Assessment of Negative Symptoms, were completed immediately following the interview. Some additional checklists about family interaction and self-care habits were included at convenient points. The interview closed with the Rochester Recovery Inventory, a measure that encouraged the subject to describe the personal effects of the illness, especially with respect to their own view of relationships with others, and beliefs about and understanding of the illness and its causes.

Modifications of this procedure were sometimes necessary. Information was obtained from one severely regressed and highly anxious subject only after moving to a park bench in front of the hospital where the subject was allowed to sit quietly and smoke. She was encouraged to volunteer whatever information she wished and efforts were made to guide the conversation by questions from the interviewer, to which she only sometimes responded. In a second interview, the subject was able to tolerate a more structured approach having discovered that the researcher could be relied upon to keep the promise of discussing only what she wished.

RESULTS

Baseline and Short-Term Follow-Up

The ISoS follow-up effort centered on all 58 subjects who were identified between August 1978 and July 1980 and passed the initial screening for the DOSMeD study. Three subjects who were subsequently dropped from the DOSMeD final incidence cohort are included in ISoS: One is included in the alive, interviewed cohort, while the other two are in the lost to follow-up cohort.

Gender and Age

At entry to the study, this cohort consisted of an almost equal gender mix—30 women (51.7%) and 28 men (48.3%). In the total original DOSMeD sample, there were 47.9% women, somewhat fewer than in Rochester. The Rochester sample who were found and interviewed almost 16 years after study entry had 18 women (54.5%) and 15 men (45.5%), suggesting a slight, nonsignificant increase in females between entry and follow-up. Overall, the Rochester sample is not far from the middle in gender distribution in comparison to the entire DOSMeD sample.

The majority of subjects (79.3%) were in the young group of those born after 1949 at the time of enrollment in the study, with 36.2% born after 1959 and 43.1% born between 1950 and 1959. The latter birth cohort is identical to that for the total original DOSMeD cohort, and in Rochester, was the most successfully interviewed 15 to 17 years later, increasing to 54.5% of the interviewed total. Interestingly, only rural Chandigarh in the DOSMeD sample had a higher percentage of followed-up subjects who had been born after 1959.

Mode of Onset

The most common mode of onset in the original Rochester cohort was "greater than one month" (41.4%), followed by "up to one month" (34.5%), with a symptomatic period of "up to one week" in only 17.2%, and 6.9% missing. The comparable figures for the total DOSMeD cohort were 32.3, 16.2, 29.8, and 21.7%. There were no major differences in mode of onset between the Rochester subjects in the follow-up group and those in the original sample. In the DOSMeD alive (interviewed at follow-up) sample, only Dublin had a lower percentage (13.5%) of acute onsets (less than one week) than did Rochester (15.2%).

Diagnosis

The grouped baseline ICD-10 diagnoses for the original sample ranked in the following order of frequency: acute schizophrenia-like (44.8%), paranoid schizophrenia (13.8%), schizoaffective (10.3%), bipolar disorder (10.3%), other psychotic but not schizophrenia (8.6%), catatonic schizophrenia (5.2%), other schizophrenia (3.4%), and nonpsychotic (3.4%). A baseline diagnosis in one of the schizophrenia categories was given to 22.4% of the original sample and to 21.2% of those who were interviewed at follow-up. By comparison, none of the other DOSMeD centers, and only Groningen (20.5%) in the entire ISoS group of centers, had a lower percentage of schizophrenia diagnoses in the original samples. This contrasts with 52.8% for the DOSMeD centers and 58.3% for all ISoS centers.

The most common baseline diagnosis in the Rochester followed-up cohort was acute schizophrenia-like symptoms (51.5%), followed by bipolar disorder (12.1%), then paranoid schizophrenia, and schizoaffective disorder (both 9.1%). The initial diagnostic categories of subjects lost to follow-up were acute schizophrenia-like symptoms (36%), paranoid schizophrenia (20%), schizoaffective (12%), other psychotic (12%), and bipolar disorder (8%). Thus, among those lost to follow-up, there were somewhat fewer who had been initially diagnosed as having schizophrenia-like symptoms and somewhat more who had been diagnosed with paranoid schizophrenia. However, given small subgroup Ns, these differences are surely not statistically significant. Only rural Chandigarh came close to having such a high percentage of the initial and followed-up samples with an initial diagnosis of acute schizophrenia-like symptoms (43.6 and 47.4%, respectively).

Course of Illness at Short-term Follow-Up

The distribution of short-term course of illness (up to 30 months) for the original Rochester sample was complete remission (41.4%), incomplete remission (44.8%), continuously psychotic (8.6%), with only 5.2% missing data. For the total DOSMeD sample, the percentages were 38.4, 29.4, 12.5, and 19.8, showing fewer incomplete remissions and more missing data, not an overall meaningful difference.

For those in the alive cohort at the 16-year follow-up, 14 (42.4%) of the 33 subjects had a course pattern of complete remission, another 14 (42.4%) had incomplete remission, and three (9.1%) were continuously psychotic. Among those not interviewed after 16 years (refusers and not found), the available data showed little difference, with 40% completely remitted,

48% incompletely remitted, and 8% continuously psychotic. Overall, those not followed up do not seem to be more likely to have had a poor early course. In the DOSMeD sample of interviewed subjects, 46.7% had a short-term course pattern of complete remission and 12.5% continuously psychotic, with only Prague and urban and rural Chandigarh having a smaller proportion of continuously psychotic subjects than Rochester.

ALIVE SUBJECTS

Overall in Rochester, 33 (56.9%) subjects or their informants were successfully interviewed, 12 (20.7%) were contacted but refused, and 13 (22.4%) were lost to follow-up, with one of these most likely deceased, though no death certificate was available.

Severity of Symptoms (Bleuler Scale)

At long-term follow-up, 31 of the 33 subjects were rated on the Bleuler Severity Scale: 17 (54.8%) were rated as recovered, five (16.1%) as having mild symptoms, seven (22.6%) as having moderate symptoms, and two (6.5%) as having severe symptoms. Thus, among subjects rated in Rochester, 70.9% were either recovered or had mild symptoms. Among the interviewed subjects in other DOSMeD centers, Dublin, Honolulu, Nottingham, and Prague had almost the same percentages of mild and recovered patients, while Moscow and urban and rural Chandigarh had more (83.8–92.3%); only Nagasaki had substantially fewer such patients (54.4%).

Global Assessment of Functioning

From the GAF-S, eight (25.9%) subjects were rated above 70, indicating only mild symptoms over the past month. Similar ratings were obtained in Dublin, Honolulu, and Nagasaki. However, 13 (42%) were rated as having relatively severe symptoms (GAF-S < 51). The remaining 10 (32.2%) ranked with moderate symptoms, with scores of 51 to 70. Thus, using this measure of recent functioning, overall impairment because of symptoms was relatively serious in the Rochester cohort. In fact, the mean GAF-S score was lower (55.8) than for any of the other treated Incidence cohorts, with the exception of Sofia (49.3).

There is clear evidence that most subjects experienced psychotic symptoms at least some of the time during the entire follow-up period. Nearly 40% of the cohort experienced episodic symptoms, 27% were reported to have continuous symptoms, and 24% had symptomatology that met neither the episodic nor continuous definition. Only two (6.1%) subjects experienced no psychotic symptoms during the entire follow-up period. Time trend data suggest improvement over time for most subjects, as 24 (72.7%) experienced the most severe symptoms during the first 5 to 6 years after initial contact. In the most recent 2 years, just over half of the cohort (51.6%) had not experienced psychotic symptoms.

Despite the lower GAF scores in the Rochester sample, over a third (34.4%) of the subjects scored as "much better" in contrast to 29.3% of the DOSMeD sample for the overall time trend. This may be a consequence of having more face-to-face interviews with subjects who had better outcomes. We surmise that of the subjects who were interviewed by telephone or for whom only an informant could be interviewed, more were likely to have more symptoms.

Reevaluation of Baseline Diagnosis

For the reevaluation of baseline diagnosis, documentation of symptoms and behaviors described in the index hospitalization were reviewed and the current ICD-10 diagnostic criteria were applied. This process involved discussion of the information and agreement on the rediagnosis by the two investigators.

Of the 33 subjects, 15 were given diagnoses of schizophrenia, five were given diagnoses of schizoaffective disorder, and six were diagnosed as having had acute schizophrenia-like symptoms. There was a strong tendency to rediagnose subjects initially given a diagnosis of acute schizophrenia-like symptoms with schizophrenia (6 of 17 [35%]). Interestingly, despite the variability over time that is usually assumed for nonschizophrenic psychoses, the number of persons initially diagnosed with bipolar disorder remained essentially the same.

Living Arrangements

Twenty-one (63.6%) subjects were living with family or friends, and eight (24.2%) were living alone. Of the three (9.1%) subjects living in supervised residences, two were in half-way houses (programs for teaching household and community living skills), and the third lived in a very low demand/low expectation facility where basic survival needs are met. Only one (3.0%)

subject was in a psychiatric hospital, where he had lived for 4 years following the death of his parents who had cared for him at home for several years. Similarly, 74% of the DOSMeD sample were living with family or friends, 15.6% lived alone, 3.3% were living in supervised housing, and 7% were in the hospital at the time of follow-up. A larger percentage of the Rochester sample lived alone because of the cultural expectation that young adults move away from their families, a feat attributable to the availability of subsidized (or otherwise affordable) housing for persons with disabilities.

In the 2 years prior to assessment, the subjects' living situations had been continuously in place. Four (12.1%) subjects were in sheltered settings throughout, and only three (9.1%) subjects spent fewer than 12 months in a hospital or other sheltered setting. In the DOSMeD total sample, 22.6% had been in a sheltered setting/hospital during the previous 2 years.

Over the entire period of 16 years, every person in the followed-up cohort spent some time in independent living, and 45.5% had lived in an independent setting (alone or with family) for more than 95% of the time. Indeed, 91% of the cohort lived in independent settings for more than 50% of the time. This was also true for 12 other centers in the total ISoS sample.

Work

In the 2-year period just prior to follow-up, 13 (40.6%) were employed, either part-time (3) or full-time (10) for most of the period. Job performance of the eight subjects continuously in full-time employment was judged to be very good. By contrast, 51% of the total DOSMeD group was employed during the 2-year period prior to interview, but the proportion employed full-time was 31.7%.

The rate of full-time employment in Rochester was comparable to centers such as Nottingham, Honolulu, Hong Kong, and Nagasaki, while other centers such as urban Chandigarh, Agra, Cali, and Moscow had considerably higher full-time employment rates. Part-time employment rates across centers range from 1.2% (urban Chandigarh) to 19.2% (Honolulu), and for "part of the period" employment, the range is 0.0% (Moscow) to 12.9% (Hong Kong). Work performance was rated good for at least 85% of all subjects who had been in their jobs for 12 months or more, at all centers except rural Chandigarh, Nagasaki, and Agra. Although the opportunity for receiving disability payments varies considerably among the centers and may account for some of the variability in employment rates, the complex pattern of full-time, part-time, and short periods of employment suggests that more complicated social and cultural factors also influence employment and employability.

Twelve (38.7%) persons in the Rochester cohort were receiving disability payments because of psychiatric illness, compared to 27.2% of the total DOSMeD sample. Five subjects were homemakers, one was a student, one was retired, and one was hospitalized. In the DOSMeD sample, 27.2% were disabled because of a psychiatric condition and 1.0% for a nonpsychiatric condition.

Social Disability

As measured by the global Disability Assessment Scale (DAS), nine (39.1%) of the cohort with available data functioned in the good to excellent range. Ten subjects were not rated. Similarly, on the Global Assessment of Functioning Scale for Disability (GAF-D), 11 (36.6%) subjects scored above 70, indicating mild to minimal disability. Three subjects (9.1%) could not be rated because of insufficient information. For the total DOSMeD alive cohort, 40.4% scored in the excellent to good range on the DAS, and 44.8% were rated above 70 on the GAF-D. For 24.2% of subjects, disability was prominent throughout the follow-up period, but for almost half, the disability was only predominant during the first third of the period. Only about 10% of the total DOSMeD sample had predominant disability throughout the period, while (similarly) upwards of half (42%) experienced the greatest amount of disability during the initial third of the period.

Violence and Suicide

Violence toward others (assault) and violence toward self (suicide attempts) were relatively infrequent. Only three (10.3%) were involved in an assault during the most recent 2 years, as was true of the DOSMeD sample (10.8%). During the entire follow-up period, six (21.4%) subjects were involved in assaults, compared to 24.2% in the DOSMeD sample. None of the assaults resulted in serious injury. Aggression directed toward objects was probably more common and more distressing to significant others, although not considered assault. For example, a family member reported that her collection of glass vases had been destroyed by her child during a time when medications were being changed. There was one suicide attempt in the Rochester sample (3.3%) in the past 2 years, and three (10.3%) in the entire follow-up period. For total DOSMeD, the figures were 4.3 and 20.3%, respectively.

Medications

During the last 2 years of follow-up, use of neuroleptics occurred in two patterns: 15 (48.4%) subjects never received neuroleptics, while another 15 received neuroleptics "most" of this period, with only one patient listed as having neuroleptics "sometimes." Three DOSMeD centers (Dublin, Nagasaki, and Prague) had a substantially lower (7.1–22.4%) portion of subjects who had never received neuroleptics during the past 2 years, while rural Chandigarh stood out as having more subjects not on neuroleptics (78.9%). Over the entire period, most of the DOSMeD centers had almost no subjects who had never been on neuroleptics, except for Honolulu, where there were 17.4% and Rochester, 12.1%. Strikingly, Rochester was midway in the percentage of those who had received neuroleptics "most" of the entire study period (39.4%), between rural Chandigarh with only 5.3% and Nagasaki with 86.0%.

Time trends of medication prescribing indicated two prevalent patterns. Most prominent was that during the first third of the follow-up period, only 18 (54.5%) of the subjects were prescribed neuroleptics. The second most frequent pattern was neuroleptic drugs prescribed throughout the follow-up period for seven (21.2%) subjects. This latter pattern was also evident in the entire DOSMeD sample, for 31.9% of the subjects.

Hospitalizations

In the last 2 years of follow-up, 26 (78.8%) of the Rochester sample spent no time in the hospital, while only four (12.1%) had lived in a hospital or supervised residence the entire time. Actually, only one (3%) was hospitalized for the entire 2-year period, and the remaining three (9.1%) lived in supervised community residences. For the total DOSMeD sample, only 5.6% spent all of the most recent 2 years in a supervised setting.

For the entire follow-up period, there were three (9.1%) persons never hospitalized and three (9.1%) who spent greater than 50% of the time in a hospital or supervised residence. More than a third (36.4%) spent less than 5% of the entire period in an institution. In the DOSMeD sample, only 4.7% spent more than 50% of the entire period in the hospital, and 24.9% were never hospitalized. Like the Rochester cohort, 36.8% of the DOSMeD sample spent less than 5% of the entire period in the hospital.

DECEASED SUBJECTS

Of the 13 subjects lost to follow-up, only one subject is thought to be deceased. Hospital records from 1989 indicate that this subject was suffering from severe, progressive kidney disease, such that imminent death was likely. Four other subjects were known to be alive at the close of the 16-year follow-up, two with evidence of psychiatric treatment during the past 6 years and two located during the last days of data collection. For the remaining six subjects, no information beyond the index admission and brief follow-up records are available. Using data from the Monroe County Case Register, Babigian and Odoroff (1969) reported that the relative risk of death at a specified age for males with schizophrenia was 1.6 that of the general population, and 1.9 in females. Thus, the lack of known deaths in this study sample appears to be a chance variation.

Rochester was unique in having no study subjects confirmed as deceased because of suicide or homicide. Kraft and Babigian (1976) found an annual suicide rate per 100,000 for schizophrenia in Monroe County to be 70, compared to 17.7 per 100,000 in the general population (adjusted for population at risk for suicide, age 15 years and older). Although much higher for persons with schizophrenia than in the general population, the suicide rate is still higher for persons with other diagnoses (e.g., 183 per 100,000 for persons with affective psychoses).

DISCUSSION

Representativeness of the Subjects Interviewed

Of the original cohort of 58 patients, 45 (77.6%) were located and contacted. This figure is close to that found in a preliminary study assessing the feasibility of long-term follow-up. Of those contacted, 33 (56.9%) subjects and/or collaterals were interviewed; another

12 (20.7%) were located and refused an interview; the remaining 13 (22.4%) could not be contacted. A comparison of those interviewed and those not interviewed indicates that demographic and diagnostic characteristics of the groups were very similar. In addition, there were very few and only minor differences between mode of onset and short-term pattern of course among the interviewed sample and the not interviewed sample, suggesting that those interviewed were reasonably representative of the original cohort. The original Rochester cohort differed from the total DOSMeD sample by having a larger proportion of patients first seen at less than age 30 and a much larger percentage of persons with schizophrenia-like symptoms.

Status of Subjects at Follow-Up

Over half (54.8%) of the 31 subjects assessed were rated as recovered on the Bleuler scale; another 16.1% had only mild symptoms. This favorable picture held true despite the fact that most subjects had experienced psychotic symptoms at some point during the follow-up period—two-thirds had either episodic or continuous symptoms throughout. Results from the GAF-S, GAF-D, and DAS assessments were, on the whole, less favorable than those from the Bleuler ratings.

Utility of Outcome Categories Used for Residence

The categories used for residence are not indicative of the functional capacity, self-sufficiency, or independence of the person. In Rochester, there are a remarkable number of choices for persons with psychiatric disabilities, and the gradations in level of independence required for various settings are considerable. For example, nursing home care requires a very low level of independence but usually also requires serious physical disability or illness. At the opposite end of the spectrum is nearly total independent living, such as supervised apartment living, with supervision consisting of staff availability by telephone and minimal direct contact. With careful planning, persons are usually placed in the sheltered community setting that most closely matches their functional capacity. However, also considered are a number of other factors such as urban/rural setting, proximity to family members, availability/need for public transportation and the like.

In our experience, persons living with family members may be at any level of symptomatology and functional capacity. It is not uncommon for psychiatric patients living with their families to be essentially recovered (except for medication), with few or no symptoms most of the time, to be employed out of the home, and to be functioning well. On the other hand, many family members provide a noninstitutional yet quite sheltered living situation for the subjects in this study. Several severely symptomatic subjects in their thirties lived with one or both parents or, if the parents were deceased, the subject was living with a sibling and his or her family. In one instance, a severely disabled subject lived at home for several years, but now resides in a psychiatric hospital since both parents are deceased. Elderly patients expressed serious concern about what would happen to their disabled adult child after their death; they did not trust institutions or institutional caregivers, and the amount of income the subject could earn (even if not totally disabled) was inadequate for obtaining decent housing.

In American culture, there are many determinants influencing accessibility to living situations, level of psychiatric symptomatology being only one. For example, one subject described living "without a home" for a few months during the cold winter season, although officially he had been placed in a halfway house. In addition, determining the "therapeutic value" of any given living situation is laden with specific cultural values and attitudes. Some families very strongly believe it is their responsibility to care for family members, while other families become intolerant, frustrated, angry, or reject a member who is symptomatic, is unable or unwilling to follow rules, or is aggressive. The values, attitudes, and beliefs of mental health system employees, who may believe that the family is too rejecting of the patient or encourages too much dependence, further complicates housing negotiations and decisions.

Utility of Categories to Describe Work

In Rochester, employment seems to mean full-time work in an unsheltered setting. Furthermore, it seems that only those who could perform well on the job and not demonstrate behavioral symptoms of psychiatric disorder were employed and worked fairly regularly.

For example, one subject with severe paranoid symptoms worked until his suspiciousness resulted in a physical fight with another employee.

Unexpected Resilience

Finally, an important finding in the Rochester cohort was the surprising degree of resilience shown by some subjects, even after several years of serious illness. The extended length of the follow-up period was essential for identifying a number of subjects as recovered, or essentially recovered, when their clinical picture 5 years into the illness trajectory suggested little chance of achieving even moderately stable community functioning. The following brief case description exemplifies this resilience and delayed recovery, coming in this instance after an early course of severe and continuous symptoms.

A male subject, now 37 years old and living alone, has been successfully managing a high-stress job in the communications industry for several years. He was first hospitalized in 1979 with psychotic symptoms, believing that he was the victim of mind control and that radio stations sent him special messages by playing certain songs. At that time, he was diagnosed with acute paranoid schizophrenia. Social stressors included dropping out of college against his parents' wishes and drug use (mainly marijuana). He was rehospitalized in 1980 with similar symptoms but diagnosed as schizoaffective. Over the next 5 years, he lived and functioned marginally, was employed only occasionally, but managed to maintain weekly contact with his mother. His family continued to pressure him to make use of his considerable intellectual ability and return to college. In 1985, at a rock concert in California, he was struck on the head during a gang fight and sustained a fractured skull, resulting in a coma for about 2 weeks. While convalescing, he had sobering discussions with his mother and vowed to turn his life around. Concurrently, his mother began to modify her long-standing career hopes for him, realizing that the most important concern was his full recovery and restoration of functioning. It was, his parents freshly understood, *his* life to lead. Soon thereafter, he began to pursue his own career goals, rather than those his parents had mapped out for him. He has been without symptoms and quite successful since that transformative experience.

This case exemplifies a pattern—seen in perhaps 12% of our cases—of a late and largely unsuspected return to good functioning, following a markedly unfavorable early illness course.

References

Babigian, H. M. (1977), The impact of community mental health centers on the utilization of services. *Arch. Gen. Psychiatry*, 34:385–394.

——Odoroff, C. L. (1969), The mortality experience of a population with psychiatric illness. *Amer. J. Psychiatry*, 126:470–480.

Kraft, D. P., & Babigian, H. M. (1976), Suicide by persons with and without psychiatric contacts. *Arch. Gen. Psychiatry*, 33:209–315.

Kramer, M. (1978), Population changes and schizophrenia, 1970–1985. In: *The Nature of Schizophrenia: New Approaches to Research and Treatment*, ed. L. C. Wynne, R. L. Cromwell, & S. Matthysse. New York: John Wiley.

Lehman, A. F., Babigian, H. M., & Reed, S. K. (1984), The epidemiology of treatment for chronic and nonchronic mental disorders. *J. Nervous & Ment. Dis.*, 172:658–666.

Liptzin, B., & Babigian, H. M. (1972), Ten years experience with a cumulative psychiatric case register. *Methods of Information in Medicine*, 11:238–242.

Miles, H. C., & Gardner, E. A. (1966), A psychiatric case register: The use of a psychiatric case register in planning community mental health services. *Arch. Gen. Psychiatry*, 14:571–580.

SECTION III.C

REDUCTION AND ASSESSMENT OF PSYCHIATRIC DISABILITY (RAPYD OR DISABILITY)

Durk Wiersma and Fokko J. Nienhuis

During the 1970s, the psychosocial consequences of psychiatric disorders like schizophrenia became a focus of systematic epidemiological research. The burden of disability on others became salient once care was transferred to community settings. With that shift in venue came growth in awareness of how such disorders could affect the social life of patients and their families. Psychiatry as a medical discipline had no simple answers. The International Pilot Study of Schizophrenia (IPSS) was aimed at assessing the prevalence of psychopathological aspects of the disorder and its diagnostic ambiguities rather than its consequences for impairment, disability, or handicap. Widely accepted concepts in the area of disability or disablement were lacking, or were only in a preliminary stage of development.

In 1976, the World Health Organization therefore initiated a Collaborative Study on the Reduction of Psychiatric Disability (RAPyD) in five European countries and one African, in order to explore the applicability, reliability, and validity of a set of instruments and procedures designed for the evaluation of functional impairments and disabilities in subjects suffering from severe psychiatric disorders (Jablensky, Schwarz, and Tomov, 1980). The study aimed at assessing psychiatric disorder in patients between 15 and 44 years of age who were living in a circumscribed catchment area and who met the criteria of a broad clinical diagnosis of schizophrenia, paranoid state, and/or other nonorganic psychosis. The first onset could be dated no more than 24 months prior to the screening. One of the instruments developed was the Disability Assessment Schedule (for a later version, see WHO-DAS, 1988), which was designed to measure disturbances in social role performance because of a diagnosable mental disorder. The instrument contains questions covering overall behavior (e.g., self-care, social withdrawal); performance in social roles like marriage, occupation, and participation in household activities; hospital ward behavior, where relevant, and an inventory of personal assets and liabilities, the first three of which were used in ISoS.

The RAPyD study included about 520 patients in seven centers who were assessed by the end of 1979 and followed up after 1 and 2 years. Regrettably, the study could not be fully implemented in some centers. Groningen, Mannheim, and Zurich have published their findings in international journals; the results of others have appeared in local and national journals. In the Dutch and German centers, the course of symptomatology did not run in synchrony with the course of disability in at least a third of the subjects, a common pattern being unfavorable social outcome with a favorable symptomatological outcome. Negative symptoms increased over time while positive symptoms stabilized. Predictions by researchers of the course of symptomatology and disability after the first assessment proved to be too optimistic.

Three centers, Groningen, The Netherlands; Mannheim, Germany; and Sofia, Bulgaria, were able to participate in ISoS. Their cohorts were traced 14 to 16 years after first assessment with relatively low rates of attrition (24, 20, and 9% lost to follow-up, respectively).

REFERENCE

Jablensky, A., Schwarz, R., & Tomov, T. (1980), WHO collaborative study on impairments and disabilities associated with schizophrenic disorders. *Acta Psychiat. Scand.*, 62(Suppl. 285):152–159.

CHAPTER 18

RAPyD: Groningen, The Netherlands

Durk Wiersma, Fokko J. Nienhuis, Cees J. Slooff, Robert Giel, and Ate de Jong

CULTURAL CONTEXT

While population growth of the Netherlands (from about 13.8 million in 1976 to over 15 million in 1990) will continue into the 21st century because of age distribution (the aging of people and the lengthening of average life expectancy which is already amongst the highest in Europe), the birthrate has been decreasing since 1963 and, in 1973, dropped below replacement level. The decrease accompanied by a high divorce rate can be regarded as an indication of a changed lifestyle in which marriage and family became less important. Since the mid-1980s, however, a growing number of marriages and a recent reduction in divorces may indicate a return to more traditional ways. The educational system is greatly accessible, and there is a very high degree of active participation by the young. Dutch is spoken and understood everywhere, although almost every region or province has a dialect or vernacular. Foreign nationals (refugees, asylum seekers, second-generation immigrants) are a small but growing (less than 5%) proportion of the Dutch population.

While the 1960s were characterized by democratization and antiauthoritarian movements, values changed starting in 1975 when economic recession refuted the idea of limitless possibilities, and society once again became more achievement oriented. People born between 1955 and 1970, who were at the beginning of their careers during the study period, are sometimes called the "lost generation" (Becker, 1992). Although the social and cultural situation in the Netherlands remained relatively favorable throughout the study period, not everyone benefited from the wealth. The number of households on long-term, minimum-level social security benefits increased nearly threefold from about 300,000 in 1980 to some 850,000 in 1989 according to a study by the Social and Cultural Planning Bureau. At the same time, rising unemployment reduced the tax base of social security from 9.9 years of labor to every year of social security benefit in 1970 to 2.9 to 1 by 1989. Unemployment was particularly high among the less educated, partly because of displacement (the more educated taking jobs usually held by the less educated). Among those 20 to 45 years old, the status of women is ambiguous: Many work (mostly part-time) outside the home but also take care of the house and the children. Increasingly women have entered the marketplace: 32% in 1976; 54% in 1990.

An increasing proportion of the population has been declared disabled. Five times the number of people received disability benefits in 1988 as in 1968. Although part of the increase could be due to sociodemographic factors and changing working conditions, new technologies, time pressure, and uncertainty about employment, much can be attributed to changes in the eligibility requirements for disability insurance, to a broadening of the concept of illness, and to increasing illness behavior (Giel, 1993). In 1970, one of every eight disabled persons was diagnosed as having a mental disorder; in 1988, one of every three. Stigma because of mental illness is still prevalent but perhaps less so than a few decades ago. Although the public is much more educated (TV and other media), general knowledge about causes and treatment of schizophrenia is limited.

In a variety of other areas, significant social change, most of which preceded the study period, can also be noted. The Dutch, formerly a religious people, have undergone substantial secularization since the mid-1960s. The number of criminal offenses more than doubled between 1975 and 1988, resulting in a growing sense of insecurity, so that in the mid-1980s, following years of relative lenience, the government began to enforce the law more strictly. Ultra right-wing racist political parties gained votes, although not at the level found in some other European countries. The consumption of alcohol rose considerably in the 1970s, but has stabilized since 1980 and has shown some decrease since 1986. Smoking became less popular as well; in 1976, about 65% of the males and 40% of the females smoked; by 1990, percentages dropped to 38 and 32%, respectively.

Cost

Most of the time, severe mental illness, such as schizophrenia, is experienced as a heavy, though difficult to quantify, burden on the family emotionally as well as with respect to its consequences for social relationships, participation in society, and occupation. Estimated direct medical costs of in- and outpatient care and medication for schizophrenia amounted to 775 million Dutch guilders in 1989, or 2% of the health care budget and about 10% of the budget for mental illness (Evers and Ament, 1995). Indirect cost (notably, production loss) has been estimated at about 70 million, not including other societal costs as non-health expenditures, legal fees, and other costs to the family. Every Dutch citizen is insured for loss of income (social benefits) and for costs of psychiatric treatment and rehabilitation (Exceptional Medical Expenses Law) including medication, out-, day-, and inpatient care and sheltered living in the community. Reimbursement for outpatient treatment is limited to a specified number of face-to-face contacts, and sometimes there is a small fee per visit. In the case of a hospital stay for more than one year, the patient receives only the money remaining after his or her social benefits pay for the treatment. The family can be compensated for the extra costs of care and support by a tax reduction.

Characteristics of the Catchment Area

The catchment area encompasses two, mainly rural, provinces, Groningen and Drenthe, with about 1 million inhabitants in an area of 5180 sq km. Most of the population is Dutch, but there is a small proportion of people from the former Dutch colonies of Indonesia and Surinam and a small proportion of guest workers from Turkey and Morocco. Part of the population belongs to Protestant and Roman Catholic religious groups. The local political system is democratic; a municipal council elected every 4 years is presided over by a mayor appointed for a 7-year term. The major city, Groningen, with 170,000 inhabitants, has many regional public and government offices and a university. Typical household composition in the catchment area is the nuclear family living in a single family dwelling or apartment. Family ties tend to be weak and intermittent, and the government is expected to assume the burden of support for disabled people. Industries include beet sugar mills, potato products, household appliance manufacturing, and chemical plants. The relative proportions of working and dependent populations continue to shift. Unemployment is rising; local industries are closing; and agriculture continues to mechanize. In general, men and women have equal employment opportunities both in the formal and in the shadow economies—for women, cleaning jobs; for men, mostly home repairs and construction.

THE MENTAL HEALTH SYSTEM

Development of Mental Health Policy

Dutch mental health care policy during the past 25 years has been a series of overlapping plans with periods of accelerated change alternating with periods of consolidation (Oldehinkel, 1997, 1998). In the early 1970s, the mental health care system could be characterized as being a wealth of organizations, entrepreneurs, and private institutions operating independently. Intra- and extramural services were not interrelated, and tasks were hardly ever specifically delegated. In general, the field was dominated by hospitals. The government, to a considerable extent, only set rules and provided funds, largely through public insurance, for a care sector that had open-ended funding. With the changing economic climate, expenditures for health care, expressed in increasing insurance fees, rose sharply.

Beginning in 1974, an active period of government planning and cost control converted health care into a more coherent system, and the key concepts of echelonization and decentralization were developed. Echelonization is a method of structuring health care according to degree of specialization and intensity of treatment so as to facilitate the substitution of less expensive kinds of care for more expensive ones. The basic echelon is directed at prevention. The first echelon consists of easily accessible services such as primary health care and district nursing. The second echelon includes specialties like mental health care. Decentralization or regionalization mandated the national government to divide the country into health care regions where local and regional authorities would have decisive power over the planning and coordination of services.

Some of the government's intentions were realized: the *Wet Ziekenhuisvoorzieningen* (Hospital Facilities Act, 1979) aimed at establishing an efficient system of hospital facilities with balanced distribution across the country (regionalization) and the *Wet Tarieven Gezondheidszorg* (Health Care Tariffs Act, 1980) aimed to regulate costs. Although expenditures for health care were cut, demand continued to grow in part because of the proportional increase in the age of the population. In 1986, government health policy shifted. *Nota 2000* (1986) concerned health itself, emphasized prevention of illness, advocated diminishing national government control, and suggested changes in financing to force insurance companies and care providers to compete for customers (patients).

In 1984, the Ministry of Welfare, Health and Culture published the *Nieuwe Nota Geestelijke Volksgezondheid (New Policy Document on Mental Health)*, which urged that mental health care be brought closer to the community, concurring with the prevailing view that inpatient care be curtailed by strengthening ambulatory mental health care and sheltered residences. In 1993, the Ministry published *Onder Anderen* (*Among Others*), which applied the idea of tailormade care to mental health: (1) keep and treat patients in the community, and (2) guarantee continuity of care through flexible responses and through integration of in-, day-, and outpatient services.

Civil rights of psychiatric patients—especially as pertains to such practices as isolating difficult patients, involuntary admission, and forced treatment—came under scrutiny in the 1960s and 1970s. In 1970, new legislation on involuntary admission (*Bijzondere Opnemingen Psychiatrische Ziekenhuizen*) was framed to replace the Insanity Act of 1884, but only became fully effective in 1994 (although its passage had changed admission and other practices long before). Patient councils were established and, beginning in 1982, patient counselors were instituted in mental hospitals. The government took steps to improve inpatient accommodations and to reduce the size of the population in a ward.

Structure of the Mental Health Services System

Mental health care in the catchment area is dominated by three mental hospitals (2000 beds) and four psychiatric units in general hospitals (175 beds) that deliver both outpatient and day care. Also, in each province there is a Regional Institute for Ambulatory Care (RIAGG) and a Regional Institute for Sheltered Accommodation (260 places); the catchment area has one addiction clinic with outpatient services. Since 1978, in- and outpatient services have become more available, and during the last 10 years, cooperation between hospitals and RIAGGs has resulted in concrete programs such as day treatment, rehabilitation, psychoeducation, intensive home care, and care coordination. Although there is no formal system for case management, such services are under development, and some have been implemented. Although some self-referral occurs, general practitioners usually refer cases to an outpatient clinic or to a RIAGG but can request inpatient admission.

With the exception of a small dip between 1982 and 1984, the annual number of admissions (including readmissions) to all psychiatric hospitals in the Netherlands has been increasing steadily from some 23,500 in 1976 to over 38,000 in 1991. On the other hand, the number of people in mental hospitals did not change much during the study period. The point prevalence decreased considerably between 1976 and 1980 mainly as a result of transfers of long-stay patients to nursing homes and to institutions for the mentally handicapped (Tholen, 1991). Increasing admission numbers combined with decreasing point prevalences implies shorter admission periods. The number of readmissions has risen more sharply than the number of admissions, and patients were also readmitted more often than formerly.

Substantial changes within psychiatric hospitals took place during the study period; wards became more open and friendly, and several innovative projects were aimed at keeping patients in the community despite being classified as needing hospital care. In 1980, the number of admissions to psychiatric units in general hospitals, a new service, approximated that to psychiatric hospitals. However, whereas the latter rose constantly, the number of admissions to psychiatric units in general hospitals decreased from 20,000 in

1980 to 17,000 in 1990. Partial hospitalization, particularly day treatment, has become increasingly popular (Wiersma, Kluiter, Nienhuis, Rüphan, & Giel, 1991, 1995). The number of entries, as well as the number of people in outpatient care at one time, has at least doubled during the past 15 years. Sheltered residences form a small but growing segment of care. Manpower (in full-time equivalents) needed to accomplish the provision of care shows a linearly increasing trend, from about 350 per 100,000 in 1980 to over 430 per 100,000 in 1989, a trend also seen in health care in general but with not as fast a rise. In 1980, 15.3% of all people employed in health care worked in the mental health care sector; in 1989, 16.9%.

PSYCHIATRIC EPIDEMIOLOGY

Oldehinkel and Giel (1995) compared first-admission rates over time for schizophrenia with those for other functional psychoses in a Dutch town of 45,000 inhabitants located in the middle of the catchment area. The mean annual rate for schizophrenia (ICD 8/9 code 295) per 100,000 for the period from 1975 to 1988 was 8.3. A broader definition of schizophrenia made no difference in the incidence rate. First admissions to intramural services showed a nonsignificant decrease for the years 1979 to 1990, an effect that seemed to disappear when all mental health services were taken into account. Diagnostic habits probably affected apparent time trends. Sytema, Micciolo, and Tansella (1996) found a 1-year prevalence of schizophrenia of 1.6 per 1000 in 1988. They followed service utilization over a 2-year period, distinguishing among inpatient, day patient, and outpatient episodes using a psychiatric case register that collected data from all kinds of mental health care facilities in the province of Drenthe (450,000 inhabitants). About three-quarters (74%) were hospitalized at least once; nearly two-thirds (63%) received outpatient care; only a minority (17%) used day patient facilities. Compared to patients in a community-based mental health system in South Verona (Italy), the Dutch schizophrenic patients used more inpatient facilities and fewer day or outpatient facilities and had fewer episodes of care.

The Groningen Center

Under the leadership of Robert Giel, the Department of Social Psychiatry at the University of Groningen soon became known for psychiatric-epidemiological research. In 1973, Giel (together with Dr. G. H. M. M. ten Horn who left the department in 1989) started a psychiatric case register that is still in use. The department has a long tradition of collaboration with the World Health Organization. Giel often acted as temporary adviser or consultant, especially in the field of transcultural psychiatry and schizophrenia, on such collaborative studies as Mental Health Services in Pilot Study Areas in Europe, Strategies for Extending Mental Health Care into Primary Care, Study on the Assessment and Reduction of Psychiatric Disability, and WHO-coordinated Multi Center Study on the Course and Outcome of Schizophrenia (ISoS). In 1982, the department was designated a WHO Collaborating Center for Training and Research in Mental Health and is currently participating in the development of the Schedules for Clinical Assessment in Neuropsychiatry (SCAN); Dr. F. J. Nienhuis represents the center on the SCAN Advisory Committee. After his retirement in 1994, Professor Giel was succeeded by Professor J. Ormel, a sociologist, psychiatric epidemiologist, and WHO consultant in multicenter studies on well-being and on psychiatric disorders in primary care.

In 1977, the department became involved in the WHO Collaborative Study on the Assessment and Reduction of Disability. In the context of this study, an incidence cohort of 83 subjects with a first lifetime episode of nonaffective functional psychosis was identified and was followed up for a period of 3 years. A 15-year follow-up of this cohort of 83 subjects forms the basis of this report. The schizophrenia research at the department is supported by a grant from the Praeventiefonds.

METHODS

Defining the ISoS Cohort

The WHO Collaborative Study on the Assessment and Reduction of Psychiatric Disability (RAPyD) was initiated in 1976 to explore the applicability, reliability, and validity of a set of instruments and procedures designed to evaluate impairments and disabilities in a population with potentially severe mental disorders (Jablensky, Schwarz, and Tomov, 1980; Canavan, Schwarz, Wiersma, Jablensky, and Biehl, 1984). The study aimed to accumulate a cohort of consecutive new patients who came from a geographically circumscribed area and who were suffering from functional psychosis of a nonaffective type. Screening criteria were: (1) age 15 to 44 years; (2) residence in Groningen or Drenthe province; (3) no evidence of organic brain disease, including epilepsy; no severe mental retardation; no severe sensory defects; and no alcohol or drug dependency; (4) presence of at least one of the following symptoms: hallucinations, delusions of the nonaffective type, bizarre or grossly inappropriate behavior, thought and speech disorder other than retardation or acceleration; and (5) recent onset of psychotic illness, that is, no more than 24 months prior to screening at the service which supplied the case. Each service extracted from its files all first admissions with a clinical diagnosis of schizophrenia (ICD 295), paranoid state (ICD 297), or other nonorganic psychosis (ICD 298.3–9) who met the criteria for residence and age. Persons with a previous history of admission or contact for other psychiatric reasons were excluded. From April 1978 to December 1979, approximately 230 patients were reported to the research team. Only one patient had not been in the hospital. A research psychiatrist did a second, on-site screening of case notes to verify that the cases selected were first episodes of nonaffective psychosis without evidence of an organic etiology. The secondary screening yielded 100 cases with a recent onset of psychotic symptoms of which 83 patients participated in the first assessment; the other 17 refused. The majority of excluded patients were chronic cases (see further Giel, Sauër, Slooff, and Wiersma, 1980; Slooff, 1984; Slooff, Giel, and Wiersma, 1982; Wiersma, Giel, de Jong, Sauër, and Slooff, 1982; Wiersma, Giel, de Jong, and Slooff, 1983, 1984, 1988; Wiersma, de Jong, Giel, and Slooff, 1983; de Jong, Giel, Slooff, and Wiersma, 1983, 1985, 1986; de Jong, Giel, ten Horn, Slooff, and Wiersma, 1983; de Jong, 1984; Giel, Wiersma, de Jong, and Slooff, 1984; de Jong, Giel, Lindeboom, Slooff, and Wiersma, 1984; Giel, de Jong, Slooff, and Wiersma, 1985; Giel, Wiersma, and de Jong, 1987; de Jong, Lubbe, and Wiersma, 1996).

The research team consisted of three psychiatrists: Drs. R. Giel, C. J. Slooff, and H. C. Sauër (who left in 1980); a sociologist/psychiatric epidemiologist, Dr. D. Wiersma (project leader); a psychologist/psychiatric epidemiologist, Dr. A. de Jong; a psychologist, Dr. F. J. Nienhuis (added to the team in 1990), and a research assistant, Mrs. E. G. Lindeboom. The three psychiatrists had all trained in the psychodynamically oriented Department of Psychiatry of the University of Groningen, and they had respectively 11, 4, and 5 years of clinical experience. The team made their own diagnostic assessment of the subjects using ICD-9 diagnostic criteria.

Case-Finding

To trace the subjects 15 years later, the team asked the Registry Offices in the cities and villages of the subjects' last known residences to check for current addresses. Of the original 83 subjects, nine had died (eight suicides), four refused contact because they did not want to be reminded of their psychotic experience, and six were untraceable because they had moved abroad, because the Registry Offices abiding by the privacy law would not release their new addresses, or because they had never registered at a new location. At the first reassessment, it emerged that one patient should not have been included, failing to meet the inclusion criteria. He was left out of further analyses and publications. In order to avoid confusion, however, we include all 83 subjects here. The follow-up cohort is 63 or 76% of the initial cohort. There are no statistically significant differences between the traced and nontraced (including all lost to follow-up) as to sex, age, and diagnosis (ICD-295 schizophrenia versus ICD-298 acute reactive psychosis). Although further details about the four respondents who refused all contact are not available, it is almost certain that they have never been chronically psychotic and that they are not currently in a mental hospital. The status of the others is completely unknown. As far as could be ascertained by telephone, through medical files, or from the 3-year assessment, adding the outcome of the 11 untraced subjects would probably not significantly change the pattern of outcome (for follow-up results, see Wiersma, Nienhuis, Giel, 1995a,b, 1996; Wiersma, Nienhuis, Slooff, Gield, and de Jong, 1997; de Jong, and Slooff, 1997; Wiersma, Nienhuis, Slooff, and Giel, 1998a,b).

Use of Study Instruments

The instruments PSE-9, SAS, and DAS were translated into Dutch and used in direct interviews. To reduce the length of the interview, the Family Interview Schedule was used in a self-report format. The Groningen Social Disabilities Schedule (Wiersma, de Jong, and Ormel, 1988; Wiersma, 1996, 1997), and two instruments for needs assessment (see Wiersma, Nienhuis, Slooff, and Giel, 1998b) were also used.

Data-Gathering Procedures

In most cases, two interviewers spent 2 to 3 hours at the respondent's location, including mental hospitals and staffed sheltered accommodation. Usually, a family or a staff member was also interviewed. For seven cases who lived outside the catchment area travel time was considerable. After written consent was obtained, the team sought additional information from mental health services on treatment and functional status during the last 10 years.

STUDY RESULTS: PATTERNS AND VARIATIONS

Baseline and Early Follow-Up

Gender and Age

At entry to the study, the cohort of 83 subjects consisted of an almost equal number of men (43) and women (40); of these, 33 men and 30 women make up the alive data cohort. Eleven subjects, mostly women, were lost to follow-up; another nine, mostly men, had died. Year of birth distribution at follow-up was similar to that at entry. The mean birth year of subjects followed up was 1953, that is, 40 years old at the time of the investigation. Age and sex distributions are quite similar to most of the other treated incidence cohorts.

Mode of Onset and Diagnosis

The distribution of mode of onset in the alive cohort is very similar to that of the total in the original study. The dead and lost-to-follow-up subjects are more frequently associated with insidious onset (>1 month)—approximately a third—compared to the alive group (21%) or the original cohort (24%), although the numbers are small.

Only 19% of the alive cohort of 63 received a baseline diagnosis of schizophrenia, using the conversions of ICD-9 to ICD-10, with half classified with hebephrenic schizophrenia. For nearly three-quarters of the alive group (73%), the baseline diagnosis in the cohort was other psychotic disorder. This distribution is quite similar to that seen both in the original study cohort and in those lost to follow-up. Although relatively rare or missing in the other two groups, acute schizophrenia-like disorder accounts for over a fifth of those who died (numbers are small). These findings differ markedly from the baseline diagnoses for the total group of treated Incidence studies (i.e., DOSMeD, Disability and Hong Kong, and Chennai [Madras] of the three invited centers). In the combined DOSMeD and Disability alive cohorts, schizophrenia accounts for over half (54%) of the total, and paranoid schizophrenia is the most prominent baseline diagnosis (at least 30%). In Hong Kong and Chennai (Madras), where initial selection criteria were different, a schizophrenia diagnosis is virtually uniform. Likewise, in the DOSMeD and Disability subsamples, schizophrenia accounts for at least half of the subjects in the dead and lost-to-follow-up groups.

The first contact "rediagnosis" for Groningen subjects looks quite different. Nearly half of the alive subjects (48%) were rediagnosed as having schizophrenia. Though most centers have higher rates of schizophrenia, the Groningen percentage is much closer to most of the centers and, indeed, much higher than the Chandigarh samples. The results of the two methods (the converted diagnosis and the first contact rediagnosis) of arriving at a diagnosis of schizophrenia according to a modern classification system (ICD-10) are so different (19 vs. 48%), that readers should be cautious in accepting either one blindly. Though other centers also show different rates of schizophrenia for the different methods, diagnostic distribution of the alive group is particularly striking in the Groningen cohort, probably reflecting the diagnostic habits of the clinicians and researchers at the time of the initial investigation (i.e., their reluctance to assign a diagnosis of schizophrenia at the time of first assessment).

Pattern of Course at Early Follow-Up

Seventeen of the 63 alive subjects (27%) had a favorable short-term (2-year) pattern of course (episodic with full remission between episodes)—very similar to the original study cohort. This compares favorably with the Disability subsample as a whole (25%), though poorly with the DOSMeD centers (47%). Both deceased subjects and those lost to follow-up for whom early course information was available (n=15) were not more likely to have had a poor early course.

ALIVE SUBJECTS

Symptomatology

Classified according to the Bleuler Severity Scale, 73% of the 63 persons in the alive cohort had recovered, 16% suffered mild or moderate symptoms, and 11% had severe symptomatology. The Groningen cohort with a higher percentage recovered appears to be (much) better off symptomatically than the other centers in the treated incidence studies although the percentage of "severe" is among the highest.

A rather different impression of current symptoms is gained from the results of the Global Assessment of Functioning Scale for Symptomatology (GAF-S). Over two-fifths of the subjects (46%) showed no significant or only mild symptoms (GAF-S scores greater than 70); but a quarter suffered from serious symptoms (GAF-S scores below 51). When mean GAF-S scores are compared, the Dutch cohort is found to be somewhat in between its counterparts in the other treated incidence cohorts—four centers much better (Chandigarh-urban, Chandigarh-rural, Moscow, Hong Kong), three centers similar (Nottingham, Prague, Chennai), and five centers much worse (Dublin, Honolulu, Nagasaki, Rochester, Sofia). The relative prominence of psychotic symptoms over time tends to conform to this latter pattern as well: 10% of the cohort subjects had prominent psychotic symptoms in all three periods which compares closely with the DOSMeD and Disability groups as a whole (9 and 12%, respectively). But for 19% of the Groningen subjects, such symptoms were never prominent, a pattern seen only in 9 and 10% of the total DOSMeD and Disability cohorts, respectively. The overall impression is that in Groningen, there are extreme cases (i.e., a very large proportion doing very well but a substantial number doing very poorly).

Course of the Illness

Fully 57% of the 63 subjects had no psychotic episode over the last 2 years of follow-up; 26% were continuously psychotic; and 16% were classified as episodic. The pattern of over half the subjects being psychosis-free while a third or fewer suffer from continuous disorder is seen in half of the treated Incidence cohorts; the contrasting cases are Dublin, Hong Kong, Mannheim, Nagasaki, Prague, Sofia, and, arguably, Honolulu. As expected, course of illness over the entire period shows a different pattern: 71% of the subjects experienced episodes of psychoses, while 22% have been continuously psychotic. Similar percentages are reported for the treated incidence sample with the exception of Dublin, Honolulu, Nagasaki, and Sofia, which report much higher percentages of continuously psychotic subjects (over 40%). For 57% of subjects, the overall trend was improvement, while for 25%, it was worsening; the latter figure is higher than most of the treated incidence cohorts but not for Nagasaki, Prague (DOSMeD), or Sofia.

Reevaluation of Baseline or First Contact Diagnosis

For all subjects, a baseline rediagnosis using DSM-III-R and ICD-10 criteria was arrived at through consensus of a diagnostic panel consisting of two psychiatrists (RG and CS) and a clinical psychologist (FN). The original assessment team had gone to great lengths to establish the first signs of the illness (particularly first psychosis) in the subjects' lives. To be able to make a diagnosis of schizophrenia according to DSM-III-R criteria, the ISoS panel used only the information related to the first 6 months from the established beginning of the illness process. The schedules (PSE-9, Past and Follow-up History Schedule, and a schedule assessing the duration of psychotic episodes and hospitalizations) used at first assessment were the main basis for diagnosis, although correspondence, files, and case notes were also used. Though complete blindness was not possible, the panel members were kept relatively blind to the outcome of individual cases.

For the alive cohort, 30 (48%) of the 63 subjects received a first-contact ICD-10 rediagnosis of schizophrenia and 24 (38%) a rediagnosis of other psychosis. Six subjects, about 10%, received a rediagnosis of bipolar disorder. The latter diagnosis occurred in many treated-incidence cohorts more frequently (even >20%). Males were more often rediagnosed as schizophrenic than females (52 vs. 43%), while the latter more frequently received the rediagnosis of other psychosis (50 vs. 27%). Diagnosis is related to mode of onset: 54% of the subjects with an acute onset received a rediagnosis of other psychosis (only 25% diagnosed with schizophrenia), while a rediagnosis of schizophrenia was given to 67 and 62% of the subjects with a subacute or insidious onset, respectively.

Living Arrangements

At the time of the follow-up assessment, most subjects were living in the community, either on their own (37%) or with their families (41%). Only 13% resided in a psychiatric hospital, while 10% lived in a supervised residence. Figures for independent living were similar in the Mannheim and Sofia cohorts as a whole, although the Groningen subjects showed a smaller tendency to be living with family and were more often living alone—probably a reflection of the cultural pattern of individualization and of the social system that ties a person's independence to income and housing. Differences are apparent in the hospital and in the supervised living arrangements of the treated incidence cohorts: Groningen, Mannheim, Honolulu, and Nagasaki provided these arrangements more than other centers. For the most part, this situation was stable for the 2 years preceding the assessment. Nearly two-thirds of the alive cohort spent all of the 2 years in an independent residence. One-third or more (33%) of the subjects spent some time in a hospital or supervised residence in the past 2 years, as was true of Honolulu, Mannheim, and Nagasaki. Males are more often found in these arrangements than females (39 vs. 27%), and on average for a longer time (15 months vs. 7 months). Over the course of the entire follow-up period, all but one female subject in the cohort lived independently in the community for some time: 84% managed to do so for over half of the period, while over half (56%) did so for more than 90% of the time.

Homelessness/Jail

None of the cohort had been homeless or vagrant or had been in jail in the preceding 2 years. Over the course of the entire follow-up period, one female and two male subjects had ever been homeless (usually for brief periods of time), and two subjects (one female and one male) had spent time in jail.

Work

Thirty percent of the subjects worked at paid jobs at some point in the past 2 years; most of them (68%) did so for at least 12 months. For those working most of the time, performance was mostly judged as good to very good. A substantially larger percentage of subjects in the other centers of the Disability and DOSMeD cohorts was employed (56%), probably a reflection of the unusually comprehensive disability benefit in the Netherlands for psychiatric disorder: Over half (54%) of the subjects received a disability pension, usually for most of the period. An additional 22% of the cohort was engaged in full-time household work with performance generally rated as good to very good. Only two female subjects were classified as students at any time in the past 2 years. None had retired.

Social Disability

With respect to overall functioning in the last month, 40% were rated poor to severe on the Disability Assessment Scale (DAS), while 52% had scores on the Global Assessment of Functioning Scale for Disability (GAF-D) lower than 51, indicating serious impairment. At the same time, 27% were rated good to excellent on the DAS and 33% scored higher than 70 on the GAF-D, indicating good functioning. The mean GAF-D in the Dutch center (56.3) is lower than in most centers reporting on treated incidence, with only Nagasaki and Rochester having a similar mean and Sofia having a much lower mean. These percentages are markedly different from the ratings of current symptomatology reviewed earlier and suggest not only that artifactual effects (different instruments) may be pertinent, but also that dimensions of recovery may vary independently. A baseline diagnosis of schizophrenia was more often associated with poorer functioning when compared to the group with other psychoses. For 30% of the alive cohort, disabilities were prominent throughout the follow-up period; for 11%, they were more prominent during the latter two-thirds of the period; while for 29%, disability was a prominent feature of only the first third. One in seven (14%) experienced no prominent disabilities at any time.

Violence

Four subjects (8%) of the 48 for whom information was available had been involved in assaults on other people in the last 2 years of follow-up. None of the assaults resulted in serious injury. Over the entire course, 12 subjects had been involved in assaults on other people. One, involving a nonfatal stabbing, resulted in the subject's being involuntarily detained in a psychiatric facility. Assault rates for the entire period are lower for the other Disability cohorts but comparable with most DOSMeD centers.

Suicide

Only one subject (2%) attempted suicide in the last 2 years of follow-up. But nearly a third (32%) of the subjects deliberately harmed themselves at some point in the entire follow-up period. For the Disability sample in Mannheim and Sofia, rates of self-harm are comparable for the entire period (26–28%). Compared to the treated Incidence cohort in Dublin (14%), the Dutch rate is higher, but lower than in Nottingham (41%).

Medication

In the past 2 years, 35 (57%) of subjects had been prescribed neuroleptics at least once, and 29 (48%) had taken them for most of the time. Twenty-six (43%) subjects had not been prescribed neuroleptics during the last 2 years of follow-up. The latter percentage is lower in the other Disability samples (22–34%) but comparable with the mean of the DOSMeD centers (38%). All subjects had been on medication at some time during the follow-up period; 26 subjects (41%) had taken neuroleptics most of the entire period. Examining time trends over the entire period reveals two patterns: For 17 subjects (27%), medication use was prominent in each third of the follow-up, while for 16 subjects (25%), the use of medication was only prominent in the first third of the follow-up period (probably reflecting initial treatment of the disorder). Figures are quite different across the treated incidence cohorts; the pattern of no prominence of medications in each of the three periods varied from 0% (Dublin, Honolulu, Rochester, Nagasaki, Chennai, Sofia) to over 30% (Chandigarh—urban and rural, Groningen), reflecting diverging attitudes and policies among centers toward prescription.

Hospitalization

Twenty-one subjects (33%) had spent some time in the hospital or supervised residence in the last 2 years of follow-up. Nearly all did so at least once during the entire follow-up period; one subject was detained on a forensic unit for 12 months. For nearly half of the subjects (46%), hospitalization was prominent in the first third of the entire period only; for 10%, it was a consistently prominent feature, a feature varying from 0% in several centers to nearly 30% in Dublin.

Gender Differences in Course and Outcome

The association of gender with course type and with symptomatology is less distinct than with disability. For example, the differences between the sexes as to the proportion of continuous or no psychosis during the last 2 years of follow-up are small. The average level of symptomatology as expressed by the GAF-S is 64 points for both sexes (i.e., mild symptoms). The average level of disability as expressed by the GAF-D is 63 for females but 50 for males. Men were assessed as much more disabled than women: 53% of the men but only 27% of women are functioning poorly (according to the DAS), and 67% of men but only 37% of women had serious impairment in social, occupational, or school functioning (according to the GAF-D). The overall time trend is much more favorable for females: 37% of the women but only 21% of men were rated as much better, and only 10% of women but 39% of men as worse or somewhat worse. The better functioning of females is also reflected in the use of neuroleptics during the past 2 years: 48% of the women did not use neuroleptic medication at all, and 45% did so most of the time, versus 38 and 50% for men, respectively.

Onset, Short-Term Course, and Rediagnosis in Relation to Long-Term Course and Outcome

Mode of onset of psychosis generally has a clear and mostly linear relationship with course, functional status, and outcome. An insidious onset of the first psychotic episode predicts a continuous course of psychosis over the most recent 2 years of follow-up among 53% of the subjects, a high level of symptomatology and disability (nearly all were rated less than 70; average about 40 GAF), and a relatively worse overall time trend (for 38% of the subjects). This pattern is the reverse for subjects with an acute onset (<1 week): generally good functioning (GAF above 65) and a favorable overall time trend. Subjects with a subacute onset occupy the middle. Medication also reflects these findings: 91% of the subjects with an insidious onset used neuroleptics most of the time during the past 2 years, while 61% with an acute onset did not use any medication at all.

A short-term pattern of continuous psychosis over the first 2 years predicts for 69% of the subjects the same pattern 13 years later. Nevertheless, one-third of the subjects with a short-term pattern of complete remission had been psychotic in the last 2 years. Generally, a rather linear relationship exists between the short-term pattern of an early course and functional status at long-term follow-up. The subjects with continuous psychosis during the first years did not fare well; almost all suffered from serious psychological and social impairments (average GAF was 43). The fully remitted subjects functioned relatively well (GAF-S 77, GAF-D 67), and the subjects with incomplete remission were in the middle (GAF-S 65, GAF-D 57).

A first contact rediagnosis of schizophrenia was common among those with short-term pattern of continuous psychosis (69% of subjects); but was much less common among those with a diagnosis of bipolar depression or other psychosis (15%). This diagnostic classification is also predictive of the long-term pattern: 45 and 17% of the subjects with schizophrenia were continuously or episodically psychotic, respectively, over the past 2 years. Differences between schizophrenia and other psychosis are apparent in functional status and course: Subjects with an early diagnosis of schizophrenia did worse than those with other psychosis: 70 vs. 42% had a GAF-S below 70 (average of 53 vs. 72), and 73 vs. 62% had a GAF-D below 70 (average of 49 vs. 63). Half of the schizophrenic subjects were rated as better on overall time trend while this was the case for 67% of those with other psychosis. Assaults (4) and suicide attempts (1) were found only among subjects with a diagnosis of schizophrenia.

DECEASED SUBJECTS

At follow-up (15 years after study entry), nine subjects were deceased. Comparison to the general population of the Netherlands shows increased death rates (SMR=8.88; for females 5.27 and for males 11.04) which are statistically significant at the 5% level. Six men and two women had committed suicide: Four were in episode; four were not; and for two, illness status is unknown. One subject died in a car accident, but it is uncertain whether it was intentional.

DISCUSSION

The description of the 15-year course of schizophrenic disorders, broadly defined by the diagnostic categories of ICD-9 (ICD 295, 297, and 298.3–9) and included in the cohort at the onset of the illness, yields a variety of patterns of course and outcome—from complete remission in 27% of the 83 subjects, to chronic psychosis (11%) or a negative syndrome after one or more episodes in 43% (Wiersma et al., 1998a). Suicide occurred in 10% of all cases. This study has demonstrated the high risk of relapse, suicide, and chronicity in this cohort.

As for representativeness, one might speculate about the sampling procedure and the inclusion criteria. All the relevant in- and outpatient psychiatric facilities in the catchment area during 21 months were screened, and all first and recent onset cases were registered. No leakage study was conducted as in the DOSMeD study, and it is possible that a small number of new cases who came solely to the attention of private practitioners, general practitioners, social workers, or the police, could have been missed; however, the total number missed is likely to be very small partly because of the organization of the Dutch system of mental health care. One could argue that the inclusion criteria were too broad, encompassing disorders too different from the narrow DSM-III-R definition of schizophrenia; half of the cohort received an initial diagnosis of other psychosis at first assessment. An examination of the possible differences in symptomatology, onset, and precipitating and predisposing factors in subjects with a diagnosis of schizophrenia (295) and with other psychosis (298) found hardly any discrepancies. The descriptions in ICD-9 were broad and not mutually exclusive which sometimes made the choice of a 295 or a 298 classification somewhat arbitrary. In those days, there was a reluctance to make the diagnosis of schizophrenia. In a reclassification exercise, all subjects were reexamined according to DSM-III-R and ICD-10 criteria using case material available at first contact. A much higher proportion was diagnosed as schizophrenic at first onset: Nearly half (48%) of those alive at follow-up received a diagnosis of schizophrenia; and 38% a diagnosis of other psychosis. This is somewhere at variance with the diagnostic distributions in the other centers.

SUMMARY

In the original cohort of 83 subjects assembled during 1978 and 1979 in the northern area of the Netherlands, men and women were equally represented, with an average age at study intake of 25 years. Fifteen years later, the follow-up effort relocated 76% of the original subjects; the alive cohort of 63 showed no apparent bias with respect to gender, age, mode of onset, baseline diagnosis, or short-term pattern of course. There were nine deaths, eight of which were attributed to suicide.

Nearly three-quarters of the alive subjects were judged to have recovered, although half still showed evidence of symptomatology and about a quarter had suffered continuously from psychotic symptoms during the last 2 years of follow-up. At least half of the subjects also showed evidence of substantial impairment in social and occupational functioning, while between a quarter and a third were rated as good or excellent in their social functioning. Those whose baseline diagnosis was reevaluated as schizophrenia were more impaired socially and symptomatically. Over 40% of the subjects were currently prescribed neuroleptic medication. The vast majority of subjects were living independently, though in a few cases the term masks the significant informal support received from family; 13% were on a long-stay ward; and 10% lived in some sort of sheltered accommodation outside the hospital. Only 30% had been employed during the past 2 years, but another 22% were engaged in full-time household work. Overall, the course of illness was rated as improving in nearly 60% of the alive subjects. Gender does not seem to have a significant effect on course or symptomatology, but women generally do better than men with respect to the level of disability: Men are much more disabled.

References

Becker, H. A. (1992), *Generations and Their Chances*. Amsterdam: Meulenhof. (In Dutch)

Canavan, K., Schwarz, R., Wiersma, D., Jablensky, A., & Biehl, H. (1984), Assessment and reduction of psychiatric disability. A selective review of legislation in seven countries participating in a WHO study. *Internat. Dig. Health Legislation*, 35(3):507–549.

Evers, S. M. A. A., & Ament, A. J. H. A. (1995), Costs of schizophrenia in the Netherlands. *Schizophr. Bull.*, 21(1):141–153.

Giel, R. (1993), The growing psychiatric morbidity. *Ned. T. Geneeskunde*, 137(27):1332–1333. (In Dutch)

——Jong, A. de, Slooff, C. J., & Wiersma, D. (1985), Social disability and chronic mental disorder. In: *The Long-Term Treatment of Functional Psychoses*, ed. T. Helgason. Cambridge, U.K.: Cambridge University Press, pp. 207–216.

——Sauër, H. C., Slooff, C. J., & Wiersma, D. (1980), On the epidemiology of functional psychoses and disability. *T. Psychiatrie*, 22:710–772. (In Dutch)

——Wiersma, D., & Jong, A. de (1987), The issue of social class and schizophrenia in the Netherlands. In: *From Social Class to Social Stress*, ed. M. C. Angermeyer. Berlin: Springer Verlag, pp. 66–81.

——,——,——Slooff, C. J. (1984), Prognosis and outcome in a cohort of patients with non-affective, functional psychosis. *Eur. Arch. Psychiatry & Neurol. Sci.*, 234:97–101.

Jablensky, A., Schwarz, R., & Tomov, T. (1980), WHO collaborative study on impairments and disabilities associated with schizophrenic disorders. *Acta Psychiatr. Scand.*, 62(Suppl. 285): 152–159.

Jong, A. de (1984), *On Psychiatric Disablement*. Thesis, University of Groningen, The Netherlands. (In Dutch)

——Giel, R., Horn, G. H. M. ten, Slooff, C. J., & Wiersma, D. (1983), Aftercare with functional psychoses: Developments in the collaboration among mental health services *T. Psychiatrie*, 25:422–439. (In Dutch)

——,——Lindeboom, E. G., Slooff, C. J., & Wiersma, D. (1984). Fould's hierarchical model of psychiatric illness in a Dutch cohort. *Psychol. Med.*, 14:647–654.

——Giel, R., Slooff, C. J., & Wiersma, D. (1983), Social disabilities as a consequence of functional psychoses. I. Design of a model for the development of social disabilities. *T. v. Soc. Gezondheidszorg*, 60:78–85. (In Dutch)

——,——,——,——(1985), Social disability and outcome in schizophrenic patients. *Brit. J. Psychiatry*, 147:621–636.

——,——,——,——(1986), Relationship between symptomatology and social disability. Empirical evidence from a follow-up study of schizophrenic patients. *Soc. Psychiatry*, 21:200–205.

——Lubbe, P. M. van der, & Wiersma, D. (1996), Social dysfunctioning in rehabilitation: Classification and assessment. In: *Handbook of Mental Health Economics and Health Policy*, Vol. 1, ed. M. Moscarelli, A. Rupp, & N. Sartorius. New York: Wiley, pp. 27–38.

Ministerie van Volksgezondheid's Gravenhage (1984), *New Policy Document on Mental Health*. The Hague: Ministerie van Volksgezondheid. (In Dutch)

Nota 2000 (1986), *On the Development of Health Policy: Facts, Reflections and Policy Intentions*. The Hague: Ministry of Welfare, Health and Culture. (In Dutch)

Oldehinkel, A. J. (1997), *Trends and Transitions in 15 Years of Psychiatric Care Utilization*. Thesis, University of Groningen, the Netherlands.

——(1998), Time trends in mental health care utilization in a Dutch area 1976–1990. *Soc. Psychiatry & Psychiatric Epidemiol.*, 33(4):181–185.

——Giel, R. (1995), Time trends in the care-based incidence of schizophrenia. *Brit. J. Psychiatry*, 167:777–782.

Slooff, C. J. (1984), *The Classification and the Course of Schizophrenic and Reactive Psychoses*. Thesis, University of Groningen, the Netherlands. (In Dutch)

——Giel, R., Wiersma, D. (1982), The classification of functional non-affective psychoses. *T. Psychiatrie*, 24: 454–469. (In Dutch)

Sytema, S., Micciolo, R., & Tansella, M. (1996), Service utilization by schizophrenic patients in Groningen and South-Verona: An event-history analysis. *Psycholog. Med.*, 26:109–119.

Tholen, A. J. (1991), *Residents or Patients? A Description of the Consequences of Chronic Psychiatric Disorders among Residents of Long-Stay Departments and Sheltered Accommodations.* Thesis, University of Groningen, the Netherlands. (In Dutch)

Wiersma, D. (1996), Measuring social disabilities in mental health. *Soc. Psychiatry & Psychiatric Epidemiol.*, 31: 101–108.

——(1997), Role functioning as a component of quality of life in mental disorders. In: *Quality of Life in Mental Disorders*, ed. H. Katschnig, H. Freeman, & N. Sartorius. New York: Wiley, pp. 43–54.

——Giel, R., Jong, A. de, Sauër, H. C., & Slooff, C. J. (1982), The social profile and the course of functional psychoses: A cohort study. *T. Psychiatrie*, 24:183–200. (In Dutch)

——,——,——Slooff, C. J. (1983), Social class and schizophrenia in a Dutch cohort. *Psychol. Med.*, 13:141–150.

——,——,——,——(1984), Chronicity of functional psychoses. *T. Psychiatrie*, 26:402–419. (In Dutch)

——(1988), Schizophrenia: Results of a cohort study with respect to cost-accounting problems of patterns of mental health care in relation to course of illness. In: *Costs and Effects of Managing Chronic Psychotic Patients*, ed. D. Schwefel, H. Zöllner, & P. Potthoff. Berlin: Springer Verlag, pp. 115–125.

——Jong, A. de, Geil, R., & Slooff, C. J. (1983), Social disabilities as a consequence of functional psychoses. II. Some results concerning the model for the development of functional psychoses. *Soc. Gezondheidszorg*, 60:168–174. (In Dutch)

——,——Kraaijkamp, H. J. M., & Ormel, J. (1990), *GSDS-II: The Groningen Social Disabilities Schedule*, 2nd ver. Rijksuniversiteit, Groningen: Department of Social Psychology.

——,——Ormel, J. (1988), The Groningen social disabilities schedule: Development, relationship with the ICIDH and psychometric properties. *Internat. J. Rehab. Res.*, 11(3):213–224.

——Kluiter, H., Nienhuis, F. J., Rüphan, M., & Giel, R. (1991), Costs and benefits of day treatment with community care as an alternative to standard hospitalization for schizophrenic patients: A randomized controlled trial in the Netherlands. *Schizophr. Bull.*, 17(3): 411–419.

——,——,——,——,——(1995), Costs and benefits of hospital and day treatment with community care of affective and schizophrenic disorders. A randomized trial with a follow-up of two years. *Brit. J. Psychiatry*, 166(Suppl. 27):52–59.

——Nienhuis, F. J., Giel, R., Jong, A. de, & Slooff, C. J. (1995a), Schizophrenia and related psychotic disorders. The 15-year course of an incidence cohort. *T. Psychiatrie*, 9:728–739. (In Dutch)

——,——,——,——,——(1995b), The assessment of need for care among persons with schizophrenia or related psychotic disorder 15 years after onset of psychosis. *T. Psychiatrie*, 10:780–789. (In Dutch)

——,——,——,——,——(1996), Assessment of the need for care 15 years after onset of a Dutch cohort of schizophrenic patients and an international comparison. *Soc. Psychiatry & Psychiatric Epidemiol.*, 31:114–121.

——,——Slooff, C. J., & Geil, R. (1998a), Natural course of schizophrenic disorders. A 15-year follow-up of a Dutch incidence cohort. *Schizophr. Bull.*, 24(1):75–85.

——,——,——,——(1998b), Stability and change in need status of patients with schizophrenic disorders over two years and a comparison between "objective" and "subjective" assessment of need for care. *Soc. Psychiatry & Psychiatric Epidemiol.*, 33:49–56.

——,——,——,——Jong, A. de (1997), Assessment of need for care among patients with schizophrenic disorders 15 and 17 years after first onset of psychosis. In: *Making Mental Health Services Rational*, ed. M. Tansella. Rome: Il Pensiero Scientifico.

Chapter 19

RAPyD: Mannheim, Germany

Wolfram an der Heiden, Bertram Krumm, Sabine Müller, Marianne Schäfer, Bettina Schwerd, and Iris Weber

CULTURAL CONTEXT

The Mannheim Field Research Center is located in the province of Baden-Württemberg in the mid-Western part of Germany. The catchment area of the study comprises Mannheim, an industrial city at the confluence of the Rhine and Neckar Rivers, the city of Heidelberg, a tourism center some 20 km from Mannheim, and the Rhine-Neckar district with a total population of about 935,000 inhabitants. Located in Mannheim are the most important industrial harbor of the province and an important railroad junction on the north/south route. The region is characterized by a massive conglomeration of industries—metal working, engine building, ship building, chemical and oil refining—as well as scattered agricultural areas cultivating mainly tobacco, hops, fruit, and vegetables. Both Mannheim and Heidelberg have high-profile universities: Heidelberg University has a long scientific tradition, having a reputation mostly in social science, medicine, and arts; the newer Mannheim University gained its reputation after World War II, especially in economics.

Since the mid-1950s, both the demand for labor by German industries and growing differences in socioeconomic development within Europe have encouraged immigration to Germany. In Western Germany, the number of "guest workers" rose from 79,600 in 1955 to 2,595,000 in 1973. A 1973 law stopped the immigration, and by 1980, the number dropped to 2,070,000 (Korte and Schmidt, 1983). The total number of foreign residents, however, increased during the period from 3,966,200 in 1973 to 4,453,300 in 1980, mainly because of the immigration of family members of resident workers, a higher birth rate, and an increasing number of political immigrants. In Mannheim, the percentage of foreign residents among the total population rose steadily from 5.0% in 1967 to 13.9% in 1980 (Weyerer and Häfner, 1992).

German unification in 1990 opened the (West) German job market to people—mostly skilled workers from the former German Democratic Republic (GDR)—thus increasing competition. At the same time, refugees by the thousands from former Eastern-bloc countries and from the war-torn former Yugoslavia fled into the catchment area. Because of the current economic crisis, big companies have cut back severely on the number of workers they employ.

The Mental Health System in The Area[1]

Mental health care in Germany in the 1950s and early 1960s was characterized by a sharp demarcation between inpatient and outpatient care. In November, 1958, there were more than 130 mental hospitals with some 99,000 beds providing mental health care in the Federal Republic of Germany (FRG) (Statistisches Bundesamt, 1960). Of all psychiatric beds, 97% were in mostly large, remote public hospitals, four of them with more than 4000 beds. Although the average length of stay was 215 days, 26% of patients stayed for more than 10 years. Outpatient psychiatric care rested almost completely with psychiatrists and psychotherapists in private practice who saw a few patients with severe mental disorders. Complementary services, such as day hospitals, supervised residences, and sheltered workshops, were almost completely lacking.

In 1965, the FRG Minister of Health convened a commission of experts to analyze the state of mental health care. In 1975, the Commission presented its

1. Drawn from Häfner and an der Heiden, 1996.

report, formulating five principles for reforming mental health care (Deutscher Bundestag, 1975):

1. For every person in need of psychiatric care, the best possible treatment in terms of effectiveness and cost must be available without undue financial and geographical barriers.
2. Physically and mentally ill individuals must be granted equal status from a legal, social, and financial point of view.
3. Psychiatric care must be integrated into the system of general health care as far as possible.
4. Inpatient psychiatric care must be organized in the form of community-based services. The intention should be to remove mentally ill persons from contact with family, society, and workplace for no longer than is necessary and to make their rehabilitation easier.
5. For socially disabled chronically ill individuals, a network of complementary services should be developed.

Subsequently, much progress was made in realizing these recommendations, both in the provision of mental health care and in enabling legislation. At the same time, the social system in Germany, which guarantees full payment for all forms of treatment and social care for anyone, favored the development of community mental health services.

In 1969, the University of Heidelberg opened a second medical school in Mannheim, and the large municipal hospital (with no psychiatry department of its own) became a teaching hospital. During this period, Mannheim had no psychiatric hospital, and those in need of psychiatric treatment were referred to a large public hospital in Wiesloch, 50km from Mannheim. Between 1973 and 1974, the clinical department of the Clinic for Social Psychiatry in Heidelberg was moved to the general hospital in Mannheim. In spring 1975, before the recommendations of the Expert Commission for Psychiatry were published, the Central Institute for Mental Health (CIMH) was founded as a teaching and research institution and as a provider of mental health care for the inhabitants of Mannheim. It found in the City of Mannheim a partner for the development of a model comprehensive community psychiatric service.

In 1975, Mannheim had one home for 19 psychiatric patients. Outpatient care was provided by psychiatrists in private practice, by a small outpatient unit at the University Department of Social Psychiatry in Heidelberg, and by general practitioners. A few social services for mentally disabled persons—for example, a sheltered workshop and facilities for mentally retarded individuals—were provided by the city or by voluntary welfare organizations. In 1982, the psychiatric day clinic with 20 places moved from Heidelberg to Mannheim.

In 1989, a social psychiatric service (which also functions as a social service agency in particular for socially disabled, chronic psychiatric patients) was implemented. By 1993, there were five sheltered homes with a total of 151 places, mainly those for chronic psychiatric illnesses. These services were supplemented by a total of 65 places in nine sheltered group homes. The complementary mental health care sector (mid-1990s) includes an additional two sheltered workshops founded in 1983, each with 60 places. The Mannheim Project for Occupational Reintegration and Rehabilitation (*Mannheimer Starthilfeprojekt*) improves occupational and social abilities under controlled conditions. Fifty companies participate in a 3-month program that prepares former patients for reintegration into the workplace (Dombrawe, 1986; Waschkowski, 1990).

As a result of the implementation of new services, especially in the outpatient and complementary sector, annual census figures for 1973 to 1980 show that the number of Mannheim inhabitants with a diagnosis of schizophrenia in psychiatric hospitals decreased steadily from 155 to 110, whereas the number of patients of the same diagnostic group in psychiatric homes nearly doubled to 100 (Häfner and an der Heiden, 1984). Of those schizophrenic patients commencing a stay of at least one year in 1980, as many as three-quarters were admitted to homes and group homes, and only one-quarter was admitted to mental hospitals (Häfner and an der Heiden, 1983). Clearly, the main burden of care for schizophrenic patients has shifted from mental hospitals to the community and to sheltered homes.

The CIMH has taken on the task of evaluating the effectiveness and efficiency of psychiatric services at different levels of care in the community mental health system in Mannheim (Häfner and Klug, 1980, 1982; Häfner and an der Heiden, 1991). In the 1970s, the evaluation was carried out using a cumulative psychiatric case register located at the Institute. Started in 1973, the register covered all contacts by Mannheim inhabitants with more than 30 mental health services in the catchment area. Although strict regulations for data protection were always observed by the Cumulative Psychiatric Case Register, the Commissioner for

Data Protection of the Bundesland of Baden Würtemberg raised legal objections, and in 1981, it was closed (Häfner and Pfeifer-Kurda, 1986).

PSYCHIATRIC EPIDEMIOLOGY

The administrative incidence of mental illness in the population of Mannheim was first investigated by Häfner, Reimann, Immich, and Martini (1969) for the year 1965. Admissions to psychiatric and nonpsychiatric hospitals, other psychiatric contacts, and all forms of welfare, such as old people's and children's homes, child guidance services, and family and marriage counseling services, were included. The 1-year incidence rate for all mental disorders in 1965 was 10.74 per 1000 population. The incidence rate for schizophrenia was 0.54 per 1000; the rate for cyclothymia and endogenous depression was 0.81 per 1000. With regard to neuroses, different forms of reaction to life events, and personality disorders, an incidence rate of 3.65 per 1000 inhabitants was found. Incidence rates for alcoholism and other forms of addiction (0.84/1000) were more concentrated in the inner city. The administrative incidence of mental disorders in the Mannheim population over 60 years was 11.17 per 1000 in 1965 (Reimann and Häfner, 1972). First contacts with all respective treatment, care, and counseling services (not including contacts with general practitioners) were included in the survey. Among all diagnoses, degenerative processes of the brain amounted to 54%, affective psychoses to 15%, acute and chronic brain syndromes to 12%, neurotic disorders to 7%, alcoholism and addiction to 6%, schizophrenia to 4%, and other nonclassified mental disorders to 2%. Older men suffer more often from brain syndromes and alcoholism compared to older women who show a higher incidence of affective psychoses and neuroses.

THE CENTER

The Central Institute of Mental Health is located in an inner city district of Mannheim. It consists of three clinical departments with a total of 202 beds: a psychiatry department (106 beds), a department for psychosomatic medicine (48 beds), and a child and adolescent department (48 beds). The psychiatry department includes an intensive care unit with 10 beds, a day clinic with 20 places, and a geriatric day clinic with 12 places. Comprehensive outpatient services are integrated into the Institute's three clinical departments, while a consulting service has been established in the city's largest general hospital. The outpatient services established a psychiatric emergency service that is staffed after normal working hours by duty physicians from the three clinical departments. Thus, crisis intervention and psychiatric emergency service are guaranteed around the clock. In addition, there are several independent departments, central facilities, and working groups, including biostatistics, clinical psychology, neuroradiology, and molecular biology. Moreover, the Institute offers postgraduate training for physicians in psychiatry, child and adolescent psychiatry, psychotherapy, and psychoanalysis, as well as for psychologists in clinical psychology. In 1980, the World Health Organization recognized the Central Institute of Mental Health as a WHO Collaborating Center for Training and Research in Mental Health.

As an independent public foundation, the Central Institute of Mental Health is supervised by an administrative board. A close connection is maintained with the University of Heidelberg; both the Rector of the University and the Dean of its Faculty for Clinical Medicine in Mannheim are members of the administrative board. Scientific counseling and control are exercised by an International Advisory board, in accord with the proposal of the Scientific Council of the FRG and the requirements for WHO Collaborating Centers. The professors at the Institute (i.e., medical directors and section leaders) are nominated by the Mannheim Faculty for Clinical Medicine in accordance with the Institute's Board of Directors, with Heidelberg University and with the Ministry of Science and Art for Baden-Würtemberg. Currently, expenses are borne by the Bundesland of Baden-Württemberg.

Methods Used in the Site

The starting point of our longitudinal follow-up study is the prospective "WHO Study on the Assessment and Reduction of Psychiatric Disability" (Jablensky, Schwarz, and Tomov, 1980), which started in 1978 in seven different centers in Europe and Africa. The Mannheim cohort was selected according to the following study criteria:

- Presence of Schneiderian first-rank symptoms (hallucinations and/or delusions of nonaffective type, and/or thought and speech disorder other

than retardation or acceleration). Note that this requirement resulted in a cohort with one of the highest percentages of ICD-10 schizophrenia diagnoses among the ISoS centers;
- Onset of illness not earlier than one year prior to index admission;
- Residence in Mannheim, Heidelberg, or the Rhine-Neckar district, and knowledge of German;
- Treatment as an in- or outpatient at one of the catchment area psychiatric hospitals;
- Age between 15 and 44 years; and
- Absence of gross organic brain disorder, severe mental and sensory disability, and drug and alcohol addiction.

Selection of the original study cohort ended with the enrollment of the 70th patient who met the criteria. Subjects were followed up for 2 years with five cross-sectional assessments at 6-month intervals (CS1-CS5). In Mannheim, they received an additional two assessments at 3 years (CS6) and at 5 years (CS7) after index-admission. Results of the first 5 years are detailed elsewhere (Schubart, Schwarz, Krumm, and Biehl, 1986; Biehl, Maurer, Schubart, Krumm, and Jung, 1986; Biehl, Maurer, Jung, Krüger, and Bauer-Schubart, 1988). Thus, at the beginning of the long-term follow-up (ISoS), data from seven cross-sectional assessments over a period of 5 years were available.

In early 1989, a 14-year follow-up of the Disability cohort was designed. To be eligible for funds from the Federal Minister of Research and Technology, preparations had to be completed by mid-1989, precisely the time when WHO was making initial preparations for the ISoS study. This tight schedule has had two major consequences: The study instruments used in Mannheim are not fully compatible with those of ISoS; and the Mannheim design differs from that used in the other ISoS Field Research Centers in that, in addition to the cross-sectional assessment at 14 years (CS8) after index admission, Mannheim subjects had assessments at 9 (CS9) and at 18 months (CS10). Also, during the prospective 18-month study, there were monthly telephone contacts with the subjects. This extended period should serve as a basis for a more valid determination of the outcome of schizophrenia.

For the sake of standardization, the study results in Mannheim are arranged so as to be, so far as possible, comparable with the presentations of the findings of the other Field Research Centers. In addition, we also present results that mirror the different set of instruments as well as the extended period of observation after the 14-year follow-up.

Defining The ISoS Cohort and Case-Finding

At the 5-year follow-up, 63 patients were still participating in the study. Three had died, four had left. All 67 living subjects had at the beginning of the study consented to allow their names and postal addresses to be retained for the purpose of reestablishing contact in the future. For the 14-year follow-up, a review of the most current postal addresses in the archives of the Central Institute yielded 14 cases. Next, the use of telephone books and city directories located another 10 persons. Letters to the remaining old postal addresses in hopes that former patients might have left forwarding addresses yielded 10 more subject locations. Next, contact with parents, relatives, or significant others was established mostly with the help of a colleague, H. Biehl, who had been involved in the first 5 study years and who knew all the subjects personally; this located 19 more. By reconstructing movement history through the residents' registration offices of different cities (eight subjects), by contacts with social psychiatric services and rehabilitation centers, and by research into the archives of other psychiatric hospitals in the area (five subjects), we clarified the fates of 13 further persons. In the end, we had valid postal addresses for 62 subjects, had information that four subjects had passed away, and knew that one person had moved abroad, address unknown. The temporal expenditure for the determination of postal addresses, approximately 140 hours, does not include travel time to different institutions. Actually establishing contact proved to be even more time-consuming; telephone calls and visits in preparation for the first contacts for the 14-year follow-up amounted to approximately 200 hours.

To summarize: Of the 70 subjects who originally participated in 1978, 56 persons agreed to participate in the long-term follow-up. Seven patients had died since the beginning of the study, six by committing suicide (of which two cases seem very probable although final evidence is lacking). Six subjects refused to participate; another one had left the catchment area and could not be traced. The following study results are based on the assessment of the 56 persons who were available at the 14-year follow-up (Häfner and an der Heiden, 1996).

According to their relatives or significant others, two of the six refusers are still symptomatic today, and three are still in outpatient treatment. Two of these subjects hold regular jobs; one has a part-time job, another indicates homemaker as an occupation. Two are married and have children; in one case an intimate partnership is presumed. None of the refusers lives in a sheltered setting, although three live with their families of origin and would be endangered socially without the help of their relatives.

Study Instruments

On November 26, 1991, approximately 9 years after the 5-year cross-sectional assessment (CS7), data collection for the 14-year follow-up began with an eighth cross-sectional assessment. At 9-month intervals (14.75 and 15.5 years after index admission), two more assessments (CS9 and CS10) were carried out. In addition to cross-sectional data collection, information on the psychopathological status, treatment, and other relevant areas was collected from year 14 (CS8) on by means of monthly telephone contacts. Whenever the telephone interview revealed signs of a relapse, the subjects were visited for further data collection.

For psychopathological signs and symptoms, the Present State Examination (PSE) by Wing, Cooper, and Sartorius (1974), plus the Brief Psychiatric Rating Schedule (BPRS) in its extended version by Lukoff, Liberman, and Neuchterlein (1986) were used. Both instruments were applied at the three main cross-sections CS8, CS9, and CS10; the BPRS was used as well in cases of relapse between scheduled interviews.

The Disability Assessment Schedule (DAS) in the German translation (DAS-M) by Jung, Krumm, Biehl, Maurer, and Bauer-Schubart (1989) was used at the three main assessment dates to assess social adaptation with respect to both general behavior and behavior in specific role areas.

The Scale for the Assessment of Negative Symptoms (SANS) by Andreasen (1989) and the Psychological Impairments Rating Schedule (PIRS) (Biehl, Maurer, Jablensky, Cooper, and Tomov, 1989) were used for recording negative symptoms and psychological impairments. Both instruments were applied at the three main cross-sections in the long-term follow-up and in addition, at contacts between the cross-sectional assessments.

The Interview for Retrospective Assessment of the Course of Schizophrenia (IRAOS-C), an adaptation of the instruments developed by Häfner and coworkers (Häfner, Riecher, Maurer et al., 1990; Häfner, Riecher-Rössler, Hambrecht et al., 1992) for the recording of characteristics and changes in both biography and illness-relevant areas was used once at year 14 (CS8). This questionnaire also recorded inpatient and outpatient supplementary treatment.

A treatment form captured detailed information on treatment, medication intake, and therapeutic and rehabilitative measures, in the data collection phase between the years 14 and 15.5 (CS8 and CS10). Besides this, an extension to the data collected through IRAOS-C, further changes with respect to housing, life, and work were recorded. This form was used at all personal and phone contacts after the 14-year follow-up.

The Scale for Telephone Assessment of Prodromal Symptoms was also implemented at all contacts in the 14-year follow-up. With reference to Pietzker et al. (1986), the prodromal symptoms—symptoms which had historically occurred before prior exacerbations—that were typical of each subject were recorded at 14 years (CS8) with the help of relatives, and their individual manifestations were noted. Subsequently, these prodromal lists set up for each individual served as checklists for the telephone interviews. In addition, the presence of Schneiderian first-rank symptoms was recorded.

STUDY RESULTS

Baseline and Early Follow-up

Gender and Age

At entry to the study, the number of the male patients (41=59%) was markedly higher than the number of females (29=41%). At the 14-year follow-up, the gender distribution was almost the same: The sample now consisted of 34 men (61%) and 22 women (39%). Today, the women are on average 41.7 years old in contrast to 38.9 years for the men. Birth year distribution at follow-up was similar to that at entry.

Diagnosis and Mode of Onset

Of the total 70 patients fulfilling the criteria for inclusion into the study, 66 patients were diagnosed with schizophrenia by their treating psychiatrists according to the discharge letter after the first hospital treatment (Schwarz, Biehl, Krumm, and Schubart, 1980); two had a diagnosis of acute paranoid reaction, and another two of neuroses. Two subjects, formerly diagnosed as neurosis and acute paranoid reaction, were identified as schizophrenic during a second hospitalization. After using the conversion tables (WHO, 1994) to convert ICD-9 diagnoses to ICD-10 diagnoses, about two-thirds (68.6%) of the original cohort was diagnosed with paranoid schizophrenia; about 14% were hebephrenic, catatonic, or other schizophrenia; 10% were schizoaffective or acute schizophrenia-like; and 7% other psychotic or nonpsychotic. The diagnostic distribution is almost identical when restricting the observation to those 56 subjects participating in the 14-year follow-up. Again, 79% received a diagnosis of schizophrenia.

There are also no differences with respect to the mode of onset between the original and the long-term cohort: There are some 37% (alive group) with insidious onset (>1 month), more than half (54%) with a mode of onset between 1 week and 1 month, and about 9% with acute onset (up to 1 week).

Pattern of Course at Early Follow-up

Almost three-quarters of the 56 subjects had incomplete remission at the end of the first 2 years, while 21% had a course characterized by complete remission. Three subjects were continuously psychotic during the 2-year period. Comparison with the data on the original cohort revealed no significant differences. A comparison between data from the 2- and 5-year cross-sectional assessments showed that about 50% of the subjects had not suffered from any acute psychotic episode (or relapse) during the preceding year (Biehl et al., 1986). The number of subjects who had been psychotic for more than 7 months in the year before follow-up assessment, however, increased from 13% at the 2-year follow-up to 32% at the 5-year follow-up.

During the first 5 years, the most frequent form of aftercare was consultation with a psychiatrist in private practice. Half a year after index admission, roughly 30 to 40% of the subjects used this form of aftercare every month up to the end of the first 5 years. The proportion of subjects in the original cohort without symptoms or medication increased over the first 2 years and reached a stable level of about one-third of the cohort until the 5-year follow-up.

ALIVE SUBJECTS

Even though we were unable to use the full set of instruments from the ISoS study, especially for ratings covering trends of psychotic symptoms and disability, medication, hospitalization, and global assessments of functioning (using the Life Chart Rating Form and the Broad Rating Schedule in ISoS), we tried to describe these areas using alternative instruments. Furthermore, whenever the other Field Research Centers described such illness characteristics as symptoms or disabilities covering the last 2 years before the long-term follow-up, we used similar information from our prospective 18-month study after the 14-year follow-up.

Symptomatology and Course of Illness

According to the Bleuler Severity Scale, 31 (56%) of the 56 subjects had recovered 14 years after index admission, 23 (42%) suffered mildly or moderately, and one patient showed severe psychotic symptoms. Taking the whole period since first contact into account, about three-quarters of the alive cohort (73%) could be classified as episodic, while one-quarter were described as neither continuous nor episodic. Only one subject suffered from a continuous disorder. A somewhat more differentiated perspective is obtained when using data from the PSE (Wing et al., 1974) and the PIRS (Biehl et al., 1989) for the assessment of symptoms and psychological impairments (Lukoff, Liberman, and Neuchterlein, 1986).

The percentage of subjects with significant ratings for each syndrome constituting the PSE-subscore DAH "delusional and hallucinatory syndromes" (at least one of the constituting signs or symptoms is clearly present; criteria according to the "syndrome check list": +, ++; Wing et al., 1974) is derived for three cross-sectional assessments: 1 year (CS3), 5 years (CS7), and 14 years (CS8) after index admission. The DAH consists of the syndromes: NS, DD, AH, PE, RE, GR, SF, VH, OH, and SC. The most often assessed symptoms—relatively independent of the time of measurement—are "delusions of reference," "sexual and fantastic delusions," and "delusions of persecution." In general, the rates are relatively low, the upper limit lying between 13 and 15%; in absolute numbers, this means a maximum of eight persons are affected at each cross-section, considering single syndromes. It is noteworthy to mention that there has been no significant change in the relative frequency of delusional syndromes and hallucinations over time (analysis of variance with repeated measurements; p=0.55). Seventeen subjects (30.4%) show significant values in at least one of the outlined syndromes at the 14-year follow-up.

Psychological impairments as operationalized by means of the PIRS show a similar result. The number of subjects with a PIRS score ≥3 (impairment at least markedly present) is relatively low. In most cases, the areas of "affective display" and "self-presentation" are affected. Even if the first impression seemed to show an increase in the number of symptomatic people up to the 14-year follow-up—especially in the areas "affective display" and "conversation"—analysis did not reveal a significant result (analysis of variance with repeated measurement; $p = .74$). Almost one-third of the subjects (30.4%) today show an impairment of some severity in at least one of the areas assessed.

Living Arrangements

At the time of follow-up assessment, four subjects (7%) were in a psychiatric hospital. Almost half of the group (48%) lived with family or friends; one-quarter (23%) resided in a (nursing) home or sheltered apartment. Twelve subjects (21%) were living alone. The high proportion of people living in supervised settings probably reflects the development of a complementary services structure in Mannheim during the past two decades. Half of the long-term cohort (52%) spent the past 2 years in an independent residence, whereas one quarter never lived independently in this period. Extending the observation to the entire follow-up period, 18% of the cohort spent more than half of the time in a hospital or in a supervised residence. In contrast, more than 55% of the subjects lived independently more than 90% of the time. None of the subjects had been homeless or vagrant during the past 2 years. Over the course of the entire follow-up period, three subjects had been homeless 11 to 25% of the time, and one person for more than 50% of the time. One subject is known to have spent at least some time in prison, but not during the last 2 years of follow-up.

A more detailed analysis covering the whole period of 14 years between index admission and long-term follow-up reveals a somewhat more dynamic picture of changes in residential and functional status over time (see Table 19.1). At index admission, 12 subjects were married; 42 subjects were single; and two subjects were divorced at this time and did not remarry. In the period between index admission and 14-year follow-up, five of the 12 married subjects got divorced and two remarried (one of whom divorced again). Twelve subjects married for the first time. Of the 14 marriages which occurred after index admission, eight were still intact at follow-up. Thirty subjects never married; five of them live with a partner, and two have an intimate relationship without sharing a home. Nineteen subjects have at least one child.

Work

With respect to the last 2 years before the 14-year follow-up, 25 (45%) subjects never held a paid full-time job and four subjects were institutionalized. Twenty-four subjects (43%) have had a full-time job at some point, the majority (29%) during the whole period, and three subjects held a part-time job. Fifteen persons (27%) were retired, all but one for the entire 2 years. Work performance in those engaged in full-time work at least 12 months was rated as good or very good in 91% of cases. At the time of the 14-year follow-up, 17 subjects (30%) held a regular job and five subjects had a job in a sheltered environment. Fifteen subjects (27%) received an early retirement pension, and 16 subjects were unemployed. The average length of unemployment in the cohort is 526 days (median: 730 days) for the last 2 years and 2032 days (median: 1431) for the whole 14-year period of observation. Fifteen subjects were never unemployed since time of first admission; for 11 subjects, the cumulated time of unemployment during this period is under 365 days; another 10 subjects had more than 10 years of unemployment.

Education/Job Training

The subjects' primary educational status rarely changed in the interval between index admission and the 14-year follow-up because most subjects had already finished primary school at the time of first admission (see Table 19.1). In contrast, there have been clear changes in secondary education and in job training opportunities in the years after first assessment. At index admission, 19 subjects had been fully trained for their jobs; two subjects had trained for two jobs. Another 19 subjects completed their training in the period between first admission and the 14-year follow-up. For eight subjects, this was their first job training; for the other five, this was their second. Six other subjects who did not have any training at the beginning of the study had the opportunity to try for at least two training certificates. At present, 17 subjects have not finished a job training program; three of them have not even begun. Two subjects who did not

TABLE 19.1 Sociodemographic Characteristics for Alive Subjects and Drop-Outs (including deaths): Changes between 1978 and 1992

	Alive Cohort (n=56)				*Drop-Outs (n=14)*	
	1978		*1992*		*1978*	
	n	*%*	*n*	*%*	*n*	*%*
Marital Status						
Single	42	75.0	30	53.6	4	28.6
Married	11	19.6	14	25.0	2	14.3
Married, but separated	1	1.8	1	1.8	1	7.1
Divorced	2	3.6	10	17.9	—	—
Widowed	—	—	1	1.8	—	—
No information	—	—	—	—	7	50.0
Living Conditions						
Living alone	13	23.2	12	21.4	1	7.1
With husband, wife, partner	13	23.2	19	33.9	3	21.4
With children alone	—	—	1	1.8	—	—
With parents	21	37.5	8	14.3	8	57.1
With relatives	2	3.6	—	—	1	7.1
With friends	5	8.9	—	—	1	7.1
Home without theraputic claim	1	1.8	3	5.4	—	—
Sheltered home, apartment	—	—	11	19.6	—	—
Other	1	1.8	2	3.6	—	—
School Education						
School education unfinished	2	3.6	3	5.4	—	—
Secondary modern school	18	32.1	20	35.7	1	7.1
Junior high school	10	17.9	11	19.6	1	7.1
Technical college	2	3.6	3	5.4	—	—
High school	18	32.1	19	33.9	4	28.6
Still in education	6	10.7	—	—	1	7.1
No information	—	—	—	—	7	50.0
Vocational Training						
No vocational training	14	25.0	17	30.4	—	—
Semiskilled	1	1.8	2	3.6	—	—
Finished apprenticeship	15	26.8	19	33.9	3	21.4
Master/craftsman	1	1.8	2	3.6	—	—
Advanced technical college	3	5.4	5	8.9	—	—
University degree	4	7.1	10	17.9	3	21.4
Pupil	6	10.7	—	—	1	7.1
Apprentice	2	3.6	—	—	1	7.1
Student	9	16.1	—	—	2	14.3
No information	1	1.8	1	1.8	4	28.6

(continued)

	Alive Cohort (n = 56)				Drop-Outs (n = 14)	
	1978		1992		1978	
	n	%	*n*	%	*n*	%
Type of Employment						
Regular job	24	42.9	17	30.4	6	42.9
Unemployed	13	23.2	16	28.6	4	28.6
Sheltered employment	—	—	5	8.9	—	—
Pensioner	—	—	15	26.8	—	—
Pupil/student	14	25.0	—	—	3	21.4
Housewife	5	8.9	3	5.4	—	—
Apprentice	—	—	—	—	1	7.1

acquire qualification, however, were taught as semi-skilled workers. Nineteen subjects ended an apprenticeship, and a further two have master's degrees. Five subjects successfully completed their education at an advanced technical college; another 10 have graduated from university.

Social Disability

Overall functioning in the last month, as measured by means of the DAS-M (Jung et al., 1989), was rated poor/very poor in almost half (48%) of the subjects, while about 30% of the cohort was judged excellent/good.

Comparing social disability at the 14-year follow-up with the situation 1 year and 5 years after index admission, showed a significant increase in the number of people affected over time (score ≥ 2; analysis of variance with repeated measurements, $p < .001$). For most items, the scores at 5 years and 14 years are similar or higher than at year 1. The most affected areas today are "underactivity" and "social withdrawal." In total, almost two-thirds (64.3%) of the subjects show a significant social disability in at least one of the areas of the DAS-M.

Violence and Suicide

For most of the subjects, no information was available about involvement in assaults. Over one-quarter (28%) of the cohort attempted suicide at some point during the 14 years; a third of those attempts had occurred in the past 2 years. Of the seven subjects who passed away during the course of the study, six committed suicide.

Medications

Thirty-seven subjects (66%) of the cohort had been prescribed neuroleptics during the past 2 years and most (55%) had taken them on a regular basis. Taking the whole period of observation into account, all but five subjects had been on neuroleptic mediation at least temporarily, more than half (55%) for most of the time since first treatment contact.

Hospitalization and Outpatient Treatment

Treatment history, as operationalized by hospital readmissions and contacts with outpatient treatment facilities, is described below.

Between 1979 and 1992, a downward trend in hospital admissions is observed from 29 in 1979 to 5 in 1992. On average, 5.7 inpatient treatment episodes are counted per subject, with a maximum of 19. For 9 subjects, the index admission is the only hospital stay during the entire period of observation.

A somewhat more differentiated picture results if outpatient treatment measures are also considered. For every month after index admission, the percentage of subjects with inpatient or outpatient contacts or without treatment was calculated. "Outpatient contacts" means the whole range of professional measures, especially contact with a psychiatrist in private practice, sheltered home, and sheltered workshop. In comparing two periods, (1) the period between the beginning of the study and the 5-year follow-up (CS1-CS7) and (2) the 18-month period after the 14-year follow-up (CS8-CS10), again there is a decrease in readmissions. But this decrease is fully compensated by an increase in outpatient and complementary measures. On average, during an 18-month period before the 5-year follow-up, 58.3% of the subjects were in contact with an inpatient or outpatient treatment facility, as compared with 58.2% in the second period.

Taking into consideration both hospital treatment and supervised residences, almost half of the cohort (48%) had spent some time as an inpatient during the last 2 years before the 14-year follow-up, with 13 subjects (23%) staying there the whole 24-month period.

DECEASED SUBJECTS

Fourteen years after inclusion into the study, seven subjects were deceased (five men, two women). One man had been discovered dead in his room. He had suffered from asthma; his inhaling device was found near his body. According to the police examination, he had died a natural death. Four subjects (three men, one woman) clearly died by suicide: One woman had cut her carotid artery; one man jumped from the top floor of the psychiatric hospital; another man jumped out of a window; and one man jumped in front of a moving train. Cause of death for one man and one woman was never fully ascertained, although the circumstances of the deaths as well as the statements of significant others render suicide rather probable.

DISCUSSION

Fourteen years after their first hospitalization with a diagnosis of schizophrenia, 56 patients of an original cohort of 70 persons could be contacted and agreed to participate in a research project on the long-term course and outcome of schizophrenia. Several persons had died in the 14-year period after first admission, six refused further participation, and one was untraceable. Already at the inception of the study, the number of men exceeded by far the number of the women—defying the expectation of equal probability between sexes of falling ill with schizophrenia, at least when applying a broad definition of schizophrenia (Lewine, Burbach, and Meltzer, 1984); however, since the inclusion criteria limited the age range to 15 to 44 years, schizophrenia of old age, which is assumed to be more common in women, was excluded.

Today, subjects are more or less isolated. Most of them (73%) are not married, and 66% do not have a stable partnership. Still, 14 subjects did marry after index admission. A far lower percentage of the cohort is married today than of the comparable age group, 30 to 60 years, in the total population (former West Germany, census December 31, 1991); 25 versus 76.6% (Statistisches Bundesamt, 1994), a difference that was already visible at index admission. In 1978, the percentage of married in the cohort was 21%, compared to 57% in the general population in the age group 15 to 44 years, the age range of the cohort (census December 31, 1978; Statistisches Bundesamt, 1980). This result reflects the often neglected fact that the onset of schizophrenia does not coincide with the time of first admission. First hospitalization instead can be looked at as the first point of culmination of a process that has been developing over several years (Häfner et al., 1994). The functional and social status of subjects at index admission already reflects the negative consequences, especially with respect to difficulties in intimate relationships, of incipient schizophrenia (Nowotny, Häfner, and Löffler, 1996).

Their educational training is to a large extent already completed by index admission. A surprisingly high number of subjects have a high-school diploma (32.1%). According to the microcensus of 1976 for Western Germany, the number of residents aged 15 to 44 with a high-school diploma is 9.5% (Statistisches Bundesamt, 1978), and those age groups with the highest rates of high-school diplomas are 20 to 24 years: 16.6%, 25 to 29 years: 13.5%. Since schizophrenia usually starts between the age of 20 and 29, the rate in our sample is still twice as high as in the same age group in the total population. An epidemiological study with 267 first onset schizophrenic patients (Häfner, an der Heinden et al., 1993; Häfner et al., 1994), conducted since 1987 in the same catchment area showed a similarly high rate (31.1%) of patients with a high-school diploma. The high level of education could be explained as a characteristic of the catchment area because Heidelberg and Mannheim, as university cities, have a high percentage of college students and are especially attractive to immigrants with a high level of education. The level of vocational training at present varies: Although almost all subjects have completed their school education, almost one-third do not have any job training certificates or secondary level education. Only 25 (45%) completed job training after index admission.

Only about one-third of the subjects are employed under normal competitive conditions. Most subjects (64.3%) are excluded from the labor market because of long-term unemployment or early retirement. However, illness and impairment may only be partially responsible. General economic development in Germany with an unemployment rate of more than 10% may play a major role here. Economic recession affects, above all, the ill, the disabled, and the poorly qualified (Franke and Prast, 1985; Kieselbach, 1995).

The agreement of psychopathological findings and impairment in psychological functioning among the different cross-sectional assessments is surprisingly high. In contrast to what one would expect, we did not find a reduction in the number of subjects with florid symptomatology over time. The trend, which nevertheless did not reach statistical significance, is more toward an increase. The same is true for impairments: Although the number of patients with impairments in affective display and conversation skills (global score) had doubled at the 14-year follow-up, a comparison of the profiles at 12 months, 5 years, and 14 years after first admission did not reveal any statistically significant change.

Social disability is somewhat different: On the one hand, the number of subjects with disabilities exceeds the number with psychological impairments and conspicuous symptomatology. Although the scales are not identical, the cut-off values were chosen to make the severity of the disorder somewhat comparable. On the other hand, the number of symptomatic people increased significantly over time. The most affected areas are underactivity and social withdrawal.

The number of inpatient readmissions per annum decreases significantly during the course of the 14 years. At the same time, the need for outpatient and complementary treatment increases so that the total need for care remains at the same level. If one further considers that the number of symptomatic subjects under no circumstances decreases, one may deduce that the number of hospital readmissions does not seem to be a valid indicator of the outcome of schizophrenia.

To sum up, the results so far show a diverse picture. In spite of a clear tendency toward the negative pole, the biographical characteristics of the sample cover the entire spectrum of possibilities: subjects who had not even begun job training and others who had received their master's degrees; subjects who today receive an early retirement pension and others who are normally employed; and some who live in a sheltered setting, while others have a stable personal relationship and live independently.

With respect to the development of psychopathology in the long run, we can make two statements; (1) The syndrome profiles at different points in time can hardly be distinguished from one another; (2) the percentage of subjects who manifest "clearly present" psychotic syndromes at the different points in time is relatively low—at a maximum of 13 to 15% per syndrome. Still, 17 subjects (30.4%) have symptomatic levels in at least one of the syndromes at the 14-year follow-up. One could conclude that after illness onset, most patients are psychopathologically inconspicuous, but also in the long-term course, no important changes should be expected. However, one has to take into account that the cross-sectional assessments are based on 4-week intervals, which are somewhat arbitrarily chosen from the point of view of the individual course of the illness. Since delusions and hallucinations are unstable over time, the probability of assessing a subject who is "in an episode" is not very high. However, to determine outcome, it is important to distinguish whether a subject who presents him- or herself now as psychopathologically inconspicuous can be considered "recovered" according to DSM-IV (APA, 1994) or as "in full remission" between episodes.

REFERENCES

American Psychiatric Association (1994), *Diagnostic and Statistical Manual of Mental Disorders*, 4th ed. (DSM-IV). Washington, DC: American Psychiatric Press.

Andreasen, N. C. (1989), Scale for the Assessment of Negative Symptoms (SANS). *Brit. J. Psychiatry*, 155(Suppl. 7):53–58.

Biehl, Maurer, K., Jung, E., Krüger, G., & Bauer-Schubart, C. (1988), Reported symptoms in schizophrenic patients within five years of onset of illness. In: *Treatment Resistance in Schizophrenia: An Approach for Research and Clinical Routine Together with a Reconaissance Paper*, ed. S. J. Dencker & F. Kulhanek. Braunschweig-Wiesbaden: Vieweg, pp. 108–118.

——, ——Jablensky, A., Cooper, J. E., & Tomov, T. (1989), The WHO Psychological Impairments Rating Schedule (WHO/PIRS). I. Introducing a new instrument for rating observed behaviour and the rationale of the psychological impairment concept. *Brit. J. Psychiatry*, 155 (Suppl. 7):68–70.

——, ——, ——Schubart, C., Krumm, B., & Jung, E. (1986), Prediction of outcome and utilization of medical services in a prospective study of first onset schizophrenics. *Eur. Arch. Psychiatry Neurol. Sci.*, 236:139–147.

Deutscher Bundestag (1975), *Report on the State of Psychiatry in the Federal Republic of Germany.* Bonn, Germany: Bonner Universitäts-buchdruckerei. (In German)

Dombrawe, H. (1986), Vocational rehabilitation for the mentally disabled: The Mannheim "Starting-Assistance" Project. *Die Rehabilitation*, 25:53–58. (In German)

Franke, H., & Prast, F. (1985), Unemployment—Facts, causes, possible solutions. *Spektrum der Wissenschaft*, 9:32–47. (In German)

Häfner, H., & an der Heiden, W. (1983), The impact of a changing system of care on patterns of utilization by schizophrenics. *Soc. Psychiatry*, 18:153–160.

——, —— (1984), An evaluation of changes in the mental health care system. In: *Psychotherapy: Macro/Micro Perspectives*, ed. U. Baumann. Göttingen, Germany: Hogrefe, pp. 52–72. (In German)

——, —— (1991), Evaluating effectiveness and cost of community care for schizophrenic patients. *Schizophr. Bull.*, 17:441–451.

——, —— (1996), The Mannheim Project. In: *Mental Health Service Evaluation*, ed. H. C. Knudsen & G. Thornicroft. Cambridge, U.K.: Cambridge University Press, pp. 82–95.

——, —— Hambrecht, M., Riecher-Rössler, A., Maurer, K., Löffler, W., & Fätkenheuer, B. (1993), A chapter in systematic schizophrenia research—The search for a causal explanation of gender differences in age at first onset. *Nervenarzt* 64:706–716. (In German)

—— Klug, J. (1980), The implementation of a community mental health care system—First results of a scientific evaluation. In: *Psychiatrie 5 Jahre nach der Enquete. Tagungsberichte*, Vol. 5, ed. H. Häfner, W. Picard, & Aktion Psychisen Kranke, e.v. Cologne, Germany: Rheinland Verlag, pp. 29–42. (In German)

——, —— (1982), The impact of an expanding community mental health service on patterns of bed usage: Evaluation of a four-year period of implementation. *Psychol. Med.*, 12:177–190.

—— Maurer, K., Löffler, W., Fätkenheuer, B., an der Heiden, W., Riecher-Rössler, A., Behrens, S., & Gattaz, W. F. (1994), The epidemiology of early schizophrenia: Influence of age and gender on onset and early course. *Brit. J. Psychiatry*, 164:29–38.

—— Pfeifer-Kurda, M. (1986), The impact of data protection laws on the Mannheim case register. In: *Psychiatric Case Registers in Public Health*, ed. G. H. M. M. ten Horn, R. Giel, W. H. Gulbinat, & J. H. Henderson. Amsterdam: Elsevier, pp. 366–371.

—— Reimann, H., Immich, H., & Martini, H. (1969), Incidence of mental disorders in Mannheim in 1965. *Soc. Psychiatry*, 4:125–135. (In German)

—— Riecher, A., Maurer, K., Meissner, S., Schmidtke, A., Fätkenheuer, B., Löffler, W., & an der Heiden, W. (1990), Instrument for the retrospective assessment of the onset of schizophrenia (IRAOS)—Development and first results. *Z. Klin. Psychol.*, 19:230–255. (In German)

—— Riecher-Rössler, A., Hambrecht, M., Maurer, K., Meissner, S., Schmidtke, A., Fätkenheuer, B., Löffler, W., & an der Heiden, W. (1992), IRAOS: An instrument for the assessment of onset and early course of schizophrenia. *Schizophr. Res.*, 6:209–223.

Jablensky, A., Schwarz, R., & Tomov, T. (1980), WHO collaborative study on impairments and disabilities associated with schizophrenic disorders. A preliminary communication: Objectives and methods. *Acta Psychiatr. Scand.*, 285(Suppl.):152–163.

Jung, E., Krumm, B., Biehl, H., Maurer, K., & Bauer-Schubart, C. (1989), *DAS—The Mannheim Scale for the Assessment of Social Disability*. Weinheim, Germany: Beltz. (In German)

Kieselbach, T. (1995), Unemployment and health. In: *Psychiatry—A Textbook for Clinical, Applied and Consultant Uses*, ed. V. Faust. Stuttgart: Fischer, pp. 501–508. (In German)

Korte, M., & Schmidt, A. (1983), *Migration and Its Social Consequences*. Göttingen, Germany: Vandenhoeck & Ruprecht. (In German)

Lewine, R. R. J., Burbach, D., & Meltzer, H. H. (1984), Effect of diagnostic criteria on the ratio of male to female schizophrenic patients. *Amer. J. Psychiatry*, 141:84–87.

Lukoff, D., Liberman, R. P., & Neuchterlein, K. H. (1986), Symptom monitoring in the rehabilitation of schizophrenic patients. *Schizophr. Bull.*, 12:578–602.

Nowotny, B., Häfner, H., & Löffler, W. (1996), The beginning schizophrenia as a break into social biography—Consequences for social disability vs. social rehabilitation. *Z. Klin. Psychol.*, 25:208–220.

Pietzker, A., Gaebel, W., Köpcke, W., Linden, M., Müller, P., Müller-Spahn, F., Schüssler, G., & Tegeler, J. (1986), The German multicenter study on the neuroleptic long-term therapy of schizophrenic patients. *Pharmacopsychiatry*, 19:161–166.

Reimann, H., & Häfner, H. (1972), Mental illness in the elderly in Mannheim—An investigation of "treated incidence." *Soc. Psychiatry*, 7:53–69. (In German)

Schubart, C., Schwarz, R., Krumm, B., & Biehl, H. (1986), *Schizophrenia and Social Adjustment*. Berlin: Springer. (In German)

Schwarz, R., Biehl, H., Krumm, B., & Schubart, C. (1980), Case-finding and characteristics of schizophrenic patients of recent onset in Mannheim. A report from the WHO collaborative study on the assessment of disability associated with schizophrenic disorder. *Acta Psychiatr. Scand.*, 285:212–219.

Statistisches Bundesamt (1960), *Statistical Yearbook 1960 for the Federal Republic of Germany*. Wiesbaden, Germany. (In German)

—— (1978), *Statistical Yearbook 1978 for the Federal Republic of Germany*. Stuttgart-Mainz: Kohlhammer. (In German)

—— (1980), *Statistical Yearbook 1980 for the Federal Republic of Germany*. Stuttgart-Mainz: Kohlhammer. (In German)

—— (1994), *Statistical Yearbook 1994 for the Federal Republic of Germany*. Stuttgart: Metzler-Poeschel. (In German)

Waschkowski, H. (1990), First experiences with the Mannheim "Starting-Assistance" Project—Five years of training on the job and rehabilitation placement for the mentally ill. *Psychiatric Prax.*, 17:66–70. (In German)

Weyerer, S. & Häfner, H. (1992), The high incidence of psychiatrically treated disorders in the inner city of Mannheim. Subceptibility of German and foreign residents. *Soc. Psychiatry Psychiatr. Epidemiol.* 27:142–146.

Wing, J. K., Cooper, J. E., & Sartorius, N. (1974), *Measurement and Classification of Psychiatric Symptoms*. London: Cambridge University Press.

World Health Organization (1994), *The ICD-10 Classification of Mental and Behavioral Disorders: Conversion Tables between ICD-8, ICD-9, and ICD-10, Revision 1*. WHO/MNH/92.16.Rev.1. Geneva, Switzerland: World Health Organization.

Chapter 20

RAPyD: Sofia, Bulgaria

Kimon Ganev, Georgi Onchev, and Plamen Ivanov

HISTORICAL, GEOGRAPHICAL, AND CULTURAL BACKGROUND

Bulgaria, with a total population of nearly 9 million, is situated in the middle of the Balkan peninsula on a territory of 110,000 sq km. The population is largely Bulgarian; Turks, the largest minority, account for about one-tenth of the population. There are also Gypsies, Jews, Armenians, and other minorities. The dominant religion is Eastern Orthodox Christianity. The official language is Bulgarian, which is also spoken by most minority group members.

The WHO Collaborating Center is located in Sofia, the largest city and the administrative and academic center of Bulgaria, comprising about 1.2 million inhabitants. The largest proportion of the population is engaged in service activities. There are also various industries, and some neighborhoods of the city are inhabited exclusively by the families of industrial workers. A significant portion of older people practices seasonal migration: They move to the villages in spring and summer, growing food and raising animals, and come back to the city during the winter.

Fifty years ago, Bulgaria was a traditional patriarchal society with extensive kinship networks as a constant source of support throughout life. Despite significant changes in this pattern during the past half-century, old traditions still have their influence, and kinship obligations can be described as strong. Even today, living in extended families—a result of both tradition and economics—is quite common. Men are more likely to occupy top positions in the labor market, whereas women have the advantage in landing less skilled jobs (e.g., secretaries, vendors). As women quit their traditional role of full-time homemakers, grandparents have taken on increased responsibilities for raising their grandchildren.

Major Changes

After 45 years of communist rule, November 10, 1989, marks the beginning of major political and economic changes which have had painful repercussions in all domains of social and personal life. A year later, the first free elections were held. The next decade of transition was characterized by rapid polarization of income distribution: About 10% of the population has an income much higher than that of the rest of the population, many of whom are living below the threshold of poverty. This development was particularly shocking because it followed years of egalitarian, socialist doctrine. Unemployment went from practically zero to 15% largely as a result of the breakdown in the public sector. The government's attempt to solve the unemployment problem by encouraging people to retire at a younger age led chiefly to an increase in the poor and dependent. Life had suddenly become uncertain, a battlefield with no clear ground rules, a place where risks had to be taken. Many experienced themselves as victims of an unjust and cruel set of circumstances. Helplessness and disillusionment reigned in the hearts of many who were not prepared psychologically to face the challenges and uncertainties of the transition period. Roughly 50,000 mostly young, active, and often well-educated Sofians emigrated to Western Europe and North America.

Mental Illness

The prevailing attitude toward mental illness is to keep it secret, not give it much thought, and to repress feelings, anxieties, and concerns. Many deny the possibility of understanding a mentally ill person and banish him or her from access to large domains of family and social life. Facing psychiatric illness provokes a serious family crisis, which often entails mobilizing close relatives to find solutions or to provide continuous care and support. Usually the family of origin assumes the bulk of the burden including financial support, care and supervision, and help seeking. It has become more difficult for people with severe mental illness to keep regular jobs, and opportunities for sheltered work are scarce. Disability pensions do not cover living expenses. The unstated belief is that mental health workers should protect the rest of society from madness by sequestering those who suffer from it. While help seeking is still channeled toward formal medical services, in the past decade, a growing number of people have gone to extrasensory healers who provide healing through the medium of unobservable "biofield" forces. Some, believing that mental health problems result from spells, resort to magical rituals; others seek treatment with herbs.

The Mental Health System in the Area

Since the mid-1990s there have been new developments in the field of mental health. The description that follows refers to the period *up to* 1995—which takes in the follow-up period of ISoS. Regulated by the Ministry of Health, the mental health system essentially has not changed since the mid-1970s despite a recent attempt to decentralize funding for large psychiatric hospitals. In 1994, inpatient hospital services were provided by university psychiatric hospitals (about 260 beds) and two psychiatric hospitals (a total of 300 beds), or 4.67 beds per 10,000 inhabitants. Some "chronic" patients were referred to other hospitals located far away from the city; other local psychiatric settings depended on community authorities. Since 1990, the overall economic crisis has cut back treatment resources (e.g., many drugs are available irregularly, if at all). Private psychiatric practice is just beginning and does not make much of a difference in the overall situation.

The main setting for outpatient care is dispensaries, each of which serves a well-defined catchment area. In the past, they tracked patients with mental illness through case registers. With the increasing awareness of human rights issues and the introduction of informed consent requirements for the registers, dispensaries are targeting more resources to genuine care and treatment of psychiatric patients. A few psychiatrists work in general health care outpatient settings, but their links with the other psychiatric services are not well established as a rule. Limited day treatment is available; two centers offer services to about 50 patients. Other forms of support for psychiatric patients (e.g., supervised residences, social support services, rehabilitation programs) are conspicuous by their absence.

The dominant paradigm of Bulgarian psychiatry can be described as "uninformed biological psychiatry." Until recently, training was characterized by a total neglect of the behavioral and human relationship aspects of psychiatric practice. Recently, psychiatry has begun to move, albeit slowly, toward a more individualized approach and to offer a larger variety of treatment.

Psychiatric Epidemiology

There have been no major epidemiological surveys on the incidence and prevalence of severe psychiatric disorders in Bulgaria. The main sources of information are clinical registers and hospital admissions (Beshkov and Gerdjikov, 1996).

Hospital Admissions

For many years, admissions to psychiatric hospitals steadily increased; however, immediately after the fall of the old regime in late 1989, there was a significant decrease in psychiatric hospital admissions, although the numbers have since somewhat risen. The halt in the upward trend of hospitalizations is especially prominent for subjects with a main diagnosis of schizophrenia, since there had been an expectation that the economic crisis would bring about larger numbers of patients seeking refuge in psychiatric hospitals. For the years 1990 to 1994, no major differences in the availability of psychiatric inpatient care could explain the lower (than expected and statistically predicted) numbers of hospital admissions.

Case Registers

The number of patients registered in psychiatric dispensaries has been rising steadily for decades. A small hesitation in the growth line occurred around the beginning of the transition period. However, the increase of registered patients soon resumed its previous pace.

THE CENTER

The WHO Collaborating Center in Sofia was established in 1984 and is currently integrated with the

National Center for Interdisciplinary Human Studies (NCIHS), founded in 1985. Although funded by the state budget, the NCIHS is a nontraditional governmental research institution: It reports to the Ministry of Health but has minimal administrative staff, does not employ research personnel, and has no laboratory or clinical facilities. Research and training activities are carried out by teams, which investigators form on an ad hoc basis, and which then contract for specific projects. The primary objective of the NCIHS is to foster research in the fields of neuroscience, behavioral science, education and child development, mental health and psychiatry, neurology, and other sciences. It also promotes interdisciplinary approaches, the use of modern research technologies, and international collaboration and free exchange of ideas (as opposed to institutional and central planning of research). The WHO Center uses the facilities, equipment, and administrative organization of NCIHS. Usually functioning with minimal staff, the WHO Center currently has only one coordinator. Its main activities in the field of mental health are to conduct research projects, to develop educational modules for mental health workers (psychiatrists, nurses, psychologists, social workers), and to assist professionals and institutions in developing service, training, and research programs. One of the research projects of the WHO Collaborating Center is the long-term course and outcome of schizophrenia (ISoS).

STUDY PROCEDURES

A sample of 121 subjects was originally selected as part of the Reduction and Assessment of Psychiatric Disability (RAPyD or Disability) study. The selection criteria were: (1) age 15 to 44; (2) residence in the defined catchment area; (3) absence of organic brain disease, severe mental retardation, severe sensory deficits, alcohol or drug dependence; (4) presence of (a) at least one of the following: hallucinations, delusions of nonaffective type, change to bizarre or grossly inappropriate behavior, thought and speech disorder other than retardation or acceleration; or (b) at least two of the following: psychomotor disorder other than simple retardation or overactivity, overwhelming fear or anxiety, marked social withdrawal, marked self-neglect; (5) clinical diagnosis of either schizophrenia (ICD-9 295), paranoid state (ICD-9 297), or other nonorganic psychosis, paranoid, or unspecified (ICD-9 298.3, 298.4, 298.8, and 298.9). The initial selection procedure included patients in various stages after onset of a severe mental illness. Subsequently, the sample was divided in two: a retrospective sample with an onset of illness more than 2 years before the initial examination, and a prospective sample with an illness onset less than 2 years prior to the initial examination. Only the latter sample was included in ISoS.

Case-Finding

The procedure for tracing subjects was: (1) Disability study documentation and medical case records were examined: (2) available information (phone numbers, addresses of subject and informants) was used to locate subject; (3) if (2) failed, neighbors were questioned for the subject's or his or her family's whereabouts; (4) if (2) and (3) failed, the address register was consulted for the subject's last known address. The average time spent locating the subject, asking his or her consent for the study, and arranging an interview with the subject and an informant, was about 4 hours. Most of this work was undertaken by a psychiatric nurse who had taken part in the initial assessment of subjects. On several occasions, it proved very important that subjects and/or relatives already knew the nurse.

Use of Study Instruments

Most of the study instruments, including the Present State Examination (PSE-9), the Disability Assessment Schedule (DAS), and the Psychological Impairments Rating Schedule (PIRS), had been translated (and back-translated) into Bulgarian for the Disability study. The Scale for the Assessment of Negative Symptoms (SANS) had also been translated previously. The new Family Interview Schedule (FIS) was translated and back-translated by two bilingual psychiatrists and tested in a few pilot interviews. No major problems were encountered.

Data-Gathering Procedures

All the interviews in the study were carried out by three psychiatrists. All but two were face-to-face; the exceptions were done by phone. About 60% of the interviews were conducted in a psychiatric setting, and the rest were carried out in subjects' and informants' homes. The average time for the subject interview was 2 hours; for the informant interview, 1.5 hours.

A search of all available medical information was done by the interviewer before and after the interview. These clinical records proved very useful, especially in completing the Life Chart Schedule (where recall problems, usually for earlier events in the study period, were common). Time proved a critical variable in the interviews. Subjects and relatives were often reluctant to continue for more than 1 hour and resisted the suggestion that the interview resume on a second occasion. Medical records saved time and enabled interview length to be within reasonable limits.

Most of the interviewees felt uncomfortable with the structured format of the FIS. They resisted choosing just one option, insisting instead of telling whole stories illustrating the item. At times, the interviewee, after finishing the personal account, suggested that the interviewer, having heard the "facts," make his own rating of the item. The implicit message was that their experience was highly emotional and much richer than suggested by the simple structured rating.

Thirty-three subjects (55% of the sample) and 32 informants (53.3%) were interviewed. Two subjects (3.3%) were dead; three subjects (5%) were lost to follow-up; eight subjects (13.3%) refused an interview; five subjects (8.3%) were not contacted because their relatives refused to allow it; nine subjects (15%) were not interviewed because of lack of sufficient resources. Some of the subjects who were not fully interviewed nevertheless had some contact with the research team. This allowed the completion of some of the ratings dependent on a face-to-face interview.

On a number of occasions, subjects' relatives turned out to be extremely reluctant to let the research team contact the subjects. The most common reason given was that a psychiatric interview would be extremely upsetting. Nine subjects were not interviewed; after they were located by the research team, a large number of phone calls, letters, home visits, and appointments failed to bring about an interview. Some of these subjects could be classified as "covert" refusers. (Note that all refusers gave consent for their medical case records to be used in the study.)

For most of the subjects who were not interviewed, good data are available from medical case records, the initial study documentation, informant interviews, and interviews with their treating psychiatrists. Overall, the quality of the information can be summarized as follows: data for all or almost all items, 33 subjects (55%); data for most the items, 15 subjects (25%); information for some of the items, nine subjects (15%); very limited information for a few items, two subjects (3.3%); completely lost to follow-up, one subject (1.7%).

RESULTS

Baseline and Short-Term Follow-Up

Gender, Age, and Status at Long-Term Follow-Up

At entry to the study, the prospective sample comprised 60 subjects (21 males and 39 females). The significant predominance of female subjects is partly explainable by peculiarities of the catchment area. The psychiatric hospital, one of the study centers, has a larger catchment area for women than for men; moreover, 10 of the women selected for the study came from the "extra" catchment area. The mean age of subjects was 27.2 at inclusion and 43.4 years at last follow-up. The mean follow-up period is 16.2 years. Fifty-five subjects were alive and traced at last follow-up in 1994. Two subjects had died (a man and a woman); both committed suicide during an episode of psychotic illness in the first 2 years after study entry. Three subjects (two men and a woman) could not be traced.

Mode of Onset

For the 55 subjects in the alive cohort, 18 subjects (32.7%) had an acute onset (up to 1 week), 21 (38.2%) had a subacute onset (from 1 week to 1 month), and 14 (25.5%) had an insidious onset (greater than 1 month); data for two subjects are missing. These figures are roughly equivalent to the two other Disability centers and are comparable to most of the ISoS centers. None of the subjects dead or lost to follow-up had an acute onset, suggesting that those with acute onset were more likely to be alive and interviewed at the 16-year follow-up.

Diagnosis

At entry to the Disability study, subjects received ICD-9 diagnoses which were converted to ICD-10 (WHO, 1994). Forty-five subjects received a baseline diagnosis of schizophrenia, and in 41 subjects, the subtype was paranoid schizophrenia. The second most prevalent diagnostic category was other psychotic disorder (8 subjects). Four subjects received a diagnosis of schizoaffective disorder, two of depression, and one subject had no diagnosis. All of the subjects dead and lost to follow-up had a baseline diagnosis of paranoid schizophrenia. This finding corroborates the evidence from most of the other centers in the ISoS study that a diagnosis of schizophrenia is associated with an elevated mortality risk.

Reevaluation of Baseline Diagnosis

The research team (three psychiatrists) who conducted the interviews reviewed all available baseline data: the medical records, interview ratings, and research notes, and assigned an ICD-10 diagnosis by consensus. For the alive cohort, 29 subjects (72.5%) with an ICD-10 baseline diagnosis of schizophrenia received the same diagnosis at reevaluation by the research team; six (15%) were rediagnosed as other psychotic disorder; three (7.5%) as affective disorder; and two (5%) as schizoaffective. The rediagnosis procedure qualified fewer subjects (34) with a diagnosis of schizophrenia (ICD-10) than the diagnoses at entry to the study simply converted to ICD-10. Of the 34 subjects rediagnosed with schizophrenia, five had another baseline diagnosis: Three were diagnosed as other psychotic disorder, one as schizoaffective, and one was without a baseline diagnosis. A substantial number of subjects (7) were rediagnosed as belonging to the group of affective disorders.

A note of caution is needed in interpreting the results of the rediagnostic procedure. On a number of occasions, it was very difficult to assess the relative prominence and duration of the affective symptoms recorded in clinical case notes. It could be that the "weight" of depressive symptoms was overestimated in the rediagnostic exercise based on clinical and research records. An indirect indication of this is that clinical and research diagnoses made at the period of the initial assessment did not detect mood disorders in the study sample to the same extent. Only two subjects included in the Disability study in Sofia received a research diagnosis of affective disorder at baseline assessment; four subjects were diagnosed with schizoaffective disorder.

Pattern of Course at Short-Term Follow-Up

Short-term follow-ups were carried out 1 and 2 years after the initial assessment. To judge from information available for 48 of the 58 subjects alive at the 2-year follow-up, short-term pattern of course varied. Eleven subjects (22.9% of subjects with available data) had continuous nonremitting psychotic symptoms. Seventeen subjects (35.4%) had various durations of psychotic symptoms followed by incomplete remissions, marked by enduring nonpsychotic symptoms. Six subjects (12.5%) experienced nonpsychotic episodes of mental illness (e.g., depression). Fourteen subjects (29.2%) had psychotic symptoms followed by complete remissions, but only one of these has been completely free from psychiatric symptoms for the follow-up period. The general trend for the short-term follow-up is that many of the subjects experienced serious psychiatric symptoms for long periods of time. However, in nearly one-third of the subjects, restoration to a symptom-free state was observed. These data suggest that slightly higher proportions of the subjects in our sample, as compared with the other two Disability centers, had severe psychiatric symptoms during the short-term follow-up period. On the whole, on short-term pattern of course, our center compares unfavorably with almost all the other ISoS centers.

Attrition of Subjects

The number of subjects of the original cohort not assessed in this study is low (two subjects dead; three lost to follow-up), making for the high success rate of 91.7% subjects traced and assessed. However, the observed trends of attrition from the study need some comment. All subjects dead and lost to follow-up had a diagnosis of schizophrenia at entry into the study; none had an acute illness onset; and none had achieved a complete remission at short-term follow-up. Evidence in the literature and subsequent analyses of our data suggest that these factors are predictors of poorer outcome. Although the numbers are small, there is a trend; subjects with characteristics predicting poorer prognosis were more likely to die or be lost to follow-up.

ALIVE SUBJECTS

Course of Illness

A very high proportion of the subjects (25, 45.5%) have had continuous psychotic symptoms for the last 2 years of follow-up, a figure which is much higher than the other two Disability centers. Only three of the

ISoS centers (Beijing, Cali, and Nagasaki) have a higher proportion of subjects with continuous psychotic symptoms. The pattern of course during those past 2 years for seven subjects (12.7%) has been episodic; 21 (38.2%) have had no psychotic symptoms and two with psychotic symptoms could not be classified as either continuous or episodic. More than half of the subjects (30, 54.5%) have had an episodic course for the entire study period, while 23 subjects (41.8%) have had continuous course. No subjects were completely free from psychotic symptoms for the entire follow-up period. In comparing the rates of continuous psychotic symptoms across centers, it becomes evident that the Sofia sample belongs in the unfavorable third of centers, with more than 40% of the subjects classified as continuously psychotic. (At the other centers, samples have fewer than 30% continuously psychotic subjects throughout the follow-up period.)

Subjects were rated by the interviewer on a scale reflecting the overall time trend of symptoms and psychosocial functioning for the entire study period. The overall trend proved to be varied. Twenty-five (45.4%) of the subjects were rated as getting at least slightly better, and 21 (38.2%) were getting at least slightly worse. Within these, the extreme categories on this item, "getting much better" was more common (21.8% of the subjects) than "getting much worse" (12.7%). The rest of the subjects showed no definite trend in their overall condition over time.

Symptoms

The Global Assessment of Functioning Scale for Symptomatology (GAF-S) provides a general estimate for symptom severity at the point of follow-up. A significant proportion of the subjects (n=12, 21.8%) had no pronounced psychiatric symptoms during the last month—GAF-S scores of at least 71. However, more than half of the subjects (29, 52.8%) exhibited serious (mostly psychotic) symptoms, with GAF-S scores lower than 51. The mean value of GAF-S ratings is 49.3. Compared with the other ISoS centers, the Sofia sample has the worst rating on symptoms, the smallest proportion of subjects with GAF-S scores greater than 70, and the highest proportion of subjects with severe psychiatric symptoms (i.e., GAF-S scores lower than 51).

The ratings on Bleuler's Severity of Symptoms Scale reveal that slightly less than half of the sample (26, 48.1%) had no psychotic symptoms at follow-up. Most of the 28 subjects with psychotic symptoms had at least "marked" psychotic symptoms (46.3% of those rated). The behavior of a large minority of the subjects (11, 20.4%) was almost completely dominated by severe psychiatric symptoms. Sofia had the highest proportion of subjects with severe psychotic symptoms, and just four of the other ISoS centers (Beijing, Dublin, Honolulu, and Nagasaki) had a lower proportion of recovered patients (28–42%).

Usually, psychotic symptoms were more prominent in the first third or first and middle thirds of the study period. This was the case for 34 (61.8%) of the subjects. The reverse pattern was observed in a much smaller proportion of the sample. Nine (16.3%) subjects have had more prominent symptoms in the last third of the follow-up period and not in the first third. The overall impression from the clinical data is that symptoms reemerge at some time after the onset of a psychotic disorder, and often are present continuously or for very considerable periods. Eight subjects (14.5%) had prominent psychotic symptoms throughout the study period. At the same time, however, a substantial proportion of the subjects was symptom-free for long periods. No one pattern of course of clinical symptoms appears to be inherently consistent with an initial diagnosis of severe psychiatric (psychotic) illness.

Living Arrangements

Thirty-eight (70.4%) subjects have lived with their families during the last month before follow-up. Only two (3.8%) were in institutions, and 14 (25.9%) were living alone. Compared with the other two Disability centers, the subjects in our sample were much more likely to live with their families and much less likely to be in supervised institutions. However, our findings are generally supported by the results of most of the other ISoS centers. The proportion of subjects living alone is roughly the same in the three Disability centers, in the European centers (minus Dublin) and in Rochester, while in the Asian and Indian centers as well as Cali it is much lower. No subjects in Sofia have been homeless or vagrant at any point in the entire follow-up period. None of the subjects has been in jail or prison.

The typical living arrangement is sharing a house with one's family. Often, the subject lives with his or

TABLE 20.1 Time in Independent Community Living in Past 2 Years of Follow-Up[a]

Independent Community Living	Family Provided Substitute for Custodial Care: Not at all	Some of the Time	Most of the Time	Total
All of the Period	26	9	5	40 (74.1%)
Most of the Period	4	4	3	11 (20.4%)
Less than Half	3	0	0	3 (5.6%)
Total	33 (61.1%)	13 (24.1%)	8 (14.8%)	54 (100%)[b]

[a] Reprinted with the permission of Munksgaard International Publishers Ltd., Copenhagen, Denmark; this table appeared originally in Ganev, K., Onchev, G., & Ivanov, P. (1998).

[b] Information on family care for one subject is missing.

her parents. Living in hospitals or supervised residences is rather uncommon. Conversely, about a quarter of the subjects in the other two Disability centers (Groningen and Mannheim) were living in supervised settings. This very significant difference cannot be explained by severity of clinical symptoms or by level of disability. In fact, subjects in Sofia have worse ratings on clinical and disability measures. A more plausible explanation involves cultural values emphasizing kinship obligations, combined with poor inpatient psychiatric treatment, and the lack of supervised residences for people with mental health problems. Additional supporting evidence is the relative brevity of the Sofia subjects' stay in hospitals. Only three subjects (5.4%) have spent more than 13 months in psychiatric institutions during the past 2 years, while another 11 subjects (20.0%) have been in the hospital for less than 12 months.

Data for the entire follow-up period confirm that Sofia subjects spent a relatively small proportion of the time in supervised residences. Only one subject (1.8%) has spent more than half of the period in a supervised residence; 12 subjects (21.8%) have been in supervised residences between 11 and 25% of the time; 18 subjects (32.7%) have spent between 6 and 10% of the time; and 24 subjects (43.6%) have spent 5% of the time or less in supervised residences. These figures compare very favorably with the other two Disability Centers whose subjects have spent significantly higher proportions of the follow-up period in supervised residences.

However, Sofia data could be misleading if interpreted at face value. Living outside psychiatric institutions cannot be equated with independent living. One of the ratings made by interviewers was whether the family provided a substitute for custodial care.

Table 20.1 presents the length of period in independent living and whether the family provided a substitute for custodial care.

A substantial proportion of subjects who have been in "independent community living" were being taken care of by their families. Relatives were a substitute for custodial care for more than a quarter of the patients who had not been in an institution during the past 2 years. Overall, nearly 40% of the families were involved to a substantial degree in providing for the subjects at follow-up.

Work

Data in this section are available for 53 subjects. More than half of the subjects have been occupied in work or household activities at least at some point during the past 2 years before follow-up assessment. Twenty-four (45.3%) have been employed and 7 (13.1%) have been engaged in full-time household activities. Thirteen subjects (24.6%) have been employed for more than 12 months of the past 2 years; the work performance for 10 of these subjects (90.9%) was rated as very good or good. Six subjects have been engaged in full-time homemaking for more than 12 months of the past 2 years; the performance of four of them (66.7%) was very good or good. Caution, however, is needed in interpreting these results. The above ratings refer only to the time when people were employed. The global evaluation of performance for the entire 2 years is good—10 (32.3%); fair—9 (29%); poor—12 (38.7%). The rest of the subjects (24, 43.6% of the 55) have not been employed or engaged in full-time homemaking. In the past 2 years, five of the subjects (all female) retired. Twenty-nine (53.7%) have been receiving a disability pension, 25 throughout the past 2 years. These findings are consonant with those of the other two Disability centers.

Social Disability

The Disability Assessment Schedule global evaluation of disability for the last month shows that nearly a third of the subjects (17, 30.9%) had excellent or good adjustment outcome; 25 (45.5%) had fair and poor adjustment; and 13 (23.6%) had very poor adjustment or severe maladjustment, results almost identical with the other two Disability centers. On this measure, the Sofia sample is situated in the medium range of the ISoS centers. The Global Assessment of Functioning Disability Scale (GAF-D) results show that although a substantial proportion of the subjects (18, 32.7%) has no or some disability at follow-up (i.e., GAF-D scores of at least 61), the lives of 20 subjects (36.4%) are heavily marked by poor functioning (GAF-D scores less than 41). The mean values on GAF-D show that the Sofia center has the poorest results across centers, although the difference is not as marked as on symptom scores.

Many subjects (23, 41.9%) tend to become worse with the passage of time; that is, disability is most prominent in the final third or in the final and middle thirds of the follow-up period. However, for a substantial proportion of the subjects (20, 36.3%) the highest ratings of disability appear in their first third or first and middle thirds of the follow-up period. The results suggest a slight trend toward increased disability with the passage of time, a finding markedly at odds with that seen in almost all other ISoS centers.

Violence and Suicide

It is the impression of the interviewers that recall and recording of "minor" assaults and "not serious" suicide attempts were rather unreliable. During the entire follow-up period, seven subjects (14% of the 50 with available data) committed assaults, and three (5.9%) committed assaults in the last 2 years. These results place Sofia in the lower half of the ISoS centers. Thirteen subjects (25.5% of the 51 alive and with available data) attempted suicide during the whole follow-up period, and four subjects (7.7%) attempted suicide during the last 2 years of the period. The proportion of suicide attempters in the Sofia sample is one of the highest, but it is roughly equivalent to that in the other two Disability centers (for the entire period especially).

Medications

All subjects took neuroleptics at some point in the follow-up period. Thirty-three subjects (60.0%) took neuroleptics for most of the time. Findings suggest that Sofia subjects take slightly more neuroleptics than the subjects in the other two Disability centers; only three ISoS centers show higher use of neuroleptics for the entire period (Dublin, Hong Kong, and Nagasaki). During the last 2 years of follow-up, 12 subjects (22.2%) did not take neuroleptics, seven subjects (13.0%) took them occasionally, and 35 subjects (64.8%) were on them for most of this period. The proportion of subjects taking neuroleptics in the sample tends to be higher than for the other two Disability centers and for most of the other ISoS centers. However, the high use of neuroleptics is not surprising because the ratings of Sofia subjects on symptom variables are highest among all study centers. For the entire period, there was a tendency for a subgroup of subjects to reduce the use of neuroleptics. Twenty-five subjects (45.5%) took more neuroleptics in the first third or in the first and second thirds of the follow-up period, while 24 subjects (43.6%) took neuroleptics during all of the follow-up period. It was quite unusual for subjects to take more neuroleptics in the final third or in the middle and final thirds of the period; only two subjects (3.6%) have had this pattern of medication.

Hospitalizations

A significant proportion of subjects has been hospitalized for psychiatric reasons in the last 2 years of follow-up (14, 25.4%). However, only three have spent more than 12 months in the hospital. The percentage is much higher in the other two Disability centers (Groningen and Mannheim) where more than half of the hospitalized subjects in the past 2 years have spent at least 13 months in the hospital. Moreover, larger proportions of those samples had been in hospitals and supervised residences during the past 2 years (one-third of the Groningen subjects and nearly half of the Mannheim subjects). Comparing the Sofia sample with the other centers, we find that six of the other centers (Agra, Beijing, Cali, Chandigarh—both urban and rural—and Chennai [Madras]) had significantly higher proportions of subjects who had not been in institutions in the past 2 years.

A large majority of Sofia subjects had been in institutions at some point in the entire follow-up period. Only five (9.1%) subjects had not been in psychiatric hospitals since inclusion in the study. Most of the subjects spent less than 25% of the time in supervised residences. Only one subject (1.8%) spent more than 25% of the period in a supervised residence. Noteworthy was the very low proportion of subjects with a long stay in institutions, comparing very favorably with the other two Disability centers where over a quarter of the subjects have spent more than 25% of the period in supervised institutions. The differences in time spent in institutions between Sofia and the other two centers of the Disability study cannot be explained by higher levels of symptoms or by social disability; on most of these outcome measures, the Sofia sample had less favorable ratings than the Groningen and Mannheim samples. Comparison of birth cohorts in Sofia showed that older subjects tend to have spent less time in institutions than younger subjects. This finding might be associated with differences in the illness course by birth cohort; differences in symptom severity and/or disability; or differences in social response to mental illness, which depend upon a subject's age. Most of the subjects spent longer periods of time in hospitals during the beginning of the follow-up period. Forty-one subjects (82% of 50 subjects with information available) had hospital admissions only in the first or the first and middle thirds of the period. Only two subjects (4%) showed the tendency to have more hospitalizations in the last third of the entire period of the study.

Prediction of Outcome by Mode of Illness Onset

Analyses used various variables as outcome predictors: gender, baseline diagnosis, mode of illness onset, and short-term course. Because of the difference in the sizes of the catchment for men and for women, analyses of the Sofia sample involving gender as a predictor of outcome could be seriously flawed. Although all of the predictor variables did explain part of the outcome variance, the outcome results only for mode of illness onset are presented here. This variable proved to be the best predictor of various dimensions of long-term outcome.

Mode of onset was defined as sudden or acute (development of symptoms within a week), subacute (within a month), and insidious (over more than one month). As data for two alive subjects are missing, findings in this section refer to the 53 subjects with available data.

Course of Illness by Mode of Onset

The course of the psychotic symptoms during the past two years of the study was strongly correlated with mode of illness onset. Subjects who had never been psychotic in the last 2 years account for two-thirds of the subjects (12) with an acute onset, 38.1% (8 subjects) of those with a subacute onset, and only 7.1% (1 subject) of those with an insidious onset. Subjects with continuous psychotic symptoms accounted for the large majority of those with an insidious onset (n=11, 78.6%), roughly half of those with subacute onset (n=11, 52.4%), and 16.7% (3 subjects) of those with acute onset. The trend is obvious: rapid illness onset is associated with greater likelihood of no psychotic symptoms for the final 2 years of a 16-year course of the disorder; slow onset is associated with high likelihood of psychotic symptoms.

Severity of Symptoms According to Mode of Illness Onset

There were pronounced differences in symptoms present at follow-up evaluation. The GAF-Symptom scores decreased significantly with slower onset of illness (i.e., subjects with more gradual illness onset tend to have more severe symptoms at the time of the follow-up). The mean GAF-Symptom values are: 60.4 for subjects with acute and sudden illness onset; 51.2 for subjects with subacute illness onset; and 32.3 for subjects with insidious illness onset. Over a third of the subjects with an acute illness onset (7, 38.9%) had no serious psychiatric symptoms at follow-up (GAF-S scores >70). The corresponding figures were 23.8% (5 subjects) for those with a subacute onset, and none of the subjects with an insidious illness onset. Very severe symptoms (GAF-S scores <31) were experienced by one subject (5.6%) with an acute illness onset, four subjects (19.1%) with a subacute onset, and eight subjects (57.1%) with an insidious onset. The general impression is that the outcome of subjects with insidious onset is extremely poor on symptom dimensions.

Social Disability According to Mode of Illness Onset

The DAS global evaluation of psychosocial adjustment at outcome shows that nine subjects (50%) with acute onset, eight subjects (38.1%) with subacute onset, and none of the subjects with insidious onset have excellent or good adjustment at the end of a 16-year follow-up. Subjects with very poor adjustment or severe maladjustment are: one subject (5.6%) with an acute onset, five subjects (23.8%) with subacute onset, and seven subjects (50%) with insidious onset. GAF-Disability scores also differ significantly according to mode of onset. The mean value of GAF-Disability is 60.5 for subjects with acute or sudden onset; 53.8 for subjects with subacute onset; and 37.9 for subjects with insidious onset. The findings suggest that more acute onset predicts better social adjustment at the end of a 16-year follow-up. This trend is well marked, although slightly less pronounced than the relationship between mode of onset and severity of symptoms at follow-up. These findings provide substantial evidence that mode of onset is a relatively strong predictor of outcome in long-term follow-up. More rapid mode of onset is significantly associated with lower levels of symptoms and disability after 16 years. These trends are robust, and the results of the other two Disability centers are in complete accord with the Sofia findings.

DECEASED SUBJECTS

At the time of follow-up two subjects (3.3%) were dead—a man and a woman. Both had committed suicide during the first 2 years after entry into the study. The suicides were committed during an exacerbation of the illness. Comparison of the sample to the general population of Sofia shows no increased death rate. The standard mortality ratio (SMR) is 1.04. This finding differs from most of the other centers where the SMRs are significantly higher than that expected for the general population.

DISCUSSION

The original cohort was assembled between 1978 and 1980 in Sofia, Bulgaria. Sixty subjects were included in the recent onset sample. The mean age of subjects at inclusion was 27.2 years. Women were nearly two-thirds of the sample because their catchment area was larger than the one for men.

Diagnosis

Inclusion criteria selected patients with functional psychotic, non-affective disorders. At entry to the study, all subjects were diagnosed with ICD-9. The conversion of ICD-9 diagnoses to ICD-10 categories was performed with the help of conversion tables. Three-quarters of the original cohort (45 subjects) received an ICD-10 diagnosis of schizophrenia. Eight subjects had a diagnosis of other psychotic disorder; four subjects had schizoaffective disorder; two had depression; and one subject had no diagnosis at entry into the study.

Sample Attrition

A large majority of the original cohort was traced and assessed: 55 of the original 60. Two subjects were dead and three were lost to follow-up. Subjects not assessed at follow-up tended to show features associated with poorer course and outcome: All had an initial diagnosis of schizophrenia, and they are more likely to have had a slower mode of onset and a more unfavorable short-term course. However, the low proportion of subjects not included in the follow-up makes it very unlikely that our findings are biased in any substantial way.

Quality of Information

Contacting subjects and their relatives and obtaining consent proved to be demanding tasks. A substantial portion of subjects and relatives were reluctant to take part in the study. The presence on the team of a psychiatric nurse who knew many of the patients and their families greatly facilitated approaching the subject and his or her family and securing his or her consent for an interview. One of the limitations of the study is that full interviews (with all the study instruments) were carried out with only 33 subjects and 32 informants. Limited contact with another eight subjects (while negotiating consent for the study and appointments) permitted the improvement of the data sets for this group. The research team used all available information in completing the study instruments including: subject and informant interviews, medical records and dispensary registers, information from treating psychiatrists, and, on a few occasions, information from neighbors. The overall impression is that each source of information contributed to the quality and comprehensiveness of the data set. If the research team had relied exclusively on data gathered in interviews, important pieces of information would have been missed or located inappropriately in time. Conversely, no major differences in data concerning the overall functioning, life circumstances, treatment history, and presence of psychotic symptoms would have resulted had we been able to interview all subjects. One exception is the lack of detailed data on psychiatric symptom profiles (full PSE-9 and PIRS) for subjects without interviews.

Informants had a peculiar difficulty with the structured format of the Family Interview Schedule—telling stories illustrating an item rather than choosing one of the options (e.g., "always," "most of the time," etc.). They experienced the interviewer's insistence upon receiving a simple answer as frustrating, so that the quality of the interview relationship suffered. In fairness, our impression is that to get a sense of how the mental illness of a family member affects the whole family, one does need to attend to the emotions and stories triggered by each specific question.

No Access Families

One of the surprising findings in the process of data collection was the refusal (or very strong reluctance) of some extremely protective relatives to allow us to contact the subject, an attitude particularly striking in the case of subjects who have had long periods of highly adaptive functioning without symptoms and without maintenance therapy. They believed that merely mentioning the issue of mental illness would very likely lead to a deterioration of the mental health of the subject. A typical pattern of coping with mental illness was denial and avoidance of any discussion of the topic. Not getting in touch with psychiatrists seemed to be ensuring—in an almost magical way—the preservation of sanity. The history of mental illness and its treatment was encapsulated (like a foreign body) rather than integrated into the history of the family. One avenue for future research, then, is the exploration of the predominant mechanisms used by patients and their relatives to cope with severe mental illness and with the stigma associated with it.

Symptoms

The pattern of course of psychotic symptoms was varied. The longitudinal unfolding of severe mental disorder in the Sofia sample cannot be associated with a specific course of symptoms. However, the results show that a very large proportion of subjects (41.8%) experienced continuous psychotic symptoms for the entire 16-year study period. Nearly half of the sample (45.5% of the subjects) had psychotic symptoms throughout the past 2 years of the study period. The opposite trend is depicted by the 38.2% of subjects who were without psychotic symptoms during the past 2 years, and the 21.8% of subjects with GAF-S scores higher than 70 at follow-up. The results suggest that Sofia subjects have continuous psychotic symptoms more frequently than subjects in similar studies (e.g., Leon, 1989; Bland, Parker, and Orn, 1976). Compared with the other ISoS centers, the Sofia sample has the worst ratings on symptom dimensions.

One likely source of bias for the longitudinal symptom ratings is our reliance on psychiatric records. Case notes tended more often to suggest the presence of continuous psychotic symptoms than did information from interviews with relatives and subjects. The advantage of clinical records for rating the course of psychotic symptoms is that symptoms are rated at many points in time and thus recall problems are circumvented. This peculiarity warrants caution when making comparisons with studies in which interviews were the only source of information. However, the unfavorable ratings of the course of psychiatric symptoms (as compared with the other centers) are confirmed by the end-point ratings of psychiatric symptoms by GAF-S, PSE-9, and PIRS, where Sofia subjects had the lowest scores.

The low mortality rate of Sofia subjects raises another issue, partially explaining the very poor symptom outcomes in the sample. One can conjecture that subjects with poor prognosis are more likely to commit suicide. Taking this into account when comparing Sophia data with other ISoS centers would result in a difference in outcome much less pronounced than is currently the case.

There was a trend toward amelioration of psychiatric symptoms in the last third of the study period. This finding seems compatible with the notion of "late recovery"; that is, the notion that there is often an improvement in the second and third decades after the onset of illness (Gross and Huber, 1986). However, it is a bit speculative to characterize these findings as evidence of late recovery.

Social Disability

Nearly a third of the subjects (30.9%) had either excellent/good adjustment as rated with DAS or (32.7%) only mild disability assessed with GAF-D (>60). The very poorly adjusted subjects were a bit less numerous

(23.6% as rated with DAS). Less than half of the subjects were working at the point of follow-up and only about a quarter of the subjects had held a job for more than 12 months in the past 2 years. On the whole, global outcome results—35.8% of the total sample worked or did household work during the past 2 years, and their performance was noted as satisfactory—tend to confirm the general finding of other long-term studies of schizophrenia that nearly a third of the subjects have good long-term outcome (Cutting, 1986; Ciompi, 1980; Huber, Gross, Schutter, and Linz, 1980). On some of the disability measures, Sofia subjects scored in the medium range of ISoS centers, while on other measures, the mean ratings were the lowest in the study. On comparison, the overall impression is the difference between Sofia and other centers is not as pronounced on social disability as it is on psychiatric symptomatology, although it ranks at or near bottom for both. The overall trend of social disability for the entire period shows that roughly equivalent proportions of subjects tended to improve (36.3%) and to deteriorate (41.9%) with the passage of time. This finding is at odds with the predominant trend on symptoms—nearly two-thirds of the subjects experienced their most severe symptoms in the first third or first and second thirds of the follow-up period. These two findings do support the relative independence of the symptom and disability dimensions of schizophrenia course and outcome. First, the predominant trends for symptoms and social disability differ significantly. While most subjects are likely to improve on symptom dimensions in the long-term course of schizophrenia, in our sample deterioration in social functioning is the most common pattern. Second, comparisons with the other ISoS centers show that while Sofia subjects have the worst outcome on both symptom dimensions and social disability, the latter is not as pronounced a difference.

Living Arrangements

In comparison with their counterparts in other ISoS cohorts, Sofia subjects tended to live more often with their families than subjects in Western centers, but less often when compared with Asian and Latin American centers. Very few subjects were living in supervised psychiatric institutions. The anomalous nature of this finding is indicated by the high rates of severe psychiatric symptoms in our sample. Our results suggest not only that kinship ties remain strong in Bulgaria, but also that families are often very much involved in the care and support of subjects with severe mental illness (Ganev, Onchev, and Ivanov, 1998). Families are a substitute for custodial care for 14 out of the 40 subjects not admitted to supervised institutions in the past 2 years of the follow-up period.

Treatment

Our data on medication use are quite in accord with the other ISoS centers: Sofia subjects had relatively high levels of neuroleptic intake. This finding agrees with the high levels of symptom severity in our sample. However, the other measure for treatment status reported here (frequency and duration of hospital admissions) stands rather apart: Sofia subjects had shorter hospital stays than expected upon comparison with the other centers (and particularly when one takes into account the high level of psychiatric symptomatology).

To judge from data on hospitalizations and use of neuroleptics, treatment had a tendency to become less intensive with time, a finding similar to the results of other studies (e.g., Eaton et al., 1992). All subjects were taking neuroleptics at some point in the follow-up period, and 60% of the subjects were on neuroleptics for most of the entire period. Only 22.2% of the subjects had not received neuroleptics during the last 2 years of follow-up. Sofia subjects were likely to have spent significantly less time in supervised residences than subjects in western centers, differences that cannot be explained by symptom severity and treatment availability. Time spent in hospitals has shown great variability across studies (e.g., Bland et al., 1976; Leon, 1989), possibly at least partly determined by local psychiatric practice and by cultural differences.

Family Involvement

Several findings can be interpreted as supporting the high degree of involvement of subjects' families in coping with mental illness. The first suggestion of this was the experience gained when contacting subjects via their relatives. On a number of occasions, we encountered strong resistance from relatives, and five subjects were not traced or interviewed because their families prevented us from doing so. Another characteristic of our sample is the high frequency of living with family as compared with Western centers; the latter usually had subjects living in supervised residences.

Families provided a substitute for custodial care for more than a third of the Sofia subjects. Correspondingly, the frequency and duration of hospitalizations are much lower than expected. The explanation that access to specialized care is the reason for the low hospitalization rates is not very likely: The catchment area of the study is a region with available psychiatric beds, and the high levels of neuroleptics prescribed by psychiatrists suggest that subjects have had access to specialists' consultations. A more plausible explanation is that kinship ties and obligations are much more important in Bulgaria than in other Western countries. One can speculate that cultural factors play an important role in developing conceptions of mental illness and in ways to cope with it. Possible avenues for exploration are studies of culture-specific beliefs and their influence on the coping mechanisms of patients and their families and of their influence in the development of mental health care systems and institutions and on the practice of specialists.

Predicting Long-Term Outcome

An attempt was made to predict long-term outcome by mode of illness onset, short-term course of illness, and diagnostic category. Mode of onset turned out to be the most robust predictor variable. Roughly the same number of patients had experienced acute, subacute, and insidious illness onset. Two-thirds of the acute onset subgroup and just one (7%) of the insidious onset subgroup had no psychotic symptoms in the last 2 years of follow-up. The large majority of the subjects of the insidious illness onset subgroup had continuous psychotic symptoms at follow-up. None of the subjects with an insidious illness onset and half of the subjects with an acute illness onset had excellent/good social adjustment at outcome. Half of the insidious onset subgroup and one (6%) of the acute onset subgroup had very poor social adjustment at outcome.

Acknowledgment This study was supported in part by a grant from the National Research Fund, Bulgaria.

References

Beshkov, N., & Gerdjikov, I. (1996), Diagnostic structure in inpatient psychiatric settings. *Bull. Bulgar. Psychiatric Assn.*, 1:4–13. (In Bulgarian)

Bland, R. C., Parker, J. H., & Orn, H. (1976), Prognosis in schizophrenia. A 10-year follow-up of first admissions. *Arch. Gen. Psychiatry*, 33:949–954.

Ciompi, L. (1980), The natural history of schizophrenia in the long-term. *Brit. J. Psychiatry*, 136:413–420.

Cutting, J. (1986), Outcome in schizophrenia: Overview. In: *Contemporary Issues in Schizophrenia*, ed. T. A. Kerr & R. P. Snaith. Washington, DC: American Psychiatric Press, pp. 433–440.

Eaton, W. W., Bilker, W., Haro, J. M., Herrman, H., Mortensen, P. B., Freeman, H., & Burgess, P. (1992), Long-term of hospitalization for schizophrenia: Part II. Change with passage of time. *Schizophr. Bull.*, 18: 229–241.

Ganev, K., Onchev, G., & Ivanov, P. (1998), A 16-year follow-up study of schizophrenia and related disorders in Sophia, Bulgaria. *Acta Psychiatr. Scand.*, 98:200–207.

Gross, G., & Huber, G. (1986), Classification and prognosis of schizophrenic disorders in light of the Bonn follow-up studies. *Psychopathology*, 19(1):50–59.

Huber, G., Gross, G., Schutter, R., & Linz, M. (1980), Longitudinal studies of schizophrenic patients. *Schizophr. Bull.*, 6(4):592–605.

Leon, C. (1989), Clinical course and outcome of schizophrenia in Cali, Colombia. A 10-year follow-up study. *J. Nerv. & Ment. Dis.*, 177(10):593–606.

World Health Organization (1994), *The ICD-10 Classification of Mental and Behavioral Disorder: Conversion Tables between ICD-8, ICD-9 and ICD-10*. Geneva: World Health Organization.

RETROSPECTIVE ANALYSIS (RA)/INVITED CENTERS

R. Thara

Although previous WHO coordinated studies (IPSS, DOSMeD, and RAPyD) encompassed a range of cultural and service settings, it was decided to strengthen the cultural diversity of ISoS by inviting three additional centers to join the study: Beijing, Hong Kong, and Chennai (Madras). These Retrospective Analysis (RA) centers had either incidence or prevalence cohorts comparable to those which had been identified in other studies, or local conditions that allowed for backward case-finding to construct a sample to be followed up using ISoS methodology. The sites were also chosen because they had at least a measure of experience with standardized assessments and epidemiological field methods.

The Beijing sample was a population-based cohort of prevalent cases originally identified in a 12-area China follow-up. This study, carried out in 1982 by the Beijing WHO Collaborating Centre for Mental Health Research and Training, was the first national epidemiological survey ever conducted in China. PSE-based data (with ICD-9 diagnoses) were generated on a large and representative population-based sample.

Hong Kong's rapid economic development over the past two decades was of special interest for the ISoS. Investigators in the Department of Psychiatry, University of Hong Kong, and Queen Mary Hospital screened all first episode cases of schizophrenia presenting between 1977 and 1978 in three treatment centers. They generated their ISoS sample by randomly selecting 100 cases.

The third invited center was the Schizophrenia Research Foundation (SCARF) in Chennai, India, a nongovernmental organization devoted to schizophrenia research, rehabilitation, and care. The original sample consisted of 100 consecutive patients (90% of whom were first episode), who attended the psychiatry department between 1981 and 1982 and who fulfilled modified Feighner and ICD-9 criteria. The PSE and other semistandardized assessments were used at intake and at the end of each year of follow-up. Ten-year assessments had already been carried out in a collaborative study with Johns Hopkins University, Baltimore, United States. This study has been one of the few prospectively conducted long-term studies of schizophrenia from this part of the world; 10-year follow-up data suggested better outcomes compared with those in "developed" settings. Female sex predicted better outcome at 5 years, but this effect was lost at 10-year follow-up when the investigators reported improving occupational functioning in men.

Clearly, comparisons among the three invited centers should be interpreted with considerable caution given the variation in case selection, but the standardization of follow-up procedures and outcome measures allows these data to contribute meaningfully to the ISoS data set.

Chapter 21

RA: Beijing, China

Changhui Chen and Yucun Shen

China, the largest developing country in the world, is now experiencing rapid change in its socioeconomic system as well as in the structure of its families and communities. These changes increase social and psychological stress and cannot but influence the mental health of individuals, possibly increasing the incidence and prevalence of mental disorders.

EPIDEMIOLOGY

Epidemiological surveys of mental disorders carried out by Chinese psychiatrists in the 1950s, 1970s, 1980s, and 1990s indicate that schizophrenia has the highest prevalence rate of all major mental disorders (Chen and Xu, 1995) including all psychoses, drug and alcohol dependencies, personality disorders, and mental retardation. Furthermore, over time, there seems to be an increasing trend in the schizophrenia prevalence rate from 0.77 to 1.13 per 1000 in the 1950s to 0.92 to 4.60 per 1000 in the 1970s, and from 5.69 per 1000 in 1982 to 6.55 per 1000 in 1993 (Chen, Zhang, and Shen, 1986a; Chen and Xu, 1995). This disorder thus merits top priority for researchers.

In the late 1950s, a door-to-door investigation of major mental disorders done by psychiatrists in various cities found a total prevalence rate for mental disorders of 1.27 to 2.82 per 1000 (Chen and Xu, 1995). These data were then used by the Health Administration as the basis of a national development plan for psychiatric institutions, professional training, and education programs.

In the mid- and late 1970s, epidemiological studies of mental disorders with large samples carried out in a majority of provinces and cities revealed a total prevalence rate for mental disorders of 6.7 to 15.6 per 1000 for urban areas and 3.2 to 16.9 per 1000 for rural areas. Of this total rate, schizophrenia ranged from 1.56 to 4.6 per 1000, manic-depressive disorder ranged from 0.002 to 0.17 per 1000, and mental retardation ranged from 1.08 to 5.0 per 1000. These results served as the basis for a national plan of prevention and treatment of mental disorders. Though the investigations in the 1970s were based on more reliable methodology, such as case-finding by various information sources in communities, comparability across studies was still very low; there were no standardized diagnostic criteria for mental disorders, no uniform definitions of mental disorders, and no uniform survey methodology with which these studies were carried out.

At the end of the 1970s and throughout the 1980s, following the inauguration of a policy of reform in China and openness toward the outside world, international exchanges were actively carried out, strongly promoting the development of psychiatric epidemiology. In June 1980, the first national seminar on epidemiological psychiatry was organized by WHO and held in Beijing with four visiting experts: E. Strömgren (Aarhus, Denmark), N. Sartorius (WHO, Geneva), A. Jablensky (WHO, Geneva), and J. E. Cooper (Nottingham, U.K.). In June 1981, a workshop on epidemiological survey methodology was also held in Beijing and attended by the heads of the 12 centers from 12 provinces and municipalities (Shen, Chen, and Zhang, 1986), who would carry out, in 1982, the first national epidemiological survey of mental disorders in China organized by the Institute of Mental Health, Beijing Medical University (WHO/Beijing Collaborating Center for Research and Training in Mental Health), and the Shanghai Mental Health Institute (WHO/Shanghai Collaborating Center for Research and Training in Mental Health). To date, it is the largest such study in the world (Cooper and Sartorius, 1996).

In addition to providing baseline data on the distribution of mental disorders in both urban and rural areas in China, this national survey introduced, in a practical way, some modern epidemiological ideas and applicable methods into the mainstream of psychiatry. In doing so, it also enhanced the comparability of Chinese epidemiological results with those of other countries. The practical experiences gained in this national survey soon bore fruit. More than 80 cities in 22 provinces subsequently carried out a wide range of studies on mental disorders including alcohol dependence, dementia, koro, drug abuse, and hyperactivity in children.

Psychiatrists from the Chinese mainland did not have the opportunity to participate in the IPSS. However, the results of the first national psychiatric epidemiological survey in China are comparable to IPSS data from other countries because the principal instruments (PSE-9, Social Disability Screening Schedule [SDSS], and ICD-9) and the procedures followed were similar to those employed in the IPSS. With regard to schizophrenia, the prevalence rate in IPSS was even higher than the rates found in Chinese psychiatric epidemiological studies.

Urban/Rural Differences

In 11 papers from the 1980s, the prevalence rate of schizophrenia in urban areas was reported as 3.15 to 6.92/1000, which was higher than that in rural areas (0.97–5.46/1000), except in Xinjian where it was reported that the rate in the rural area (2.8/1000) was much higher than that in the urban area (1.76/1000). A similar trend was also reported in the papers from the 1970s describing large sample size investigations (Chen and Xu, 1995).

Gender Differences

In most of the papers from the 1970s, the prevalence rate of schizophrenia for females (1.44–5.7/1000) was higher than that for males (1.2–4.73/1000). However, one report found a contrary result: The rate for males (2.68/1000) was higher than that for females (1.44/1000) (Li and Shen, 1982). Additionally, the report of a multiple stepwise regression analysis of factors contributing to a good prognosis of schizophrenia found that the first three contributing factors were the availability of family care, fewer relapses, and effective medication (Li, Chen, and Zhang, 1987).

Two retrospective studies, in Shanghai (Liu, Li, Wang, Ju, and Zue, 1980) and in Sichun (Liu, Huang, Zhang, Zhang, and Hu, 1980), with a survey period of 10 years or more, reported annual average incidence rates of 0.22/1000 (0.14–0.33/1000) and 0.35/1000 (0.24–0.49/1000), respectively. A prospective study on the incidence rate of schizophrenia from 1975 to 1981 in Beijing's rural communities, where the Institute of Mental Health, Beijing Medical University, has had a community mental health program since 1974, reported an annual average incidence rate of 0.11/1000 (0.07–0.16/1000) (Chen et al., 1984). Differences among the incidence rates reported may possibly stem from variation in the methodologies applied in the various studies.

Building upon the baseline data from the first national epidemiological survey of mental disorders in 12 areas in 1982, a follow-up study, the second epidemiological survey of mental disorders, was carried out in 1993 in seven of the original 12 areas surveyed in 1982: Beijing, Daqing, Hunan, Jiling, Liaoning, Nanjing, and Shanghai (Zhang et al., 1998; Chen et al., 1998). This study yielded valuable data on the long-term course of severe mental disorders in China, especially schizophrenia. Since the 1993 survey used the same methods as the 1982 survey, the data were highly comparable. The results of the 1993 survey showed that schizophrenia had a lifetime prevalence rate of 6.55 per 1000, slightly higher than that originally reported for these seven areas in the 1982 survey (5.65/1000) (Zhang et al., 1998; Chen et al., 1998), though the difference was not statistically significant. This trend holds when a comparison is made between urban and rural areas and between males and females. However, when the data are standardized with the data of the 1982 census and compared by individual areas, one of the seven areas had a very significantly higher rate in 1993 than in 1982 ($p < .0001$). Increases were found in the mean age of the patients and in the number of patients with either a course over 10 years or age 60+ years. The increase in life expectancy in the prior 11 years, a benefit of the significant improvement in health services, may contribute to the increase in the lifetime prevalence rate of schizophrenia.

ISoS is a naturalistic, longitudinal follow-up study that rests upon previous WHO-coordinated epidemiological surveys carried out by collaborating centers from different countries. Since China was not involved in any of them, Beijing's ISoS program, which includes eight urban centers, is based on the 1982 national epidemiological survey of mental disorders (Shen, 1986; Chen, Zhang, and Shen, 1986a,b; Shen, Chen, and Zhang, 1986).

Cultural Context

The cultural context of the eight urban areas chosen for ISoS is very similar, so that the following description of west Beijing is generally applicable to all. Because of reforms and open policies initiated in 1978, collective enterprises, individual businesses, and domestic-foreign joint investment ventures are flourishing. Most people, however, are employed by state-owned enterprises or by administrative bodies and live on their own wages or on retirement pensions. Area leaders usually come from the lower administrative levels of agencies-enterprises and from professional ranks. The area provides sufficient conveniences for people's daily lives so that the population is significantly increasing. Migrant laborers from rural areas flow in and serve as housekeepers, run stores, or become street peddlers. In the last decade, economic crime has increased significantly. Women and men are equal in society and must have equal opportunities for employment, but businesses prefer employing male over female graduates. Even though a woman is employed, she generally also has more housekeeping and child care responsibility, as well as more kinship obligations, than a man. The Han nationality accounts for the majority of the population, followed by Hui and Man minorities. People have their choice of religion, but no church has yet been established locally in this area of Beijing.

Typically, resident families are nuclear; however, steady increases in life expectancy have resulted in more aged people in families. As average income has increased, the living conditions of most people have improved significantly. In these urban areas, education is compulsory until age 16, and most children complete their junior middle school course. In the last decade, alcohol dependence has increased.

People who are employed view time in strictly linear fashion, seeing the rushed pace of everyday life, while the retired elderly, by contrast, view time in cyclical fashion without time-pressure, seeing the relaxed pace of daily life. A majority of people believe that death means the end of life; however, some aged and poorly educated people may still believe that doing good for others when alive will be rewarded in future life.

Persons with mental illness are generally cared for by family members, usually with support from their relatives, friends, and colleagues. Most people recognize that the suffering of mentally ill people is not preordained but is mainly caused by negative sociopsychological stress. Prevention and alleviation of suffering through modern medicine is stressed; however, a few may believe that mental illness is related to spirit possession. Madness is generally viewed as a disorder, but most people regard such suffering as shameful, and worry that sufferers will be looked down upon or will lose their jobs. Many, particularly the young and their families, would prefer that no one know of their illness.

THE MENTAL HEALTH SYSTEM IN THE EIGHT AREAS

In recent years, the mental health policy developed by the government has been favorable to mentally ill persons, stressing prevention first, then early identification and early treatment with rehabilitation. A new law safeguarding handicapped persons includes mentally disabled persons. Psychiatric or psychotherapy/psychological counseling units have been set up in general hospitals. In addition, those with severe mental disabilities are expected to continue receiving services at no charge, while those with mild disabilities are provided with an appropriate work opportunity. Unfortunately, the practical implementation of this policy varies depending upon economic conditions in the government or collective agencies where the patients are employed.

In the surveyed area in Beijing, for example, there are five general hospitals, one with a psychiatric unit, and one psychiatric hospital with 100 beds, the Institute of Mental Health Care of the Western Urban District. Additionally, Beijing Municipal Institute of Mental Health Care supervises a system of community mental health services and home-beds which provides medication and/or rehabilitation in the home and regular visits by primary health workers. In general, mental health services are more available today in this area as well as in other cities than they were 15 years ago. For example, there are community-based psychiatric rehabilitation services in Shanghai including psychiatric clinics in primary general hospitals, "guardianship networks" operated by nonprofessional volunteers, and work therapy stations promoting rehabilitation and preventing psychosocial deterioration of mental patients.

Several models of payment for mental health services coexist: payment by government, partial payment by government or collective agency (employer), private payment, and a combination of the three resources. For patients with transient financial difficulties, some subsidy is available from the employer. For patients with low income or without relatives, the local administration either provides the necessary social support or sends them to social welfare institutions. It is much the same for the seven other areas surveyed.

CENTERS AND STUDY AREAS

The Chinese ISoS study team includes 20 psychiatrists from eight participating psychiatric institutions and study centers (Shen and Wang, 1985).

1. Beijing

Institute of Mental Health, Beijing Medical University—General sponsor: Professor Yucun Shen; Professors Changhui Chen, principal investigator, Zhang Weixi, and Li Shuren. Designated a WHO Collaborating Center in 1982, the Institute of Mental Health, Beijing Medical University, with research departments in biological and social psychiatry, coordinated ISoS in China; three professors of psychiatric epidemiology were the principal investigators for the national epidemiological surveys of mental disorders in 1982 and in 1993. Beijing, the capital of China, is the nation's political, cultural, and communication center, one of the world's famous ancient cities but one which has been notably modernized. Urban area: a section of the west part of Beijing containing some of the oldest residential areas, with 33 neighborhood committees. Commerce, service, and a few industrial plants are the essential economic activities (population 82,992).

2. Shanghai

Shanghai Mental Health Institute, since 1982, a WHO/Shanghai Collaborating Center for Research and Training in Mental Health—Drs. Qu Gangya and Meng Guorong, chief investigator. Shanghai, regarded as a socially, economically, and industrially well-developed city with only 7% illiteracy, is also one of the biggest cities in the world with a population of about 12 million. Urban area: two communities in the southwest of the city, including an area noted for religious groups with strong local traditions of stability (population 106,900).

3. Nanjing

Brain Hospital of Nanjing—Drs. Luo Kailin, Zhang Zhongying, chief investigator, and Ying Zhifeng. Nanjing, the capital of Jianshu Province, a large city of about 3 million people in the mid-southeast of China, is in a region of hills, lakes, and rivers bordering the Yangtse River. Urban area: three streets in the northwest of the city (population 111,281).

4. Shenyang

The Office of Prevention and Cure of Mental Disorders—Drs. Zai Zhiping, chief investigator, and Liu Guangzhi (Liaoning Provincial Psychiatric Hospital). Shenyang, the Capital of Liaoning Province, is a large industrial city of about 4 million people some 500 km northeast of Beijing, with agricultural surroundings noted for the production of ginseng. Urban area: four streets of the city (population 126,190).

5. Siping

Psychiatric Hospital of Jiling Province—Dr. Zhai Zhibin, chief investigator. Siping, a medium-sized and newly developing industrial city of Jiling Province in the northeastern part of China, is situated on the edge of a fertile plain sometimes referred to as the "granary" of China. Urban area: four streets of Siping city (population 106,286).

6. Daqing

The Third Hospital of Daqing City—Drs. Wang Jingrong and Wang Deping, chief investigators. Daqing is a new city in the northeast of China developed to exploit oil. Many of the population are, therefore, recent immigrants but not predominantly from any particular location. The rural surroundings are flat and only moderately prosperous; the whole area is noted for its long and very cold winters. Urban area: a southern section of Daqing occupied by drilling and oil exploration company employees containing six street agencies (population 102,293).

7. Changsha

Psychiatric Hospital of Hunan Province—Drs. Tu Jian, chief investigator, and Cao Huaguang. Changsha, the capital of Hunan Province, is a medium-sized city in the midsouthern part of China of considerable historical and political importance. Urban area: five streets in the western part of Changsha (population 90,744).

8. Chengdu

Department of Psychiatry, The West China University of Medical Sciences—Professors Xiang Mengze, Guo Lanting, chief investigator, and Drs. Wang Guangxin and Liu Guoqing. Chengdu, the capital of Sichuan Province, is a large city of about 2 million people in the western part of China, at the foot of the mountainous plateau of central Asia. It has been an important trading and political center for more than 2000 years. Urban area: the area of the central street leading from the city center to the suburbs (population 82,540).

METHODS

Defining the ISoS Cohort

In the 1982 survey, five criteria defined the study areas (Shen and Wang, 1985): (1) relatively stable population; (2) no major economic and/or cultural changes in the last few years; (3) population mainly of Han origin (as Han nationality accounts for 94% of the population, bias that might have resulted from more diverse sociocultural backgrounds was avoided); (4) well-developed community organizations and adequate mental health services; and (5) total population of at least 80,000 to 100,000 to provide an adequate sampling frame. Each study center had to be able to include a rural and an urban sample, each of 500 households. Patients residing in acute or long-stay psychiatric hospitals or wards were also included in this survey. For urban area sampling, neighborhood committees were used as the primary sampling unit. From all the neighborhood committees in each study area, 10 were selected as being of typical socioeconomic status for that area. A random sample of 50 families was then taken from each of these selected neighborhood committees, resulting in 500 households from each urban area.

The screening schedule for psychosis, which was used for the key informant interview, was filled in after discussions with heads of the local administration, public security officers, the public health unit, and neighborhood and village leaders, as well as with the heads of all the households comprising the survey sample. A family member of those subjects with scores of 2 or more on the screening schedule for psychosis was questioned about the subject's history. The interviewer entered the information into a history record, and the subject was assessed with the PSE-9 and diagnosed using ICD-9 criteria. The following four general requirements for defining a current case had to be met before a diagnosis could be made: (1) Symptoms as specified for each diagnostic category had to be present; (2) symptoms had to be sufficiently marked as to have a detectable effect upon some aspect of the subject's life such as everyday activities, performance at work, or academic achievements; (3) these effects must have been detectable for a significant length of time, as specified for schizophrenia; and (4) none of the exclusion criteria listed for schizophrenia was applicable. At the same time, 10% of all those over the age of 15 who had negative scores on the Psychosis Screening Schedule were interviewed with the PSE-9 in order to check for false negative cases. The survey diagnosis, given to each subject by the study area teams, was a consensus diagnosis, arrived at by the team after discussion of all the survey information.

In 1994, the ISoS cohort was defined as those persons living in the eight urban communities who were diagnosed with schizophrenia in the first national epidemiological survey of mental disorders in 1982, a total of 89 patients.

Use of Study Instruments

In March 1992, principal investigators from the eight centers attended a course in Beijing given by Drs. Glynn Harrison from the United Kingdom and Lee Wing Ho Peter from Hong Kong on the application of the 13 ISoS field survey instruments. After the final versions of the instruments were received on May 20, 1993, a process of translation into Chinese and back-translation into English and rechecking was implemented. The schedules were then printed in a handbook for field investigators. In September 1993, eight field investigators, one from each center, gathered in Beijing for more training to ensure reliability among the eight Chinese centers. The training covered 11 instruments (BIS, PSE-9, SAS, DAS, LCS, BII, FIS, PIRS, SANS, BRS, and DSS), and assessments were performed on 10 schizophrenic patients. Of the 691 items in the instruments, 665 items (96.2%) were higher than 0.7 on both ICC and pairwise agreement rates. The remaining 26 items below 0.7 were rechecked, item by item, and necessary steps for improvement were suggested. For the intercenter reliability assessment, the principal investigator, Professor Changhui Chen Institute of Mental Health, Beijing Medical University, rated the videotaped interviews from the United Kingdom, Hong Kong, and India; her scores were sent to WHO. Two background Information Schedules, Local Area Profile Schedule and Mental Health Treatment System Survey, were completed for each of the eight areas.

Data-Gathering Procedures

Using information from historical records of the 1982 survey, the neighborhood committee where the patient had been living was asked for a current address. Then, investigators made contact with a family member. If a formal consent was given by the subject, investigators went to interview the subject and an informant. At the same time, the 1982 case record of the patient was carefully read as a reference.

STUDY RESULTS: BASELINE AND EARLY FOLLOW-UP

In 1982, 89 cases in the eight urban areas were diagnosed with schizophrenia using ICD-9. In 1994, of these 89 cases, 58 were alive, 20 were dead, and 11 were lost, one because of a changed diagnosis from schizophrenia to depression.

Gender and Age

In the original cohort of 89 schizophrenic patients, there was an almost equal number of men (45) and women (44); in 1994 at the start of ISoS, the alive follow-up cohort had an equal number of men (29) and women (29). Age distribution at follow-up was not significantly different from that at entry. The mean birth year for the alive cohort was 1942, while that for everyone at entry was 1940. No differences in gender or age for the alive cohort are found when compared with the entire cohort at entry in 1982.

Mode of Onset and Diagnosis

Sixty-nine percent of the alive cohort of 58 had an insidious onset of schizophrenia, and 29% had either subacute (25.9%) or acute/sudden (3.4%) onset and one (1.7%) unknown. Similarly, 73% of the total 89 patients had insidious onset, and 26% had subacute or acute/sudden onset. Using the conversion of baseline ICD-9 to ICD-10 diagnoses, all 58 of the alive cohort are classified with schizophrenia.

TABLE 21.1 Severity of Symptoms (Bleuler) for Dead and Lost Cohorts[a]

		Dead		*Lost*	
		N	%	N	%
Available	Bleuler: Severity of Psychotic Symptoms				
	1. Severe	12	60.0	6	75.0
	2. Moderate	8	40.0	1	12.5
	3. Mild	0	0.0	0	0.0
	4. Recovered	0	0.0	1	12.5
Missing	Not supplied	0	—	1	—
	9. Unknown	0	—	2	—
Available		20	100.0	8	72.7
Missing		0	0.0	3	27.3
Total		20	100.0	11	100.0

[a] For the dead and lost-to-follow-up cohorts, the severity of symptoms is rated in the period for which information is available. The rating best describes most of the period.

Severity of Symptoms

Of the 31 subjects who had died (20) or were lost to follow-up (11), Bleuler ratings were possible for 20 of the dead and 8 of the lost (Table 21.1). All the dead were assessed with severe or moderate symptoms; while 87.5% of the lost were assessed with such symptoms. One of the 8 lost (12.5%) was assessed as having recovered.

Early Follow-Up

No 1- or 5-year follow-up studies were conducted.

ALIVE SUBJECTS

Symptomatology

Rating by the Bleuler scale showed that of the 58 in the alive cohort, 37.9% had recovered, 44.9% suffered mildly or moderately from symptoms, and 17.2% had severe symptomatology. Overall ratings of the alive cohort appear to be better than those who were dead or lost to follow-up (so far as they can be compared). Measured by the Global Assessment of Functioning Scale for Symptomatology (GAF-S) in the past month, almost half (48.2%) of the 58 subjects had no significant symptoms or only mild symptoms (score > 60). Fewer than one-third (29.2%) suffered from serious symptoms (score < 51). In this respect, Beijing cohort subjects were slightly worse than the total Invited subsample, GAF-S mean scores 59.7 (SD=23.6) vs. 64.8 (SD=22.8). By gender, 55.1% of men had no significant or only mild symptoms (score > 60), much better than women (41.3%); while 31% of men suffered from severe symptoms (score < 51), slightly worse than women (27.4%). The GAF-S mean scores show a similar trend: Men had a higher mean (61.8) than women (57.6). Comparable figures of the total Invited subsample show a more favorable outcome (mean scores: 63.4 for men and 66.3 for women). For GAF-S assessment by mode of onset, there is a pattern of decreasing mean score among the three modes of onset: 82.5 for acute onset (up to 1 week; N=2), 71.5 for subacute onset (up to 1 month; N=15), and 53.4 for insidious onset (greater than 1 month; N=40), indicating the more acute onset, the more favorable the outcome. However, no such pattern is found in the total Invited subsample.

Time Trend

The trend of psychotic symptoms shows that 8.6% of the 58 alive subjects had prominent psychotic symptoms in all three periods, compared with 3.9% for the total Invited subsample. For 19%, such symptoms were never prominent, as compared with 6.8% for the total Invited subsample. For 48.3% of the 58 subjects, the overall time trend was much better or somewhat better, while for 25.9%, it was somewhat worse or worse. However, the eight subjects (13.8%) listed as "other" in the Beijing sample were, in fact, recovered at the time of the follow-up interview. Their scores on both GAF-S and Global Assessment of Functioning-Disability (GAF-D) were 83 to 90 (mean score=89). Therefore, improvement in the Beijing sample is 62.1% (48.3%+13.8%), higher than that for the Invited subsample as a whole (56.8%). Including the recovered cases in "other," rather than in "much better," was a question of judgment; "recovery," as seen in clinical practice, means that the patient has returned to normal, quite different from "much better." For overall time trend by gender, 41.3% of the men and 55.2% of the women had improved, while 27.5% of men and 24.1% of the women were worsening. Comparable figures of the total Invited subsample also show a favorable outcome for women (improvement: 50% of men vs. 63.5% of women and worsening: 25% of men vs. 16.3% of women).

Course of the Illness

In the last 2 years of follow-up, 34.5% of the 58 subjects had no psychotic episode; 51.7% were continuously psychotic; and 6.9% were classified as episodic. Compared with figures for the total Invited subsample, the percentage of no psychotic episodes in the 58 subjects is lower (34.5% vs. 47.5%), while the percentage of continuously psychotic is higher (51.7% vs. 33.8%). For the course of illness over the entire period, there seems to be a different pattern: In the 58 subjects, the figures for no psychotic episodes and of continuously psychotic are 19 and 50%, respectively, higher than the corresponding figures in the total Invited subsample (5.9% and 26.7%, respectively). With respect to course type by gender, 38% of men had no psychotic episodes and 48% were continuously psychotic over the past 2 years, both slightly better than that of women (31 and 55%, respectively).

Reevaluation of Baseline Diagnosis

Reevaluation of clinical status at baseline showed all 58 alive subjects to be diagnosed with schizophrenia using either ICD-9 or ICD-10, almost the same diagnosis distribution as in the 89-person entry cohort.

Residential and Functional Status

In the last month of follow-up, most subjects (81.0%) were living with their families, but a few were living on their own (6.9%). Only 10.3% were in the hospital, and 1.7% lived in a supervised residence. The residential pattern is similar to that of the total Invited subsample. In the past 2 years, the residential trend was rather stable: 91.4% were in independent living, very similar to that of the total Invited subsample (94.2%). For those in independent living >12 months, the figures were 89.7% of the former against 92.2% of the latter. By gender, data show an almost equal average number of months of independent living for men and for women (23.0 months vs. 23.9 months). In the entire period, nearly 95% (55 subjects) of the alive cohort had ever been in independent living situations in the community. For those 55 subjects, 7.3% lived independently in the community for some time (<50%), and 12.7% managed to do so for over half of the period (but less than 90%), while 80% did so for more than 90% of the time. In this respect, women did better (mean=95.2) than men (mean=89.0), although the effect was not pronounced in the Invited subsample.

Homelessness and Jail

One female has been homeless, but no one has been in jail in the most recent 2 years. Over the course of the entire follow-up period, only that one woman had been homeless, and only one man had been in jail. These low rates were similar in the other Invited centers. Historically in China, cultural tradition decrees that a patient with a long-term disabling mental condition be cared for by family who provide him or her with the essentials of daily life, including medication, and prevent the patient from leaving the family home. This may be the reason why there are so few homeless persons with schizophrenia in China.

Social Disability

In the GAF-D measurements for overall social functioning in the past month, 39.6% had scores lower than 51, indicating serious impairment in social functioning, slightly worse than the total Invited subsample (32.7%). At the time, 32.8% scored higher than 80 on the GAF-D, indicating good functioning, slightly better than the total Invited subsample (28.8%). By gender, 37.9% of men scored lower than 51, somewhat less than the 41.3% of women with such scores; 34.5% of men scored lower than 51, somewhat less than the 41.3% of women with such scores; 34.5% of men scored higher than 80 (compared with 31% of women), indicating that social functioning of men is better than women (mean=62.9 for men vs. mean=58.3 for women). By contrast, in the Invited subsample as a whole, female subjects scored better with regard to social functioning than did males (means of 63.3 and 61.3, respectively). By mode of onset, there is a pattern of decrease in mean score among the three modes of onset: 82.5 for acute onset (up to 1 week), 73.8 for subacute onset (up to 1 month), and 53.8 for insidious onset (greater than 1 month), indicating that more acute onset is associated with more favorable social functioning; however, no such pattern is found in the Invited subsample as a whole. To describe trend of disability, the entire follow-up period was divided into three parts. In all thirds, 6.9% of the alive cohort had prominent disabilities; and in the middle and most recent thirds, 5.2% had prominent disabilities; while 51.7% had prominent disabilities for the first third. Almost one-fifth (19%) experienced no time-specific prominent disabilities.

Work

Of the alive cohort, 27.6% (11 men, 5 women) had worked at paid jobs at some point in the last 2 years of follow-up; most of them (68.8%) did so for at least 12 months. For those working full-time and more than 12 months, performance was judged as good to very good. A large percentage of subjects in the total Invited subsample was employed (44%), the majority of them (73.6%) working for at least 12 months. In the total Invited subsample, 90% of those working full-time and more than 12 months were judged as having good to very good performance. Additionally, 34.5% of the cohort (vs. 31.7% of the total Invited) was engaged in full-time household work, and 78% of those performing household work for the entire 2 years were rated as having good to very good performance. In the last 2 years, 41.4% were retired (22 cases retired more than 12 months, and two cases retired less than 12 months). More women were retired than men (45 vs. 38%). Fewer than one-fifth of the alive subjects (19%) were receiving a disability pension, and most of them (91%) for more than 12 months.

Violence

Of the 58 follow-up subjects, 19% (4 men, 7 women) had been involved in assaults on other people in the last 2 years of follow-up, resulting in only mild harm by seven subjects and moderate injury by four subjects. Over the entire period, 32.8% (12 men, 7 women) had been involved in assaults on other people, resulting in mild harm by 11 cases (57.9%, 7 men and 4 women), moderate injury by seven cases (36.8%, 4 men and 3 women), and severe injury by one man (5.3%). Assault rates are slightly higher than the total Invited subsample (12.2% in the past 2 years: 11.1% of men vs. 13.3% of women, and 28.5% in the entire period).

Only one man (1.7% of the 58 subjects) attempted suicide in the past 2 years, and six subjects (10.3%, 5 men and 1 woman) attempted suicide in the entire period. Suicide rates are slightly lower than those for the Invited subsample as a whole (3.9% in the last 2 years and 13.9% in the entire period).

Treatment Status—Medications

In the last 2 years, 32.8% of the 58 subjects had been prescribed neuroleptics at some time, 37.9% for most of the time, and 29.3% had taken no neuroleptics. In the entire period, 51.7% of the 58 subjects had been on medication at some time; 39.7% for most of the entire period; and 8.6% had no neuroleptics. Both in the last 2 years and in the entire period, figures for medication for most of the time are lower than for the total Invited subsample. Of those taking no medication in the past 2 years, six subjects had recovered; four subjects were viewed by their families as having no need for continuous medication since they were able to do some work; five subjects without insight stopped medication by themselves; and two had no resources for obtaining medication. An examination of time trends reveals three patterns: For 13 subjects (22.4%), medication use was prominent in each third of the follow-up period, while for 35 subjects (60.3%), the use of medication was only prominent in the first third, and for four subjects (6.9%), the use of medication was not prominent in any third.

Hospitalization

In the last 2 years of follow-up, eight subjects (13.8%) had hospital admissions; six patients were in the hospital for more than 12 months; and two patients were in for less than 12 months. For mean hospitalization time by gender, there were six males for 16 months and two females for 24 months. In the entire period, 26 subjects (45%) were admitted at least once to a psychiatric hospital, of whom 16 were men and 10 were women. Comparable figures for the total Invited subsample are 16.1% for the past 2 years and 66% in the entire period. For three subjects (5.2%), hospital admissions were prominent features in each third, 18 subjects (31%) had admissions in the first third, and one subject (1.7%) stayed in a hospital only in the recent third, suggesting a significantly decreasing trend for hospitalization. For percentage of hospitalization time in the entire period, six subjects (10%) were in the hospital less than 5% of the time, and six subjects (10%) were in the hospital more than 50% of the time, quite different from the total Invited subsample (38% and 4%, respectively). Because Beijing results were based on a prevalence sample in the 1982 epidemiological survey of eight urban areas and the hospitalization of patients, they could not but differ from incidence samples from the Invited centers.

Second, social stigma (against mental patients, especially those suffering from schizophrenia) usually drives a family to care for the patient at home, rather than to have a hospitalization, particularly for new onset and young patients. Because of this, the majority of patients in psychiatric institutions usually have severe symptoms and so need longer hospitalization.

Clinical Assessment—PSE-140

The total mean PSE score for 55 subjects assessed completely in 1994 is 16.5, not significantly different from that of 1982 (17.5). However, the percentage of subjects scoring 1 or more for 44 items of PSE (eliminating nonspecific symptoms) decreased in 1994 (Table 21.2), especially for the items of visual hallucinations, preoccupation with delusions and hallucinations, and acting out delusions, suggesting that most of the positive symptoms are somewhat decreased 12 years later. (Note, however, that the original PSEs were administered to a prevalence cohort that was, on average, 13 years into illness course, dating from the emergence of psychotic symptoms. Hence, the two PSEs are assessments of symptoms in the mid- and late stages of the disorder to date, when less discordance might be expected.) Cases with a GAF-D score of good to fairly good functioning (61–90) have a lower PSE mean score, 7.5, than that of those with moderate impairment or worse (1–60) whose mean score is 25.2, showing a close correlation between the two assessments.

Clinical Assessment—DAS

In 1994, 22.2 to 48.1% of 56 patients assessed completely were found with moderate or severe social disability (Table 21.3). A comparison of the data in 1994 with the data collected by SDSS, a similar instrument provided by WHO for the 1982 survey, shows that except for the item of self care which had a higher score, the scores for the remaining seven items were generally lower,

TABLE 21.2 Comparison of the Percent of Subjects Scoring 1 or More in 44 Items of PSE between 1982 and 1994 (N=55)

Number: Item	*1982 %*	*1994 %*
Affect:		
23: Depressed mood	5.3	3.8
27: Morning depression	3.6	1.9
37: Early waking	1.8[a]	11.1[a]
41: Expansive mood	1.8	0.0
42: Ideomotor pressure	1.8	0.0
43: Grandiose ideas and actions	1.8	0.0
Subjective Thought Disorder		
55: Thought insertion	0.0	1.9
56: Thought broadcast	3.6	0.0
57: Thought echo	1.8	0.0
58: Thought withdrawal	3.6	0.0
59: Thoughts being read	7.3	7.4
Hallucinations		
62: Voices in third person	12.7	11.2
63: Voices speaking to subject	14.5	11.2
64: Dissociative hallucinations	1.8	1.9
66: Visual hallucinations	10.9[a]	0.0[a]
68: Olfactory hallucinations	5.4	0.0
69: Delusion of smell	0.0	0.0
70: Other hallucinations	9.1	3.7
Delusions		
49: Delusional mood	7.3	1.9
71: Control	7.2	5.6

Number: Item	*1982 %*	*1994 %*
72: Reference	29.0	22.2
73: Delusional misinterpretation	14.5	13.0
74: Persecution	18.2	31.5
75: Assistance	10.9	1.9
76. Grandiose abilities	7.3	1.9
77: Grandiose identity	3.6	0.0
78: Religious	3.6	0.0
79: Paranormal	1.8	0.0
80: Physical forces	9.1	3.7
81: Alien forces	5.5	1.9
82: Primary delusions	7.3	7.5
83: Subcultural	1.8	0.0
84: Morbid jealousy	10.9	13.0
86: Sexual	0.0	0.0
87: Fantastic	3.6	0.0
88: Guilt	0.0	0.0
89: Appearance	3.6	0.0
90: Depersonalization	0.0	0.0
91: Hypochondriacal	3.6	0.0
92: Catastrophe	0.0	0.0
93: Systematization of delusions	56.3	40.8
94: Evasiveness	20.0	27.9
95: Preoccupation with delusions or hallucinations	70.9[b]	40.8[b]
96: Acting out of delusions	63.6[a]	44.5[a]

[a] $p<0.05$

[b] $p<0.01$

suggesting some improvement in 1994. The total mean scores are 11.3 for DAS in 1994 and 10.0 for SDSS in 1982. In 1994, a very significant difference was found between the mean score of 3.9 for good outcome (GAF-D score ≥ 60) and that of 18.3 for poor outcome (GAF-D score $= 1 < 61$ ($p < 0.0001$), also showing a close correlation between the two assessments.

DECEASED SUBJECTS

At the time of the 12-year follow-up, 20 subjects (10 men, 10 women) were deceased, including two subjects (10%) who committed suicide by drug overdoses (a man, aged 30, and a woman, aged 34, at the time of death). For the 18 who died naturally (9 men and 9 women), 17 subjects died of physical diseases (respiratory, cardio-cerebral-vascular, digestive and urinary systems disorders, and infectious disease) and one died of unknown causes. At the time of their deaths, four (21.1%) were well/in remission, 11 (57.9%) were in partial remission, four (21.1%) were in an episode of illness, and the condition of one case is unknown. Among the 20 dead, the mean age of death is 56.6 years for men and 59 years for women. Of the 20 subjects, 65% died between 1980 and 1989, the other 35% died in the pe-

TABLE 21.3 Disability Scores over Time: Minimum or No Dysfunction vs. Moderate and Severe

	DAS					SDSS				
	1994 (scores 0–5)					1982 (scores 0–2)				
Items	N	*(0–1)%*	N	*(2–5)%*	*8/9**	N	*(0)%*	N	*(1–2)%*	*8/9*
Overall Dysfunctional Behavior										
Social withdrawal	37	66.1	19	33.9		28	50.9	27	49.1	
Self-care	36	64.3	20	35.7		38	69.1	17	30.9	
Dysfunction in Social Roles										
Participation in household activities	34	69.4	15	30.6	7	27	49.1	28	50.9	
Marital/affective	27	73.0	10	27.0	19	32	66.7	16	33.3	7
Marital/sexual	19	63.3	11	36.7	26					
Parental	28	77.8	8	22.2	20	31	63.3	18	36.7	6
Sexual/with others	12	63.2	7	36.8	37					
Social contacts	31	63.3	18	36.7	7	28	51.9	26	48.1	1
Work performance	14	51.9	13	48.1	29	23	44.2	29	55.7	3
Interest in getting job	18	60.0	12	40.0	26					
Information	29	59.2	20	40.8	7	29	52.7	26	47.3	

* 8/9 = Missing or not applicable.

riod 1990 to 1994. The Standardized Mortality Rate (SMR) for the total Beijing cohort is 2.97 (male = 3.37, female = 2.59), higher than that of Chennai (Madras) (total = 1.90, male = 1.73 and female = 2.11), but lower than that of Hong Kong (total = 5.76, male = 7.16 and female = 3.78). The much higher SMR for Hong Kong may be due essentially to the difference in rates of suicide. The comparable figure for suicide of the total Invited subsamples (38%) is much higher than that of the current Chinese deceased cohort (10%).

CONCLUSIONS

The original cohort of 89 persons diagnosed with schizophrenia was assembled in 1982 in eight cities in China. Men and women were equally represented, with an average age at study entry of 42 years for both sexes. Twelve years later, 89% (58 alive, 20 dead and one changed diagnosis) of the original subjects were located; no apparent bias was found with respect to gender, age, mode of onset, or baseline diagnosis for the 58 alive, though the Bleuler scores of the dead or lost cases evaluated by their informants showed much higher deteriorization (combing severe and moderate rankings) than those of the alive cohort. At follow-up, all but one subject received a rediagnosis of schizophrenia (ICD-10); one had a diagnosis change from schizophrenia to depression.

At follow-up, more than one-third of the alive subjects were judged to have recovered (Bleuler), although half still showed evidence of continuous psychotic symptoms during the past 2 years. Just over half of the subjects showed evidence, too, of moderate and severe impairment in social functioning, while one third were rated as good or excellent in their social functioning. Thirty-eight percent of the subjects are currently prescribed neuroleptic medication. The vast majority of subjects were living on their own (i.e., not hospitalized); almost 14% were in a hospital or in a supervised residence during the past 2 years. Only 28% had been employed during those 2 years, but another 31% were engaged in full-time household work. Overall, the course of illness was rated as improving in nearly half.

Gender seems to have some effect on course and/or symptomatology: Women have a more continuous course; and women were more disabled than men.

In 1994, the scores of most items on the PSE and DAS are generally lower than in 1982, suggesting, in general, symptomatic improvement and more favorable social functioning for most subjects 12 years later.

This supports, at least indirectly, the good outcomes in most followed-up subjects suggested by the GAF-S and GAF-D assessments.

Since some significant differences are found among sample sources, the results from the Beijing cohort and those of Hong Kong and Chennai are often not comparable. The results from China were based on an epidemiological follow-up cohort in eight urban communities, while the samples of Hong Kong and Chennai were patients who had come to a clinic. The various sources of sampling would undoubtedly bring about many differences. Taking birth year as an example, the subjects of birth years 1920 to 1939 make up 48.3% of the Beijing alive cohort, but only 12.9% and 1.3% of the Hong Kong and Chennai subjects, respectively. Therefore, care must be exercised when comparison of the results in China are made either with the total Invited subsample or with Hong Kong or Chennai separately.

References

Chen, C. H., Shen, Y. C., Xi, T. M., Tian, Y. H., & Wei, C. S. (1984), Incidence and prevalence rate of schizophrenia in community mental health service from 1975–1981. *Chin. J. Neurol. & Psychiatry*, 17(6):321–324. (In Chinese)

——, ——Zhang, W. X., Li, S. R., Huang, Y. Q., Wang, J. R., Wang, D. P., Tu, J., Ning, Z. X., Fu, L. M., Ji, L. P., Liu, Z. G., Wu, H. M., Luo, K. L., Zhai, S. T., Yan, H. Q., & Meng, G. R. (1998), Epidemiological survey of schizophrenia in seven areas of China. *Chin.J. Neurol. & Psychiatry*, 31(2):72–74. (In Chinese)

——Xu, C. L. (1995), The development of psychiatric epidemiology in China. In: *Overall Development of Modern Neurology and Psychiatry in China*, ed. X. S. Chen & S. H. Chen. Beijing: Chinese Publishing House of Science and Technology, pp. 171–185. (In Chinese)

——Zhang, W. X., & Shen, Y. C. (1986a), Analysis of epidemiological data of schizophrenia. *Chin. J. Neurol. & Psychiatry*, 19(2):73–76. (In Chinese)

——, ——, ——(1986b), Data analysis of an epidemiological study on mental disorders, drug and alcohol dependence and personality disorders. *Chin. J. Neurol. & Psychiatry*, 19(2):70–72. (In Chinese)

Cooper, J. E., & Sartorius, N. (1996), Editors' preface. In: *Mental Disorders in China*, ed. J. E. Cooper & N. Sartorius. London: Gaskell Royal College of Psychiatrists.

Li, C. P., & Shen, Y. C. (1982), Review: Psychiatric epidemiology of some provinces and cities in recent years. *Chin. J. Neurol. & Psychiatry*, 15(2):120–125. (In Chinese)

Li, S. R., Chen, C. H., & Zhang, W. X. (1987), A computer analysis of multiple steps regression for the possible factors contributed to the prognosis of schizophrenia. *Chin. Ment. Health J.*, 1(4):180–182. (In Chinese)

Liu, J. Q., Li, S. L., Wang, C. H., Ju, D. C., & Zue, Y. X. (1980), An epidemiological investigation of mental disorders in Xuhui district of Shanghai. *Chin. J. Neurol. & Psychiatry*, 13(1):1–6. (In Chinese)

Liu, X. H., Huang, M. S., Zhang, R. S., Zhang, Y. P., & Hu, G. C. (1980), An epidemiological survey of psychoses in Sichuan Province. *Chin. J. Neurol. & Psychiatry*, 13(1)7–9. (In Chinese)

Shen, Y. C. (1986), Investigation on the prevalence of various mental disorders and analysis of the data. *Chin. J. Neurol. & Psychiatry*, 19(2):80–82. (In Chinese)

——Chen, C. H., Zhang, W. X. (1986), An epidemiological investigation on mental disorders in 12 regions of China. Methodology and data analysis. *Chin. J. Neurol. & Psychiatry*, 19(2):65–69. (In Chinese)

——Wang, C. H., Eds. (1985), *Manual of Epidemiology of Psychiatric Disorders*. Beijing: People's Publishing House. (In Chinese)

Zhang, W. X., Shen, Y. C., Li, S. R., Chen, C. H., Huang, Y. Q., Wang, J. R., Wang, D. P., Tu, J., Ning, Z. X., Fu, L. M., Ji, L. P., Liu, Z. G., Wu, H. M., Luo, K. L., Zhai, S. T., Yan, H. Q., & Meng, G. R. (1998), Epidemiological investigation of mental disorders in seven areas of China. *Chin. J. Neurol & Psychiatry*, 31(2):69–71. (In Chinese)

Chapter 22

RA: Hong Kong

Peter W. H. Lee, F. Lieh-Mak, K. Y. Mak, Amy S. M. Fung, M. C. Wong, and Julia Lam

The present study reports on results of a 15-year follow-up of first onset schizophrenic patients in Hong Kong. Since this covers a period of rapid economic growth, the results may cast some light on the relationship between a country's economic status and the outcome of schizophrenia.

CULTURAL CONTEXT

Hong Kong, one of the last of the British Crown colonies, reverted to Chinese sovereignty in July 1997. For the duration of the study, however, Hong Kong had a British-appointed Governor, a civil service of predominantly Chinese origin but with an overrepresentation of British in the top ranks, appointed members of the Executive Council, and a predominantly elected Legislative Council. Hong Kong consists of four relatively distinct geographic areas, namely Hong Kong Island, a group of outlying islands nearby, Kowloon peninsula, and parts of the New Territories adjoining Mainland China. Ninety-five percent of the population is Chinese and Cantonese speaking, with an ever-increasing number of residents speaking English as well. The literacy rate is over 90%.

The past 40 years of development have seen two major trends in Hong Kong: first, a dramatic increase in population from less than 2 million before 1950 to over 6 million to date; and second, a rapid increase in industrial and commercial enterprises. New towns are being built, while rural lands are becoming increasingly impoverished. With rapid urbanization, living conditions have become harsher and more competitive. The population is more mobile with increased interpersonal distance, a growing trend toward more perfunctory and instrumental human relationships outside of the family, and a growing predominance of individualist and capitalistic concerns over the traditional Chinese communal and collectivistic ideals.

Politically, Hong Kong has enjoyed one of the most stable systems in the world. When the return of Hong Kong to Mainland China became imminent, however, various degrees of ambivalence showed themselves. While many Chinese are happy about reunion with the Motherland, which promised to strengthen their ethnic Chinese identity, many have been fearful and mistrust the Mainland Chinese regime. Emigration increased, often resulting in disrupted family structures with the major bread-winner remaining in Hong Kong while other members of the family relocated to satisfy the residency requirements for obtaining citizenship in other countries. Not uncommonly, the weak, sickly, elderly and, all too often, mentally ill persons in the family were abandoned to the care of society.

MENTAL HEALTH SERVICES IN HONG KONG

Mental health services have traditionally been part of overall medical and health services in Hong Kong. The first white paper presented at the Legislative Council, *Development of Medical Services in Hong Kong*, was issued in 1964. In 1974, another white paper, *Further Development of Medical and Health Services in Hong Kong*, enunciated the basic principle "to safeguard and promote the general public health of the community as a whole and ensure the provision of medical and personal health facilities for the people of Hong Kong including particularly that large section of the community which relies on subsidized medical attention." The Hong Kong government has so far succeeded in providing heavily subsidized health services for the entire population. In mental health, the government is primarily responsible for the provision of outpatient and hospital treatment services. Since its inception, the health service has placed emphasis on specialized psychiatric inpatient services and on mental health services units in general hospitals, but the range of psychiatric services also includes psychiatric outpatient clinics, day patient units, residential care, and community psychiatric rehabilitation services. In 1996, there were 4683 psychiatric inpatient beds provided by 10 psychiatric and general hospitals. Apart from government-run facilities, services are also provided by nongovernmental organizations to symptomatic and former mental patients through outreach services, halfway houses, supervised residences, counseling, and occupational rehabilitation services. A small but active private sector provides care to the more affluent.

STUDIES OF SCHIZOPHRENIA IN THE CHINESE

Although there have been few systematic studies on the prevalence and outcome of schizophrenia among the Chinese, in general, and in Hong Kong, in particular, there is little doubt that the largest portion of available mental health resources has been deployed in caring for patients with schizophrenia. For example, in 1994, over 50% of the mental health bed hospital discharges were schizophrenic and psychotic patients (Hong Kong Department of Health, 1994–1995). Song (1985) provided findings on the Minnesota Multiphasic Personality Inventory (MMPI) indicating that compared to American norms, the Chinese profile was elevated in factors for schizophrenia and depression—"emotionally more reserved, introverted, fond of tranquillity, overly considerate, socially overcautious, habituated to self-restraint. . . ." Tseng, Lin, and Yeh (1995) noted that although it is difficult to describe the Chinese culture or character without overgeneralizing, a number of common cultural threads remain salient: a harmonious attitude toward nature, an emphasis on balance and conservation for optimal health, the family as the basic resource of support, an emphasis on humanistic and interpersonal orientation characterized by mutual interdependency and harmony, and practical and dynamic adjustment in life situations emphasizing the middle way and flexibility.

Using a symptom checklist (Langner's scale), Millar (1979) in a biosocial survey conducted between 1973 and 1976 found that 25% of males and 37% of females had personal distress or psycho-physiological disturbances; however, specific diagnoses and validated screenings by clinicians were not available. Chen et al. (1993) conducted perhaps the only systematic community mental health survey in a relatively well-delineated group of residents in the Shatin area (population about 200,000). Using a two-stage design consisting of an initial case screening phase and a subsequent case identification phase, 12,000 subjects were studied. The lifetime prevalence rate of schizophrenia (defined by the investigators as "the proportion of individuals in the population, who have ever been ill, alive on a given day") was 0.12 ± 0.06 for males and 0.13 ± 0.06 for females. The lifetime prevalence of schizophreniform disorder was 0.06 ± 0.04 for males and 0.05 ± 0.04 for females.

Lo and Lo (1977) reported findings on a 10-year follow-up study of 133 patients between the ages of 14 to 60 living in Hong Kong, who had experienced their first psychiatric episode in 1965. Successful evaluation of outcomes was performed on 82 of the patients, with a follow-up rate of 62%. Of those successfully followed up, 21% were in lasting remission; 44% had remissions and relapses with no or only mild personality deterioration; 22% had remissions and relapses with moderate personality deterioration and/or residual psychotic symptoms; and 12% had continuing illness with persistent or incapacitating symptoms during a good part of the follow-up period. The number of hospital admissions and the total lengths of stay were in direct relationship to the four categories of outcomes, with poorer outcome associated with longer hospital stay. A number of good prognostic indicators were noted: female gender, shorter duration of illness, acute onset, predominant symptom groups other than disturbances of emotion and volition, and presence of a supportive relative. The study assessed patients only on broad outcome categories and made no attempt to evaluate specific levels of functioning in important domains of the patients' lives.

Lee, Lieh-Mak, Yu, and Spinks (1991) reported on the cross-sectional outcome of all schizophrenic patients (153 patients) who were being actively followed in the outpatient clinic of Queen Mary Hospital between July and December 1987. Twenty-two percent of the subjects had been ill for less than 3 years, 30% for 3 to 6 years, 16% for 7 to 9 years, and 32% for 10 years or more. Lee and his colleagues reported detailed breakdowns on levels of functioning in different life domains. Control of symptoms was most favorable with about 90% of the subjects being free of psychotic symptoms. Psychosocial deficits, however, were enduring and significant in a large proportion of the subjects: Over 60% lived a relatively isolated and celibate life; only 46% were fully employed, while the rest were employed only part of the time or not at all. Over 50% were rated as having a relatively empty life; 10% had a "vegetative existence." Subjects engaged predominantly in passive activities, while those involving self-discipline, social interaction, and self-initiative occurred much less frequently. Reevaluation after one year showed that except for symptomatic outcome, which tended to fluctuate across individuals, the outcome patterns in other areas were highly consistent over time, indicating a relative persistence of most of the identified psychosocial disabilities.

Several limitations of the Hong Kong studies reviewed here should be noted. First, the patients studied attended a single clinic and may not be representative of the entire schizophrenic population in Hong Kong. Second, Lo and Lo's follow-up study made predominant use of global outcome measures, and assessed status at initial presentation and at subsequent follow-up evaluations was not presented with clarity. Third, Lee et al.'s study was a cross-sectional study and did not differentiate outcome by duration of illness.

Since the 1940s, mental illness in Taiwan, another Chinese population, has been systematically studied. In the 1980s, structured interview schedules were deployed as case-finding tools to arrive at clinical diagnoses of mental disorders in large community samples and to provide more reliable estimates of prevalence. The Taiwan Psychiatric Epidemiology Project conducted by Yeh (1985; Yeh, Hwu, Chang, and Yeh, 1990) used a multistage random and stratified method for interviewing participants to determine DSM-III diagnoses. Lin (1985) studied inhabitants over 65 years of age in a small town and provided ICD-9 diagnoses. Similarly, Cheng (1985, 1988) and Rin, Hung, and Tseng (1987) studied different populations in Taiwan and arrived at prevalence of various psychiatric disorders using ICD-9 diagnoses. A review by Yeh, Hwu, and Lin (1995) found the prevalence rate of psychotic disorders in Taiwan to be 3.1/1000, and the rate of schizophrenia to be 1.4/1000. Various Taiwanese subgroups may be delineated: Taiwanese (Chinese people who had immigrated to Taiwan at the end of the Ming dynasty some four centuries ago); Mainlanders (Chinese who had migrated to Taiwan after the communist takeover of China in 1949); and in-migrants (Taiwanese who moved from other parts of Taiwan into the surveyed community). Even among different subgroups within a relatively clearly demarcated geographical region, different rates and types of mental disorders are apparent. For example, the original residents were found to have higher rates of manic-depressive psychoses and mental deficiency, while psychoneuroses were more prevalent among Mainlanders (16.9/1000 compared with 6 to 12/1000 in other subgroups). Although the reasons for such differences remain obscure, such findings indicate that even among ethnically homogeneous Chinese, diversity is the rule, and the prevalence and outcome of mental disorders may differ greatly from one subgroup to another.

HONG KONG CENTER

The researchers conducting ISoS are affiliated with the University Psychiatric Unit (92 beds) at Queen Mary Hospital, the first psychiatric unit in Hong Kong attached to a general hospital and a teaching unit of the University of Hong Kong. The unit accepts patients referred from Accidents and Emergency Departments on Hong Kong island, from outpatient departments, from other units of Queen Mary Hospital, from private practitioners, and from government subsidized hospitals. Between 1977 and 1978, when subjects were first recruited, the University Psychiatric Unit at Queen Mary Hospital was the only one on the island with psychiatric inpatient beds. The others, Hong Kong Psychiatric Center and the then newly opened Chaiwan Psychiatric Center, provided outpatient or day treatment services. When admission was required, patients went to either Castle Peak Hospital in the New Territories or Kwai Chung Hospital on the Kowloon side.

The research study team was co-led by the head and consultant clinical psychologist and the head and professor of psychiatry and supported by a consultant psychiatrist in rehabilitation psychiatry, a senior medical officer in psychiatry, a senior clinical psychologist, and a full-time research assistant majoring in psychology.

THE STUDY

Aims

The aims of this research project were to: (1) determine the course and outcome of schizophrenia over a 15-year period in a representative sample of Hong Kong Chinese; (2) identify predictors of outcome; (3) contribute to the development and refinement of valid and reliable instruments to diagnose and assess the course and outcome of schizophrenia and to record changes in symptoms and levels of disability over time, with a view in particular toward their applicability in the local setting; (4) provide reliable data for cross-cultural comparison, particularly with another Chinese sample studied in Beijing; and (5) obtain reliable indicators for understanding the long-term needs of schizophrenic patients and for promoting better rehabilitation and treatment.

Subject Recruitment

Extensive amounts of time and manpower were spent locating the subjects with first onset of schizophrenic illness between 1977 and 1978. All relevant patient files were reviewed in the then operating centers on Hong Kong island: University Psychiatric Unit at Queen Mary Hospital, David Trench Psychiatric Center, and Chaiwan Psychiatric Center. The files of all 797 patients who had been seen in 1977 and 1978 with a first onset diagnosis of schizophrenia were accessed, and 100 patients were randomly drawn from this pool. Each selected patient's file was then reviewed by the study team to determine whether the patient satisfied the ICD-9 criteria for a diagnosis of schizophrenia. When a patient did not meet the criteria, another case was randomly drawn from the pool of potential subjects, until the target of 100 subjects was reached.

As there were enormous socioeconomic changes and much mobility of the population during the past 15 years and because subjects selected for inclusion in the study may have been followed up in any of the psychiatric clinics located anywhere within Hong Kong island, Kowloon, or the New Territories, contacts were made with all mental health services and clinics in Hong Kong. Approval was obtained from the consultant psychiatrist in charge of mental health services in Hong Kong for contacts with the patients and/or their family members to obtain the patient's whereabouts and vital status. Hong Kong does not have a central location register for its citizens, and the early patient files did not record the subjects' unique identity card numbers. As identical names are common among the Chinese, the subjects' names were always checked against their ages before inclusion. The extensive mobility of the Hong Kong population and the continuous development of new towns resulted in many of the subjects being untraceable either because they had discontinued treatment some years ago or because they had moved. As expected, a number of subjects had moved to Mainland China (as resources are cheaper and living demands are less stringent), or had emigrated to other countries because of the impending sociopolitical changes. Some of the untraceable subjects might also have died.

Instruments

Key words on the study instruments that required direct administering to the subjects or to informants were translated into "spoken" Cantonese. Researchers held several meetings where standardized forms of questions and wordings were discussed, agreed upon, tape recorded, and then transcribed. The wording thus generated was clinically relevant, colloquially appropriate in the usual style of the indigenous spoken language. The translated versions were then back-translated into English. The emphasis of the exercise was not on getting the wordings exactly right, but rather on retaining the original meaning of the instruments.

In reviews of video recorded interviews, researchers standardized interviewing styles, use of specific wordings and questioning techniques and established reliability in scoring and in coding the patients' responses. Areas of unreliability were resolved through consensus and with the explicit agreement that the "outlier" raters would abide by the majority view. Satisfactory reliability in assessing and rating psychological and recovery status was achieved within the local research team through blind ratings of video recorded patient interviews. Subsequent data processing by the Collaborating Center at the Nathan Kline Institute led to further analyses and finally to the smoothing out of major differences among raters.

Data Collection

First, the research assistant located the target patient's files and ascertained his or her whereabouts. Then, the patient's file was reviewed by a member of the research team who confirmed the diagnosis. Only unambiguous cases of schizophrenia or of the schizophrenic group of disorders at onset in 1977 to 1978 were included in the follow-up study. Through the rediagnosis, seven potential subjects were rejected on the basis that the ICD-9 diagnostic criteria for schizophrenia were not fulfilled. Target subjects were traced via their medical history records in all the mental health clinics and psychiatric hospitals in Hong Kong, Kowloon, and the New Territories. In cases where subjects were not easily traceable (e.g., those who had defaulted on their follow-up treatment), two registered letters were sent to their last known addresses inviting them to participate. The research assistant also followed up by phone. If subjects declined, the reasons were noted, and they were then asked to think about the invitation for a further period. Two months later, the research team again contacted the subject. Two of the subjects were enlisted through this process. If a subject's whereabouts were unknown, the relative's last known addresses and phone number were used, and the subject's present whereabouts sought so far as resources allowed. After the target subjects were ascertained as available, the researcher and a research assistant generally saw the patient and the informant either in the current clinic at the time when he or she returned for a follow-up visit, in the person's home, or in some other place (e.g., in a fast food shop) preferred by the subject. Each subject and informant assessment took an average of 3 to 4 hours.

RESULTS

Baseline and Early Follow-Up

Gender and Age

The randomly selected cohort of 100 schizophrenic subjects consisted of an almost equal number of men (51) and women (49). On follow-up, 33 men and 37 women were alive, 11 had died, and the 19 subjects who were lost to follow-up had been lost to clinical attention or treatment personnel for at least 10 years. Birth year distribution at follow-up is similar to that at entry; mean birth year is 1952.

Mode of Onset and Diagnosis

The distribution of mode of onset in the alive cohort is similar to that in the original sample. The dead cohort has more subjects with insidious onset (>1 month)—approximately 82% compared to 66% of the alive and 63% of the lost to follow-up, although the numbers affected in the dead and lost cohorts are small (9 and 12, respectively). However, when data in the missing category are excluded, the dead and the lost to follow-up cohort has a population with predominantly insidious onset (100 and 92%, respectively). Insidious onset has been found to be a predictor of worse outcome generally, implying that the alive group of subjects may be biased toward having a better outcome. Almost all subjects (69 of 70) of the alive cohort received a baseline diagnosis of schizophrenia using the conversion of ICD-9 to ICD-10.

Pattern of Course at Early Follow-Up

Twenty-two of the 70 (31%) alive subjects had a favorable short-term (2-year) pattern of course (episodic, with full remissions between episodes). Deceased subjects and those lost to follow-up for whom early course information was available (n=25) were more likely to have had a poor early course. Only 20% of the subjects who had died or were lost to follow-up were assessed as having a complete remission, while 8% of these subjects, in contrast to none of the subjects who were successfully followed up, were rated as having a continuous psychotic illness.

Alive Subjects

Symptomatology

Classified according to the Bleuler Severity Scale, 53% of the 70 persons in the alive cohort had recovered, 27% suffered mild symptoms, 13% suffered moderate symptoms, and 7% had severe symptomatology. Combining the percentages of subjects who had recovered and those with only mild symptoms, the Hong Kong cohort may be classified as among those cohorts with relatively better symptomatic outcome.

About three-quarters (71%) of the subjects showed no significant (or only mild) symptoms as measured by the Global Assessment of Functioning Scale for Symptomatology (with GAF-S scores >60). Fourteen percent suffered from serious symptoms (with GAF-S scores < 51). When the GAF-S scores are compared, Hong Kong subjects are found to be among the cohorts with better outcome. The relative prominence of psychotic symptoms over time also conforms to this pattern. Four percent of the subjects had prominent psychotic symptoms in all three periods, while for another 4%, such symptoms were never prominent.

Overall, for 61% of the subjects psychotic symptoms were prominent for the initial period, while for 33% of the subjects psychotic symptoms were prominent in the most recent period of follow-up.

Course of the Illness

At the time of assessment, 44% of the 70 subjects had no psychotic episodes over the past 2 years; 36% were continuously psychotic; and 16% were classified as episodic. This pattern of almost half or more of the subjects being psychosis-free is also seen in many of the treated incidence samples (urban and rural Chandigarh, Honolulu, Moscow, Nottingham, Rochester, Groningen, and Chennai [Madras]. As expected, course of illness over the entire period shows a different pattern: 60% had an episodic course, 27% had a continuous psychotic course, and 12% had a neither continuous nor episodic course. For 46% of the subjects, the overall trend was improvement, while for 26%, it was worsening.

Reevaluation of Baseline Diagnosis

Reevaluation of clinical status at baseline showed that 96% were diagnosed with schizophrenia; one was diagnosed as acute schizophrenia-like and two as other psychosis.

Living Arrangements

At the time of the follow-up assessment, most subjects were living in the community, either on their own (7%), or with family (79%). Only 9% resided in a psychiatric hospital, while 6% lived in a supervised residence not on hospital grounds. Figures for independent living were similar to the other centers as a whole. For prevalence of psychiatric hospitalization, which varies somewhat across different centers, Hong Kong ranks in the middle.

For the most part, this situation was stable for the 2 years preceding the assessment. Only a few (less than 5%) of those who spent some time in independent living arrangements spent less than 12 months there; 86% spent all of those 2 years in an independent residence. About one-fifth (21%) of the subjects spent some time in a hospital or supervised residence in the past 2 years. For living arrangements, the majority of both males and females lived in the community. Over the course of the entire follow-up period, each subject lived independently in the community for some time. Ninety-four percent of the subjects managed to do so for the majority of the period, while only 6% did so for less than 10 years over the entire period. In terms of hospitalization, 57% of the subjects had been hospitalized at least once over the entire 15-year period. Only one female subject had been homeless or vagrant (for less than 6 months in the preceding 2 years) in the entire follow-up period. No subject had ever spent any time in jail. Low rates of homelessness and jail were common throughout the ISoS centers.

Social Disability

With respect to overall functioning in the last month (as measured by the GAF-disability rating), 31% had GAF-D scores lower than 51, indicating serious impairment. At the same time, 14% of the subjects scored 80 and higher on the GAF-D, indicating good functioning. Six of the 70 (9%) subjects had disabilities that were prominent throughout the follow-up period; 10 (14%) subjects had disabilities that were more prominent during the last third of the period, while for another 30 (43%) subjects, disabilities were prominent only during the first third of the period. Six out of the 70 (9%) subjects experienced no prominent disabilities at any time.

Work

Fifty-six percent of the subjects worked at paid jobs at some point in the last 2 years of follow-up; more than half of those who worked (67%) did so for at least 12 months. For those working most of the time, performance was judged mostly as good to very good (89%). Another 16% was engaged in full-time homemaking for the entire period, and their performance for the most part was rated as good (73%). None of the subjects was classified as being a student at any time in the past 2 years, and only three subjects had retired. The majority of these subjects (70%) had not received any disability pension. Fifteen subjects (21%) had received disability pensions for the entire period.

Violence

Eight percent of the subjects (2 men, 3 women) had been involved in assaults that can be characterized as transient and short-lived outbursts of aggression toward other people in the last 2 years of follow-up (e.g., a single punch or pushing). None of the assaults resulted in serious injury. Over the entire course, one-third of the cohort (22 subjects) had been involved in assaults on other people. Two subjects (3%) attempted a nonfatal suicide in the past 2 years, and an additional seven subjects (10%) deliberately harmed themselves at some point in the follow-up period.

Medications

In the last 2 years, all but two subjects had been prescribed neuroleptics; 94% were on them for most of the time. Ninety-six percent were on regular medication during most of the entire 15-year period. An examination of time trends reveals three major patterns: For 23%, medication use was prominent throughout the follow-up period; for 36%, medication had a decreasing trend throughout the period; and for yet another 10%, medication use was more prominent in the last third of the follow-up period.

Hospitalization

Fifty-five subjects (79%) spent no time in a hospital or a supervised residence in the past 2 years of follow-up. Of the subjects who had been in these settings, nine were there for one year or more. Forty subjects (57%) were admitted to a psychiatric ward at least once during the entire follow-up period. Of these, 18 subjects (26%) were admitted once or twice, five subjects (7%) were admitted three times, and 17 subjects (24%) were admitted four or more times including nine (13%) who had 10 or more admissions. For 40% of the subjects, hospital admissions were prominent events only in the first part of the entire period; for 13% of the subjects, hospital admission became prominent only during the later third of the period. No subjects had hospital admission as a prominent event during all phases of the follow-up period.

Sex Differences in Outcome

Females generally have a more benign course compared with their male counterparts. Where 51% of the females were not psychotic at follow-up, only 34% of the males were not psychotic. In contrast, 41% of the males had been continuously psychotic compared with only 32% of the females. Further breakdown of the data also indicates that females generally had better outcomes compared to their male counterparts. (see Table 22.1).

TABLE 22.1 Comparison of Males vs. Females on Different Outcome Indicators

	Males %	*Females* %
1. Course Type: Past 2 Years		
Continuous	41	32
Not psychotic	34	51
2. GAF Disability Score: Past Month		
Below 61	42	32
61–70	12	16
71–80	36	32
81 and above	9	19
Mean	60	66
3. Overall Time Trend		
Much better/somewhat better	38	54
Same	28	24
Somewhat worse/worse	34	21
4. Assaults: Past 2 years	7	9
5. Suicidal Attempts: Past 2 Years	3	3

DECEASED SUBJECTS

At the time of the 15-year follow-up, 11 subjects (8 males and 3 females) were deceased. Of these, nine had committed suicide (four by jumping from heights, three were drowned after jumping into the sea, one had a drug overdose, and one hanged himself); one subject, whose body was found in the countryside, died of cardiac arrest; and one died of unknown causes. Half of the subjects were determined to be in an episode of illness at the time of their deaths; three subjects were in partial remission; and two subjects were noted in the case notes as being well. So far as can be ascertained, the subjects committed suicide mostly in depressed states of mind (e.g., frustration over work, over interpersonal relationships, and over the chronicity of their illness). A strong feeling of inferiority with depressive mood was commonly noted.

DISCUSSION

The Representativeness of the Study Cohort

The subjects were from a geographically distinct area consisting entirely of Hong Kong Island and can be regarded as representative of a group of schizophrenic patients with first onset of illness 15 years ago. Because of the recruitment process, the only potential subjects who might have been missed are those patients who presented themselves in the private sector. However, because private psychiatric services were very limited during that period (fewer than five psychiatrists were in private practice); these potential subjects comprise only a very small minority of the schizophrenic population in Hong Kong.

The Status of the Subjects at Follow-Up

Subjects can be roughly classified into three groups according to outcome status at follow-up. About 14% of the subjects who scored 80 or more points on the GAF-D scale were functioning free from psychotic symptoms and comparable to other Hong Kong residents with similar backgrounds as if they had never been ill. The only characteristic which would identify them as having had a psychiatric illness was that they are most likely still on prescribed neuroleptic medication and attending a psychiatric outpatient clinic two to three times per year. Another 15% of the subjects who had GAF-D scores below 40 remained clearly and persistently incapacitated in their social and occupational roles as well as in their symptom status. A middle group of schizophrenic subjects, comprising the majority of the cases, had varied outcomes and were marginally functional. Some were able to hold jobs over the most recent 2 years, although their performance may not have been optimal and the duration of their employment varied. Socially, they tend to be relatively isolated: 56% of the subjects remained single, and another 7% were either separated or divorced. The majority stayed with their families and required varying degrees of support from relatives. Their mental status, symptom level, and need for psychiatric hospitalization fluctuated depending on environmental stresses, compliance with medication, degree of interpersonal difficulties, and available support. The picture that emerges clearly echoes Strauss and Carpenter's (1972, 1974) and Ciompi's (1980) assertion that outcome in schizophrenia is not characterized by a homogeneous overall process but instead can be highly variable and heterogeneous.

Comparison of 15-Year Outcome Findings with Previous Findings

The subjects' outcomes 15 years after onset were generally similar to previous findings on outcomes of persons with schizophrenia in Hong Kong. However, it is difficult to reconcile various methods of classifying outcomes. For example, Bleuler's system and the Global Assessment of Functioning for Symptomatology (GAF-S) are based primarily on symptomatic level. Evidence indicates that psychotic symptoms are relatively easier to control. Eighty percent of subjects were rated as having recovered or having only mild symptoms on Bleuler's scale, and only 14% scored below 50 on the GAF-S scale. Positive symptom control alone, however, may give rise to an overly optimistic view of outcome, as is illustrated by ratings of subjects' outcome on the GAF-Disability scale with 31% of the subjects scoring below 50, and only 14% scoring 80 or better. When the patient's real life adjustment in various aspects of psychosocial functioning is examined, the picture that emerges indicates that while symptomatic outcome was favorable, social disability, and suboptimal real-life adjustment problems may remain prominent in about half of the patients.

Comparison with Other Countries

Although it is difficult to compare outcomes across studies where good versus bad outcome is clearly defined differently, it is worth remarking that our findings compare favorably with those of Tsoi and Wong (1991) in Singapore, who found slightly more than 30% of their follow-up cohort to be fully recovered (working and not receiving treatment). Note, however, that the treatment philosophy in Hong Kong is that regardless of their symptomatic status, schizophrenic patients are followed up and maintained on neuroleptic medications for prolonged periods of time. Hence, our subjects cannot be directly equated with subjects in Singapore where "not receiving treatment" was used as one of the criteria.

The earlier report of Lo and Lo (1977), which found that 65% of the Hong Kong schizophrenic patients whom they followed up had full and lasting remission (or despite relapses, showed only mild or no deterioration), seems to portray a better outcome picture than our present findings. However, as psychosocial functions were not systematically assessed, it is hard to compare our data with theirs. On symptomatic control alone, 53% of our subjects were rated as recovered on Bleuler's scale, and 71% of patients scored above 60 on the GAF-S scale. Our subjects' outcome 15 years from Lo and Lo's (1977) study would thus indicate at least a comparable picture. Likewise, our findings are comparable to those of Murphy and Raman (1971) for Mauritian subjects in that 60% were noted to be functioning normally 12 years after onset, and with those of Thara and Eaton (1996) where 65% of subjects were symptom free at the end of the 10-year follow-up study.

Comparing data from the Hong Kong, Singapore, and Indian studies with other WHO Collaborating Centers in the West indicates that a comparable and perhaps slightly higher percentage of Asian schizophrenic patients are free from active psychotic symptoms at follow-up. The reported outcomes in Asia are slightly better than those reported in a British (Mason et al., 1995; Harrison, Croudace, Mason, Glazebrook, and Medley, 1996) and a Dutch sample (Wiersma, Nienhuis, Slooff, and Giel, 1998). Whereas 53% of the patients in Hong Kong and a comparable 53% of the patients followed up in Chennai are free from psychotic symptoms, only 17% of patients in the English sample and 27% of the Dutch sample are free from psychotic symptoms over the long-term course of 13 to 15 years. Also, 54% of the subjects in Hong Kong were employed compared to 37% in the Nottingham sample. However, such comparisons are necessarily imprecise and need to be interpreted with caution, as clearly different standards of care are provided in different countries, and different definitions of "recovery" are employed by different researchers. The Nottingham research team, for example, defines "recovery" as meaning that "the subject is alive at follow-up with no symptoms, no disability and on no treatment" (Mason et al., 1995); while the Dutch team (Wiersma et al., 1998) defines "complete remission" as "no symptoms; no care." The Hong Kong sample, despite relatively higher symptom-free status and more employment, is clearly different from the other samples in that continuing care is still provided (although probably more because of prevailing treatment practice than because of the actual clinical needs of the subjects).

It is also worth noting that Hong Kong, despite being a relatively developed city, retains a schizophrenic population with perhaps better outcome when compared with the other developed countries. Good outcome is also consistent over a long period of time extending from Lo and Lo's (1977) study, when Hong Kong was less developed, to the present time when Hong Kong's economy compares favorably with most developed Western countries. The previous notion that schizophrenic patients in developed countries tend to have a poorer outcome than in developing countries (Leff, Sartorius, Jablensky, Korten, and Ernberg, 1992) may need to be considered more carefully in light of the current data.

Several factors unique to Hong Kong may be relevant. Vigorous follow-up of schizophrenic patients has been an explicit mental health policy since 1984. Compared to patients elsewhere, patients in Hong Kong have the highest active treatment and follow-up rates. More than 90% of our subjects were still actively followed up after 15 years and maintained on neuroleptic medications, compared to only 51% in Chennai and 58% in Nottingham. As a result, the average default rate of psychiatric follow-up is only 16%. Hong Kong also has a heavily subsidized health care system funded by the government's general revenue. Eighty percent of psychiatric inpatients do not have to pay for their medications, medical services, or hospitalization. Forty-five percent of psychiatric outpatients also received their treatment free of charge. In addition to direct services, Hong Kong also employs an equally heavily subsidized network of community-based services for mentally ill persons, e.g., the Community Chest in Hong Kong supports a substantial number of nongovernment mental health agencies.

The vast majority of our subjects have also been staying with their families from whom they receive different levels of support. Our data indicate that 85% of the patients were still living at home with their families 15 years after having developed schizophrenia. Despite its rapid economic development, the structure of the Chinese traditional family and its values have not changed. It is plausible that the extended family provides what are, in effect, surrogate hospital services and other kin-based psychosocial support supplementing the already easily available psychiatric and community support. The average length of stay for psychiatric admissions had been reduced dramatically from 60 days before 1991 to 40 days after 1991. The stability of family support, the continuity of care, and the continuous availability of psychotropic medications for our patients, we believe, is vitally linked to favorable outcomes.

Sex Differences in Outcome

It is apparent that females generally have a more favorable outcome than their male counterparts. This is clearly reflected in the women's marital status and overall improving time trend and symptom status. This finding appears to be consistent across different cultures and levels of economic development.

SUMMARY

The study cohort (51 males and 49 females) is a random sample of 100 subjects from first onset cases of schizophrenia seen during 1977 and 1978 in the psychiatric outpatient clinics on Hong Kong island. Men and women were equally represented, with an average age at illness onset of 27 years. At 15-year follow-up, 70% of the original subjects were located. While showing no apparent bias with respect to gender, age, or baseline diagnosis, the follow-up cohort tends to have more acute modes of onset when compared to the dead and the lost to follow-up group. Short-term pattern of course was also slightly poorer for the deceased and for those lost to follow-up.

At the time of follow-up, about half of the subjects were judged to have recovered, although another 36% still showed evidence of continuous symptomatology during the last 2 years. Thirty-one percent of the subjects showed evidence, too, of significant impairment in social and occupational functioning, in contrast to about 14% of the subjects rated as good. Almost all subjects were currently on prescribed neuroleptic medications. Eighty percent of the subjects had not spent any time in a mental hospital for treatment in the most recent 2 years. The vast majority of the subjects are living in the community, mostly with family. About half of the subjects had been employed for varying periods of time during the past 2 years, and another 16% were engaged in full-time household work. Overall, the course of the illness was rated as improving in almost half of the subjects.

The long-term life course of schizophrenia is still fraught with difficulties and unresolved challenges. While relatively few patients are bothered by psychotic symptoms, marginal or suboptimal psychosocial adjustment is still common. Even though patients are generally living in the community, their dependence on family support is still paramount. Our data suggest that instead of generalizing on developed versus developing countries as being instrumental in promoting a better or worse outcome in schizophrenia, more clearly delineated factors such as continuity and availability of care, family, and community resources, and traditional roles of male versus females seem to be equally pertinent considerations.

Acknowledgments The study is funded by a research grant award by the Hong Kong Research Grants Council. The authors would also like to express their grateful thanks to Dr. P. S. Sham, Dr. H. K. Cheung and their colleagues in the mental health services in Hong Kong for their kind help in tracing patients for the study.

References

Chen, C. N., Wong, J., Lee, N., Chan-Ho, M. W., Lau, J. T. F., & Fung, M. (1993), The Shatin community mental health survey in Hong Kong II. Major findings. *Arch. Gen. Psychiatry*, 50:125–133.

Cheng, T. A. (1985), A pilot study of mental disorders in Taiwan. *Psycholog. Med.*, 15:195–203.

——(1988), A community study of minor psychiatric morbidity. *Psycholog. Med.*, 18:953–968.

Ciompi, L. (1980), Catamnestic long-term study on the course of life and aging of schizophrenics. *Schizophr. Bull.*, 6(4):606–618.

Harrison, G., Croudace, T., Mason, P., Glazebrook, C., & Medley, I. (1996), Predicting the long-term outcome of schizophrenia. *Psycholog. Med.*, 26:697–705.

Hong Kong Department of Health (1994–1995), *Annual Report 1994/95*. Hong Kong: Hong Kong Government Press.

Hong Kong Government (1964), *White Paper: Development of Medical Services in Hong Kong*. Hong Kong: Hong Kong Government Press.

——(1974), *White Paper: Further Development of Medical Services in Hong Kong*. Hong Kong: Hong Kong Government Press.

Lee, P. W. H., Lieh-Mak, F., Yu, K. K., & Spinks, J. A. (1991), Patterns of outcome in schizophrenia in Hong Kong. *Acta Psychiatr. Scand.*, 84:346–352.

Leff, J., Sartorius, N., Jablensky, A., Korten, A., & Ernberg, G. (1992), The international pilot study of schizophrenia: Five-year follow-up findings. *Psycholog. Med.*, 22: 131–145.

Lin, T. Y. (1985), Mental disorders and psychiatry in Chinese culture: Characteristic features and major issues. In: *Chinese Culture and Mental Health*, ed. W. S. Tseng & D. Y. H. Wu. Orlando, FL: Academic Press, pp. 367–388.

Lo, W. H., & Lo, T. (1977), A ten-year follow-up study of Chinese schizophrenics in Hong Kong. *Brit. J. Psychiatry*, 131:63–66.

Mason, P., Harrison, G., Glazebrook, C., Medley, I., Dalkin, T., & Croudace, T. (1995), Characteristics of outcome in schizophrenia at 13 years. *Brit. J. Psychiatry*, 167:596–603.

Millar, S. (1979), *Hong Kong Human Ecology Programme: The Biosocial Survey in Hong Kong*. Canberra: Centre for Resource and Environmental Studies, Australian National University.

Murphy, H. B. M., & Raman, A. C. (1971), The chronicity of schizophrenia in indigenous tropical peoples: Results of a twelve-year follow-up survey in Mauritius. *Brit. J. Psychiatry*, 118:489–497.

Rin, H., Hung, M. G., & Tseng, M. C. (1987), Prevalence of elderly dementias in Taipei area. *Proc. Ann. Meeting Chin. Soc. Neurol. & Psychiatry*, p. 24.

Song, W. Z. (1985), A preliminary study of the character traits of the Chinese. In: *Chinese Culture and Mental Health*, ed. W. S. Tseng & D. Y. H. Wu. Orlando, FL: Academic Press, pp. 47–55.

Strauss, J. P., & Carpenter, W. T., Jr. (1972), The prediction of outcome in schizophrenia: I. Characteristics of outcome. *Arch. Gen. Psychiatry*, 27:739–746.

——, ——(1974), The prediction of outcome of schizophrenia: II. Relationships between predictor and outcome variables. *Arch. Gen. Psychiatry*, 31:37–42.

Thara, R., & Eaton, W. S. (1996), Outcome of schizophrenia: The Madras longitudinal study. *Austral. & New Z. J. Psychiatry*, 30(4):516–522.

Tseng, W. S., Lin, T. Y., & Yeh, E. K. (1995), Chinese societies and mental health. In: *Chinese Societies and Mental Health*, ed. T. Y. Lin, W. S. Tseng, & E. K. Yeh. Oxford: Oxford University Press, pp. 3–18.

Tsoi, W. F., & Wong, K. E. (1991), A 15-year follow-up study of Chinese schizophrenic patients. *Acta Psychiatr. Scand.*, 84:217–220.

Wiersma, D., Nienhuis, F. J., Slooff, C. J., & Giel, R. (1998), Natural course of schizophrenic disorders. A 15-years follow-up of a Dutch incidence cohort. *Schizophr. Bull.*, 24(1):75–85.

Yeh, E. K. (1985), Sociocultural changes and prevalence of mental disorders in Taiwan. In: *Chinese Culture and Mental Health*, ed. W. S. Teng & Y. H. Wu. New York: Academic Press, pp. 265–284.

——Hwu, H. G., Chang, L. Y., & Yeh, Y. L. (1990), Lifetime prevalence of cognitive impairment by Chinese-modified NIMH diagnostic interview schedule among the elderly in Taiwan community. *J. Neurolinguistics*, 5:83–104.

——, ——Lin, T. Y. (1995), Mental disorders in Taiwan: Epidemiological studies of community population. In: *Chinese Societies and Mental Health*, ed. T. Y. Lin, W. S. Tseng, & E. K. Yeh. Oxford: Oxford University Press, pp. 247–265.

CHAPTER 23

RA: Chennai (Madras), India

R. Thara, S. Rajkumar, and A. Albert Joseph

CULTURAL CONTEXT

Chennai (Madras) is the fourth largest city in India, the second most populous country in the world, with a population of nearly 980 million. Chennai and its suburbs contain about 5.5 million people. A port city, Chennai is the seat of south Indian culture and the capital of the state of Tamil Nadu bordering the southeast coast of the country. For the past 30 years, the state has been ruled only by regional political parties that have no base outside the state. A matter of political contention has been the relationship between the central government and the states, and the struggle for greater autonomy for states continues. Hindus constitute about 80% of the population with Christians and Muslims accounting for the rest; religious groups generally coexist in harmony. There is an air of cultural homogeneity. The literacy rate in the city of Chennai is quite high, nearly 82%, while in the state of Tamil Nadu it is 62.7%. The decennial growth rate in the population of Tamil Nadu from 1981 to 1991 was 15.4%, which is less than the national growth rate of 24%. There are 974 women for every 1000 men in the state.

Until the late 1970s, most families in Chennai were joint or extended. Now, there is a distinct trend toward nuclear families. Women enjoy much higher status here than in many other parts of the country, with a labor force participation rate of nearly 30%. While conventionally in families where both parents work, grandparents have looked after the children, this pattern is also changing with the change in family configuration. The increase in the number of nuclear families, especially in urban areas, has served to deprive grandparents of the role of caring for their grandchildren. As a sequel to this, the need for *crèches* to look after the children of working mothers is on the increase.

Chennai has witnessed a great deal of migration since independence 50 years ago. Migration from rural to urban areas was at its peak in the late 1970s and has shown a modest decline since then. Most of those who migrate seek jobs in small industries or in the film industry, which is very active in Chennai. Intraurban mobility is seen among construction workers, daily wage earners, and nomadic Gypsies. About 20 to 25% of the population lives in slums, many of whose residents are relatively recent migrants to the city.

The major events from 1980 to follow-up assessment have been:

1980 The local state government was dismissed, and the President's rule was imposed with administration by bureaucrats.

1984 The Pope visited, and Catholic identity reemerged. (Early Christianity is associated with Chennai—St. Thomas, one of Jesus's disciples, is buried here. Also, there are several educational institutions run by Christian missionaries.)

1984 The government launched the popular "noon meal scheme" which provided free lunch at school for poor children, an effective incentive for attendance. Since then, many other Indian states have followed suit. A number of Balwadi centers, which give children in urban areas access to education, were also opened.

1987 Actor-turned-politician, Chief Minister M. G. Ramachandran died. His charisma was so overpowering to the masses that a spate of suicides followed.

Sri Lankan problems: Tamil Nadu has experienced repercussions; for example, increases in drug abuse and crime rates, stemming from the politico-ethnic strife between the Sri Lankan government and the Tamil militants. Thousands of Tamils have immigrated, leaving their families, wealth, and belongings, and are accommodated in refugee camps all over the state.

1989 The withdrawal of the Indian army from Sri Lanka resulted in an increased influx of Sri Lankan refugees.

1991 Former Prime Minister Rajiv Gandhi was murdered at Sriperumbudur, near Chennai, after a political meeting. A woman, a living bomb, garlanded him, exploded, and killed him, herself, and 10 others. There followed long-reaching sociopolitical consequences.

1994 Tamil Nadu, in an official policy on the handicapped, became the first state in the country to place the disability caused by mental illness on a par with other disabilities.

1996 The government of Ms. Jayalalitha, voted into power in 1991 by a huge margin over the main opposition party, was totally routed in the elections of 1996, an event widely understood to be a protest both against the widespread corruption that had infiltrated every aspect of public life and against an autocratic manner of functioning in a democratic state. It was evident that even the illiterate poor are sensitive to such issues and cannot be swayed by the power of money.

1992–1997 Economic liberalization measures during this period attracted many foreign investments into the country. Some were in the health sector, which in the past 10 years has seen a proliferation of private hospitals, many of them financed by nonresident Indians; some are corporate and have gone public. There has also been a commendable increase in the number of nongovernmental organizations (NGOs) that have devoted themselves to drug abuse and alcoholism, suicide prevention, schizophrenia, and destitute mentally ill persons. With increasing trends of urbanization and the break-up of joint families, the number of residential facilities for elderly citizens is also on the increase.

Beliefs about Mental Illness

A recently completed study on explanatory models of mental illness in a rural community in the state of Tamil Nadu (Thara, Islam, and Padmavati, 1997) shows that these are largely dependent on the proximity to and the availability of mental health services. In remote villages where services are not available, the magicoreligious model is predominant. The first contact for 90% of mentally ill persons seeking help in such places is still with religious institutions or the traditional healer. Closer to the city, the sociomedical model becomes more evident. Much of the suffering in life, including that caused by mental illness, is seen as "preordained," a result of past misdeeds or "karma" (the Hindu belief that one reaps the fruits of deeds done in previous lives). The onus of caregiving rests largely with the family as there are few institutions that can provide for persons with persistent mental illness on a lifelong basis, and no public disability benefits have been accorded them.

Linguistic Characteristics of the Culture

Tamil, an ancient language, is spoken in south India, especially in Tamil Nadu, parts of Sri Lanka, Malaysia, and Singapore. Although several dialects of the language can be seen in various parts of the state, the language itself has enough richness to convey mental illness in all its subtleties. Mental illness has been referred to even in the ancient scriptures, and some great works such as *Thirukkural* include descriptions of several types of emotional states such as depression, anxiety, fears, and psychotic symptoms. A popular form of treatment that emerged in the 15th century A.D. was known as Siddha Vaidhya, which follows the "tridosha" (three types of body humors) theory and contains descriptions of clinical syndromes corresponding to schizophrenia, mania, and depression. "Kirukku" (lunacy), recognized by the practitioners of Siddha Vaidya in Tamil Nadu, is similar in description to schizophrenia, and is believed to have 18 subtypes (Namboodri, 1986). Other south Indian languages and Hindi are also spoken, but the medium of instruction in most schools is English.

Impact of Mental Health Issues on Society

Over 95% of mentally ill persons live with their families. Research done at the Schizophrenia Research Foundation (SCARF) and at other centers reveals a high degree of burden on caregivers: financial, physical, and particularly emotional. Compounding this is social stigma, most prevalent in middle and higher income groups. Marriages are still largely arranged, and marital prospects provoke much anxiety in many families with mentally ill members. The magicoreligious explanatory models, still widely prevalent especially in rural areas, might mitigate stigma to a certain extent, but when events like marriage are involved, the matter is still tricky. It is also the bane of this society that should a young woman become mentally ill after marriage, she is very often sent back to her parents' home for treatment.

Although the government of India passed legislation in January 1996 recognizing disability caused by mental illness, at the time of ISoS follow-up there was as yet no job reservations ("set-aside" positions) in the organized sector of employment. SCARF research has shown that patients from lower and lower-middle classes are able to find jobs in the unorganized (informal) sector, but those from higher income groups and the literate have problems. In some cases, disclosure of mental illness to potential employees has had disastrous consequences.

Among mental disorders, concern regarding alcohol and drug abuse especially among youth has caused the government to set up several counseling centers. Another priority area is AIDS, with its physical, emotional, and social sequelae, which is increasing in alarming proportions. Tamil Nadu is one of the states which has shown great concern for this issue, and there are several NGOs working in this area.

MENTAL HEALTH SYSTEM

Organization, Policies, and Changes in the Mental Health System Since the Mid-1970s

In India, health care is essentially a state government concern, although the central government forms policies which, to an extent, impact state level programs. The state of Tamil Nadu, like the adjoining state of Kerala, has an excellent mental health care infrastructure. Mental health facilities are available at all district headquarters, and psychiatric outpatient departments are found in almost all general hospitals. There are also a few voluntary NGOs which offer mental health care. The state-run hospitals provide medical treatment free of cost. Nevertheless, improvement is needed in mental health care delivery in the rural areas. Although the National Mental Health Program envisaged the integration of mental health with primary care, this has not been adopted uniformly by all the states, and there are few primary health centers that have the trained personnel and medication to handle mental illnesses.

Structure of the Mental Health Services System

In the city of Chennai at the time of this follow-up study, the following primary services offer mental health care:

1. A large Institute of Mental Health (previously called the Madras Mental Hospital), about 150 years old, caters to patients from all over the state of Tamil Nadu and from neighboring states. It has 2000 inpatient beds, an outpatient clinic, and some special clinics.
2. The four general hospitals each has a psychiatric outpatient department. While much liaison psychiatry work is done here, each has fewer than 20 inpatient beds. The Institute of Mental Health and departments of psychiatry attached to general hospitals are run by the state government.
3. Some inexpensive and many expensive private hospitals offer psychiatric treatment, catering mainly to middle and higher income groups.
4. A few NGOs offer specialized care in schizophrenia, alcohol and drug abuse, and suicide. Some run halfway homes and sheltered workshops. Most, however, deal with mental retardation.
5. There are about 125 psychiatrists in private practice.
6. Traditional and religious healers: Native systems of medicine such as Ayurveda and Siddha offer treatment. More commonly used are the magicoreligious healers, who are the first contact for over 60% of mentally ill persons in the city and for 90% in rural areas. All people, irrespective of their religious faith, seek help from places of worship; in and around Chennai, priests in selected temples (Hindu) and durghas (Muslim) offer specialized psychiatric care.

Financial Support

Primarily, two categories of patients utilize mental health services. The first group hails from lower and lower-middle economic classes and avails itself of free services offered in the state-run institutions and by some NGOs. Middle and higher-income patients opt for private treatment where they have to pay for professional services and other forms of treatment as well as for medicines. There is no insurance coverage for mental illness and no social security benefits for mentally disabled persons. Many families with chronically mentally ill members are heavily burdened by the costs of treatment.

PSYCHIATRIC EPIDEMIOLOGY IN INDIA

A number of epidemiological studies have been conducted in India since 1970. One of the most relevant to ISoS is the Study of Functional Psychoses in an Urban Community (SOFPUC) at Chennai (Padmavati, Rajkumar, Narendra, Manohar, and Kamath, 1988), a multistage census survey of a population of over 100,000 screened using the Indian Psychiatric Survey Schedule (Kapur, Kapur, and Carstairs, 1974) and the Present State Examination (PSE; Wing, Cooper, and Sartorius, 1974). The prevalence rate of schizophrenia was estimated at 2.62 per 1000 cases (265 cases in a population of 101,229). The age-corrected prevalence was 3.96 per 1000. Prior prevalence studies found rates ranging from 2.6 to 3.4 per 1000, after age correction (Surya, Datta, and Krishna, 1964; Dube, 1970; Elnager, Maitra, and Rao, 1971; Verghese, Beig, and Sensemen, 1973; Sethi, Gupta, Mahendru, and Kumari, 1974; Thacore, Gupta, and Suriya, 1975; Nandi, Ajmany et al., 1976; Nandi, Mukerjee et al., 1980). Comparability across these studies is limited by such factors as differing sample sizes (ranging from 674 to 101,229), methods and diagnostic criteria, which range from the researcher's own case definitions to standardized criteria. Lack of facilities in most parts of the country has limited application of computerized diagnostic systems.

There appears to be no consistent rural-urban difference in frequency of illness, nor have clear pockets of high or low prevalence been demonstrated. A pattern of increased prevalence of schizophrenia in the rural area contiguous to a major city in north India has been reported (Sethi et al., 1974) in a community survey of adjoining rural, semirural, and urban areas. A prevalence rate of 2.58 per 1000 was estimated in the rural areas as compared to 2.03 per 1000 in the nearby urban-industrial area, but this difference was not statistically significant. A higher prevalence rate was found in the urban slums of Chennai by the SOFPUC study.

Incidence rates for schizophrenia in India have been consistently higher than those from the developed countries. Significant studies in India have been conducted in West Bengal (Nandi et al., 1976), Chandigarh (Varma, 1989), and Chennai (Rajkumar and Thara, 1989; Rajkumar, Padmavati, and Thara, 1993). The paucity of incidence studies in India is due probably to the absence of demarcated catchment areas for health service delivery, to an absence of case registers, and to the high cost of conducting such studies (Indian Council of Medical Research, 1990). In a community survey in West Bengal that used a screening schedule and a consensus clinical diagnosis, the estimated incidence rate of schizophrenia was 0.93 per 1000. However, inference is limited because only one new case of schizophrenia was seen during the study period. In Chandigarh, one of the centers of the WHO DOSMeD study, the incidence rate was 0.38 per 1000 in the urban region and 0.44 per 1000 in the rural population. The study design was a methodologically refined, extended case-finding approach, which included first service contact cases as well as those seeking traditional or religious treatment. The estimation of incidence of schizophrenia in the slums of Chennai involved a door-to-door survey of the population at risk (a population of 25,661 that excluded all prevalence cases and all children below 15 years of age). A leakage study undertaken to obviate underreporting involved scrutinizing the records of nearby mental health facilities, general practitioners, private psychiatrists, traditional and faith healers for new cases during the study period. The incidence rate was 0.35 per 1000. The authors recommended the use of both community surveys and an extended case-finding "leakage" method for estimating total incidence rates (Indian Council of Medical Research, 1990).

Gender differences have not been consistent. The SOFPUC study did not find any gender variations in incidence of schizophrenia; however, in rural Chandigarh, a higher rate was found in women (0.48 per 1000) than in men (0.37 per 1000).

THE CENTER

The Schizophrenia Research Foundation (SCARF), India, a premier voluntary, nonprofit, nongovernmental center carried out the ISoS at Chennai. The tripartite objectives of SCARF are research, care and rehabilitation, awareness, and training. Established in 1984, SCARF has gained credibility nationally and internationally and has been designated a WHO Collaborating Center for Mental Health

Research and Training. A Board of Management comprised of mental health professionals, prominent citizens, and philanthropists meets four times a year to oversee the functioning of the organization. Professional staff includes the director and four other psychiatrists, nine psychiatric social workers, two clinical psychologists, one statistician-cum-computer manager, and two workshop supervisors. Administrative staff includes one controller (finance and administration), one chief administrative officer, two accountants, three clerical officers, three drivers, and four support staff.

A day treatment center offers psychosocial rehabilitation programs (vocational and occupational training, social skills, training, group therapy, and cognitive retraining) for nearly 60 men and 15 women. Work with families is a high priority, and family group sessions are held regularly. The education of 30 children whose fathers are so disabled that they cannot work is being supported by SCARF. There is also an active outpatient department open 7 days a week. Poor patients receive medication free. Apart from the main center in the city of Chennai, SCARF operates two residential rehabilitation centers on the outskirts of the city. These house 55 women and elderly in one and 20 men in the other, all of them mentally disabled. There are also three community outreach programs, two in rural areas and one in the city slums.

Research

Research is aimed primarily at improving SCARF programs and at better understanding patients and their families. SCARF has forged research links with other national and international centers. Some important research projects are:

Collaborations in India

1. WHO South East Asia Regional Office—A project to study "Family Burden in Schizophrenia" has been completed.
2. Indian Council of Social Scientific Research (ICSSR)—A project on disability in schizophrenia has been completed.
3. With the National Institute for Mental Health and Neurosciences, Bangalore: Participated in multisite drug trials. Some SCARF staff have undergone training programs related to the National Mental Health Programme and SCAN conducted at NIMHANS.
4. Maintenance medication in schizophrenia funded by Searle, India.
5. Risperidone in schizophrenia funded by Johnson & Johnson.

Collaborations Outside India

1. WHO-Geneva-ISoS; WHO-SATIS—a multisite study to assess satisfaction with mental health services, and the Cross-Cultural Applicability Research (CAR) jointly with NIMH, United States, in the field of disabilities, impairments, and handicaps.
2. Johns Hopkins University, Baltimore, United States—A collaborative study on outcome of schizophrenia funded by the U.S. NIMH has been completed (Thara, Henrietta, Joseph, Rajkumar, and Eaton, 1994; Eaton, Thara, Freeman, Melton, and Liang, 1995; Thara and Eaton, 1996; Thara and Srinivasan, 1997a,b; Srinivasan, and Thara 1997; Eaton, Thara, Federman, and Tien, 1998).
3. Crichton Royal Hospital, Dumfries, Scotland—A study on abnormal involuntary movements in elderly mentally ill persons, cognitive functions, and estimations of lipid peroxide in patients with schizophrenia (McCreadie, Thara, Kamath et al., 1996; McCreadie, Latha, Thara, Padmavati, and Ayankaran, 1997).
4. International Development Research Centre, Canada, sponsored a 5-year study on community mental health in a rural population.
5. Central Institute of Mental Health, Mannheim, Germany—A comparison of coping strategies used by schizophrenic patients in Madras and Mannheim (Kumar, Thara, and Rist, 1994).
6. Douglas Hospital and Research Centre, Montreal, Canada—Two studies (a) on "Turning Point," (b) on people seeking religious treatment for mental illness.

While SCARF is the center conducting ISoS, the patients included were first seen at the Department of Psychiatry, Government General Hospital, and Madras Medical College where the first 7-year follow-up was conducted. Under the leadership of Dr. S. Rajkumar, the department was very active in research on schizophrenia and dementia and participated in several international projects. When

Dr. Thara (P.I.) shifted to SCARF, the research was moved there.

METHODS USED AT THE SITE

Defining the ISoS Cohort and Case-Finding

The sample consisted of 100 consecutive patients who fulfilled ICD-9 and modified Feighner's criteria for schizophrenia (Verghese et al., 1985; Thara and Rajkumar, 1990) and who attended the psychiatry outpatient department at the Madras Medical College and Government General Hospital between 1981 and 1982. They were recruited for the 5-year multicenter follow-up study on "Factors Affecting the Course and Outcome of Schizophrenia," coordinated by the Indian Council of Medical Research (ICMR, 1988). Ninety of the 100 were first episode cases making first contact with a treatment facility. Dr. Thara, Senior Research Officer in the study, continued to follow up this cohort with funding from the Schizophrenia Research Foundation so that, by the beginning of the ISoS study, the sample was already being followed. Some who were not under active treatment and were not coming to the facility regularly responded either to letters or to home visits and cooperated with the interviewers. In three cases, where the patients had moved outside the city of Chennai, the research staff traveled to their homes. Those who had changed residence and had not informed SCARF were impossible to follow up; there are no movement registers in Chennai nor is it mandatory for people who move to inform the post office. In urban areas, where living space is expensive and hard to come by, mentally ill people are not well tolerated; very often the house owner on receiving complaints from neighbors and co-tenants will urge the family to move. Despite this, the rate of follow-up is good. Difficulties were faced only with three patients, all of them young, unmarried women. Their families resented the visits of the research staff since they feared that word about mental illness would become common knowledge and jeopardize the women's prospects for marriage.

Use of Study Instruments

Some of the instruments, such as the PSE and the DAS, had already been translated into Tamil. Most of the others were not translated since time and resources were not available, and all patients/families were interviewed by the same investigator.

Data-Gathering Procedures

As this was being done on a continuous basis, the data already obtained needed only to be collated and transcribed.

STUDY RESULTS: PATTERNS AND VARIATIONS

Baseline and Short-Term Follow-Up

Gender and Age

The original sample had an almost equal distribution of men and women aged 15 to 45 years. There was no gender difference in the age of onset. Over 60% were unmarried at inclusion. None of the patients lived alone; about 80% lived in nuclear families and the rest in joint or extended households. As is usually true of the population using the facilities of a state-run hospital, almost the entire cohort hailed from middle and lower socioeconomic groups. Very few had a university education, but none was illiterate. Most of the men were employed, unskilled and skilled labor predominating among the occupational categories. Prevalence of drug and alcohol abuse was low. Of the original cohort, 77 were alive and could be assessed at the end of the follow-up period; 14 were lost to follow-up and nine had died. The characteristics of the alive cohort were almost similar to the entire sample, with the number of men and women being almost equal. The age distribution of the alive cohort, whose mean birth year was 1958, was no different from that of the entire sample. Those who died had a slightly lower mean birth year.

Mode of Onset and Diagnosis

Nearly 60% of those in the alive cohort had an insidious onset of illness (>1 month), which was similar to that of the entire sample. All the subjects who died and over 60% of those who were lost to follow-up also had an insidious onset of illness. Paranoid schizophrenia was the predominant diagnostic category in the original sample as well as in each of the cohorts—alive, dead, and lost to follow-up. All of the Madras alive cohort received a diagnosis of schizophrenia when the baseline diagnoses were converted to ICD-10 format. All but one of the nonmissing cases for Beijing and Hong Kong also had an ICD-10 converted diagnosis of schizophrenia. This was not the case in all of the other non-invited centers, where converted diagnoses for the original cohorts ranged from 85% schizophrenia in Nagasaki to 20% schizophrenia in Groningen; nine centers had 50% or less.

Pattern of Course at Early Follow-Up

Forty-five of the alive subjects (58%) had a good short-term course, having remitted completely. Another 24 (31%) had an incomplete remission, and only eight had continuous illness. This pattern is strikingly similar to that of the original cohort. The dead and drop-out groups, however, had higher rates of continuing psychosis and incomplete remission.

ALIVE SUBJECTS

Symptomatology

The Bleuler scale, which classified the severity of psychotic symptoms at the end of the 12-year follow-up period, revealed that 58% of subjects were totally recovered, 30% had mild to moderate psychotic symptoms, while only 12% had severe symptoms. This was not very much different from Chandigarh urban and rural. The Global Assessment of Functioning Scale for current symptomatology (GAF-S) reflected a similar pattern. Forty-eight subjects (62.4%) were either not or only mildly symptomatic (GAF-S score of over 70). The mean GAF-S score was 65.2, which was not too different from that of the Invited centers but was lower than that of the other three Indian cohorts (Agra, 76; Chandigarh, 71 urban; 77, rural).

Course of Illness

As might be expected given the symptomatology findings, 78% of the subjects had an episodic course of illness since first treatment contact. Only seven (9%) were continuously ill, and the remaining 13% had a course which could be classified as neither continuous nor episodic. This pattern was similar to that of the Chandigarh cohorts, but quite different from that of the other two Invited centers. Fifty percent of the Beijing sample and 27% of the Hong Kong cohort were continuously ill during the entire study period. With respect to time trends, over 90% were intensely psychotic during the first one-third of the follow-up period with a decline in intensity over the rest of the period; overall, 41.6% were much better at the time of follow-up, 31.2% somewhat better, and 16% remained the same, while only 10.4% were worse or somewhat worse. Over the last 2 years, over half (61%) of the cohort experienced no psychotic episodes, and equal numbers experienced either continuous illness (18%) or short psychotic episodes (17%).

Reevaluation of Baseline Diagnosis

At the time of inclusion of the subjects into the original study, two criteria were used: ICD-9 for schizophrenia and Feighner's criteria (with the minimum duration of illness modified from 6 months to 3 months). Reevaluation of diagnosis was undertaken by a psychiatrist who had never been involved in the study. All 77 cases were diagnosed with schizophrenia when both ICD-10 and DSM-IV were used.

Residential and Functional Status

At the time of assessment, 73 (94.8%) of the subjects lived with their families. (Three other subjects, one in the hospital and the other two in residential rehabilitation facilities, were in touch with their families.) This is strikingly similar to the other two Indian centers where most subjects were in independent community living for the greater part of the follow-up period. Note, however, what makes this "independence" possible: For 38 of the 47 subjects (81%) on whom information was available, informants reported that the family had provided a substitute for institutional or custodial care for "most" of the last 2 years of the follow-up period. Over the course of the follow-up, none of the subjects had been homeless, vagrant, or jailed. The total amount of time spent in the hospital during the entire follow-up period was less than all of the other centers, except for the other Indian centers, and Cali: 30% had never been hospitalized, and 56%

were in the hospital for less than 5% of the follow-up period. Only one of the subjects spent over 50% of the time in the hospital.

Work

In the 2 years prior to assessment, 29 subjects (37.7%) had been employed continuously for the 24 months; another four had some full-time employment, while three had only worked part-time. Forty subjects, mostly women, were unemployed in the formal sector. The work performance of 87% of the group working at least 12 months was rated as good or very good; the Hong Kong sample had a similar work profile. Another 28 subjects (70% of those formally unemployed) were engaged for the entire 2 years in household work. Their performance, however, was not as good as those who worked outside the home, with 12 (43%) rated as being poor or very poor. The samples in the other two invited centers had a good household work rating in three-quarters of the subjects. None in the Chennai sample had retired from work. None received disability benefits. In the 2 years prior to assessment, 36 had been formally employed, 28 were in full-time household work, 12 were unemployed, and one was in an institution.

Social Disability

Functioning in the last month of follow-up was assessed using the DAS and the GAF-D. Of the 75 who were rated on the DAS, 35 (46.7%) subjects had a good to excellent rating, 13 (17%) were rated as fair, and the remaining 27 (36%) as poor to severe. On the GAF-D, 39 (50.7%) had scores higher than 71 indicating rather good functioning, 16 (20.8%) scored from 51 to 70, with the remaining 22 (28.6%) rated as functioning poorly. Most of the cohort (87%) had the maximum disability in the first third of the follow-up period, while six had equally severe disability in the first and last thirds of the entire period.

Violence and Suicide

At the time of assessment, only eight of the 75 subjects for whom information was available had engaged in assaultive behavior in the last 2 years. When the entire period was considered, this figure went to 16 (20.8%). Five had made suicide attempts in the past 2 years, and 13 in the entire 12 years. None of these was of a serious nature.

Medications

In the last 2 years of follow-up, half the Chennai sample was off neuroleptics; 16% took them at times and 35% for most of the time. During the entire follow-up period, 43% were on neuroleptics sometimes, and 57% for most of the time. When the trend of medication during the entire period was examined, for 86.5% the use of medication was prominent in the first third of the follow-up period only, while 7% had equally prominent medication in all three time periods.

Hospitalization

At the time of assessment, sixty-seven subjects (87%) had not been hospitalized during the past 2 years. Ten had been either hospitalized or placed in a supervised residence. During the entire follow-up period, 23 (30%) had never been hospitalized, 48 (62%) for less than 10% of the time and the remaining six for over 10%. In 92% of the 63 subjects for whom information was available, hospitalization was prominent in the first third of the follow-up period only.

DECEASED SUBJECTS

Nine patients had died during the follow-up period: four men and five women. There was little gender difference in the mean ages at death. Six of those who died were young (less than 40 years of age); five died of natural causes; four committed suicide. The events preceding death for two subjects were chronic fever with dehydration in a young girl who was hospitalized following a diagnosis of enteric fever, and a suspected rupture of an aortic aneurysm in a man who had no previous history of illness. Another middle-aged man's death was not known until a few weeks after the event, and his daughter knew only that he had been suffering from recurrent abdominal pain but had not wanted to have medical treatment. One patient, who was psychotic at the time of his death, went to the top floor of his apartment building and fell, possibly accidentally. Two, a man and a woman, consumed insecticide and died before they could be taken to the hospital; there were no suicide notes. One woman doused herself with kerosene and set herself on fire. Another death was by hanging. At the time of death, four were in an episode of illness, two in partial remission, and three in total remission. The death rate of the cohort is higher than the rate in the general population which is 7 per 1000 for all ages, but the difference is not statistically significant. If only the age group 25 to 45 (to which most of the sample belonged) is considered, the age-specific rate of death in the local population is only 3.5 per 1000. Hence, the age-adjusted death rate in the cohort could be considerably higher and, indeed, the standardized mortality ratio is calculated to be 1.9.

DISCUSSION

The intake cohort of 100 subjects was assembled in 1981 to 1982, and can be held to be representative of the middle and lower economic population, characteristic of persons seeking state-run, general hospital services in Chennai. The cohort, therefore, excludes higher income, more literate persons who generally visit private psychiatric facilities. The subjects were predominantly first onset schizophrenia patients of an active outpatient psychiatry department of a general hospital in Chennai; men and women are represented fairly evenly, and most were younger than 35 at entry. Treatment was provided free. Follow-up was prospective, and at the end of 12 years, the alive cohort fell into the following groups: One group had continued treatment (those with periodic relapses or who were continuously ill) reporting to the SCARF fairly regularly (n=21); a second group (n=53) responded well to letters sent to them and was keen to maintain contact with the center; many of them were off medication or were in treatment at another facility; and a third, small group (n=3) resented contact with the research team and consisted mainly of young women who married after the onset of illness and who feared rejection from the spouse's family. Of those lost to follow-up, five were early drop-outs, seven had emigrated outside the catchment area, one refused to cooperate, and one went missing.

Follow-up was fraught with difficulties. Since there are no movement registers, it was impossible to trace a subject unless he or she chose to remain in contact with the facility. Despite this, follow-up of the cohort was quite good because it was a regularly and prospectively followed-up sample, and the presence of the same investigator over the entire 12-year period provided the continuity that is often critical in follow-up exercises.

A comparison of the three groups (alive, dead, lost to follow-up) did not reveal significant differences in their clinical state or course of illness. There does not seem to be bias affecting the alive cohort.

The outcome at the end of 12 years was essentially good: Over half (58%) were rated as fully recovered, according to the Bleuler scale; another 30% had only mild to moderate symptoms. The mean GAF-S score was 65.2, which indicates an essentially nonpsychotic nature of the clinical profile and is almost identical to the score for the entire ISoS sample (65.1). The mean GAF-D score was 63. Only eight of the men were unemployed, another indicator of good psychosocial functioning, especially when one considers that there are, as yet, no specific welfare measures for this disability group. Women had a better pattern of course and lower disability scores. All of them lived with families, with no homelessness or jail sentences.

In the last 2 years of follow-up, 61% of the sample was not psychotic, 18% had continuous illness, and 17% had short psychotic episodes. The pattern of course during the entire period was also favorable in most cases: 30% had never been in the hospital, and 56% spent less than 5% of the time there. As is natural for first onset cases that form the bulk of this sample (90%), the severity of symptoms was greatest in the early part of the follow-up period and tended to stabilize thereafter. Three-quarters of the sample were considered to have improved in their overall course of symptoms and in disability severity.

Rates of hospitalization during the entire follow-up period were low, reflecting not severity of illness, but rather the types of resources available (Verghese et al., 1985; Rajkumar and Thara, 1989; Thara and Rajkumar, 1990). In a country like India, where the number of hospital beds is low for 7 to 8 million people with severe mental illness, hospitalization cannot be considered an indicator of the severity of either the initial episode or the subsequent relapses. Since admission into a mental health facility, especially into a mental hospital, carries a good deal of stigma, many families are willing to care for the subjects at home, even if this results in disruption of family life and routines. In addition, psychiatric care is not covered by insurance, further compounding the family's problems. At the same time, the sociocultural context in which all of the subjects live—primarily with families—greatly enhances medication compliance.

The concept of "independent community living" as applied to developed countries is not applicable to the Indian situation. Most people suffering from schizophrenia live with their families, and the level of dependence on families varies. Those subjects who are unemployed are totally dependent on their families. (In many instances, normal young women awaiting marriage are also totally dependent on the families, since they are not expected to support themselves.) There are virtually no facilities that cater exclusively to those with chronic mental illness. Reluctance of landlords to rent them apartments and hostility and intolerance of neighbors, particularly those living in crowded tenements in urban areas, are predominant factors in accounting for internal migration of mentally ill persons.

Many of the men in the sample were forced to fend for themselves, since unemployment among the middle and lower income groups is synonymous with abject poverty; however, the motivation to find work is quite high. Some change jobs quite often. Although much is expected from the family, it is equally important for mentally ill persons from lower economic groups to maintain a certain degree of "wellness" in order to keep their jobs, to care for their families, and to live up to their role expectations to a reasonable extent. They may know little about the illness, its characteristics, social ramifications, and disabilities, but they do appreciate the need to continue medication since it enables them to resume and maintain productive activity. During the initial stages, many of them sought traditional/religious treatment, sometimes concomitantly with medical treatment, but as the years rolled by, they have come to rely primarily on medication and on the support of the research team.

SUMMARY

On most parameters, the characteristics of the sample were similar to that of the other two Invited centers (Beijing and Hong Kong) and, in fact, to the entire ISoS sample.

ISoS is one of the few prospective, follow-up studies using standardized assessment tools done in the region. The fact that 90% of subjects were first onset cases adds to its merit.

References

Dube, K. C. (1970), A study of prevalence and biological variables in mental illness in a rural and urban community in Uttar Pradesh, India. *Acta Psychiatr. Scand.*, 46:327.

Eaton, W. W., Thara, R., Federman, E., Melton, B., & Liang, K. Y. (1995), Structure and course of positive and negative symptoms in schizophrenia. *Arch. Gen. Psychiatry*, 52:127–134.

——, ——, ——Tien, A. (1998), Remission and relapse in schizophrenia: The Madras longitudinal study. *J. Nerv. & Ment. Dis.*, 186(6):357–363.

Elnager, M. N., Maitra, P., & Rao, M. N. (1971), Mental health in an Indian rural community. *Brit. J. Psychiatry*, 118:499–503.

Indian Council of Medical Research (1988), *Multicentered Collaborative Study of Factors Associated with the Course and Outcome of Schizophrenia—Final Report.* New Delhi: Indian Council of Medical Research.

——(1990), *Final Report of the Longitudinal Study of Functional Psychoses in an Urban Community.* New Delhi: Indian Council of Medical Research.

Kapur, R. L., Kapur, M., & Carstairs, G. M. (1974), Indian psychiatric survey schedule (IPSS). *Soc. Psychiatry*, 9: 61–69.

Kumar, S., Thara, R., & Rist, F. (1994), Coping with symptoms of schizophrenia—A cross-cultural comparison. *Ind. J. Soc. Psychiatry*, 10(1–4):4–10.

McCreadie, R. G., Latha, S., Thara, R., Padmavathi, R., & Ayankaran, J. R. (1997), Poor memory, negative symptoms and abnormal movements in never treated Indian schizophrenic patients. *Brit. J. Psychiatry*, 171:360–363.

——Thara, R., Kamath, S., Padmavathy, R., Latha, S., Mathruboothan, N., & Menon, M. S. (1996), Abnormal movements in never medicated Indian patients with schizophrenia. *Brit. J. Psychiatry*, 168:221–226.

Namboodri, V. M. D., (1986), *Ancient Indian Systems in Schizophrenia: Historical Trends.* Madras: SCARF.

Nandi, D. N., Ajmany, S., Ganguli, H. H., Banerjee, G., Boral, G. C., Gosh, A., & Sarkar, S. (1976), Psychiatric disorders in rural community in West Bengal. An epidemiological study. *Ind. J. Psychiatry*, 17:87–90.

——Mukerjee, S. P., Boral, G. C., Banerjee, G., Ghosh, A., Sarkar, S., & Ajmany, S. (1980), Socio-economic status and mental morbidity in certain tribes and castes in India—A cross cultural study. *Brit. J. Psychiatry*, 136: 73–85.

Padmavati, R., & Rajkumar, S. (1989), Prevalence and incidence of schizophrenia. In: *The Natural History of Schizophrenia*, ed. S. Rajkumar, R. Thara, V. Nagaswami. Madras: Schizophrenia Research Foundation.

——, ——Narendra, K., Manohar, A., & Kamath, S. (1988), Prevalence of schizophrenia in an urban community in Madras. *Ind. J. Psychiatry*, 30(3):233–239.

Rajkumar, S., Padmavati, R., & Thara, R. (1993), Incidence of schizophrenia in an urban community in Madras. *Ind. J. Psychiatry*, 35(1):18–21.

——Thara, R. (1989), Factors affecting relapse in schizophrenia. *Schizophr. Res.*, 2:403–409.

Sethi, B. B., Gupta, S. C., Mahendru, R. K., & Kumari, P. (1974), Mental health and urban life. A study of 850 families. *Brit. J. Psychiatry*, 124:243–246.

Srinivasan, T. N., & Thara, R. (1997), How do men with schizophrenia fare at work?—Results of a longitudinal study from Madras. *Schizophr. Res.*, 25:149–154.

Surya, N. C., Datta, S. P., & Krishna, R. G. (1964), Mental morbidity in Pondicherry (1962–1963). *Trans. All Ind. Inst. Ment. Health,* Bangalore, A:50–61.

Thacore, V. R., Gupta, S. C., & Suriya, M. (1975), Psychiatric morbidity in a North Indian community. *Brit. J. Psychiatry,* 126:364–369.

Thara, R., & Eaton, W. W. (1996), Ten-year outcome of schizophrenia—The Madras longitudinal study. *Austral. & N. Z. J. Psychiatry,* 30:482–488.

——Henrietta, M., Joseph, A., Rajkumar, S., & Eaton, W. W. (1994), Ten-year course of schizophrenia—The Madras longitudinal study. *Acta Psychiatr. Scand.,* 1: 329–336.

——Islam, A., & Padmavati, R. (1997), Management of psychosocial problems in a rural community in India. In: *Proceedings of the Third Asia & Pacific Conference on the Social Sciences & Medicine,* Vol. 2. Perth, Australia: Edith Cowan University.

——Rajkumar, S. (1990), A study of sample attrition in follow-up of schizophrenia. *Ind. J. Psychiatry,* 32(3):217–222.

——Srinivasan, T. N. (1997a), Outcome of marriage in schizophrenia. *Soc. Psychiatry & Psychiatric Epidemiology,* 32:416–420.

——, ——(1997b), Marriage and gender in schizophrenia. *Ind. J. Psychiatry,* 1:64–69.

Varma, V. K. (1989), *Final Report of the Determinants of Outcome of Severe Mental Disorders: A Seven-Year Follow-Up Study.* New Delhi: Indian Council of Medical Research.

Verghese, A., Beig, A., & Sensemen, C. A. (1973), A social and psychiatric study of a representative group of families in Vellore town. *Ind. J. Med. Res.,* 61:608–620.

——Dube, K. C., John, J., Menon, D. K., Menon, M. S., Rajkumar, S., Richard, J., Sethi, B. B., Trivedi, J. K., & Wig, N. N. (1985), Factors associated with course and outcome of schizophrenia. *Ind. J. Psychiatry,* 27: 201–204.

Wing, J. K., Cooper, J. E., & Sartorius, N. (1974), *The Measurement and Classification of Psychiatric Symptoms.* Cambridge, U.K.: Cambridge University Press.

Conclusion

Kim Hopper, Glynn Harrison, Aleksandar Janca, Norman Sartorius, and Durk Wiersma

ISoS spanned roughly the last quarter of the 20th century, during which time schizophrenia and related disorders continued to exact great costs and cause untold suffering throughout the world (World Bank, 1993; Rupp and Keith, 1993). Suggestive reports that incidence may be declining in the developed world have yet to be confirmed (Jablensky, 1995). Conversely, if anything the incidence of such disorders is increasing in developing countries, as public health advances ensure that more people survive childhood and early adolescence (Sugar, Kleinman, and Heggenbougen, 1994). Worldwide, the burden of neuropsychiatric disorders (a measure combining mortality and disability)—estimated at 10.5% of the total global disease load in 1990—is projected to increase to 14.7% over the next two decades (Murray and Lopez, 1996, 1997; Ustun, 1999).

Substantial gains have been made in our understanding of brain structure and functioning, in neuropharmacology, in family education techniques, psychosocial interventions, and the improvisations of supportive work—in all the manifold tools and strategies of rehabilitation, some ingeniously adapted to cultural circumstances and resource scarcity (as recent reports from China suggest [Phillips, Pearson, and Wang, 1994])—as well as in our appreciation of the role that individuals can play in the day-to-day management of their own illnesses (Davidson and Strauss, 1992; Shore, 1993; Andreasen, 1994). Even in resource-rich countries, however, the gap between hard-won knowledge and common practice remains large, and is often skewed in ways that mimic larger social inequalities (Lehman, Steinwachs, and the Survey Co-Investigators of the PORT Project, 1998). Evidence has steadily accumulated, too, that specific environmental factors in the immediate life-world of the afflicted individual (whether these be features of ward routine, sources of persistent stress, disruptive life events, hostile/critical family atmosphere, or accommodating social space) play a significant role in the likelihood of relapse or persistence of disability. These targeted inquiries have yet to be productively enmeshed with ethnographic documentation in ways that would allow for deeper understanding of the particular sociocultural features of contexts that promote recovery (Day et al., 1987; Corin, 1990; Jenkins and Karno, 1992; Miklowitz, 1994; Desjarlais, Eisenberg, Good, and Kleinman, 1995; Bebbington, 1996).

Most important of all, the premise that a deteriorating course was a signature feature of schizophrenia—with us since the earliest taxonomic efforts of Kraepelin (Berrios and Hauser, 1988)—is now widely questioned.[1] As the earlier WHO studies had suggested and others since have corroborated, the course of schizophrenia is not "hard-wired" into the diagnosis itself; rather, it is a developmental product of continuing interaction of disease process, treatment, local environment, and the active agency of the person. Heterogeneity in outcome—across subjects in research studies, across domains of symptoms and social functioning within subjects—has become accepted clinical principle in many quarters, with profound implications for both rehabilitation and outcome assessment (Carpenter and Kirkpatrick, 1988; Harding, Zubin, and Strauss, 1992; Warner, 1994; de Jong, van der Lubbe, & Wiersma,

1. Interestingly, the older emphasis on deteriorating course is more discernible in the DSM-IV nomenclature than in the ICD-10 scheme, which places greater emphasis on Schneiderian first-rank symptoms at the present time (McGee, Swanson, Jones, and Frances, 1996, p. 10).

1996; Fenton, 1996; Davidson and McGlashan, 1997).

SOME HIGHLIGHTS

Though the picture of course and outcome of schizophrenia and related psychoses assembled here is by no means consistent, a number of salient findings merit note:

- Overall recovery: Judged by clinical ratings of overall status and functioning, the long-term outcome for over half of ISoS subjects was quite good. Even when potential biases in follow-up are taken into account and adjustments are made to produce the most conservative estimates of recovery, the ISoS results rank among the most favorable long-term outcomes to date.
- The predictive value of early course of illness: Two-year course (viz., percent time psychotic) was confirmed as the most robust predictor of symptom and functioning for the DOSMeD cohort, though unspecified cultural variables also play a role. Even so, for a fifth of ISoS subjects, poor early course of illness was coupled with later recovery.
- Diagnostic stability: The vast majority of ISoS subjects (88%) retained their baseline diagnosis of schizophrenia spectrum in later "lifetime" assessments. Diagnostic stability was observed far more frequently for schizophrenia than for either schizoaffective disorder or acute schizophrenia. Proportions of diagnostic change were virtually identical in the incidence and prevalence cohorts of ISoS.
- Mortality: ISoS confirms that persons diagnosed with schizophrenia and related psychoses are at increased risk of death in both developed and developing countries, with elevated standardized mortality ratios (SMRs) especially marked in industrialized centers. Infectious diseases, however, did not figure highly in such elevations for this largely pre-AIDS pandemic cohort.
- Developed versus developing differential: Consistent with the earlier findings of IPSS and DOSMeD, course and outcome for subjects in the developing centers were more favorable than for their developed world counterparts. Most of the difference registers early on, in the initial two years of illness (Jablensky et al., 1992). But even for subjects whose early course was poor, the likelihood of later recovery favors those in the developing centers (42 vs. 33%) (see Hopper and Wanderling, 2000, for further analysis).
- Work: As expected, employment (including household work) was more often reported for subjects in developing centers. Overall, over half the ISoS cohort was working at follow-up. And when one looks at the likelihood of working in persons for whom symptoms and/or disabilities continue to present substantial problems, little difference was found between developing and developed centers—in both, nearly 20% of those meeting the symptom and/or disability criteria had worked most of the last 2 years of follow-up.
- Homelessness: Although a pronounced feature at the intersection of severe mental illness and poverty in many Western cities in the 1980s to 1990s, homelessness proved rare in those traced in ISoS. Only 16 subjects (out of 1005) were ever homeless during the last 2 years of follow-up.[2]
- Comorbidity: Likewise, comorbid conditions—especially substance abuse—so common as accompaniments of psychiatric disorders among some North American and European cohorts (Kessler, 1995; Batel, 2000), were less significant findings here.[3]

THE ROLE OF CULTURE

Statements about the role of culture in prior WHO studies of course and outcome have been carefully hedged, and for good reason. The sustained inquiry and customized tools needed to take the measure of "local moral worlds" were conspicuous by their absence in these epidemiological investigations. What documentation there was of individual field sites tended to be impressionistic, unsystematic, enlivened with local color and, reassuringly, riddled with inconsistencies. So mixed a picture was bound to disappoint those seeking evidence of "communities of recovery"—stigma-free havens, blessed by forgiving beliefs in the

2. Because those lost to follow-up were more likely to be younger men with poorer short-term outcomes, the estimates of homelessness may be biased downward, as this group is most susceptible to such extreme dislocation.

3. Significant current drug or alcohol use was documented for only 5.8% of the ISoS follow-up group. This may reflect the timing of the early phase of illness for the ISoS cohorts (treated incidence especially), which occurred as hallucinogenic use was tapering off and preceded the secular upturn in stimulant drug use among psychiatric patients. For the DOSMeD cohort, drug use at baseline was concentrated in two U.S. and one Danish center; alcohol problems were concentrated in three European and one U.S. center (Jablensky et al., 1992, pp. 41–42). Local market conditions clearly play a role as well (Warner, Taylor, Wright, Sloat, Springett, Arnold, and Weinberg, 1994).

other-worldly origins of psychiatric disorder, and ready stores of supportive kin and accommodating work. No doubt, a determined reading of the portraits of "traditional" societies contained in the early IPSS reports could find passages describing places where subsistence economies prevailed, extended families were the norm, and magiocoreligious explanations of madness held sway. But such selective reading would have to ignore inconvenient and neighboring text demonstrating that the locus of such environs was as likely shantytown as village, that closely configured families could be tyrannical as well as supportive, and that local practitioners found "superstition" to be as exasperating as it was exculpatory. Hence, the sensibly considered tone to the pointed observations on culture made by these authors.

Fifteen years later, we still lack even the limited cultural data collected early on by the DOSMeD substudies that would make for modest comparative analysis.[4] Nor have we made substantial analytic headway in resolving the "dilemma of context" (Scharfstein, 1989): devising appropriate means for assessing the influence of cultural variables that take into account the contexts within which such variables acquire meaning and exert effect (Hopper, 1991, p. 313; Edgerton and Cohen, 1994, p. 228). The earlier observation of Jablensky and colleagues is thus doubly chastening: that although a strong case for the importance of cultural factors in course and outcome seems eminently reasonable, we have yet to "penetrate in sufficient depth below the surface on which the impact of the [hypothesized] factor was established" (1992, p. 89). Nonetheless, even the relatively crude measures of center environs collected in ISoS by straightforward survey questionnaires showed predictive promise (Siegel et al., Chapter 4, this volume).

None of this is to suggest that the influence of culture is too unstable or evanescent to be measured. Rather, in line with recent anthropological thinking (see Rosaldo, 1989; Bourdieu and Wacquant, 1992; Ware and Kleinman, 1992; Ortner, 1999; Lopez and Guarnaccia, 2000), it is to urge that the most fruitful course is to seek the telltale imprint of culture locally, at the level of documented practice, rather than ecologically, at the level of reputed habitat. "Family" offers one such domain of everyday practice.

HOW FAMILY FIGURES

Close examination of individual center chapters yields dividends forgone in more aggregated analyses. Consider how the operation of the "same" factor—family involvement—varied across study sites, as suggested by some observations on its role in mediating course and outcome:

- In Chandigarh, very favorable outcome results were once again obtained, which some have attributed (at least in part) to the lack of emotional overinvolvement and paucity of critical comments, coupled with steady support, in family environs (Leff et al., 1987).
- In Sofia, where generally poor results—high levels of symptoms and social disability coupled with low hospitalization—were obtained, investigators found families serving as surrogates for custodial care for 39% of subjects. Resource scarcity in times of political instability accounts for some of this; but investigators also attribute it to unspecified "cultural" factors encouraging high levels of family involvement in ongoing care (Ganev, Onchev, and Ivanov, 1998).
- The available follow-up cohort in Moscow may be biased toward better outcome because some of those with poor early course may have had no means of staying put. Lacking local kin ties and alternative sources of support in the event of job loss, when they experienced relapse and rehospitalization, they had no option but to leave the city and return home to family in the provinces (Tsirkin, chapter 14, this volume).

With respect to teasing out the cultural variation in such groupings as "developing" centers, however, we are not quite so hamstrung in ISoS as had been the case in IPSS and DOSMeD. Owing to logistical difficulties encountered in mounting another follow-up study, only the original Chandigarh-treated incidence cohorts (urban and rural) appear in ISoS. Coupled with the addition of the Chennai (Madras) cohort, this makes for a relatively culturally homogeneous grouping of Indian subjects—albeit one that spans the developmental space from ancient imperial city to modern planned community to agricultural village. While this restricts the generalizability of the finding on the differential advantage conferred by "developing" country status, it simplifies the cultural question. One might, that is, le-

4. We have baseline "expressed emotion" (EE) data on the relatives of 78 subjects in Chandigarh, but have no data more recent and none at all for any other participating research center. Aarhus, which had participated in the early EE study, was unable to participate in the follow-up.

gitimately inquire into salient characteristics of the Indian subcontinent in ways that would be foreclosed were members of the group spread all over the globe.

Take, for example, the extraordinary engagement of Indian families in the course of treatment. From the initial deliberations over whether to seek help, to taking care of basic needs and medication adherence during hospitalization, to everyday support after release, including monitoring of medications and functioning—family participation is well documented as a distinctive feature of the ethnopsychiatry practiced in that country (Nunley, 1998).[5] Earlier styles of family interaction documented in the DOSMeD substudies (Wig, Menon, Bedi, Ghosh et al., 1987; Wig, Menon, Beddi, Leff et al., 1987) are thus an obvious candidate for further longitudinal research. As the measurement problems posed by "expressed emotion" in those studies illustrate,[6] useful constructs will have to be embedded in everyday practice and observed over time for their meaning as "variables" to be interpretable. But the pragmatics of family communication hardly exhaust the range of potential family influence. Narrative accounts from Chennai, drawn up as part of ISoS and now being analyzed, suggest that the high cultural value placed upon responsible rearing of children can provide a powerful motivation for women not to let their illness interfere with their mothering.

In this regard, the "developed" and "developing" center groups in ISoS offer rather disparate pictures of the differential impact of psychotic disorder on matrimonial prospects. The likelihood of marriage for members of the Indian cohort at the time of follow-up was 73% (71% male, 74% female); for the developed centers, it was 38% (28% male, 48% female). More striking still is that the differential marital rates hold even when unfavorable early illness course is taken into account. The odds of marriage for an Indian woman with poor 2-year course decline somewhat, but are still 2:1; for her developed world counterpart, they are 2:3. Comparable figures for men are 3:2 versus 1:4.[7]

Anthropologists have come to appreciate the stubborn particularities of the "local" and the interconnected nature of the "contextual" in studies of other worlds. The objects of such study—"cultures" in action—are often notable for the lack of binding coherence that was once thought to be an anthropological staple of sojourns "elsewhere."[8] For their part, clinicians have shown renewed interest in the "intricacy of the ordinary" in devising successful programs of aftercare (Sørenson, 1994). So although the precise mechanisms through which culture exerts its influence remain obscure, this much should be clear: The heedless acts and "mind-forg'd manacles" that make madness at once the most public and the most private of afflictions are not simply things of its own making (MacDonald, 1981; Porter, 1987). What we observe, measure, contend with, and treat is not nature's mischief alone, but the work of culture too.

That dual provenance not only opens the door to a host of potentially therapeutic interventions and contrivances—suppose the remedial features of reliably salutary family environments could be identified: How might they be replicated in settings where kinship no longer provides the essential armature of support? It also ratifies the importance of the active agency of the afflicted person in managing the illness, an asset that earlier generations of psychiatric practitioners were rarely taught to value (Strauss, 1992). In some places this has translated into a shift in the therapeutic practice of even "tenacious" case management from aggressive aftercare to negotiated treated regimens (Diamond, 1996). And although still confined to a relatively few countries, the vigorous flourishing of self-help movements in mental health in the closing decades of the 20th century should be noted as well (Carling, 1995).

5. Such intensive "compensatory support mechanisms," available through extended kin over long periods of time, can also mean that seriously disordered members of the family may never seek treatment, as was found for nearly a third of persons diagnosed with schizophrenia in a 1985–1986 community survey in Madras (Padmavathi, Rajkumar, and Srinivasan, 1998).

6. Among the methodological difficulties encountered were the validity of assessing "emotion" from verbal material only (Kleinman, 1988), and scaling problems that arose from having to recalibrate ratings of "overinvolvement" in this most familially engaged culture (Nunley, 1998).

7. A closely documented study (monthly assessments over 10 years) of marital outcome in the Chennai (Madras) cohort supports this impression (Thara and Srinivasan, 1997). Its authors underscore the importance of duty (*dharma*) and presence of children in this predominantly Hindu culture, especially in explaining the high marital success for women (even for those whose homemaking skills are impaired; see Srinivasan and Thara, 1999). This success is the more striking given the persistent stigma attached to mental illness, especially with respect to marriage (Thara and Srinivasan, 2000).

8. The sustained documentary efforts of traditional ethnography commonly reveal beliefs and practices to be highly variable, often internally inconsistent, situation-dependent and riven by class, gender, ethnic, religious, and other structural divisions (Ortner, 1995).

The varieties of madness and its unruly course have long been reckoned among the toll of "social suffering" (Kleinman, Das, and Lock, 1997) worldwide. Knowledge, tested practice, social acceptance, and political will are needed to reduce this toll. The combined results of the WHO-Collaborative studies of schizophrenia will contribute, we hope, to at least the first of these factors.

References

Andreasen, N. C. (1994), *Schizophrenia: From Mind to Molecule*. Washington, DC: American Psychiatric Press.

Batel, P. (2000), Addiction and schizophrenia. *Eur. Psychiatry*, 15:115–122.

Bebbington, P. (1996), The economic significance of social factors influencing the outcome of schizophrenia. In: *Handbook of Mental Health Economics and Health Policy*, Vol. 1, *Schizophrenia*, ed. M. Moscarelli, A. Rupp, & N. Sartorius. New York: Wiley, pp. 65–78.

Berrios, G. E., & Hauser, R. (1982), The early development of Kraepelin's ideas on classification. *Psycholog. Med.*, 18:813–821.

Bourdieu, P., & Wacquant, L. J. D. (1992), *An Invitation to Reflexive Sociology*. Chicago: University of Chicago Press.

Carling, P. (1995), *Return to Community*. New York: Guilford Press.

Carpenter, W. T., & Kirkpatrick, B. (1988), The heterogeneity of the long-term course of schizophrenia. *Schizophr. Bull.*, 14:645–652.

Corin, E. E. (1990), Facts and meaning in psychiatry: An anthropological approach to the life-world of schizophrenia. *Culture, Med. & Psychiatry*, 14:153–188.

Davidson, L., & McGlashan, T. H. (1997), The varied outcomes of schizophrenia. *Can. J. Psychiatry*, 42:34–43.

——Strauss, J. S. (1992), Sense of self in recovery from severe mental illness. *Brit. J. Med. Psychology*, 65:131–145.

Day, R., Nielsen, J. A., Korten, A., Ernberg, G., Dube, K. C., Gebhart, J., Jablensky, A., Leon, C., Marsella, A., Olatawura, M., Sartorius, N., Strömgren, E., Takahashi, R., Wig, N., & Wynne, L. C. (1987), Stressful life events preceding the acute onset of schizophrenia. A cross-national study from the World Health Organization. *Culture, Med., & Psychiatry*, 11:123–205.

de Jong, A., van der Lubbe, P. M., & Wiersma, D. (1996), Social dysfunctioning in rehabilitation: Classification and assessment. In: *Handbook of Mental Health Economics and Health Policy*, Vol. 1, ed. M. Moscarelli, A. Rupp, & N. Sartorius. New York: Wiley, pp. 27–38.

Desjarlais, R., Eisenberg, L., Good, B., & Kleinman, A. (1995), *World Mental Health: Problems and Priorities in Low-Income Countries*. New York: Oxford University Press.

Diamond, R. J. (1996), Coercion and tenacious treatment in the community: Applications to the real world. In: *Coercion and Aggressive Community Treatment*, ed. D. L. Dennis & J. Monahan. New York: Plenum.

Edgerton, R., & Cohen, A. (1994), Culture and schizophrenia: The DOSMD challenge. *Brit. J. Psychiatry*, 164:222–231.

Fenton, W. S. (1996), Longitudinal course and outcome of schizophrenia. In: *Handbook of Mental Health Economics and Health Policy*, Vol. 1, ed. M. Moscarelli, A. Rupp, & N. Sartorius. New York: Wiley, pp. 79–91.

Ganev, K., Onchev, G., & Ivanov, P. (1998), A 16-year follow-up study of schizophrenia and related disorders in Sofia, Bulgaria. *Acta Psychiatr. Scand.*, 98:200–207.

Harding, C. M., Zubin, J., & Strauss, J. S. (1992), Chronicity in schizophrenia: Revisited. *Brit. J. Psychiatry*, 161 (Suppl. 18):27–37.

Hopper, K. (1991), Some old questions for the new cross-cultural psychiatry. *Med. Anthropol. Quart.*, 5 (new series):299–330.

——Wanderling, J. (2000), Revisiting the developed versus developing country distinction in course and outcome in schizophrenia: Results from ISoS, the WHO collaborative followup project. *Schizophr. Bull.*, 26(4): 835–846.

Jablensky, A. (1995), Schizophrenia: Recent epidemiologic issues. *Epidemiol. Rev.*, 17:10–20.

——Sartorius, N., Ernberg, G., Anker, M., Korten, A., Cooper, J. E., Day, R., & Bertelsen, A. (1992), Schizophrenia: Manifestations, incidence and course in different cultures. A World Health Organization ten-country study. *Psycholog. Med.* (Monogr. Suppl. 20): 1–97.

Jenkins, J. H., & Karno, M. (1992), The meaning of "expressed emotion": Theoretical issues raised by cross-cultural research. *Amer. J. Psychiat.*, 149(1):9–21.

Kessler, R. C. (1995), Epidemiology of psychiatric comorbidity. In: *Textbook in Psychiatric Epidemiology*, ed. M. T. Tsuang, M. Tohen, & G. E. P. Zahner. New York: Wiley, pp. 179–197.

Kleinman, A. (1988), *Rethinking Psychiatry*. New York: Free Press.

——Das, V., Lock, M., eds. (1997), *Social Suffering*. Berkeley: University of California Press.

Leff, J., Wig, N. N., Ghosh, A., Bedi, H., Menin, D. K., Kuipers, L., Korten, A., Ernberg, G., Day, R., Sartorius, N., & Jablensky, A. (1987), Influence of relatives' expressed emotion on the course of schizophrenia in Chandigarh. *Brit. J. Psychiatry*, 151:166–173.

Lehman, A. F., Steinwachs, D. M., & the Survey Co-Investigators of the PORT Project (1998), Patterns of usual care for schizophrenia: Initial results from the schizophrenia patient outcomes research team (PORT) client survey. *Schizophr. Bull.*, 24:1–10.

Lopez, S. R., & Guarnaccia, P. J. J. (2000), Cultural psychopathology: Uncovering the social world of mental illness. *Ann. Rev. Psychol.*, 51:571–598.

MacDonald, M. (1981), *Mystical Bedlam*. New York: Cambridge University Press.

McGee, M., Swanson, C., Jones, C., & Frances, A. (1996), Diagnosis: The DSM-IV approach to schizophrenia. In: *Handbook of Mental Health Economics and Health Policy*, Vol. 1, *Schizophrenia*, ed. M. Moscarelli, A. Rupp, & N. Sartorius. New York: Wiley, pp. 3–13.

Miklowitz, D. J. (1994), Family risk indicators in schizophrenia. *Schizophr. Bull.*, 20:137–149.

Murray, C. J., & Lopez, A. D. (1996), *The Global Burden of Disease*. Cambridge, MA: Harvard University Press.
——(1997), Alternative projections of mortality and disability by cause, 1990–2020: Global Burden of Disease Study. *Lancet*, 349:1498–1504.
Nunley, M. (1998), The involvement of families in Indian psychiatry. *Culture, Med., & Psychiatry*, 22:317–353.
Ortner, S. B. (1995), Resistance and the problem of ethnographic refusal. *Compar. Stud. in Soc. & Hist.*, 37: 179–193.
——ed. (1999), *The Fate of "Culture": Geertz and Beyond*. Berkeley: University of California Press.
Padmavathi, R., Rajkumar, S., & Srinivasan, T. N. (1998), Schizophrenic patients who were never treated—A study in an Indian urban community. *Psycholog. Med.*, 28:1113–1117.
Phillips, M. R., Pearson, V., Wang, R., eds. (1994), Psychiatric rehabilitation in China. *Brit. J. Psychiatry*, 165(Suppl. 24).
Porter, R. (1987), *Mind-Forg'd Manacles*. London: Athlone.
Rosaldo, R. (1989), *Culture and Truth*. Boston: Beacon.
Rupp, A., & Keith, S. (1993), The costs of schizophrenia: Assessing the burden. *Psychiat. Clin. N. A.*, 16:413–423.
Scharfstein, B.-A. (1989), *The Dilemma of Context*. New York: New York University Press.
Shore, D., ed. (1993), Special Report: Schizophrenia 1993. *Schizophr. Bull.*, 19(2).
Sørenson, T. (1994), The intricacy of the ordinary. *Brit. J. Psychiatry*, 23(Suppl):108–114.
Srinivasan, T. N., & Thara, R. (1999), The long-term homemaking functioning of women with schizophrenia. *Schizophr. Res.*, 35:97–98.
Strauss, J. S. (1992), The person—key to understanding mental illness: Towards a new dynamic psychiatry, III. *Brit. J. Psychiatry*, 18(Suppl.):19–26.
Sugar, J. A., Kleinman, A., & Heggenbougan, K. (1994), Social and behavioral pathologies. In: *Health and Social Change in International Perspective*, ed. L. C. Chen, A. Kleinman, & N. C. Ware. Boston: Harvard School of Public Health, pp. 51–84.
Thara, R., & Srinivasan, T. N. (1997), Outcome of marriage in schizophrenia. *Soc. Psychiatry & Psychiatric Epidemiol.*, 32:416–420.
——(2000), How stigmatizing is schizophrenia in India? *Internat. J. Soc. Psychiatry*, 46:135–141.
Ustun, T. B. (1999), The global burden of mental disorders. *Amer. J. Pub. Health*, 89:1315–1318.
Ware, N. C., & Kleinman, A. (1992), Culture and somatic experience. The social course of illness in neurasthenia and chronic fatigue syndrome. *Psychosom. Med.*, 54:546–560.
Warner, R. (1994), *Recovery from Schizophrenia: Psychiatry and Political Economy*, 2nd ed. New York: Routledge.
——Taylor, D., Wright, J., Sloat, A., Springett, G., Arnold, S., & Weinberg, H. (1994), Substance use among the mentally ill. *Amer. J. Orthopsychiatry*, 64:30–38.
Wig, N. N., Menon, D. K., Bedi, H., Ghosh, A., Kuipers, L., Leff, J., Korten, A., Day, R., Sartorius, N., Ernberg, G., & Jablensky, A. (1987), Expressed emotion and schizophrenia in North India. I. Cross-cultural transfer of ratings of relatives' expressed emotion. *Brit. J. Psychiatry*, 151:156–160.
——, ——, ——Leff, J., Kuipers, L., Ghosh, A., Day, R., Korten, A., Ernberg, G., Sartorius, N., & Jablensky, A. (1987), Expressed emotion and schizophrenia in North India. 2. Distribution of expressed emotion components among relatives of schizophrenia patients in Aarhus and Chandigarh. *Brit. J. Psychiatry*, 151:160–165.
World Bank (1993), *World Development Report: Investing in Health*. New York: Oxford University Press.

Appendices — Tabular Material

Appendix A

Baseline and Short-Term Follow-Up

TABLE A.1 Baseline and Short-Term Demographic and Clinical Description: Alive Cohort—by Center

	Chandigarh Urban		*Chandigarh Rural*		*Dublin*		*Honolulu*		*Moscow*		*Nagasaki*		*Nottingham*		*Prague DOSMeD*		*Rochester*	
	N	%	N	%	N	%	N	%	N	%	N	%	N	%	N	%	N	%
Gender																		
Male	43	53.8	16	42.1	18	48.6	14	53.8	19	36.5	29	50.9	57	66.3	27	34.2	15	45.5
Female	37	46.3	22	57.9	19	51.4	12	46.2	33	63.5	28	49.1	29	33.7	52	65.8	18	54.5
Birth Year																		
1920–1929	1	1.2	0	0.0	0	0.0	0	0.0	7	13.5	1	1.8	2	2.3	1	1.3	1	3.0
1930–1939	5	6.3	4	10.5	4	10.8	1	3.8	16	30.8	5	8.8	15	17.4	11	13.9	0	0.0
1940–1949	16	20.0	5	13.2	13	35.1	5	19.2	12	23.1	5	8.8	17	19.8	23	29.1	3	9.1
1950–1959	40	50.0	15	39.5	13	35.1	12	46.2	12	23.1	29	50.9	35	40.7	38	48.1	18	54.5
1960–1969	18	22.5	14	36.8	7	18.9	8	30.8	5	9.6	17	29.8	17	19.8	6	7.6	11	33.3
Grouped Mode of Onset																		
Sudden (IPSS overnight)	0	0.0	0	0.0	0	0.0	0	0.0	0	0.0	0	0.0	0	0.0	0	0.0	0	0.0
Slow (IPSS > 24 hours)	0	0.0	0	0.0	0	0.0	0	0.0	0	0.0	0	0.0	0	0.0	0	0.0	0	0.0
Up to 1 week	36	45.0	27	71.1	5	13.5	5	19.2	15	28.8	16	28.1	20	23.3	26	32.9	5	15.2
Up to 1 month	12	15.0	5	13.2	5	13.5	5	19.2	11	21.2	12	21.1	18	20.9	12	15.2	12	36.4
Greater 1 month	19	23.7	3	7.9	22	59.5	11	42.3	26	50.0	25	43.9	37	43.0	18	22.8	14	42.4
Other/missing	13	16.2	3	7.9	5	13.5	5	19.2	0	0.0	4	7.0	11	12.8	23	29.1	2	6.1
Baseline Diagnosis Converted to ICD-10																		
Paranoid schizophrenia	11	13.8	2	5.3	7	18.9	10	38.5	33	63.5	14	24.6	38	44.2	28	35.4	3	9.1
Hebephrenic schizophrenia	1	1.2	0	0.0	12	32.4	0	0.0	2	3.8	33	57.9	12	14.0	2	2.5	0	0.0
Catatonic schizophrenia	3	3.8	5	13.2	0	0.0	0	0.0	0	0.0	1	1.8	1	1.2	0	0.0	2	6.1
Residual schizophrenia	0	0.0	0	0.0	0	0.0	2	7.7	0	0.0	0	0.0	0	0.0	2	2.5	0	0.0
Undiff. schizophrenia	0	0.0	0	0.0	0	0.0	0	0.0	0	0.0	0	0.0	0	0.0	0	0.0	0	0.0
Other schizophrenia	12	15.0	3	7.9	1	2.7	1	3.8	2	3.8	4	7.0	3	3.5	8	10.1	2	6.1
Schizoaffective	0	0.0	0	0.0	11	29.7	1	3.8	0	0.0	1	1.8	3	3.5	13	16.5	3	9.1

Acute schizolike	28	35.0	18	47.4	5	13.5	5	19.2	8	15.4	3	5.3	3	3.5	4	5.1	17	51.5
Bipolar	3	3.8	1	2.6	1	2.7	1	3.8	0	0.0	0	0.0	10	11.6	0	0.0	4	12.1
Depression	12	15.0	7	18.4	0	0.0	3	11.5	0	0.0	0	0.0	8	9.3	0	0.0	0	0.0
Other psychotic	5	6.3	2	5.3	0	0.0	1	3.8	0	0.0	0	0.0	5	5.8	13	16.5	2	6.1
Other nonpsychotic	5	6.3	0	0.0	0	0.0	1	3.8	7	13.5	1	1.8	3	3.5	5	6.3	0	0.0
Missing/unknown	0	0.0	0	0.0	0	0.0	1	3.8	0	0.0	0	0.0	0	0.0	4	5.1	0	0.0
Grouped Baseline Diagnoses																		
Schizophrenia	27	33.8	10	26.3	20	54.1	13	50.0	37	71.2	52	91.2	54	62.8	40	50.6	7	21.2
Non-schizophrenia/missing	53	66.3	28	73.7	17	45.9	13	50.0	15	28.8	5	8.8	32	37.2	39	49.4	26	78.8
Grouped Short-Term Pattern of Course																		
Complete remission	46	57.5	28	73.7	13	35.1	6	23.1	10	19.2	16	28.1	50	58.1	45	57.0	14	42.4
Incomplete remission	21	26.2	10	26.3	17	45.9	8	30.8	31	59.6	20	35.1	20	23.3	12	15.2	14	42.4
Continuously psychotic	3	3.8	0	0.0	5	13.5	5	19.2	8	15.4	19	33.3	13	15.1	5	6.3	3	9.1
Other/missing	10	12.5	0	0.0	2	5.4	7	26.9	3	5.8	2	3.5	3	3.5	17	21.5	2	6.1
Short-Term Follow-up Time																		
0, missing (baseline)	6	7.5	0	0.0	0	0.0	1	3.8	0	0.0	1	1.8	2	2.3	16	20.3	0	0.0
1–17 months (1 year)	2	2.5	1	2.6	2	5.4	6	23.1	2	3.8	6	10.5	2	2.3	2	2.5	15	45.5
18–30 months (2 year)	72	90.0	37	97.4	35	94.6	19	73.1	50	96.2	50	87.7	82	95.3	61	77.2	18	54.5
5 year	0	0.0	0	0.0	0	0.0	0	0.0	0	0.0	0	0.0	0	0.0	0	0.0	0	0.0
Total	80	100.0	38	100.0	37	100.0	26	100.0	52	100.0	57	100.0	86	100.0	79	100.0	33	100.0
Birth Year N	80		38		37		26		52		57		86		79		33	
19xx Mean	53.03		54.92		50.76		54.73		42.85		54.47		50.13		49.56		56.55	
STD	8.10		8.48		8.69		7.10		11.06		8.83		10.24		8.29		7.13	

(continued)

TABLE A.1 *(continued)*

	Agra		*Cali*		*Prague IPSS*		*Groningen*		*Mannheim*		*Sofia*		*Beijing*		*Hong Kong*		*Chennai (Madras)*	
	N	%	N	%	N	%	N	%	N	%	N	%	N	%	N	%	N	%
Gender																		
Male	39	63.9	37	51.4	18	41.9	33	52.4	34	60.7	18	32.7	29	50.0	33	47.1	39	50.6
Female	22	36.1	35	48.6	25	58.1	30	47.6	22	39.3	37	67.3	29	50.0	37	52.9	38	49.4
Birth Year																		
1920–1929	4	6.6	2	2.8	9	20.9	0	0.0	0	0.0	0	0.0	9	15.5	0	0.0	0	0.0
1930–1939	24	39.3	16	22.2	8	18.6	4	6.3	3	5.4	8	14.5	19	32.8	9	12.9	1	1.3
1940–1949	18	29.5	41	56.9	23	53.5	7	11.1	14	25.0	11	20.0	14	24.1	12	17.1	5	6.5
1950–1959	15	24.6	13	18.1	3	7.0	43	68.3	33	58.9	25	45.5	10	17.2	42	60.0	36	46.8
1960–1969	0	0.0	0	0.0	0	0.0	9	14.3	6	10.7	11	20.0	6	10.3	7	10.0	35	45.5
Grouped Mode of Onset																		
Sudden (IPSS overnight)	32	52.5	9	12.5	9	20.9	0	0.0	0	0.0	0	0.0	0	0.0	0	0.0	0	0.0
Slow (IPSS > 24 hours)	29	47.5	63	87.5	32	74.4	0	0.0	0	0.0	0	0.0	0	0.0	0	0.0	0	0.0
Up to 1 week	0	0.0	0	0.0	0	0.0	28	44.4	5	8.9	18	32.7	2	3.4	2	2.9	21	27.3
Up to 1 month	0	0.0	0	0.0	0	0.0	21	33.3	30	53.6	21	38.2	15	25.9	22	31.4	9	11.7
Greater 1 month	0	0.0	0	0.0	0	0.0	13	20.6	21	37.5	14	25.5	40	69.0	46	65.7	46	59.7
Other/missing	0	0.0	0	0.0	2	4.7	1	1.6	0	0.0	2	3.6	1	1.7	0	0.0	1	1.3
Baseline Diagnosis Converted to ICD-10																		
Paranoid schizophrenia	5	8.2	10	13.9	8	18.6	4	6.3	35	62.5	36	65.5	36	62.1	47	67.1	40	51.9
Hebephrenic schizophrenia	1	1.6	17	23.6	1	2.3	6	9.5	4	7.1	1	1.8	8	13.8	2	2.9	5	6.5
Catatonic schizophrenia	8	13.1	11	15.3	0	0.0	0	0.0	1	1.8	1	1.8	1	1.7	3	4.3	12	15.6
Residual schizophrenia	0	0.0	4	5.6	0	0.0	1	1.6	0	0.0	0	0.0	4	6.9	1	1.4	7	9.1
Undiff. schizophrenia	0	0.0	0	0.0	0	0.0	0	0.0	0	0.0	0	0.0	6	10.3	0	0.0	0	0.0
Other schizophrenia	13	21.3	2	2.8	4	9.3	1	1.6	4	7.1	2	3.6	3	5.2	16	22.9	13	16.9
Schizoaffective	6	9.8	5	6.9	5	11.6	1	1.6	6	10.7	4	7.3	0	0.0	0	0.0	0	0.0
Acute schizolike	6	9.8	20	27.8	4	9.3	2	3.2	1	1.8	0	0.0	0	0.0	1	1.4	0	0.0

Bipolar	10	16.4	0	0.0	4	9.3	0	0.0	0	0.0	0	0.0	0	0.0	0	0.0	0	0.0
Depression	11	18.0	0	0.0	11	25.6	0	0.0	0	0.0	2	3.6	0	0.0	0	0.0	0	0.0
Other psychotic	0	0.0	0	0.0	5	11.6	46	73.0	2	3.6	8	14.5	0	0.0	0	0.0	0	0.0
Other nonpsychotic	1	1.6	3	4.2	1	2.3	1	1.6	3	5.4	0	0.0	0	0.0	0	0.0	0	0.0
Missing/unknown	0	0.0	0	0.0	0	0.0	1	1.6	0	0.0	1	1.8	0	0.0	0	0.0	0	0.0
Grouped Baseline Diagnosis																		
Schizophrenia	27	44.3	44	61.1	13	30.2	12	19.0	44	78.6	40	72.7	58	100.0	69	98.6	77	100.0
Non-schizophrenia/missing	34	55.7	28	38.9	30	69.8	51	81.0	12	21.4	15	27.3	0	0.0	1	1.4	0	0.0
Grouped Short-Term Pattern of Course																		
Complete remission	45	73.8	21	29.2	16	37.2	17	27.0	12	21.4	14	25.5	0	0.0	22	31.4	45	58.4
Incomplete remission	5	8.2	26	36.1	12	27.9	31	49.2	41	73.2	21	38.2	0	0.0	48	68.6	24	31.2
Continuously psychotic	6	9.8	13	18.1	5	11.6	13	20.6	3	5.4	11	20.0	0	0.0	0	0.0	8	10.4
Other/missing	5	8.2	12	16.7	10	23.3	2	3.2	0	0.0	9	16.4	58	100.0	0	0.0	0	0.0
Short-Term Follow-up Time																		
0, missing (baseline)	0	0.0	0	0.0	0	0.0	1	1.6	0	0.0	3	5.5	58	100.0	0	0.0	0	0.0
1–17 months (1 year)	0	0.0	0	0.0	0	0.0	3	4.8	0	0.0	6	10.9	0	0.0	0	0.0	0	0.0
18–30 months (2 year)	8	13.1	2	2.8	0	0.0	59	93.7	56	100.0	46	83.6	0	0.0	70	100.0	77	100.0
5 Year	53	86.9	70	97.2	43	100.0	0	0.0	0	0.0	0	0.0	0	0.0	0	0.0	0	0.0
Total	61	100.0	72	100.0	43	100.0	62	100.0	56	100.0	55	100.0	58	100.0	70	100.0	77	100.0
Birth Year N	61		72		43		63		56		55		58		70		77	
19xx Mean	41.48		43.69		38.74		53.00		51.91		51.67		41.81		51.53		57.60	
STD	7.76		6.27		8.31		6.90		6.49		8.09		12.35		8.07		6.27	

TABLE A.2 Baseline and Short-Term Demographic and Clinical Description: Dead Cohort—by Center

	Chandigarh Urban		*Chandigarh Rural*		*Dublin*		*Honolulu*		*Moscow*		*Nagasaki*		*Nottingham*		*Prague DOSMeD*		*Rochester*	
	N	%	N	%	N	%	N	%	N	%	N	%	N	%	N	%	N	%
Gender																		
Male	8	57.1	7	70.0	6	75.0	4	100.0	4	40.0	4	57.1	5	55.6	3	27.3	0	—
Female	6	42.9	3	30.0	2	25.0	0	0.0	6	60.0	3	42.9	4	44.4	8	72.7	0	—
Birth Year																		
Missing	0	0.0	0	0.0	0	0.0	0	0.0	0	0.0	0	0.0	0	0.0	0	0.0	0	—
1901–1919	0	0.0	0	0.0	0	0.0	0	0.0	0	0.0	0	0.0	0	0.0	0	0.0	0	—
1920–1929	1	7.1	3	30.0	1	12.5	1	25.0	3	30.0	0	0.0	0	0.0	3	27.3	0	—
1930–1939	0	0.0	3	30.0	0	0.0	0	0.0	3	30.0	1	14.3	3	33.3	1	9.1	0	—
1940–1949	5	35.7	3	30.0	2	25.0	0	0.0	3	30.0	1	14.3	4	44.4	3	27.3	0	—
1950–1959	3	21.4	1	10.0	4	50.0	3	75.0	1	10.0	2	28.6	2	22.2	4	36.4	0	—
1960–1969	5	35.7	0	0.0	1	12.5	0	0.0	0	0.0	3	42.9	0	0.0	0	0.0	0	—
Grouped Mode of Onset																		
Sudden (IPSS overnight)	0	0.0	0	0.0	0	0.0	0	0.0	0	0.0	0	0.0	0	0.0	0	0.0	0	—
Slow (IPSS > 24 hours)	0	0.0	0	0.0	0	0.0	0	0.0	0	0.0	0	0.0	0	0.0	0	0.0	0	—
Up to 1 week	8	57.1	6	60.0	0	0.0	0	0.0	5	50.0	3	42.9	1	11.1	3	27.3	0	—
Up to 1 month	1	7.1	1	10.0	2	25.0	1	25.0	1	10.0	0	0.0	1	11.1	3	27.3	0	—
Greater 1 month	4	28.6	2	20.0	4	50.0	2	50.0	4	40.0	1	14.3	7	77.8	2	18.2	0	—
Other/missing	1	7.1	1	10.0	2	25.0	1	25.0	0	0.0	3	42.9	0	0.0	3	27.3	0	—
Baseline Diagnosis Converted to ICD-10																		
Paranoid schizophrenia	5	35.7	2	20.0	1	12.5	1	25.0	9	90.0	0	0.0	5	55.6	1	9.1	0	—
Hebephrenic schizophrenia	0	0.0	0	0.0	2	25.0	0	0.0	0	0.0	4	57.1	0	0.0	0	0.0	0	—
Catatonic schizophrenia	1	7.1	0	0.0	0	0.0	0	0.0	0	0.0	0	0.0	0	0.0	1	9.1	0	—
Residual schizophrenia	0	0.0	0	0.0	1	12.5	0	0.0	0	0.0	1	14.3	0	0.0	0	0.0	0	—

Undiff. schizophrenia	0	0.0	0	0.0	0	0.0	0	0.0	0	0.0	0	0.0	0	0.0	0	0.0	0	—
Other schizophrenia	3	21.4	2	20.0	1	12.5	1	25.0	0	0.0	1	14.3	0	0.0	0	0.0	0	—
Schizoaffective	0	0.0	0	0.0	0	0.0	1	25.0	0	0.0	0	0.0	2	22.2	1	9.1	0	—
Acute schizolike	2	14.3	2	20.0	3	37.5	0	0.0	1	10.0	1	14.3	0	0.0	1	9.1	0	—
Bipolar	2	14.3	2	20.0	0	0.0	0	0.0	0	0.0	0	0.0	0	0.0	0	0.0	0	—
Depression	1	7.1	1	10.0	0	0.0	0	0.0	0	0.0	0	0.0	1	11.1	0	0.0	0	—
Other psychotic	0	0.0	1	10.0	0	0.0	1	25.0	0	0.0	0	0.0	0	0.0	7	63.6	0	—
Other nonpsychotic	0	0.0	0	0.0	0	0.0	0	0.0	0	0.0	0	0.0	1	11.1	0	0.0	0	—
Missing/unknown	0	0.0	0	0.0	0	0.0	0	0.0	0	0.0	0	0.0	0	0.0	0	0.0	0	—
Grouped Baseline Diagnosis																		
Schizophrenia	9	64.3	4	40.0	5	62.5	2	50.0	9	90.0	6	85.7	5	55.6	2	18.2	0	—
Non-schizophrenia/missing	5	35.7	6	60.0	3	37.5	2	50.0	1	10.0	1	14.3	4	44.4	9	81.8	0	—
Grouped Short-Term Pattern of Course																		
Complete remission	4	28.6	6	60.0	0	0.0	1	25.0	0	0.0	0	0.0	3	33.3	4	36.4	0	—
Incomplete remission	5	35.7	2	20.0	6	75.0	2	50.0	9	90.0	2	28.6	4	44.4	4	36.4	0	—
Continuously psychotic	5	35.7	2	20.0	1	12.5	1	25.0	1	10.0	3	42.9	2	22.2	1	9.1	0	—
Other/missing	0	0.0	0	0.0	1	12.5	0	0.0	0	0.0	2	28.6	0	0.0	2	18.2	0	—
Short-Term Follow-up Time																		
0, missing (baseline)	0	0.0	0	0.0	1	12.5	0	0.0	0	0.0	2	28.6	0	0.0	2	18.2	0	—
1–17 months (1 year)	2	14.3	2	20.0	0	0.0	0	0.0	6	60.0	2	28.6	1	11.1	1	9.1	0	—
18–30 months (2 year)	12	85.7	8	80.0	7	87.5	4	100.0	4	40.0	3	42.9	8	88.9	8	72.7	0	—
5 year	0	0.0	0	0.0	0	0.0	0	0.0	0	0.0	0	0.0	0	0.0	0	0.0	0	—
Total	14	100.0	10	100.0	8	100.0	4	100.0	10	100.0	7	100.0	9	100.0	11	100.0	0	—
Birth Year N	14		10		8		4		10		7		9		11			
19xx Mean	52.36		37.70		49.38		46.50		36.20		54.71		44.33		44.91			
STD	10.10		10.85		9.91		13.10		9.17		11.07		9.95		12.21			

(*continued*)

TABLE A.2 *(continued)*

	Agra		*Cali*		*Prague IPSS*		*Groningen*		*Mannheim*		*Sofia*		*Beijing*		*Hong Kong*		*Chennai (Madras)*	
	N	%	N	%	N	%	N	%	N	%	N	%	N	%	N	%	N	%
Gender																		
Male	20	46.5	9	75.0	10	21.7	7	77.8	5	71.4	1	50.0	11	55.0	8	72.7	4	44.4
Female	23	53.5	3	25.0	36	78.3	2	22.2	2	28.6	1	50.0	9	45.0	3	27.3	5	55.6
Birth Year																		
Missing	0	0.0	0	0.0	0	0.0	0	0.0	0	0.0	0	0.0	0	0.0	0	0.0	1	11.1
1901–1919	0	0.0	0	0.0	0	0.0	0	0.0	0	0.0	0	0.0	3	15.0	0	0.0	0	0.0
1920–1929	6	14.0	1	8.3	14	30.4	0	0.0	0	0.0	0	0.0	7	35.0	0	0.0	0	0.0
1930–1939	16	37.2	6	50.0	15	32.6	1	11.1	2	28.6	1	50.0	5	25.0	1	9.1	1	11.1
1940–1949	17	39.5	5	41.7	15	32.6	1	11.1	0	0.0	0	0.0	2	10.0	3	27.3	2	22.2
1950–1959	4	9.3	0	0.0	2	4.3	7	77.8	3	42.9	1	50.0	3	15.0	6	54.5	2	22.2
1960–1969	0	0.0	0	0.0	0	0.0	0	0.0	2	28.6	0	0.0	0	0.0	1	9.1	3	33.3
Grouped Mode of Onset																		
Sudden (IPSS overnight)	21	48.8	0	0.0	10	21.7	0	0.0	0	0.0	0	0.0	0	0.0	0	0.0	0	0.0
Slow (IPSS > 24 hours)	22	51.2	12	100.0	36	78.3	0	0.0	0	0.0	0	0.0	0	0.0	0	0.0	0	0.0
Up to 1 week	0	0.0	0	0.0	0	0.0	3	33.3	1	14.3	0	0.0	0	0.0	0	0.0	0	0.0
Up to 1 month	0	0.0	0	0.0	0	0.0	3	33.3	5	71.4	1	50.0	1	5.0	0	0.0	0	0.0
Greater 1 month	0	0.0	0	0.0	0	0.0	3	33.3	1	14.3	1	50.0	19	95.0	9	81.8	9	100.0
Other/missing	0	0.0	0	0.0	0	0.0	0	0.0	0	0.0	0	0.0	0	0.0	2	18.2	0	0.0
Baseline Diagnosis Converted to ICD-10																		
Paranoid schizophrenia	7	16.3	5	41.7	13	28.3	1	11.1	6	85.7	2	100.0	17	85.0	2	18.2	5	55.6
Hebephrenic schizophrenia	2	4.7	2	16.7	1	2.2	1	11.1	1	14.3	0	0.0	1	5.0	0	0.0	0	0.0
Catatonic schizophrenia	10	23.3	0	0.0	0	0.0	0	0.0	0	0.0	0	0.0	0	0.0	0	0.0	1	11.1
Residual schizophrenia	0	0.0	1	8.3	2	4.3	0	0.0	0	0.0	0	0.0	1	5.0	0	0.0	1	11.1
Undiff. schizophrenia	0	0.0	0	0.0	0	0.0	0	0.0	0	0.0	0	0.0	1	5.0	0	0.0	0	0.0
Other schizophrenia	13	30.2	0	0.0	4	8.7	0	0.0	0	0.0	0	0.0	0	0.0	0	0.0	2	22.2

Schizoaffective	3	7.0	0	0.0	8	17.4	0	0.0	0	0.0	0	0.0	0	0.0	0	0.0	0	0.0
Acute schizolike	2	4.7	4	33.3	0	0.0	2	22.2	0	0.0	0	0.0	0	0.0	0	0.0	0	0.0
Bipolar	3	7.0	0	0.0	4	8.7	0	0.0	0	0.0	0	0.0	0	0.0	0	0.0	0	0.0
Depression	3	7.0	0	0.0	7	15.2	0	0.0	0	0.0	0	0.0	0	0.0	0	0.0	0	0.0
Other psychotic	0	0.0	0	0.0	6	13.0	4	44.4	0	0.0	0	0.0	0	0.0	0	0.0	0	0.0
Other nonpsychotic	0	0.0	0	0.0	1	2.2	1	11.1	0	0.0	0	0.0	0	0.0	0	0.0	0	0.0
Missing/unknown	0	0.0	0	0.0	0	0.0	0	0.0	0	0.0	0	0.0	0	0.0	*9	81.8	0	0.0
Grouped Baseline Diagnosis																		
Schizophrenia	32	74.4	8	66.7	20	43.5	2	22.2	7	100.0	2	100.0	20	100.0	2	18.2	9	100.0
Non-schizophrenia/missing	11	25.6	4	33.3	26	56.5	7	77.8	0	0.0	0	0.0	0	0.0	*9	81.8	0	0.0
Grouped Short-Term Pattern of Course																		
Complete remission	23	53.5	2	16.7	12	26.1	2	22.2	0	0.0	0	0.0	0	0.0	2	18.2	1	11.1
Incomplete remission	6	14.0	2	16.7	14	30.4	3	33.3	6	85.7	0	0.0	0	0.0	7	63.6	6	66.7
Continuously psychotic	9	20.9	5	41.7	6	13.0	2	22.2	1	14.3	0	0.0	0	0.0	0	0.0	1	11.1
Other/missing	5	11.6	3	25.0	14	30.4	2	22.2	0	0.0	2	100.0	20	100.0	2	18.2	1	11.1
Short-Term Follow-up Time																		
0, missing (baseline)	0	0.0	1	8.3	6	13.0	1	11.1	0	0.0	2	100.0	20	100.0	3	27.3	1	11.1
1–17 months (1 year)	0	0.0	0	0.0	0	0.0	3	33.3	2	28.6	0	0.0	0	0.0	0	0.0	1	11.1
18–30 months (2 year)	18	41.9	0	0.0	5	10.9	5	55.6	5	71.4	0	0.0	0	0.0	8	72.7	7	77.8
5 year	25	58.1	11	91.7	35	76.1	0	0.0	0	0.0	0	0.0	0	0.0	0	0.0	0	0.0
Total	43	100.0	12	100.0	46	100.0	9	100.0	7	100.0	2	100.0	20	100.0	11	100.0	9	100.0
Birth Year N	43		12		46		9		7		2		20		11		8	
19xx Mean	38.65		37.42		35.39		53.00		52.43		47.00		30.70		51.36		54.50	
STD	8.00		6.96		8.19		7.42		10.06		14.14		12.38		7.23		9.52	

*Cases known to be ICD-9 Schizophrenia (subtype missing)

TABLE A.3 Baseline and Short-Term Demographic and Clinical Description: Lost to Follow-up Cohort by Center

	Chandigarh Urban		*Chandigarh Rural*		*Dublin*		*Honolulu*		*Moscow*		*Nagasaki*		*Nottingham*		*Prague DOSMeD*		*Rochester*	
	N	%	N	%	N	%	N	%	N	%	N	%	N	%	N	%	N	%
Gender																		
Male	40	65.6	4	57.1	12	54.5	23	56.1	6	60.0	29	56.9	3	75.0	13	46.4	13	52.0
Female	21	34.4	3	42.9	10	45.5	18	43.9	4	40.0	22	43.1	1	25.0	15	53.6	12	48.0
Birth Year																		
Missing	0	0.0	0	0.0	0	0.0	0	0.0	0	0.0	0	0.0	0	0.0	0	0.0	0	0.0
1901–1919	0	0.0	0	0.0	0	0.0	0	0.0	0	0.0	0	0.0	0	0.0	0	0.0	0	0.0
1920–1929	2	3.3	0	0.0	2	9.1	0	0.0	0	0.0	0	0.0	0	0.0	1	3.6	3	12.0
1930–1939	3	4.9	0	0.0	0	0.0	0	0.0	1	10.0	1	2.0	0	0.0	1	3.6	1	4.0
1940–1949	8	13.1	0	0.0	10	45.5	9	22.0	2	20.0	14	27.5	1	25.0	10	35.7	4	16.0
1950–1959	37	60.7	4	57.1	7	31.8	22	53.7	5	50.0	22	43.1	1	25.0	12	42.9	7	28.0
1960–1969	11	18.0	3	42.9	3	13.6	10	24.4	2	20.0	14	27.5	2	50.0	4	14.3	10	40.0
Grouped Mode of Onset																		
Sudden (IPSS overnight)	0	0.0	0	0.0	0	0.0	0	0.0	0	0.0	0	0.0	0	0.0	0	0.0	0	0.0
Slow (IPSS > 24 hours)	0	0.0	0	0.0	0	0.0	0	0.0	0	0.0	0	0.0	0	0.0	0	0.0	0	0.0
Up to 1 week	16	26.2	6	85.7	3	13.6	8	19.5	6	60.0	9	17.6	0	0.0	7	25.0	5	20.0
Up to 1 month	2	3.3	0	0.0	7	31.8	1	2.4	0	0.0	9	17.6	0	0.0	2	7.1	8	32.0
Greater 1 month	10	16.4	0	0.0	9	40.9	7	17.1	4	40.0	8	15.7	3	75.0	10	35.7	10	40.0
Other/missing	33	54.1	1	14.3	3	13.6	25	61.0	0	0.0	25	49.0	1	25.0	9	32.1	2	8.0
Baseline Diagnosis Converted to ICD-10																		
Paranoid schizophrenia	14	23.0	0	0.0	8	36.4	12	29.3	5	50.0	17	33.3	2	50.0	8	28.6	5	20.0
Hebephrenic schizophrenia	0	0.0	0	0.0	0	0.0	1	2.4	1	10.0	17	33.3	0	0.0	0	0.0	0	0.0
Catatonic schizophrenia	4	6.6	1	14.3	0	0.0	0	0.0	0	0.0	1	2.0	0	0.0	1	3.6	1	4.0
Residual schizophrenia	0	0.0	0	0.0	0	0.0	0	0.0	0	0.0	0	0.0	0	0.0	0	0.0	0	0.0
Undiff. schizophrenia	0	0.0	0	0.0	0	0.0	0	0.0	0	0.0	0	0.0	0	0.0	0	0.0	0	0.0

Other schizophrenia	11	18.0	2	28.6	0	0.0	8	19.5	0	0.0	5	9.8	0	0.0	2	7.1	0	0.0
Schizoaffective	0	0.0	0	0.0	6	27.3	6	14.6	0	0.0	0	0.0	0	0.0	2	7.1	3	12.0
Acute schizolike	17	27.9	4	57.1	5	22.7	5	12.2	1	10.0	1	2.0	1	25.0	2	7.1	9	36.0
Bipolar	3	4.9	0	0.0	2	9.1	1	2.4	0	0.0	0	0.0	0	0.0	0	0.0	2	8.0
Depression	6	9.8	0	0.0	1	4.5	2	4.9	0	0.0	1	2.0	0	0.0	0	0.0	0	0.0
Other psychotic	4	6.6	0	0.0	0	0.0	4	9.8	0	0.0	6	11.8	0	0.0	10	35.7	3	12.0
Other nonpsychotic	2	3.3	0	0.0	0	0.0	2	4.9	3	30.0	3	5.9	1	25.0	1	3.6	2	8.0
Missing/unknown	0	0.0	0	0.0	0	0.0	0	0.0	0	0.0	0	0.0	0	0.0	2	7.1	0	0.0
Grouped Baseline Diagnosis																		
Schizophrenia	29	47.5	3	42.9	8	36.4	21	51.2	6	60.0	40	78.4	2	50.0	11	39.3	6	24.0
Non-schizophrenia/missing	32	52.5	4	57.1	14	63.6	20	48.8	4	40.0	11	21.6	2	50.0	17	60.7	19	76.0
Grouped Short-Term Pattern of Course																		
Complete remission	17	27.9	4	57.1	9	40.9	1	2.4	2	20.0	8	15.7	2	50.0	12	42.9	10	40.0
Incomplete remission	7	11.5	2	28.6	5	22.7	3	7.3	5	50.0	11	21.6	0	0.0	6	21.4	12	48.0
Continuously psychotic	5	8.2	0	0.0	2	9.1	2	4.9	2	20.0	9	17.6	1	25.0	1	3.6	2	8.0
Other/missing	32	52.5	1	14.3	6	27.3	35	85.4	1	10.0	23	45.1	1	25.0	9	32.1	1	4.0
Short-Term Follow-up Time																		
0, missing (baseline)	30	49.2	0	0.0	4	18.2	24	58.5	0	0.0	21	41.2	1	25.0	9	32.1	1	4.0
1–17 months (1 year)	5	8.2	1	14.3	3	13.6	10	24.4	9	90.0	9	17.6	0	0.0	0	0.0	8	32.0
18–30 months (2 year)	26	42.6	6	85.7	15	68.2	7	17.1	1	10.0	21	41.2	3	75.0	19	67.9	16	64.0
5 year	0	0.0	0	0.0	0	0.0	0	0.0	0	0.0	0	0.0	0	0.0	0	0.0	0	0.0
Total	61	100.0	7	100.0	22	100.0	41	100.0	10	100.0	51	100.0	4	100.0	28	100.0	25	100.0
Birth Year N	61		7		22		41		10		51		4		28		25	
19xx Mean	52.62		58.43		49.27		54.80		53.80		53.96		55.00		50.57		52.08	
STD	8.26		3.60		10.96		6.39		7.19		7.31		9.20		7.94		12.32	

(continued)

TABLE A.3 *(continued)*

	Agra		*Cali*		*Prague IPSS*		*Groningen*		*Mannheim*		*Sofia*		*Beijing*		*Hong Kong*		*Chennai (Madras)*	
	N	%	N	%	N	%	N	%	N	%	N	%	N	%	N	%	N	%
Gender																		
Male	26	72.2	10	23.3	15	41.7	3	27.3	2	28.6	2	66.7	5	45.5	10	52.6	8	57.1
Female	10	27.8	33	76.7	21	58.3	8	72.7	5	71.4	1	33.3	6	54.5	9	47.4	6	42.9
Birth Year																		
Missing	0	0.0	1	2.3	0	0.0	0	0.0	0	0.0	0	0.0	0	0.0	0	0.0	0	0.0
1901–1919	0	0.0	0	0.0	0	0.0	0	0.0	0	0.0	0	0.0	1	9.1	0	0.0	0	0.0
1920–1929	2	5.6	5	11.6	6	16.7	0	0.0	0	0.0	0	0.0	0	0.0	0	0.0	0	0.0
1930–1939	14	38.9	16	37.2	11	30.6	0	0.0	1	14.3	0	0.0	1	9.1	1	5.3	1	7.1
1940–1949	17	47.2	17	39.5	18	50.0	1	9.1	2	28.6	0	0.0	4	36.4	4	21.1	1	7.1
1950–1959	3	8.3	4	9.3	1	2.8	8	72.7	4	57.1	3	100.0	5	45.5	10	52.6	8	57.1
1960–1969	0	0.0	0	0.0	0	0.0	2	18.2	0	0.0	0	0.0	0	0.0	4	21.1	4	28.6
Grouped Mode of Onset																		
Sudden (IPSS overnight)	17	47.2	3	7.0	1	2.8	0	0.0	0	0.0	0	0.0	0	0.0	0	0.0	0	0.0
Slow (IPSS > 24 hours)	19	52.8	39	90.7	35	97.2	0	0.0	0	0.0	0	0.0	0	0.0	0	0.0	0	0.0
Up to 1 week	0	0.0	0	0.0	0	0.0	4	36.4	0	0.0	0	0.0	0	0.0	0	0.0	2	14.3
Up to 1 month	0	0.0	0	0.0	0	0.0	2	18.2	4	57.1	3	100.0	5	45.5	1	5.3	3	21.4
Greater 1 month	0	0.0	0	0.0	0	0.0	4	36.4	3	42.9	0	0.0	6	54.5	12	63.2	9	64.3
Other/missing	0	0.0	1	2.3	0	0.0	1	9.1	0	0.0	0	0.0	0	0.0	6	31.6	0	0.0
Baseline Diagnosis Converted to ICD-10																		
Paranoid schizophrenia	3	8.3	5	11.6	15	41.7	0	0.0	7	100.0	3	100.0	6	54.5	0	0.0	7	50.0
Hebephrenic schizophrenia	0	0.0	1	2.3	1	2.8	2	18.2	0	0.0	0	0.0	4	36.4	0	0.0	2	14.3
Catatonic schizophrenia	4	11.1	2	4.7	0	0.0	1	9.1	0	0.0	0	0.0	0	0.0	0	0.0	1	7.1
Residual schizophrenia	0	0.0	1	2.3	0	0.0	0	0.0	0	0.0	0	0.0	0	0.0	0	0.0	2	14.3
Undiff. schizophrenia	0	0.0	0	0.0	0	0.0	0	0.0	0	0.0	0	0.0	1	9.1	0	0.0	0	0.0

Other schizophrenia	8	22.2	1	2.3	1	2.8	0	0.0	0	0.0	0	0.0	0	0.0	0	0.0	2	14.3
Schizoaffective	8	22.2	2	4.7	7	19.4	0	0.0	0	0.0	0	0.0	0	0.0	0	0.0	0	0.0
Acute schizo-like	2	5.6	5	11.6	0	0.0	0	0.0	0	0.0	0	0.0	0	0.0	0	0.0	0	0.0
Bipolar	7	19.4	3	7.0	2	5.6	0	0.0	0	0.0	0	0.0	0	0.0	0	0.0	0	0.0
Depression	3	8.3	9	20.9	8	22.2	0	0.0	0	0.0	0	0.0	0	0.0	0	0.0	0	0.0
Other psychotic	0	0.0	2	4.7	2	5.6	7	63.6	0	0.0	0	0.0	0	0.0	0	0.0	0	0.0
Other nonpsychotic	1	2.8	12	27.9	0	0.0	1	9.1	0	0.0	0	0.0	0	0.0	0	0.0	0	0.0
Missing/unknown	0	0.0	0	0.0	0	0.0	0	0.0	0	0.0	0	0.0	0	0.0	*19	100.0	0	0.0
Grouped Baseline Diagnosis																		
Schizophrenia	15	41.7	10	23.3	17	47.2	3	27.3	7	100.0	3	100.0	11	100.0	0	0.0	14	100.0
Non-schizophrenia/missing	21	58.3	33	76.7	19	52.8	8	72.7	0	0.0	0	0.0	0	0.0	*19	100.0	0	0.0
Grouped Short-Term Pattern of Course																		
Complete remission	18	50.0	11	25.6	11	30.6	2	18.2	0	0.0	0	0.0	0	0.0	3	15.8	6	42.9
Incomplete remission	5	13.9	11	25.6	9	25.0	4	36.4	7	100.0	2	66.7	0	0.0	11	57.9	6	42.9
Continuously psychotic	7	19.4	9	20.9	8	22.2	2	18.2	0	0.0	0	0.0	0	0.0	2	10.5	2	14.3
Other/missing	6	16.7	12	27.9	8	22.2	3	27.3	0	0.0	1	33.3	11	100.0	3	15.8	0	0.0
Short-Term Follow-up Time																		
0, missing (baseline)	0	0.0	6	14.0	4	11.1	1	9.1	0	0.0	0	0.0	11	100.0	3	15.8	0	0.0
1–17 months (1 year)	0	0.0	0	0.0	0	0.0	5	45.5	0	0.0	1	33.3	0	0.0	0	0.0	9	64.3
18–30 months (2 year)	11	30.6	0	0.0	2	5.6	5	45.5	7	100.0	2	66.7	0	0.0	16	84.2	5	35.7
5 year	25	69.4	37	86.0	30	83.3	0	0.0	0	0.0	0	0.0	0	0.0	0	0.0	0	0.0
Total	36	100.0	43	100.0	36	100.0	11	100.0	7	100.0	3	100.0	11	100.0	19	100.0	14	100.0
Birth Year N	36		42		36		11		7		3		11		19		14	
19xx Mean	39.81		39.31		38.94		54.73		48.29		55.33		45.91		53.42		56.36	
STD	6.96		7.63		7.75		4.58		8.79		2.08		11.41		7.21		7.37	

*cases known to be ICD-9 Schizophrenia (subtype missing)

TABLE A.4 Baseline and Short-Term Demographic and Clinical Description: Original Study Cohort—by Center

	Chandigarh Urban		*Chandigarh Rural*		*Dublin*		*Honolulu*		*Moscow*		*Nagasaki*		*Nottingham*		*Prague DOSMeD*		*Rochester*	
	N	%	N	%	N	%	N	%	N	%	N	%	N	%	N	%	N	%
Gender																		
Male	91	58.7	27	49.1	36	53.7	41	57.7	29	40.3	62	53.9	65	65.7	43	36.4	28	48.3
Female	64	41.3	28	50.9	31	46.3	30	42.3	43	59.7	53	46.1	34	34.3	75	63.6	30	51.7
Birth Year																		
Missing	0	0.0	0	0.0	0	0.0	0	0.0	0	0.0	0	0.0	0	0.0	0	0.0	0	0.0
1901–1919	0	0.0	0	0.0	0	0.0	0	0.0	0	0.0	0	0.0	0	0.0	0	0.0	0	0.0
1920–1929	4	2.6	3	5.5	3	4.5	1	1.4	10	13.9	1	0.9	2	2.0	5	4.2	4	6.9
1930–1939	8	5.2	7	12.7	4	6.0	1	1.4	20	27.8	7	6.1	18	18.2	13	11.0	1	1.7
1940–1949	29	18.7	8	14.5	25	37.3	14	19.7	17	23.6	20	17.4	22	22.2	36	30.5	7	12.1
1950–1959	80	51.6	20	36.4	24	35.8	37	52.1	18	25.0	53	46.1	38	38.4	54	45.8	25	43.1
1960–1969	34	21.9	17	30.9	11	16.4	18	25.4	7	9.7	34	29.6	19	19.2	10	8.5	21	36.2
Grouped Mode of Onset																		
Sudden (IPSS overnight)	0	0.0	0	0.0	0	0.0	0	0.0	0	0.0	0	0.0	0	0.0	0	0.0	0	0.0
Slow (IPSS > 24 hours)	0	0.0	0	0.0	0	0.0	0	0.0	0	0.0	0	0.0	0	0.0	0	0.0	0	0.0
Up to 1 week	60	38.7	39	70.9	8	11.9	13	18.3	26	36.1	28	24.3	21	21.2	36	30.5	10	17.2
Up to 1 month	15	9.7	6	10.9	14	20.9	7	9.9	12	16.7	21	18.3	19	19.2	17	14.4	20	34.5
Greater than 1 month	33	21.3	5	9.1	35	52.2	20	28.2	34	47.2	34	29.6	47	47.5	30	25.4	24	41.4
Other/missing	47	30.3	5	9.1	10	14.9	31	43.7	0	0.0	32	27.8	12	12.1	35	29.7	4	6.9
Baseline Diagnosis Converted to ICD-10																		
Paranoid schizophrenia	30	19.4	4	7.3	16	23.9	23	32.4	47	65.3	31	27.0	45	45.5	37	31.4	8	13.8
Hebephrenic schizophrenia	1	0.6	0	0.0	14	20.9	1	1.4	3	4.2	54	47.0	12	12.1	2	1.7	0	0.0
Catatonic schizophrenia	8	5.2	6	10.9	0	0.0	0	0.0	0	0.0	2	1.7	1	1.0	2	1.7	3	5.2
Residual schizophrenia	0	0.0	0	0.0	1	1.5	2	2.8	0	0.0	1	0.9	0	0.0	2	1.7	0	0.0
Undiff. schizophrenia	0	0.0	0	0.0	0	0.0	0	0.0	0	0.0	0	0.0	0	0.0	0	0.0	0	0.0

Other schizophrenia	26	16.8	7	12.7	2	3.0	10	14.1	2	2.8	10	8.7	3	3.0	10	8.5	2	3.4
Schizoaffective	0	0.0	0	0.0	17	25.4	8	11.3	0	0.0	1	0.9	5	5.1	16	13.6	6	10.3
Acute schizo-like	47	30.3	24	43.6	13	19.4	10	14.1	10	13.9	5	4.3	4	4.0	7	5.9	26	44.8
Bipolar	8	5.2	3	5.5	3	4.5	2	2.8	0	0.0	0	0.0	10	10.1	0	0.0	6	10.3
Depression	19	12.3	8	14.5	1	1.5	5	7.0	0	0.0	1	0.9	9	9.1	0	0.0	0	0.0
Other psychotic	9	5.8	3	5.5	0	0.0	6	8.5	0	0.0	6	5.2	5	5.1	30	25.4	5	8.6
Other nonpsychotic	7	4.5	0	0.0	0	0.0	3	4.2	10	13.9	4	3.5	5	5.1	6	5.1	2	3.4
Missing/unknown	0	0.0	0	0.0	0	0.0	1	1.4	0	0.0	0	0.0	0	0.0	6	5.1	0	0.0
Grouped Baseline Diagnosis																		
Schizophrenia	65	41.9	17	30.9	33	49.3	36	50.7	52	72.2	98	85.2	61	61.6	53	44.9	13	22.4
Nonschizophrenia/missing	90	58.1	38	69.1	34	50.7	35	49.3	20	27.8	17	14.8	38	38.4	65	55.1	45	77.6
Grouped Short-Term Pattern of Course																		
Complete remission	67	43.2	38	69.1	22	32.8	8	11.3	12	16.7	24	20.9	55	55.6	61	51.7	24	41.4
Incomplete remission	33	21.3	14	25.5	28	41.8	13	18.3	45	62.5	33	28.7	24	24.2	22	18.6	26	44.8
Continuously psychotic	13	8.4	2	3.6	8	11.9	8	11.3	11	15.3	31	27.0	16	16.2	7	5.9	5	8.6
Other/missing	42	27.1	1	1.8	9	13.4	42	59.2	4	5.6	27	23.5	4	4.0	28	23.7	3	5.2
Short-Term Follow-up Time																		
0, missing (baseline)	36	23.2	0	0.0	5	7.5	25	35.2	0	0.0	24	20.9	3	3.0	27	22.9	1	1.7
1–17 months (1 year)	9	5.8	4	7.3	5	7.5	16	22.5	17	23.6	17	14.8	3	3.0	3	2.5	23	39.7
18–30 months (2 year)	110	71.0	51	92.7	57	85.1	30	42.3	55	76.4	74	64.3	93	93.9	88	74.6	34	58.6
5 year	0	0.0	0	0.0	0	0.0	0	0.0	0	0.0	0	0.0	0	0.0	0	0.0	0	0.0
Total	155	100.0	55	100.0	67	100.0	71	100.0	72	100.0	115	100.0	99	100.0	118	100.0	58	100.0
Birth Year N	155		55		67		71		72		115		99		118		58	
19xx Mean	52.81		52.24		50.10		54.31		43.44		54.26		49.80		49.36		54.62	
STD	8.30		10.93		9.50		7.24		11.31		8.26		10.28		8.68		9.87	

TABLE A.4 (*continued*)

	Agra		*Cali*		*Prague IPSS*		*Groningen*		*Mannheim*		*Sofia*		*Beijing*		*Hong Kong*		*Chennai (Madras)*	
	N	%	N	%	N	%	N	%	N	%	N	%	N	%	N	%	N	%
Gender																		
Male	85	60.7	56	44.1	43	34.4	43	51.8	41	58.6	21	35.0	45	50.6	51	51.0	51	51.0
Female	55	39.3	71	55.9	82	65.6	40	48.2	29	41.4	39	65.0	44	49.4	49	49.0	49	49.0
Birth Year																		
Missing	0	0.0	1	0.8	0	0.0	0	0.0	0	0.0	0	0.0	0	0.0	0	0.0	1	1.0
1901–1919	0	0.0	0	0.0	0	0.0	0	0.0	0	0.0	0	0.0	4	4.5	0	0.0	0	0.0
1920–1929	12	8.6	8	6.3	29	23.2	0	0.0	0	0.0	0	0.0	16	18.0	0	0.0	0	0.0
1930–1939	54	38.6	38	29.9	34	27.2	5	6.0	6	8.6	9	15.0	25	28.1	11	11.0	3	3.0
1940–1949	52	37.1	63	49.6	56	44.8	9	10.8	16	22.9	11	18.3	20	22.5	19	19.0	8	8.0
1950–1959	22	15.7	17	13.4	6	4.8	58	69.9	40	57.1	29	48.3	18	20.2	58	58.0	46	46.0
1960–1969	0	0.0	0	0.0	0	0.0	11	13.3	8	11.4	11	18.3	6	6.7	12	12.0	42	42.0
Grouped Mode of Onset																		
Sudden (IPSS overnight)	70	50.0	12	9.4	20	16.0	0	0.0	0	0.0	0	0.0	0	0.0	0	0.0	0	0.0
Slow (IPSS > 24 hours)	70	50.0	114	89.8	103	82.4	0	0.0	0	0.0	0	0.0	0	0.0	0	0.0	0	0.0
Up to 1 week	0	0.0	0	0.0	0	0.0	35	42.2	6	8.6	18	30.0	2	2.2	2	2.0	23	23.0
Up to 1 month	0	0.0	0	0.0	0	0.0	26	31.3	39	55.7	25	41.7	21	23.6	23	23.0	12	12.0
Greater 1 month	0	0.0	0	0.0	0	0.0	20	24.1	25	35.7	15	25.0	65	73.0	67	67.0	64	64.0
Other/mission	0	0.0	1	0.8	2	1.6	2	2.4	0	0.0	2	3.3	1	1.1	8	8.0	1	1.0
Baseline Diagnosis Converted to ICD-10																		
Paranoid schizophrenia	15	10.7	20	15.7	36	28.8	5	6.0	48	68.6	41	68.3	59	66.3	49	49.0	52	52.0
Hebephrenic schizophrenia	3	2.1	20	15.7	3	2.4	9	10.8	5	7.1	1	1.7	13	14.6	2	2.0	7	7.0
Catatonic schizophrenia	22	15.7	13	10.2	0	0.0	1	1.2	1	1.4	1	1.7	1	1.1	3	3.0	14	14.0
Residual schizophrenia	0	0.0	6	4.7	2	1.6	1	1.2	0	0.0	0	0.0	5	5.6	1	1.0	10	10.0

(*continued*)

Undiff. schizophrenia	0	0.0	0	0.0	0	0.0	0	0.0	0	0.0	0	0.0	8	9.0	0	0.0	0	0.0
Other schizophrenia	34	24.3	3	2.4	9	7.2	1	1.2	4	5.7	2	3.3	3	3.4	16	16.0	17	17.0
Schizoaffective	17	12.1	7	5.5	20	16.0	1	1.2	6	8.6	4	6.7	0	0.0	0	0.0	0	0.0
Acute schizolike	10	7.1	29	22.8	4	3.2	4	4.8	1	1.4	0	0.0	0	0.0	1	1.0	0	0.0
Bipolar	20	14.3	3	2.4	10	8.0	0	0.0	0	0.0	0	0.0	0	0.0	0	0.0	0	0.0
Depression	17	12.1	9	7.1	26	20.8	0	0.0	0	0.0	2	3.3	0	0.0	0	0.0	0	0.0
Other psychotic	0	0.0	2	1.6	13	10.4	57	68.7	2	2.9	8	13.3	0	0.0	0	0.0	0	0.0
Other nonpsyhotic	2	1.4	15	11.8	2	1.6	3	3.6	3	4.3	0	0.0	0	0.0	0	0.0	0	0.0
Missing/unknown	0	0.0	0	0.0	0	0.0	1	1.2	0	0.0	1	1.7	0	0.0	*28	28.0	0	0.0
Grouped Baseline Diagnosis																		
Schizophrenia	74	52.9	62	48.8	50	40.0	17	20.5	58	82.9	45	75.0	89	100.0	71	71.0	100	100.0
Non-schizophrenia/missing	66	47.1	65	51.2	75	60.0	66	79.5	12	17.1	15	25.0	0	0.0	*29	29.0	0	0.0
Grouped Short-Term Pattern of Course																		
Complete remission	86	61.4	34	26.8	39	31.2	21	25.3	12	17.1	14	23.3	0	0.0	27	27.0	52	52.0
Incomplete remission	16	11.4	39	30.7	35	28.0	38	45.8	54	77.1	23	38.3	0	0.0	66	66.0	36	36.0
Continuously psychotic	22	15.7	27	21.3	19	15.2	17	20.5	4	5.7	11	18.3	0	0.0	2	2.0	11	11.0
Other/missing	16	11.4	27	21.3	32	25.6	7	8.4	0	0.0	12	20.0	89	100.0	5	5.0	1	1.0
Short-Term Follow-up Time																		
0, missing (baseline)	0	0.0	7	5.5	10	8.0	3	3.6	0	0.0	5	8.3	89	100.0	6	6.0	1	1.0
1–17 months (1 year)	0	0.0	0	0.0	0	0.0	11	13.3	2	2.9	7	11.7	0	0.0	0	0.0	10	10.0
18–30 months (2 year)	37	26.4	2	1.6	7	5.6	69	83.1	68	97.1	48	80.0	0	0.0	94	94.0	89	89.0
5 year	103	73.6	118	92.9	108	86.4	0	0.0	0	0.0	0	0.0	0	0.0	0	0.0	0	0.0
Total	140	100.0	127	100.0	125	100.0	83	100.0	70	100.0	60	100.0	89	100.0	100	100.0	100	100.0
Birth Year N	140		126		125		83		70		60		89		100		99	
Mean	40.18		41.63		37.57		53.23		51.60		51.70		39.82		51.87		57.17	
STD	7.68		7.18		8.21		6.65		7.10		8.05		13.14		7.79		6.71	

*Cases known to be ICD-9 Schizophrenia (subtype missing).

Appendix B

Course and Outcome for Alive Cohort

TABLE B.1 Course Type: Past 2 Years Alive Cohort—by Center

		Chandigarh Urban		*Chandigarh Rural*		*Dublin*		*Honolulu*		*Moscow*		*Nagasaki*		*Nottingham*		*Prague DOSMeD*		*Rochester*	
		N	%	N	%	N	%	N	%	N	%	N	%	N	%	N	%	N	%
Available	Course Type: Past 2 yrs.																		
	1: Episodic: <6 Mos.	7	8.8	3	7.9	7	19.4	2	7.7	14	26.9	9	16.1	9	10.6	29	37.7	2	6.5
	2: Continuous	15	18.8	3	7.9	16	44.4	11	42.3	3	5.8	31	55.4	23	27.1	15	19.5	10	32.3
	3: Neither Cont. / Epi.	7	8.8	5	13.2	2	5.6	0	0.0	0	0.0	2	3.6	3	3.5	1	1.3	3	9.7
	4: Not Psychotic	51	63.8	27	71.1	11	30.6	13	50.0	35	67.3	14	25.0	50	58.8	32	41.6	16	51.6
	5: Psych. in Period*	0	0.0	0	0.0	0	0.0	0	0.0	0	0.0	0	0.0	0	0.0	0	0.0	0	0.0
Missing	9: Unknown	0	—	0	—	1	100.0	0	—	0	—	1	100.0	1	100.0	2	100.0	2	100.0
Available		80	100.0	38	100.0	36	97.3	26	100.0	52	100.0	56	98.2	85	98.8	77	97.5	31	93.9
Missing		0	0.0	0	0.0	1	2.7	0	0.0	0	0.0	1	1.8	1	1.2	2	2.5	2	6.1
Total		80	100.0	38	100.0	37	100.0	26	100.0	52	100.0	57	100.0	86	100.0	79	100.0	33	100.0

		Agra		*Cali*		*Prague IPSS*		*Groningen*		*Mannheim*		*Sofia*		*Beijing*		*Hong Kong*		*Chennai (Madras)*	
		N	%	N	%	N	%	N	%	N	%	N	%	N	%	N	%	N	%
Available	Course Type: Past 2 yrs.																		
	1: Episodic: <6 Mos.	11	18.3	2	2.8	8	19.0	10	16.1	11	20.0	7	12.7	4	6.9	11	15.9	13	16.9
	2: Continuous	8	13.3	43	59.7	6	14.3	16	25.8	3	5.5	25	45.5	30	51.7	25	36.2	14	18.2
	3: Neither Cont./Epi.	3	5.0	1	1.4	0	0.0	1	1.6	1	1.8	2	3.6	4	6.9	3	4.3	3	3.9
	4: Not Psychotic	38	63.3	26	36.1	28	66.7	35	56.5	19	34.5	21	38.2	20	34.5	30	43.5	47	61.0
	5: Psych. in Period*	0	0.0	0	0.0	0	0.0	0	0.0	21	38.2	0	0.0	0	0.0	0	0.0	0	0.0
Missing	9: Unknown	1	100.0	0	—	1	100.0	1	100.0	1	100.0	0	—	0	—	1	100.0	0	—
Available		60	98.4	72	100.0	42	97.7	62	98.4	55	98.2	55	100.0	58	100.0	69	98.6	77	100.0
Missing		1	1.6	0	0.0	1	2.3	1	1.6	1	1.8	0	0.0	0	0.0	1	1.4	0	0.0
Total		61	100.0	72	100.0	43	100.0	63	100.0	56	100.0	55	100.0	58	100.0	70	100.0	77	100.0

* Note that this category does not appear on the LCS schedule. The April 1996 listings for correcting the database allowed this code if the case was psychotic in the period but it was impossible to use codes 1 to 3.

TABLE B.2 Course Type: Since First Contact Alive Cohort—by Center

		Chandigarh Urban		*Chandigarh Rural*		*Dublin*		*Honolulu*		*Moscow*		*Nagasaki*		*Nottingham*		*Prague DOSMeD*		*Rochester*	
		N	%	N	%	N	%	N	%	N	%	N	%	N	%	N	%	N	%
Available	Course Type: Since 1st																		
	1: Episodic: <2 Yrs.	60	75.0	30	78.9	16	45.7	6	24.0	41	78.8	21	37.5	59	68.6	59	77.6	13	39.4
	2: Continuous	12	15.0	4	10.5	16	45.7	11	44.0	3	5.8	25	44.6	21	24.4	10	13.2	9	27.3
	3: Neither Cont./Epi.	7	8.8	4	10.5	3	8.6	0	0.0	4	7.7	10	17.9	6	7.0	2	2.6	8	24.2
	4: Not Psychotic	1	1.2	0	0.0	0	0.0	8	32.0	4	7.7	0	0.0	0	0.0	5	6.6	2	6.1
	5: Psych. in Period	0	0.0	0	0.0	0	0.0	0	0.0	0	0.0	0	0.0	0	0.0	0	0.0	1	3.0
Missing	.: Not Supplied	0	—	0	—	0	0.0	1	100.0	0	—	0	0.0	0	—	0	0.0	0	—
	8: Not Applicable	0	—	0	—	0	0.0	0	0.0	0	—	0	0.0	0	—	0	0.0	0	—
	9: Unknown	0	—	0	—	2	100.0	0	0.0	0	—	1	100.0	0	—	3	100.0	0	—
Available		80	100.0	38	100.0	35	94.6	25	96.2	52	100.0	56	98.2	86	100.0	76	96.2	33	100.0
Missing		0	0.0	0	0.0	2	5.4	1	3.8	0	0.0	1	1.8	0	0.0	3	3.8	0	0.0
Total		80	100.0	38	100.0	37	100.0	26	100.0	52	100.0	57	100.0	86	100.0	79	100.0	33	100.0

		Agra		*Cali*		*Prague IPSS*		*Groningen*		*Mannheim*		*Sofia*		*Beijing*		*Hong Kong*		*Chennai (Madras)*	
		N	%	N	%	N	%	N	%	N	%	N	%	N	%	N	%	N	%
Available	Course Type: Since 1st																		
	1: Episodic: <2 Yrs.	19	31.7	4	5.6	22	51.2	45	71.4	41	73.2	30	54.5	11	19.0	40	59.7	60	77.9
	2: Continuous	8	13.3	42	58.3	6	14.0	14	22.2	1	1.8	23	41.8	29	50.0	18	26.9	7	9.1
	3: Neither Cont./Epi.	2	3.3	2	2.8	4	9.3	4	6.3	14	25.0	2	3.6	7	12.1	8	11.9	10	13.0
	4: Not Psychotic	31	51.7	24	33.3	11	25.6	0	0.0	0	0.0	0	0.0	11	19.0	1	1.5	0	0.0
	5: Psych. in Period	0	0.0	0	0.0	0	0.0	0	0.0	0	0.0	0	0.0	0	0.0	0	0.0	0	0.0
Missing	.: Not Supplied	0	0.0	0	—	0	—	0	—	0	—	0	—	0	—	0	0.0	0	—
	8: Not Applicable	0	0.0	0	—	0	—	0	—	0	—	0	—	0	—	1	33.3	0	—
	9: Unknown	1	100.0	0	—	0	—	0	—	0	—	0	—	0	—	2	66.7	0	—
Available		60	98.4	72	100.0	43	100.0	63	100.0	56	100.0	55	100.0	58	100.0	67	95.7	77	100.0
Missing		1	1.6	0	0.0	0	0.0	0	0.0	0	0.0	0	0.0	0	0.0	3	4.3	0	0.0
Total		61	100.0	72	100.0	43	100.0	63	100.0	56	100.0	55	100.0	58	100.0	70	100.0	77	100.0

TABLE B.3A Global Assessment of Functioning (GAF) Scale—Symptoms: Past Month Alive Cohort—by Center

		Chandigarh Urban		*Chandigarh Rural*		*Dublin*		*Honolulu*		*Moscow*		*Nagasaki*		*Nottingham*		*Prague DOSMeD*		*Rochester*	
		N	%	N	%	N	%	N	%	N	%	N	%	N	%	N	%	N	%
Available	GAF Scale: Symptoms																		
	1–10	1	1.2	0	0.0	0	0.0	1	3.8	0	0.0	0	0.0	0	0.0	0	0.0	0	0.0
	11–20	1	1.2	0	0.0	1	2.9	0	0.0	0	0.0	2	3.5	0	0.0	3	4.0	0	0.0
	21–30	4	5.0	1	2.7	3	8.6	2	7.7	1	1.9	6	10.5	8	9.4	3	4.0	4	12.9
	31–40	1	1.2	1	2.7	4	11.4	5	19.2	2	3.8	6	10.5	19	22.4	2	2.7	7	22.6
	41–50	5	6.3	0	0.0	2	5.7	3	11.5	2	3.8	2	3.5	5	5.9	1	1.3	2	6.5
	51–60	8	10.0	5	13.5	7	20.0	3	11.5	9	17.3	14	24.6	8	9.4	18	24.0	5	16.1
	61–70	11	13.8	5	13.5	8	22.9	5	19.2	8	15.4	10	17.5	8	9.4	21	28.0	5	16.1
	71–80	11	13.8	8	21.6	3	8.6	2	7.7	3	5.8	6	10.5	12	14.1	11	14.7	2	6.5
	81–90	38	47.5	17	45.9	7	20.0	5	19.2	27	51.9	11	19.3	25	29.4	16	21.3	6	19.4
Missing	. : Not Supplied	0	—	0	0.0	0	0.0	0	—	0	—	0	—	0	0.0	0	0.0	0	0.0
	99: Unknown	0	—	1	100.0	2	100.0	0	—	0	—	0	—	1	100.0	4	100.0	2	100.0
Available		80	100.0	37	97.4	35	94.6	26	100.0	52	100.0	57	100.0	85	98.8	75	94.9	31	93.9
Missing		0	0.0	1	2.6	2	5.4	0	0.0	0	0.0	0	0.0	1	1.2	4	5.1	2	6.1
Total		80	100.0	38	100.0	37	100.0	26	100.0	52	100.0	57	100.0	86	100.0	79	100.0	33	100.0

(continued)

TABLE B.3A (*continued*)

		Agra		*Cali*		*Prague IPSS*		*Groningen*		*Mannheim*		*Sofia*		*Beijing*		*Hong Kong*		*Chennai (Madras)*	
		N	%	N	%	N	%	N	%	N	%	N	%	N	%	N	%	N	%
Available	GAF Scale: Symptoms																		
	1–10	1	1.6	0	0.0	0	0.0	0	0.0	0	—	0	0.0	0	0.0	0	0.0	2	2.6
	11–20	1	1.6	0	0.0	0	0.0	0	0.0	0	—	4	7.3	1	1.7	1	1.4	4	5.2
	21–30	2	3.3	11	15.5	0	0.0	8	12.7	0	—	9	16.4	9	15.5	3	4.3	7	9.1
	31–40	3	4.9	3	4.2	1	2.6	5	7.9	0	—	9	16.4	6	10.3	4	5.7	7	9.1
	41–50	2	3.3	7	9.9	2	5.1	3	4.8	0	—	7	12.7	1	1.7	2	2.9	1	1.3
	51–60	1	1.6	14	19.7	3	7.7	9	14.3	0	—	9	16.4	13	22.4	10	14.3	3	3.9
	61–70	5	8.2	14	19.7	4	10.3	9	14.3	0	—	5	9.1	4	6.9	14	20.0	5	6.5
	71–80	7	11.5	10	14.1	8	20.5	7	11.1	0	—	7	12.7	6	10.3	10	14.3	13	16.9
	81–90	39	63.9	12	16.9	21	53.8	22	34.9	0	—	5	9.1	18	31.0	26	37.1	35	45.5
Missing	. : Not Supplied	0	—	0	0.0	0	0.0	0	—	56	100.0	0	—	0	—	0	—	0	—
	99: Unknown	0	—	1	100.0	4	100.0	0	—	0	0.0	0	—	0	—	0	—	0	—
Available		61	100.0	71	98.6	39	90.7	63	100.0	0	0.0	55	100.0	58	100.0	70	100.0	77	100.0
Missing		0	0.0	1	1.4	4	9.3	0	0.0	56	100.0	0	0.0	0	0.0	0	0.0	0	0.0
Total		61	100.0	72	100.0	43	100.0	63	100.0	56	100.0	55	100.0	58	100.0	70	100.0	77	100.0

TABLE B.3B (GAF) Scale—Symptoms: Past Month Alive Cohort—by Center

		Chandigarh Urban	*Chandigarh Rural*	*Dublin*	*Honolulu*	*Moscow*	*Nagasaki*	*Nottingham*	*Prague DOSMeD*	*Rochester*
Total	N	80	37	35	26	52	57	85	75	31
	Mean	71.10	77.38	59.97	58.15	73.46	59.23	61.05	65.16	55.84
	STD	20.23	15.34	19.84	20.97	16.95	20.69	21.69	17.82	20.55
		Agra	*Cali*	*Prague IPSS*	*Groningen*	*Mannheim*	*Sofia*	*Beijing*	*Hong Kong*	*Chennai (Madras)*
Total	N	61	71	39	63	0	55	58	70	77
	Mean	76.03	61.56	77.87	63.87	—	49.33	59.69	68.74	65.16
	STD	21.96	18.65	14.07	22.72	—	20.39	23.63	17.69	25.78

TABLE B.4 Severity of Psychotic Symptoms, Bleuler Scale: Past Month Alive Cohort—by Center

		Chandigarh Urban		*Chandigarh Rural*		*Dublin*		*Honolulu*		*Moscow*		*Nagasaki*		*Nottingham*		*Prague DOSMeD*		*Rochester*	
		N	%	N	%	N	%	N	%	N	%	N	%	N	%	N	%	N	%
Available	Bleuler: Severity of Psychotic Symptoms																		
	1: Severe	4	5.0	0	0.0	4	11.4	1	3.8	1	1.9	7	12.3	4	4.7	8	10.4	2	6.5
	2: Moderate	9	11.3	6	15.8	7	20.0	6	23.1	3	5.8	19	33.3	19	22.4	15	19.5	7	22.6
	3: Mild	14	17.5	9	23.7	11	31.4	8	30.8	9	17.3	15	26.3	10	11.8	9	11.7	5	16.1
	4: Recovered	53	66.3	23	60.5	13	37.1	11	42.3	39	75.0	16	28.1	52	61.2	45	58.4	17	54.8
Missing	. : Not Supplied	0	—	0	—	0	0.0	0	—	0	—	0	—	0	0.0	1	50.0	1	50.0
	9: Unknown	0	—	0	—	2	100.0	0	—	0	—	0	—	1	100.0	1	50.0	1	50.0
Available		80	100.0	38	100.0	35	94.6	26	100.0	52	100.0	57	100.0	85	98.8	77	97.5	31	93.9
Missing		0	0.0	0	0.0	2	5.4	0	0.0	0	0.0	0	0.0	1	1.2	2	2.5	2	6.1
Total		80	100.0	38	100.0	37	100.0	26	100.0	52	100.0	57	100.0	86	100.0	79	100.0	33	100.0

		Agra		*Cali*		*Prague IPSS*		*Groningen*		*Mannheim*		*Sofia*		*Beijing*		*Hong Kong*		*Chennai (Madras)*	
		N	%	N	%	N	%	N	%	N	%	N	%	N	%	N	%	N	%
Available	Bleuler: Severity of Psychotic Symptoms																		
	1: Severe	7	11.5	8	11.1	2	5.0	7	11.1	1	1.8	11	20.4	10	17.2	5	7.1	9	11.7
	2: Moderate	6	9.8	17	23.6	5	12.5	4	6.3	13	23.6	14	25.9	15	25.9	9	12.9	13	16.9
	3: Mild	1	1.6	6	8.3	4	10.0	6	9.5	10	18.2	3	5.6	11	19.0	19	27.1	10	13.0
	4: Recovered	47	77.0	41	56.9	29	72.5	46	73.0	31	56.4	26	48.1	22	37.9	37	52.9	45	58.4
Missing	. : Not Supplied	0	—	0	—	3	100.0	0	—	1	100.0	1	100.0	0	—	0	—	0	—
	9: Unknown	0	—	0	—	0	0.0	0	—	0	0.0	0	0.0	0	—	0	—	0	—
Available		61	100.0	72	100.0	40	93.0	63	100.0	55	98.2	54	98.2	58	100.0	70	100.0	77	100.0
Missing		0	0.0	0	0.0	3	7.0	0	0.0	1	1.8	1	1.8	0	0.0	0	0.0	0	0.0
Total		61	100.0	72	100.0	43	100.0	63	100.0	56	100.0	55	100.0	58	100.0	70	100.0	77	100.0

TABLE B.5 Trend of Psychotic Symptoms: Entire Period Alive Cohort—by Center

		Chandigarh Urban		*Chandigarh Rural*		*Dublin*		*Honolulu*		*Moscow*		*Nagasaki*		*Nottingham*		*Prague DOSMeD*		*Rochester*	
		N	%	N	%	N	%	N	%	N	%	N	%	N	%	N	%	N	%
Available	Trend of Psychotic Symptoms																		
	XXX	21	26.2	11	28.9	0	0.0	0	0.0	8	15.4	1	1.8	0	0.0	2	2.7	0	0.0
	XX1[a]	2	2.5	2	5.3	0	0.0	3	11.5	0	0.0	7	12.3	0	0.0	6	8.0	0	0.0
	X1X	0	0.0	2	5.3	2	5.7	4	15.4	0	0.0	1	1.8	0	0.0	5	6.7	2	6.1
	X11	0	0.0	0	0.0	0	0.0	1	3.8	1	1.9	5	8.8	0	0.0	0	0.0	0	0.0
	1XX	52	65.0	20	52.6	19	54.3	14	53.8	29	55.8	29	50.9	59	68.6	52	69.3	24	72.7
	1X1	2	2.5	3	7.9	1	2.9	2	7.7	4	7.7	5	8.8	6	7.0	7	9.3	0	0.0
	11X	0	0.0	0	0.0	5	14.3	2	7.7	3	5.8	6	10.5	2	2.3	2	2.7	4	12.1
	111	3	3.8	0	0.0	8	22.9	0	0.0	7	13.5	3	5.3	19	22.1	1	1.3	3	9.1
Missing	MMM	0	—	0	—	2	100.0	0	—	0	—	0	—	0	—	4	100.0	0	—
Available		80	100.0	38	100.0	35	94.6	26	100.0	52	100.0	57	100.0	86	100.0	75	94.9	33	100.0
Missing		0	0.0	0	0.0	2	5.4	0	0.0	0	0.0	0	0.0	0	0.0	4	5.1	0	0.0
Total		80	100.0	38	100.0	37	100.0	26	100.0	52	100.0	57	100.0	86	100.0	79	100.0	33	100.0

(continued)

TABLE B.5 *(continued)*

		Agra		*Cali*		*Prague IPSS*		*Groningen*		*Mannheim*		*Sofia*		*Beijing*		*Hong Kong*		*Chennai (Madras)*	
		N	%	N	%	N	%	N	%	N	%	N	%	N	%	N	%	N	%
Available	Trend of Psychotic Symptoms																		
	XXX	1	2.4	9	12.5	1	2.4	12	19.0	0	—	0	0.0	11	19.0	3	4.3	0	0.0
	XX1	6	14.6	5	6.9	3	7.1	1	1.6	0	—	8	14.5	3	5.2	11	15.7	0	0.0
	X1X	5	12.2	3	4.2	2	4.8	3	4.8	0	—	2	3.6	2	3.4	9	12.9	0	0.0
	X11	0	0.0	3	4.2	0	0.0	2	3.2	0	—	1	1.8	2	3.4	4	5.7	0	0.0
	1XX	21	51.2	48	66.7	32	76.2	32	50.8	0	—	29	52.7	31	53.4	32	45.7	72	93.5
	1X1	1	2.4	2	2.8	0	0.0	5	7.9	0	—	2	3.6	3	5.2	5	7.1	5	6.5
	11X	1	2.4	0	0.0	3	7.1	2	3.2	0	—	5	9.1	1	1.7	3	4.3	0	0.0
	111	6	14.6	2	2.8	1	2.4	6	9.5	0	—	8	14.5	5	8.6	3	4.3	0	0.0
Missing	MMM	20	100.0	0	—	1	100.0	0	—	56	100.0	0	—	0	—	0	—	0	—
Available		41	67.2	72	100.0	42	97.7	63	100.0	0	0.0	55	100.0	58	100.0	70	100.0	77	100.0
Missing		20	32.8	0	0.0	1	2.3	0	0.0	56	100.0	0	0.0	0	0.0	0	0.0	0	0.0
Total		61	100.0	72	100.0	43	100.0	63	100.0	56	100.0	55	100.0	58	100.0	70	100.0	77	100.0

[a] The number "1" designates that third of the entire period when variable was most prominent (where the leftmost position represents the earliest third). Where it appears in more than one time slot, the variable was considered to be equally prominent in the designated periods.

TABLE B.6 Overall Illness Trajectory: Entire Period Alive Cohort—by Center

		Chandigarh Urban		*Chandigarh Rural*		*Dublin*		*Honolulu*		*Moscow*		*Nagasaki*		*Nottingham*		*Prague DOSMeD*		*Rochester*	
		N	%	N	%	N	%	N	%	N	%	N	%	N	%	N	%	N	%
Available	Overall Time Trend																		
	1: Much Better	13	16.2	17	44.7	14	40.0	11	42.3	15	28.8	13	22.8	31	36.0	17	21.8	11	34.4
	2: Somewhat Better	10	12.5	5	13.2	12	34.3	9	34.6	15	28.8	7	12.3	17	19.8	17	21.8	9	28.1
	3: Same	22	27.5	7	18.4	6	17.1	1	3.8	20	38.5	18	31.6	33	38.4	9	11.5	11	34.4
	4: Somewhat Worse	4	5.0	2	5.3	3	8.6	4	15.4	2	3.8	13	22.8	5	5.8	26	33.3	0	0.0
	5: Much Worse	3	3.8	0	0.0	0	0.0	0	0.0	0	0.0	6	10.5	0	0.0	8	10.3	0	0.0
	6: Other	28	35.0	7	18.4	0	0.0	1	3.8	0	0.0	0	0.0	0	0.0	1	1.3	1	3.1
Missing	9: Unknown	0	—	0	—	2	100.0	0	—	0	—	0	—	0	—	1	100.0	1	100.0
Available		80	100.0	38	100.0	35	94.6	26	100.0	52	100.0	57	100.0	86	100.0	78	98.7	32	97.0
Missing		0	0.0	0	0.0	2	5.4	0	0.0	0	0.0	0	0.0	0	0.0	1	1.3	1	3.0
Total		80	100.0	38	100.0	37	100.0	26	100.0	52	100.0	57	100.0	86	100.0	79	100.0	33	100.0

		Agra		*Cali*		*Prague IPSS*		*Groningen*		*Mannheim*		*Sofia*		*Beijing*		*Hong Kong*		*Chennai (Madras)*	
		N	%	N	%	N	%	N	%	N	%	N	%	N	%	N	%	N	%
Available	Overall Time Trend																		
	1: Much Better	8	13.1	21	29.2	13	31.0	18	28.6	0	—	12	21.8	15	25.9	12	17.4	32	41.6
	2: Somewhat Better	3	4.9	5	6.9	15	35.7	18	28.6	0	—	13	23.6	13	22.4	20	29.0	24	31.2
	3: Same	14	23.0	27	37.5	5	11.9	11	17.5	0	—	9	16.4	7	12.1	18	26.1	13	16.9
	4: Somewhat Worse	3	4.9	11	15.3	5	11.9	11	17.5	0	—	14	25.5	7	12.1	11	15.9	7	9.1
	5: Much Worse	2	3.3	5	6.9	2	4.8	5	7.9	0	—	7	12.7	8	13.8	8	11.6	1	1.3
	6: Other	31	50.8	3	4.2	2	4.8	0	0.0	0	—	0	0.0	8	13.8	0	0.0	0	0.0
Missing	9: Unknown	0	—	0	—	1	100.0	0	—	56	100.0	0	—	0	—	1	100.0	0	—
Available		61	100.0	72	100.0	42	97.7	63	100.0	0	0.0	55	100.0	58	100.0	69	98.6	77	100.0
Missing		0	0.0	0	0.0	1	2.3	0	0.0	56	100.0	0	0.0	0	0.0	1	1.4	0	0.0
Total		61	100.0	72	100.0	43	100.0	63	100.0	56	100.0	55	100.0	58	100.0	70	100.0	77	100.0

TABLE B.7 Current Living Arrangements: Past Month Alive Cohort—by Center

		Chandigarh Urban		*Chandigarh Rural*		*Dublin*		*Honolulu*		*Moscow*		*Nagasaki*		*Nottingham*		*Prague DOSMeD*		*Rochester*	
		N	%	N	%	N	%	N	%	N	%	N	%	N	%	N	%	N	%
Available	Current Living Location																		
	1: Hospital	2	2.5	0	0.0	0	0.0	3	11.5	1	1.9	19	33.3	3	3.5	5	6.3	1	3.0
	2: Sup. Res./Other Inst.	0	0.0	0	0.0	3	8.1	5	19.2	0	0.0	0	0.0	1	1.2	4	5.1	3	9.1
	4: Family/Friends	73	91.3	37	97.4	30	81.1	14	53.8	37	71.2	35	61.4	57	66.3	57	72.2	21	63.6
	5: Alone	5	6.3	1	2.6	4	10.8	4	15.4	14	26.9	3	5.3	24	27.9	13	16.5	8	24.2
	6: Other	0	0.0	0	0.0	0	0.0	0	0.0	0	0.0	0	0.0	1	1.2	0	0.0	0	0.0
Missing	9: Unknown	0	—	0	—	0	—	0	—	0	—	0	—	0	—	0	—	0	—
Available		80	100.0	38	100.0	37	100.0	26	100.0	52	100.0	57	100.0	86	100.0	79	100.0	33	100.0
Missing		0	0.0	0	0.0	0	0.0	0	0.0	0	0.0	0	0.0	0	0.0	0	0.0	0	0.0
Total		80	100.0	38	100.0	37	100.0	26	100.0	52	100.0	57	100.0	86	100.0	79	100.0	33	100.0

		Agra		*Cali*		*Prague IPSS*		*Groningen*		*Mannheim*		*Sofia*		*Beijing*		*Hong Kong*		*Chennai (Madras)*	
		N	%	N	%	N	%	N	%	N	%	N	%	N	%	N	%	N	%
Available	Current Living Location																		
	1: Hospital	0	0.0	1	1.4	1	2.3	8	12.7	4	7.1	1	1.9	6	10.3	6	8.6	1	1.3
	2: Sup. Res./Other Inst.	0	0.0	0	0.0	4	9.3	6	9.5	13	23.2	1	1.9	1	1.7	4	5.7	2	2.6
	4: Family/Friends	58	95.1	66	91.7	27	62.8	26	41.3	27	48.2	38	70.4	47	81.0	55	78.6	73	94.8
	5: Alone	2	3.3	4	5.6	11	25.6	23	36.5	12	21.4	14	25.9	4	6.9	5	7.1	0	0.0
	6: Other	1	1.6	1	1.4	0	0.0	0	0.0	0	0.0	0	0.0	0	0.0	0	0.0	1	1.3
Missing	9: Unknown	0	—	0	—	0	—	0	—	0	—	1	100.0	0	—	0	—	0	—
Available		61	100.0	72	100.0	43	100.0	63	100.0	56	100.0	54	98.2	58	100.0	70	100.0	77	100.0
Missing		0	0.0	0	0.0	0	0.0	0	0.0	0	0.0	1	1.8	0	0.0	0	0.0	0	0.0
Total		61	100.0	72	100.0	43	100.0	63	100.0	56	100.0	55	100.0	58	100.0	70	100.0	77	100.0

TABLE B.8 Living Arrangements—Independent: Past 2 Years Alive Cohort—by Center

		Chandigarh Urban		*Chandigarh Rural*		*Dublin*		*Honolulu*		*Moscow*		*Nagasaki*		*Nottingham*		*Prague DOSMeD*		*Rochester*	
		N	%	N	%	N	%	N	%	N	%	N	%	N	%	N	%	N	%
Available	Months Independent Living																		
	. Never	1	1.2	0	0.0	2	5.6	8	30.8	0	0.0	14	24.6	2	2.3	0	0.0	4	12.1
	<=12 Months	1	1.2	0	0.0	1	2.8	0	0.0	0	0.0	2	3.5	0	0.0	1	1.3	0	0.0
	13–23 Months	3	3.8	2	5.3	7	19.4	3	11.5	10	19.2	11	19.3	15	17.4	26	33.3	3	9.1
	24 Months	75	93.8	36	94.7	26	72.2	15	57.7	42	80.8	30	52.6	69	80.2	51	65.4	26	78.8
Missing	Unknown	0	—	0	—	1	100.0	0	—	0	—	0	—	0	—	1	100.0	0	—
Available		80	100.0	38	100.0	36	97.3	26	100.0	52	100.0	57	100.0	86	100.0	78	98.7	33	100.0
Missing		0	0.0	0	0.0	1	2.7	0	0.0	0	0.0	0	0.0	0	0.0	1	1.3	0	0.0
Total		80	100.0	38	100.0	37	100.0	26	100.0	52	100.0	57	100.0	86	100.0	79	100.0	33	100.0

		Agra		*Cali*		*Prague IPSS*		*Groningen*		*Mannheim*		*Sofia*		*Beijing*		*Hong Kong*		*Chennai (Madras)*	
		N	%	N	%	N	%	N	%	N	%	N	%	N	%	N	%	N	%
Available	Months Independent Living																		
	. Never	2	3.3	0	0.0	2	4.7	12	19.0	13	23.2	2	3.6	5	8.6	6	8.6	1	1.3
	<=12 Months	0	0.0	0	0.0	2	4.7	2	3.2	3	5.4	1	1.8	1	1.7	3	4.3	0	0.0
	13–23 Months	2	3.3	3	4.2	6	14.0	7	11.1	11	19.6	11	20.0	3	5.2	6	8.6	9	11.7
	24 Months	57	93.4	69	95.8	33	76.7	42	66.7	29	51.8	41	74.5	49	84.5	55	78.6	67	87.0
Missing	Unknown	0	—	0	—	0	—	0	—	0	—	0	—	0	—	0	—	0	—
Available		61	100.0	72	100.0	43	100.0	63	100.0	56	100.0	55	100.0	58	100.0	70	100.0	77	100.0
Missing		0	0.0	0	0.0	0	0.0	0	0.0	0	0.0	0	0.0	0	0.0	0	0.0	0	0.0
Total		61	100.0	72	100.0	43	100.0	63	100.0	56	100.0	55	100.0	58	100.0	70	100.0	77	100.0

TABLE B.9 Living Arrangements—Institution: Past 2 Years SET 1: Alive Cohort—by Center

		Chandigarh Urban		*Chandigarh Rural*		*Dublin*		*Honolulu*		*Moscow*		*Nagasaki*		*Nottingham*		*Prague DOSMeD*		*Rochester*	
		N	%	N	%	N	%	N	%	N	%	N	%	N	%	N	%	N	%
Available	Months in Hospital/ Supervised																		
	Residence																		
	. Never	76	95.0	38	100.0	26	72.2	16	61.5	42	80.8	30	52.6	69	80.2	53	67.9	26	78.8
	≤ 12 Months	2	2.5	0	0.0	8	22.2	3	11.5	10	19.2	12	21.1	15	17.4	25	32.1	3	9.1
	13–23 Months	1	1.2	0	0.0	0	0.0	1	3.8	0	0.0	2	3.5	1	1.2	0	0.0	0	0.0
	24 Months	1	1.2	0	0.0	2	5.6	6	23.1	0	0.0	13	22.8	1	1.2	0	0.0	4	12.1
Missing	Not Supplied	0	—	0	—	1	100.0	0	—	0	—	0	—	0	—	1	100.0	0	—
Available		80	100.0	38	100.0	36	97.3	26	100.0	52	100.0	57	100.0	86	100.0	78	98.7	33	100.0
Missing		0	0.0	0	0.0	1	2.7	0	0.0	0	0.0	0	0.0	0	0.0	1	1.3	0	0.0
Total		80	100.0	38	100.0	37	100.0	26	100.0	52	100.0	57	100.0	86	100.0	79	100.0	33	100.0

		Agra		*Cali*		*Prague IPSS*		*Groningen*		*Mannheim*		*Sofia*		*Beijing*		*Hong Kong*		*Chennai (Madras)*	
		N	%	N	%	N	%	N	%	N	%	N	%	N	%	N	%	N	%
Available	Months in Hospital/ Supervised																		
	Residence																		
	. Never	59	96.7	70	97.2	33	76.7	42	66.7	29	51.8	41	74.5	50	86.2	55	78.6	67	87.0
	≤ 12 Months	2	3.3	2	2.8	6	14.0	8	12.7	12	21.4	11	20.0	2	3.4	6	8.6	9	11.7
	13–23 Months	0	0.0	0	0.0	2	4.7	1	1.6	2	3.6	1	1.8	1	1.7	3	4.3	0	0.0
	24 Months	0	0.0	0	0.0	2	4.7	12	19.0	13	23.2	2	3.6	5	8.6	6	8.6	1	1.3
Missing	Not Supplied	0	—	0	—	0	—	0	—	0	—	0	—	0	—	0	—	0	—
Available		61	100.0	72	100.0	43	100.0	63	100.0	56	100.0	55	100.0	58	100.0	70	100.0	77	100.0
Missing		0	0.0	0	0.0	0	0.0	0	0.0	0	0.0	0	0.0	0	0.0	0	0.0	0	0.0
Total		61	100.0	72	100.0	43	100.0	63	100.0	56	100.0	55	100.0	58	100.0	70	100.0	77	100.0

TABLE B.10 Living Arrangements—Homeless: Past 2 Years Alive Cohort—by Center

		Chandigarh Urban		*Chandigarh Rural*		*Dublin*		*Honolulu*		*Moscow*		*Nagasaki*		*Nottingham*		*Prague DOSMeD*		*Rochester*	
		N	%	N	%	N	%	N	%	N	%	N	%	N	%	N	%	N	%
Available	Months Homeless or Vagrant																		
	. Never	79	98.8	36	94.7	34	91.9	24	92.3	52	100.0	57	100.0	85	98.8	76	97.4	33	100.0
	≤ 12 Months	1	1.2	2	5.3	3	8.1	1	3.8	0	0.0	0	0.0	1	1.2	2	2.6	0	0.0
	13–23 Months	0	0.0	0	0.0	0	0.0	1	3.8	0	0.0	0	0.0	0	0.0	0	0.0	0	0.0
	24 Months	0	0.0	0	0.0	0	0.0	0	0.0	0	0.0	0	0.0	0	0.0	0	0.0	0	0.0
Missing	Unknown	0	—	0	—	0	—	0	—	0	—	0	—	0	—	1	100.0	0	—
Available		80	100.0	38	100.0	37	100.0	26	100.0	52	100.0	57	100.0	86	100.0	78	98.7	33	100.0
Missing		0	0.0	0	0.0	0	0.0	0	0.0	0	0.0	0	0.0	0	0.0	1	1.3	0	0.0
Total		80	100.0	38	100.0	37	100.0	26	100.0	52	100.0	57	100.0	86	100.0	79	100.0	33	100.0

		Agra		*Cali*		*Prague IPSS*		*Groningen*		*Mannheim*		*Sofia*		*Beijing*		*Hong Kong*		*Chennai (Madras)*	
		N	%	N	%	N	%	N	%	N	%	N	%	N	%	N	%	N	%
Available	Months Homeless or Vagrant																		
	. Never	59	96.7	72	100.0	43	100.0	63	100.0	56	100.0	55	100.0	57	98.3	69	98.6	77	100.0
	≤ 12 Months	0	0.0	0	0.0	0	0.0	0	0.0	0	0.0	0	0.0	1	1.7	1	1.4	0	0.0
	13–23 Months	0	0.0	0	0.0	0	0.0	0	0.0	0	0.0	0	0.0	0	0.0	0	0.0	0	0.0
	24 Months	2	3.3	0	0.0	0	0.0	0	0.0	0	0.0	0	0.0	0	0.0	0	0.0	0	0.0
Missing	Unknown	0	—	0	—	0	—	0	—	0	—	0	—	0	—	0	—	0	—
Available		61	100.0	72	100.0	43	100.0	63	100.0	56	100.0	55	100.0	58	100.0	70	100.0	77	100.0
Missing		0	0.0	0	0.0	0	0.0	0	0.0	0	0.0	0	0.0	0	0.0	0	0.0	0	0.0
Total		61	100.0	72	100.0	43	100.0	63	100.0	56	100.0	55	100.0	58	100.0	70	100.0	77	100.0

TABLE B.11 Living Arrangements—Jail: Past 2 Years Alive Cohort—by Center

		Chandigarh Urban		*Chandigarh Rural*		*Dublin*		*Honolulu*		*Moscow*		*Nagasaki*		*Nottingham*		*Prague DOSMeD*		*Rochester*	
		N	%	N	%	N	%	N	%	N	%	N	%	N	%	N	%	N	%
Available	Months in Jail or Prison																		
	. Never	80	100.0	38	100.0	36	97.3	24	92.3	52	100.0	56	98.2	85	98.8	78	100.0	33	100.0
	≤ 12 Months	0	0.0	0	0.0	1	2.7	2	7.7	0	0.0	1	1.8	1	1.2	0	0.0	0	0.0
Missing	Unknown	0	—	0	—	0	—	0	—	0	—	0	—	0	—	1	100.0	0	—
Available		80	100.0	38	100.0	37	100.0	26	100.0	52	100.0	57	100.0	86	100.0	78	98.7	33	100.0
Missing		0	0.0	0	0.0	0	0.0	0	0.0	0	0.0	0	0.0	0	0.0	1	1.3	0	0.0
Total		80	100.0	38	100.0	37	100.0	26	100.0	52	100.0	57	100.0	86	100.0	79	100.0	33	100.0

		Agra		*Cali*		*Prague IPSS*		*Groningen*		*Mannheim*		*Sofia*		*Beijing*		*Hong Kong*		*Chennai (Madras)*	
		N	%	N	%	N	%	N	%	N	%	N	%	N	%	N	%	N	%
Available	Months in Jail or Prison																		
	. Never	61	100.0	72	100.0	43	100.0	63	100.0	56	100.0	55	100.0	58	100.0	70	100.0	77	100.0
	≤ 12 Months	0	0.0	0	0.0	0	0.0	0	0.0	0	0.0	0	0.0	0	0.0	0	0.0	0	0.0
Missing	Unknown	0	—	0	—	0	—	0	—	0	—	0	—	0	—	0	—	0	—
Available		61	100.0	72	100.0	43	100.0	63	100.0	56	100.0	55	100.0	58	100.0	70	100.0	77	100.0
Missing		0	0.0	0	0.0	0	0.0	0	0.0	0	0.0	0	0.0	0	0.0	0	0.0	0	0.0
Total		61	100.0	72	100.0	43	100.0	63	100.0	56	100.0	55	100.0	58	100.0	70	100.0	77	100.0

TABLE B.12 Living Arrangements—Independent: Entire Period Alive Cohort—by Center

		Chandigarh Urban		*Chandigarh Rural*		*Dublin*		*Honolulu*		*Moscow*		*Nagasaki*		*Nottingham*		*Prague DOSMeD*		*Rochester*	
		N	%	N	%	N	%	N	%	N	%	N	%	N	%	N	%	N	%
Available	% Time Independent Living																		
	. Never	0	0.0	0	0.0	0	0.0	3	12.0	0	0.0	1	1.8	0	0.0	0	0.0	0	0.0
	≤ 50%	2	2.5	0	0.0	0	0.0	4	16.0	0	0.0	12	21.4	1	1.2	1	1.3	3	9.1
	51–90%	0	0.0	0	0.0	4	11.1	5	20.0	3	5.8	16	28.6	8	9.3	16	20.3	9	27.3
	91–95%	3	3.8	0	0.0	12	33.3	2	8.0	17	32.7	11	19.6	23	26.7	28	35.4	6	18.2
	96–100%	75	93.8	38	100.0	20	55.6	11	44.0	32	61.5	16	28.6	54	62.8	34	43.0	15	45.5
Missing	Not Supplied	0	—	0	—	1	100.0	1	100.0	0	—	1	100.0	0	—	0	—	0	—
Available		80	100.0	38	100.0	36	97.3	25	96.2	52	100.0	56	98.2	86	100.0	79	100.0	33	100.0
Missing		0	0.0	0	0.0	1	2.7	1	3.8	0	0.0	1	1.8	0	0.0	0	0.0	0	0.0
Total		80	100.0	38	100.0	37	100.0	26	100.0	52	100.0	57	100.0	86	100.0	79	100.0	33	100.0

		Agra		*Cali*		*Prague IPSS*		*Groningen*		*Mannheim*		*Sofia*		*Beijing*		*Hong Kong*		*Chennai (Madras)*	
		N	%	N	%	N	%	N	%	N	%	N	%	N	%	N	%	N	%
Available	% Time Independent Living																		
	. Never	1	1.6	0	0.0	1	2.3	1	1.6	1	1.8	0	0.0	3	5.2	0	0.0	0	0.0
	≤ 50%	0	0.0	1	1.4	3	7.0	9	14.3	12	21.4	1	1.8	4	6.9	1	1.4	1	1.3
	51–90%	1	1.6	1	1.4	12	27.9	18	28.6	12	21.4	12	21.8	7	12.1	17	24.3	5	6.5
	91–95%	0	0.0	0	0.0	0	0.0	7	11.1	13	23.2	18	32.7	6	10.3	9	12.9	5	6.5
	96–100%	59	96.7	70	97.2	27	62.8	28	44.4	18	32.1	24	43.6	38	65.5	43	61.4	66	85.7
Missing	Not Supplied	0	—	0	—	0	—	0	—	0	—	0	—	0	—	0	—	0	—
Available		61	100.0	72	100.0	43	100.0	63	100.0	56	100.0	55	100.0	58	100.0	70	100.0	77	100.0
Missing		0	0.0	0	0.0	0	0.0	0	0.0	0	0.0	0	0.0	0	0.0	0	0.0	0	0.0
Total		61	100.0	72	100.0	43	100.0	63	100.0	56	100.0	55	100.0	58	100.0	70	100.0	77	100.0

TABLE B.13 Living Arrangements—Institution: Entire Period Alive Cohort—by Center

		Chandigarh Urban		*Chandigarh Rural*		*Dublin*		*Honolulu*		*Moscow*		*Nagasaki*		*Nottingham*		*Prague DOSMeD*		*Rochester*	
		N	%	N	%	N	%	N	%	N	%	N	%	N	%	N	%	N	%
Available	% Time in Hospital/ Supervised Residence																		
	. Never	52	65.0	33	86.8	6	16.7	6	24.0	1	1.9	6	10.5	5	5.8	9	11.4	3	9.1
	≤ 5%	24	30.0	5	13.2	15	41.7	5	20.0	31	59.6	11	19.3	50	58.1	26	32.9	12	36.4
	6–10%	2	2.5	0	0.0	12	33.3	3	12.0	17	32.7	11	19.3	23	26.7	28	35.4	7	21.2
	11–25%	0	0.0	0	0.0	2	5.6	4	16.0	3	5.8	7	12.3	6	7.0	14	17.7	6	18.2
	26–50%	0	0.0	0	0.0	1	2.8	3	12.0	0	0.0	9	15.8	1	1.2	2	2.5	2	6.1
	>50%	2	2.5	0	0.0	0	0.0	4	16.0	0	0.0	13	22.8	1	1.2	0	0.0	3	9.1
Missing	Not Supplied	0	—	0	—	1	100.0	1	100.0	0	—	0	—	0	—	0	—	0	—
Available		80	100.0	38	100.0	36	97.3	25	96.2	52	100.0	57	100.0	86	100.0	79	100.0	33	100.0
Missing		0	0.0	0	0.0	1	2.7	1	3.8	0	0.0	0	0.0	0	0.0	0	0.0	0	0.0
Total		80	100.0	38	100.0	37	100.0	26	100.0	52	100.0	57	100.0	86	100.0	79	100.0	33	100.0

		Agra		*Cali*		*Prague IPSS*		*Groningen*		*Mannheim*		*Sofia*		*Beijing*		*Hong Kong*		*Chennai (Madras)*	
		N	%	N	%	N	%	N	%	N	%	N	%	N	%	N	%	N	%
Available	% Time in Hospital/ Supervised Residence																		
	. Never	58	95.1	57	79.2	19	44.2	2	3.2	0	0.0	5	9.1	32	55.2	15	21.4	23	29.9
	≤ 5%	2	3.3	13	18.1	8	18.6	26	41.3	18	32.1	19	34.5	6	10.3	28	40.0	43	55.8
	6–10%	0	0.0	0	0.0	0	0.0	7	11.1	13	23.2	18	32.7	7	12.1	9	12.9	5	6.5
	11–25%	1	1.6	1	1.4	12	27.9	12	19.0	8	14.3	12	21.8	5	8.6	10	14.3	4	5.2
	26–50%	0	0.0	0	0.0	1	2.3	6	9.5	7	12.5	0	0.0	2	3.4	7	10.0	1	1.3
	>50%	0	0.0	1	1.4	3	7.0	10	15.9	10	17.9	1	1.8	6	10.3	1	1.4	1	1.3
Missing	Not Supplied	0	—	0	—	0	—	0	—	0	—	0	—	0	—	0	—	0	—
Available		61	100.0	72	100.0	43	100.0	63	100.0	56	100.0	55	100.0	58	100.0	70	100.0	77	100.0
Missing		0	0.0	0	0.0	0	0.0	0	0.0	0	0.0	0	0.0	0	0.0	0	0.0	0	0.0
Total		61	100.0	72	100.0	43	100.0	63	100.0	56	100.0	55	100.0	58	100.0	70	100.0	77	100.0

TABLE B.14 Living Arrangements—Homeless: Entire Period Alive Cohort—by Center

		Chandigarh Urban		*Chandigarh Rural*		*Dublin*		*Honolulu*		*Moscow*		*Nagasaki*		*Nottingham*		*Prague DOSMeD*		*Rochester*	
		N	%	N	%	N	%	N	%	N	%	N	%	N	%	N	%	N	%
Available	% Time Homeless or Vagrant																		
	. Never	73	91.3	34	89.5	32	88.9	16	64.0	52	100.0	56	98.2	84	97.7	76	96.2	32	97.0
	≤ 5%	7	8.8	4	10.5	4	11.1	4	16.0	0	0.0	1	1.8	0	0.0	1	1.3	1	3.0
	6–10%	0	0.0	0	0.0	0	0.0	0	0.0	0	0.0	0	0.0	2	2.3	1	1.3	0	0.0
	11–25%	0	0.0	0	0.0	0	0.0	4	16.0	0	0.0	0	0.0	0	0.0	1	1.3	0	0.0
	26–50%	0	0.0	0	0.0	0	0.0	1	4.0	0	0.0	0	0.0	0	0.0	0	0.0	0	0.0
	>50%	0	0.0	0	0.0	0	0.0	0	0.0	0	0.0	0	0.0	0	0.0	0	0.0	0	0.0
Missing	Not Supplied	0	—	0	—	1	100.0	1	100.0	0	—	0	—	0	—	0	—	0	—
Available		80	100.0	38	100.0	36	97.3	25	96.2	52	100.0	57	100.0	86	100.0	79	100.0	33	100.0
Missing		0	0.0	0	0.0	1	2.7	1	3.8	0	0.0	0	0.0	0	0.0	0	0.0	0	0.0
Total		80	100.0	38	100.0	37	100.0	26	100.0	52	100.0	57	100.0	86	100.0	79	100.0	33	100.0

		Agra		*Cali*		*Prague IPSS*		*Groningen*		*Mannheim*		*Sofia*		*Beijing*		*Hong Kong*		*Chennai (Madras)*	
		N	%	N	%	N	%	N	%	N	%	N	%	N	%	N	%	N	%
Available	% Time Homeless or Vagrant																		
	. Never	60	98.4	72	100.0	43	100.0	60	95.2	52	92.9	55	100.0	57	98.3	69	98.6	77	100.0
	≤ 5%	0	0.0	0	0.0	0	0.0	2	3.2	0	0.0	0	0.0	0	0.0	1	1.4	0	0.0
	6–10%	0	0.0	0	0.0	0	0.0	0	0.0	0	0.0	0	0.0	1	1.7	0	0.0	0	0.0
	11–25%	0	0.0	0	0.0	0	0.0	1	1.6	3	5.4	0	0.0	0	0.0	0	0.0	0	0.0
	26–50%	0	0.0	0	0.0	0	0.0	0	0.0	0	0.0	0	0.0	0	0.0	0	0.0	0	0.0
	>50%	1	1.6	0	0.0	0	0.0	0	0.0	1	1.8	0	0.0	0	0.0	0	0.0	0	0.0
Missing	Not Supplied	0	—	0	—	0	—	0	—	0	—	0	—	0	—	0	—	0	—
Available		61	100.0	72	100.0	43	100.0	63	100.0	56	100.0	55	100.0	58	100.0	70	100.0	77	100.0
Missing		0	0.0	0	0.0	0	0.0	0	0.0	0	0.0	0	0.0	0	0.0	0	0.0	0	0.0
Total		61	100.0	72	100.0	43	100.0	63	100.0	56	100.0	55	100.0	58	100.0	70	100.0	77	100.0

TABLE B.15 Living Arrangements—Jail: Entire Period Alive Cohort—by Center

		Chandigarh Urban		*Chandigarh Rural*		*Dublin*		*Honolulu*		*Moscow*		*Nagasaki*		*Nottingham*		*Prague DOSMeD*		*Rochester*	
		N	%	N	%	N	%	N	%	N	%	N	%	N	%	N	%	N	%
Available	% Time in Jail or Prison																		
	. Never	77	96.3	38	100.0	33	91.7	20	80.0	52	100.0	55	96.5	83	96.5	78	98.7	32	97.0
	≤ 5%	2	2.5	0	0.0	2	5.6	2	8.0	0	0.0	2	3.5	2	2.3	0	0.0	0	0.0
	6–10%	1	1.2	0	0.0	0	0.0	0	0.0	0	0.0	0	0.0	0	0.0	0	0.0	0	0.0
	11–25%	0	0.0	0	0.0	1	2.8	2	8.0	0	0.0	0	0.0	1	1.2	0	0.0	1	3.0
	26–50%	0	0.0	0	0.0	0	0.0	1	4.0	0	0.0	0	0.0	0	0.0	0	0.0	0	0.0
	>50%	0	0.0	0	0.0	0	0.0	0	0.0	0	0.0	0	0.0	0	0.0	1	1.3	0	0.0
Missing	Not Supplied	0	—	0	—	1	100.0	1	100.0	0	—	0	—	0	—	0	—	0	—
Available		80	100.0	38	100.0	36	97.3	25	96.2	52	100.0	57	100.0	86	100.0	79	100.0	33	100.0
Missing		0	0.0	0	0.0	1	2.7	1	3.8	0	0.0	0	0.0	0	0.0	0	0.0	0	0.0
Total		80	100.0	38	100.0	37	100.0	26	100.0	52	100.0	57	100.0	86	100.0	79	100.0	33	100.0

		Agra		*Cali*		*Prague IPSS*		*Groningen*		*Mannheim*		*Sofia*		*Beijing*		*Hong Kong*		*Chennai (Madras)*	
		N	%	N	%	N	%	N	%	N	%	N	%	N	%	N	%	N	%
Available	% Time in Jail or Prison																		
	. Never	61	100.0	72	100.0	43	100.0	61	96.8	55	98.2	55	100.0	57	98.3	70	100.0	77	100.0
	≤ 5%	0	0.0	0	0.0	0	0.0	1	1.6	0	0.0	0	0.0	1	1.7	0	0.0	0	0.0
	6–10%	0	0.0	0	0.0	0	0.0	1	1.6	1	1.8	0	0.0	0	0.0	0	0.0	0	0.0
	11–25%	0	0.0	0	0.0	0	0.0	0	0.0	0	0.0	0	0.0	0	0.0	0	0.0	0	0.0
	26–50%	0	0.0	0	0.0	0	0.0	0	0.0	0	0.0	0	0.0	0	0.0	0	0.0	0	0.0
	>50%	0	0.0	0	0.0	0	0.0	0	0.0	0	0.0	0	0.0	0	0.0	0	0.0	0	0.0
Missing	Not Supplied	0	—	0	—	0	—	0	—	0	—	0	—	0	—	0	—	0	—
Available		61	100.0	72	100.0	43	100.0	63	100.0	56	100.0	55	100.0	58	100.0	70	100.0	77	100.0
Missing		0	0.0	0	0.0	0	0.0	0	0.0	0	0.0	0	0.0	0	0.0	0	0.0	0	0.0
Total		61	100.0	72	100.0	43	100.0	63	100.0	56	100.0	55	100.0	58	100.0	70	100.0	77	100.0

TABLE B.16 Disability Assessment Scale—Global Evaluation: Past Month Alive Cohort—by Center

		Chandigarh Urban		*Chandigarh Rural*		*Dublin*		*Honolulu*		*Moscow*		*Nagasaki*		*Nottingham*		*Prague DOSMeD*		*Rochester*	
		N	%	N	%	N	%	N	%	N	%	N	%	N	%	N	%	N	%
Available	Global Evaluation																		
	0: Excellent	12	17.6	6	19.4	0	0.0	6	23.1	2	3.8	6	10.7	12	14.0	0	0.0	4	17.4
	1: Good	31	45.6	16	51.6	6	28.6	6	23.1	8	15.4	8	14.3	21	24.4	5	27.8	5	21.7
	2: Fair	18	26.5	6	19.4	6	28.6	9	34.6	23	44.2	9	16.1	22	25.6	6	33.3	7	30.4
	3: Poor	6	8.8	1	3.2	5	23.8	3	11.5	17	32.7	19	33.9	18	20.9	7	38.9	2	8.7
	4: Very Poor	0	0.0	1	3.2	3	14.3	1	3.8	2	3.8	12	21.4	8	9.3	0	0.0	3	13.0
	5: Severe	1	1.5	1	3.2	1	4.8	1	3.8	0	0.0	2	3.6	5	5.8	0	0.0	2	8.7
Missing	. : Not Supplied	11	91.7	6	85.7	12	75.0	0	—	0	—	1	100.0	0	—	16	26.2	9	90.0
	9: No Rating	1	8.3	1	14.3	4	25.0	0	—	0	—	0	0.0	0	—	45	73.8	1	10.0
Available		68	85.0	31	81.6	21	56.8	26	100.0	52	100.0	56	98.2	86	100.0	18	22.8	23	69.7
Missing		12	15.0	7	18.4	16	43.2	0	0.0	0	0.0	1	1.8	0	0.0	61	77.2	10	30.3
Total		80	100.0	38	100.0	37	100.0	26	100.0	52	100.0	57	100.0	86	100.0	79	100.0	33	100.0

		Agra		*Cali*		*Prague IPSS*		*Groningen*		*Mannheim*		*Sofia*		*Beijing*		*Hong Kong*		*Chennai (Madras)*	
		N	%	N	%	N	%	N	%	N	%	N	%	N	%	N	%	N	%
Available	Global Evaluation																		
	0: Excellent	19	31.7	6	9.0	2	11.8	8	12.9	9	16.1	5	9.1	1	8.3	18	56.3	26	34.7
	1: Good	17	28.3	29	43.3	3	17.6	9	14.5	8	14.3	12	21.8	2	16.7	2	6.3	9	12.0
	2: Fair	12	20.0	25	37.3	7	41.2	20	32.3	12	21.4	10	18.2	1	8.3	7	21.9	13	17.3
	3: Poor	7	11.7	6	9.0	4	23.5	12	19.4	14	25.0	15	27.3	3	25.0	2	6.3	15	20.0
	4: Very Poor	2	3.3	1	1.5	0	0.0	10	16.1	13	23.2	12	21.8	4	33.3	3	9.4	9	12.0
	5: Severe	3	5.0	0	0.0	1	5.9	3	4.8	0	0.0	1	1.8	1	8.3	0	0.0	3	4.0
Missing	. : Not Supplied	0	0.0	4	80.0	3	11.5	1	100.0	0	—	0	—	46	100.0	38	100.0	2	100.0
	9: No Rating	1	100.0	1	20.0	23	88.5	0	0.0	0	—	0	—	0	0.0	0	0.0	0	0.0
Available		60	98.4	67	93.1	17	39.5	62	98.4	56	100.0	55	100.0	12	20.7	32	45.7	75	97.4
Missing		1	1.6	5	6.9	26	60.5	1	1.6	0	0.0	0	0.0	46	79.3	38	54.3	2	2.6
Total		61	100.0	72	100.0	43	100.0	63	100.0	56	100.0	55	100.0	58	100.0	70	100.0	77	100.0

TABLE B.17A Global Assessment of Functioning (GAF) Scale—Disability: Past Month Alive Cohort—by Center

		Chandigarh Urban		*Chandigarh Rural*		*Dublin*		*Honolulu*		*Moscow*		*Nagasaki*		*Nottingham*		*Prague DOSMeD*		*Rochester*	
		N	%	N	%	N	%	N	%	N	%	N	%	N	%	N	%	N	%
Available	GAF Scale: Disability																		
	1–10	1	1.2	0	0.0	0	0.0	0	0.0	0	0.0	0	0.0	0	0.0	0	0.0	0	0.0
	11–20	0	0.0	0	0.0	0	0.0	0	0.0	0	0.0	1	1.8	2	2.3	1	1.3	0	0.0
	21–30	3	3.8	0	0.0	1	2.9	1	3.8	1	1.9	4	7.0	2	2.3	3	4.0	2	6.7
	31–40	5	6.3	2	5.4	2	5.7	1	3.8	4	7.7	10	17.5	11	12.8	10	13.3	9	30.0
	41–50	2	2.5	0	0.0	8	22.9	4	15.4	4	7.7	13	22.8	17	19.8	15	20.0	5	16.7
	51–60	11	13.8	5	13.5	8	22.9	7	26.9	8	15.4	6	10.5	7	8.1	11	14.7	3	10.0
	61–70	11	13.8	5	13.5	6	17.1	4	15.4	11	21.2	5	8.8	7	8.1	5	6.7	0	0.0
	71–80	11	13.8	9	24.3	5	14.3	3	11.5	11	21.2	6	10.5	12	14.0	12	16.0	4	13.3
	81–90	36	45.0	16	43.2	5	14.3	6	23.1	13	25.0	12	21.1	28	32.6	18	24.0	7	23.3
Missing	. : Not Supplied	0	—	0	0.0	0	0.0	0	—	0	—	0	—	0	—	0	0.0	0	0.0
	99: Unknown	0	—	1	100.0	2	100.0	0	—	0	—	0	—	0	—	4	100.0	3	100.0
Available		80	100.0	37	97.4	35	94.6	26	100.0	52	100.0	57	100.0	86	100.0	75	94.9	30	90.9
Missing		0	0.0	1	2.6	2	5.4	0	0.0	0	0.0	0	0.0	0	0.0	4	5.1	3	9.1
Total		80	100.0	38	100.0	37	100.0	26	100.0	52	100.0	57	100.0	86	100.0	79	100.0	33	100.0

		Agra		Cali		Prague IPSS		Groningen		Mannheim		Sofia		Beijing		Hong Kong		Chennai (Madras)	
		N	%	N	%	N	%	N	%	N	%	N	%	N	%	N	%	N	%
Available	GAF Scale: Disability																		
	1–10	1	1.6	0	0.0	0	0.0	0	0.0	0	—	0	0.0	0	0.0	0	0.0	3	3.9
	11–20	0	0.0	0	0.0	0	0.0	0	0.0	0	—	0	0.0	0	0.0	1	1.4	2	2.6
	21–30	5	8.2	3	4.2	1	2.6	6	9.5	0	—	5	9.1	6	10.3	3	4.3	6	7.8
	31–40	3	4.9	5	7.0	2	5.1	12	19.0	0	—	15	27.3	9	15.5	9	12.9	4	5.2
	41–50	2	3.3	7	9.9	2	5.1	15	23.8	0	—	13	23.6	8	13.8	9	12.9	7	9.1
	51–60	2	3.3	12	16.9	4	10.3	6	9.5	0	—	4	7.3	7	12.1	4	5.7	7	9.1
	61–70	3	4.9	18	25.4	3	7.7	3	4.8	0	—	6	10.9	3	5.2	10	14.3	9	11.7
	71–80	8	13.1	13	18.3	8	20.5	7	11.1	0	—	6	10.9	6	10.3	24	34.3	9	11.7
	81–90	37	60.7	13	18.3	19	48.7	14	22.2	0	—	6	10.9	19	32.8	10	14.3	30	39.0
Missing	. : Not Supplied	0	—	0	0.0	0	0.0	0	—	56	100.0	0	—	0	—	0	—	0	—
	99: Unknown	0	—	1	100.0	4	100.0	0	—	0	0.0	0	—	0	—	0	—	0	—
Available		61	100.0	71	98.6	39	90.7	63	100.0	0	0.0	55	100.0	58	100.0	70	100.0	77	100.0
Missing		0	0.0	1	1.4	4	9.3	0	0.0	56	100.0	0	0.0	0	0.0	0	0.0	0	0.0
Total		61	100.0	72	100.0	43	100.0	63	100.0	56	100.0	55	100.0	58	100.0	70	100.0	77	100.0

TABLE B.17B (GAF) Scale—Disability: Past Month Alive Cohort—by Center

		Chandigarh Urban	*Chandigarh Rural*	*Dublin*	*Honolulu*	*Moscow*	*Nagasaki*	*Nottingham*	*Prague DOSMeD*	*Rochester*
Total	N	80	37	35	26	52	57	86	75	30
	Mean	70.83	77.38	61.31	63.85	69.13	56.26	63.28	60.87	55.17
	STD	19.81	14.58	17.28	15.97	16.42	21.18	20.44	20.90	22.23
		Agra	*Cali*	*Prague IPSS*	*Groningen*	*Mannheim*	*Sofia*	*Beijing*	*Hong Kong*	*Chennai (Madras)*
Total	N	61	71	39	63	0	55	58	70	77
	Mean	74.56	65.58	74.54	56.29	—	51.51	60.60	62.84	63.12
	STD	23.06	16.05	17.43	22.11	—	18.42	22.54	18.42	24.42

TABLE B.18 Trend of Disability: Entire Period Alive Cohort—by Center

		Chandigarh Urban		*Chandigarh Rural*		*Dublin*		*Honolulu*		*Moscow*		*Nagasaki*		*Nottingham*		*Prague DOSMeD*		*Rochester*	
		N	%	N	%	N	%	N	%	N	%	N	%	N	%	N	%	N	%
Available	Trend of Disability																		
	XXX	22	27.5	12	31.6	0	0.0	1	3.8	32	61.5	1	1.8	9	10.5	4	5.2	1	3.0
	XX1[a]	4	5.0	0	0.0	4	11.4	7	26.9	2	3.8	4	7.0	11	12.8	22	28.6	1	3.0
	X1X	0	0.0	2	5.3	2	5.7	5	19.2	1	1.9	1	1.8	3	3.5	8	10.4	5	15.2
	X11	0	0.0	0	0.0	0	0.0	3	11.5	4	7.7	8	14.0	5	5.8	7	9.1	0	0.0
	1XX	46	57.5	22	57.9	12	34.3	9	34.6	9	17.3	22	38.6	34	39.5	33	42.9	16	48.5
	1X1	2	2.5	2	5.3	1	2.9	0	0.0	0	0.0	4	7.0	1	1.2	0	0.0	1	3.0
	11X	0	0.0	0	0.0	6	17.1	1	3.8	1	1.9	5	8.8	2	2.3	2	2.6	1	3.0
	111	6	7.5	0	0.0	10	28.6	0	0.0	3	5.8	12	21.1	21	24.4	1	1.3	8	24.2
Missing	MMM	0	—	0	—	2	100.0	0	—	0	—	0	—	0	—	2	100.0	0	—
Available		80	100.0	38	100.0	35	94.6	26	100.0	52	100.0	57	100.0	86	100.0	77	97.5	33	100.0
Missing		0	0.0	0	0.0	2	5.4	0	0.0	0	0.0	0	0.0	0	0.0	2	2.5	0	0.0
Total		80	100.0	38	100.0	37	100.0	26	100.0	52	100.0	57	100.0	86	100.0	79	100.0	33	100.0

		Agra		*Cali*		*Prague IPSS*		*Groningen*		*Mannheim*		*Sofia*		*Beijing*		*Hong Kong*		*Chennai (Madras)*	
		N	%	N	%	N	%	N	%	N	%	N	%	N	%	N	%	N	%
Available	Trend of Disability																		
	XXX	2	4.8	18	25.0	1	2.4	9	14.3	0	—	0	0.0	11	19.0	6	8.6	0	0.0
	XX1	5	11.9	12	16.7	5	11.9	3	4.8	0	—	20	36.4	6	10.3	10	14.3	1	1.3
	X1X	4	9.5	3	4.2	2	4.8	4	6.3	0	—	1	1.8	1	1.7	8	11.4	0	0.0
	X11	0	0.0	4	5.6	1	2.4	7	11.1	0	—	3	5.5	3	5.2	5	7.1	1	1.3
	1XX	22	52.4	31	43.1	28	66.7	18	28.6	0	—	18	32.7	30	51.7	30	42.9	67	87.0
	1X1	1	2.4	2	2.8	0	0.0	2	3.2	0	—	2	3.6	3	5.2	1	1.4	6	7.8
	11X	2	4.8	0	0.0	2	4.8	1	1.6	0	—	2	3.6	0	0.0	4	5.7	1	1.3
	111	6	14.3	2	2.8	3	7.1	19	30.2	0	—	9	16.4	4	6.9	6	8.6	1	1.3
Missing	MMM	19	100.0	0	—	1	100.0	0	—	56	100.0	0	—	0	—	0	—	0	—
Available		42	68.9	72	100.0	42	97.7	63	100.0	0	0.0	55	100.0	58	100.0	70	100.0	77	100.0
Missing		19	31.1	0	0.0	1	2.3	0	0.0	56	100.0	0	0.0	0	0.0	0	0.0	0	0.0
Total		61	100.0	72	100.0	43	100.0	63	100.0	56	100.0	55	100.0	58	100.0	70	100.0	77	100.0

[a] The number "1" designates that third of the entire period when variable was most prominent (where the leftmost position represents the earliest third). Where it appears in more than one time slot, the variable was considered to be equally prominent in the designated periods.

TABLE B.19A Paid Employment: Past 2 Years Alive Cohort—by Center

		Chandigarh Urban		*Chandigarh Rural*		*Dublin*		*Honolulu*		*Moscow*		*Nagasaki*		*Nottingham*		*Prague DOSMeD*		*Rochester*	
		N	%	N	%	N	%	N	%	N	%	N	%	N	%	N	%	N	%
Available	Months Employed Full-Time																		
	. Inst.	0	0.0	0	0.0	0	0.0	0	0.0	0	0.0	1	1.8	0	0.0	0	0.0	0	0.0
	. Never	29	36.3	21	55.3	24	64.9	12	46.2	19	36.5	33	57.9	47	54.7	34	43.6	19	59.4
	[a] Part-time Only	1	1.2	1	2.6	5	13.5	5	19.2	2	3.8	4	7.0	7	8.1	12	15.4	3	9.4
	≤ 12 Months	2	2.5	1	2.6	3	8.1	3	11.5	0	0.0	4	7.0	3	3.5	4	5.1	1	3.1
	13–23 Months	3	3.8	1	2.6	0	0.0	0	0.0	10	19.2	3	5.3	4	4.7	5	6.4	0	0.0
	24 Months	43	53.8	14	36.8	5	13.5	6	23.1	20	38.5	12	21.1	25	29.1	21	26.9	8	25.0
	Unknown Months	2	2.5	0	0.0	0	0.0	0	0.0	1	1.9	0	0.0	0	0.0	2	2.6	1	3.1
Missing	Unknown	0	—	0	—	0	—	0	—	0	—	0	—	0	—	1	100.0	1	100.0
Available		80	100.0	38	100.0	37	100.0	26	100.0	52	100.0	57	100.0	86	100.0	78	98.7	32	97.0
Missing		0	0.0	0	0.0	0	0.0	0	0.0	0	0.0	0	0.0	0	0.0	1	1.3	1	3.3
Total		80	100.0	38	100.0	37	100.0	26	100.0	52	100.0	57	100.0	86	100.0	79	100.0	33	100.0

		Agra		*Cali*		*Prague IPSS*		*Groningen*		*Mannheim*		*Sofia*		*Beijing*		*Hong Kong*		*Chennai (Madras)*	
		N	%	N	%	N	%	N	%	N	%	N	%	N	%	N	%	N	%
Available	Months Employed Full-Time																		
	. Inst.	0	0.0	0	0.0	0	0.0	0	0.0	4	7.1	0	0.0	3	5.2	0	0.0	1	1.3
	. Never	34	55.7	23	31.9	21	48.8	44	69.8	25	44.6	29	54.7	39	67.2	31	44.3	40	51.9
	[a] Part-time Only	1	1.6	11	15.3	7	16.3	5	7.9	3	5.4	9	17.0	2	3.4	4	5.7	3	3.9
	≤ 12 Months	0	0.0	7	9.7	2	4.7	1	1.6	5	8.9	2	3.8	3	5.2	9	12.9	3	3.9
	13–23 Months	1	1.6	2	2.8	1	2.3	2	3.2	2	3.6	3	5.7	1	1.7	7	10.0	1	1.3
	24 Months	25	41.0	29	40.3	12	27.9	11	17.5	16	28.6	10	18.9	10	17.2	19	27.1	29	37.7
	Unknown Months	0	0.0	0	0.0	0	0.0	0	0.0	1	1.8	0	0.0	0	0.0	0	0.0	0	0.0
Missing	Unknown	0	—	0	—	0	—	0	—	0	—	2	100.0	0	—	0	—	0	—
Available		61	100.0	72	100.0	43	100.0	63	100.0	56	100.0	53	96.4	58	100.0	70	100.0	77	100.0
Missing		0	0.0	0	0.0	0	0.0	0	0.0	0	0.0	2	3.6	0	0.0	0	0.0	0	0.0
Total		61	100.0	72	100.0	43	100.0	63	100.0	56	100.0	55	100.0	58	100.0	70	100.0	77	100.0

[a] The number "1" designates that third of the entire period when variable was most prominent (where the leftmost position represents the earliest third). Where it appears in more than one time slot, the variable was considered to be equally prominent in the designated periods.

TABLE B.19B Work Performance (if employed full-time for at least 12 months): Past 2 Years Alive Cohort—by Center

		Chandigarh Urban		*Chandigarh Rural*		*Dublin*		*Honolulu*		*Moscow*		*Nagasaki*		*Nottingham*		*Prague DOSMeD*		*Rochester*	
		N	%	N	%	N	%	N	%	N	%	N	%	N	%	N	%	N	%
Available	Work Performance																		
	1, 2: Good-Very Good	41	89.1	10	66.7	4	80.0	6	100.0	28	93.3	10	76.9	27	100.0	21	87.5	8	100.0
	3, 4: Poor-Very Poor	5	10.9	5	33.3	1	20.0	0	0.0	2	6.7	3	23.1	0	0.0	3	12.5	0	0.0
Missing	. : Not Supplied	0	—	0	—	0	—	0	—	0	—	1	50.0	0	0.0	0	0.0	0	—
	8: Not Applic.	0	—	0	—	0	—	0	—	0	—	0	0.0	0	0.0	0	0.0	0	—
	9: Unknown	0	—	0	—	0	—	0	—	0	—	1	50.0	2	100.0	2	100.0	0	—
Available		46	100.0	15	100.0	5	100.0	6	100.0	30	100.0	13	86.7	27	93.1	24	92.3	8	100.0
Missing		0	0.0	0	0.0	0	0.0	0	0.0	0	0.0	2	13.3	2	6.9	2	7.7	0	0.0
Total		46	100.0	15	100.0	5	100.0	6	100.0	30	100.0	15	100.0	29	100.0	26	100.0	8	100.0

		Agra		*Cali*		*Prague IPSS*		*Groningen*		*Mannheim*		*Sofia*		*Beijing*		*Hong Kong*		*Chennai (Madras)*	
		N	%	N	%	N	%	N	%	N	%	N	%	N	%	N	%	N	%
Available	Work Performance																		
	1,2: Good-Very Good	21	84.0	27	90.0	13	100.0	12	92.3	10	90.9	10	90.9	11	100.0	23	88.5	26	86.7
	3,4: Poor-Very Poor	4	16.0	3	10.0	0	0.0	1	7.7	1	9.1	1	9.1	0	0.0	3	11.5	4	13.3
Missing	. : Not Supplied	1	100.0	0	0.0	0	—	0	—	0	0.0	2	100.0	0	—	0	—	0	—
	8: Not Applic.	0	0.0	1	100.0	0	—	0	—	0	0.0	0	0.0	0	—	0	—	0	—
	9: Unknown	0	0.0	0	0.0	0	—	0	—	7	100.0	0	0.0	0	—	0	—	0	—
Available		25	96.2	30	96.8	13	100.0	13	100.0	11	61.1	11	84.6	11	100.0	26	100.0	30	100.0
Missing		1	3.8	1	3.2	0	0.0	0	0.0	7	38.9	2	15.4	0	0.0	0	0.0	0	0.0
Total		26	100.0	31	100.0	13	100.0	13	100.0	18	100.0	13	100.0	11	100.0	26	100.0	30	100.0

TABLE B.20A Household Work: Past 2 Years Alive Cohort—by Center

		Chandigarh Urban		Chandigarh Rural		Dublin		Honolulu		Moscow		Nagasaki		Nottingham		Prague DOSMeD		Rochester	
		N	%	N	%	N	%	N	%	N	%	N	%	N	%	N	%	N	%
Available	Months Full-Time Housework																		
	. Inst.	0	0.0	0	0.0	0	0.0	0	0.0	0	0.0	1	1.8	0	0.0	0	0.0	0	0.0
	. Never	58	72.5	16	42.1	28	75.7	21	80.8	50	96.2	43	75.4	68	79.1	52	66.7	26	81.3
	≤12 Months	0	0.0	0	0.0	0	0.0	1	3.8	0	0.0	3	5.3	2	2.3	6	7.7	1	3.1
	13–23 Months	0	0.0	0	0.0	3	8.1	1	3.8	0	0.0	3	5.3	3	3.5	5	6.4	0	0.0
	24 Months	22	27.5	22	57.9	6	16.2	3	11.5	2	3.8	7	12.3	13	15.1	14	17.9	5	15.6
	Unknown Months	0	0.0	0	0.0	0	0.0	0	0.0	0	0.0	0	0.0	0	0.0	1	1.3	0	0.0
Missing	Unknown	0	—	0	—	0	—	0	—	0	—	0	—	0	—	1	100.0	1	100.0
Available		80	100.0	38	100.0	37	100.0	26	100.0	52	100.0	57	100.0	86	100.0	78	98.7	32	97.0
Missing		0	0.0	0	0.0	0	0.0	0	0.0	0	0.0	0	0.0	0	0.0	1	1.3	1	3.0
Total		80	100.0	38	100.0	37	100.0	26	100.0	52	100.0	57	100.0	86	100.0	79	100.0	33	100.0

		Agra		Cali		Prague IPSS		Groningen		Mannheim		Sofia		Beijing		Hong Kong		Chennai (Madras)	
		N	%	N	%	N	%	N	%	N	%	N	%	N	%	N	%	N	%
Available	Months Full-Time Housework																		
	. Inst.	0	0.0	0	0.0	0	0.0	0	0.0	4	7.1	0	0.0	3	5.2	0	0.0	1	1.3
	. Never	39	63.9	54	75.0	25	58.1	49	77.8	50	89.3	47	87.0	35	60.3	54	77.1	47	61.0
	≤12 Months	1	1.6	3	4.2	2	4.7	1	1.6	1	1.8	1	1.9	1	1.7	1	1.4	0	0.0
	13–23 Months	0	0.0	2	2.8	0	0.0	0	0.0	0	0.0	1	1.9	0	0.0	4	5.7	1	1.3
	24 Months	21	34.4	13	18.1	16	37.2	12	19.0	1	1.8	5	9.3	18	31.0	11	15.7	28	36.4
	Unknown Months	0	0.0	0	0.0	0	0.0	1	1.6	0	0.0	0	0.0	1	1.7	0	0.0	0	0.0
Missing	Unknown	0	—	0	—	0	—	0	—	0	—	1	100.0	0	—	0	—	0	—
Available		61	100.0	72	100.0	43	100.0	63	100.0	56	100.0	54	98.2	58	100.0	70	100.0	77	100.0
Missing		0	0.0	0	0.0	0	0.0	0	0.0	0	0.0	1	1.8	0	0.0	0	0.0	0	0.0
Total		61	100.0	72	100.0	43	100.0	63	100.0	56	100.0	55	100.0	58	100.0	70	100.0	77	100.0

TABLE B.20B Household Work Performance (if full-time for at least 12 months): Past 2 Years Alive Cohort—by Center

		Chandigarh Urban		*Chandigarh Rural*		*Dublin*		*Honolulu*		*Moscow*		*Nagasaki*		*Nottingham*		*Prague DOSMeD*		*Rochester*	
		N	%	N	%	N	%	N	%	N	%	N	%	N	%	N	%	N	%
Available	Housework Performance																		
	1, 2: Good–Very Good	19	86.4	22	100.0	7	77.8	2	50.0	2	100.0	5	55.6	16	100.0	15	88.2	5	100.0
	3, 4: Poor–Very Poor	3	13.6	0	0.0	2	22.2	2	50.0	0	0.0	4	44.4	0	0.0	2	11.8	0	0.0
Missing	.: Not Supplied	0	—	0	—	0	—	0	—	0	—	0	0.0	0	—	1	50.0	0	—
	8: Not Applic.	0	—	0	—	0	—	0	—	0	—	0	0.0	0	—	0	0.0	0	—
	9: Unknown	0	—	0	—	0	—	0	—	0	—	1	100.0	0	—	1	50.0	0	—
Available		22	100.0	22	100.0	9	100.0	4	100.0	2	100.0	9	90.0	16	100.0	17	89.5	5	100.0
Missing		0	0.0	0	0.0	0	0.0	0	0.0	0	0.0	1	10.0	0	0.0	2	10.5	0	0.0
Total		22	100.0	22	100.0	9	100.0	4	100.0	2	100.0	10	100.0	16	100.0	19	100.0	5	100.0

		Agra		*Cali*		*Prague IPSS*		*Groningen*		*Mannheim*		*Sofia*		*Beijing*		*Hong Kong*		*Chennai (Madras)*	
		N	%	N	%	N	%	N	%	N	%	N	%	N	%	N	%	N	%
Available	Housework Performance																		
	1, 2: Good–Very Good	19	90.5	11	78.6	13	92.9	11	91.7	0	—	4	66.7	14	77.8	11	73.3	16	57.1
	3, 4: Poor–Very Poor	2	9.5	3	21.4	1	7.1	1	8.3	0	—	2	33.3	4	22.2	4	26.7	12	42.9
Missing	.: Not Supplied	0	—	0	0.0	1	50.0	0	—	0	0.0	0	—	0	—	0	—	0	0.0
	8: Not Applic.	0	—	1	100.0	0	0.0	0	—	0	0.0	0	—	0	—	0	—	1	100.0
	9: Unknown	0	—	0	0.0	1	50.0	0	—	1	100.0	0	—	0	—	0	—	0	0.0
Available		21	100.0	14	93.3	14	87.5	12	100.0	0	0.0	6	100.0	18	100.0	15	100.0	28	96.6
Missing		0	0.0	1	6.7	2	12.5	0	0.0	1	100.0	0	0.0	0	0.0	0	0.0	1	3.4
Total		21	100.0	15	100.0	16	100.0	12	100.0	1	100.0	6	100.0	18	100.0	15	100.0	29	100.0

TABLE B.21 Retired: Past 2 Years Alive Cohort—by Center

		Chandigarh Urban		*Chandigarh Rural*		*Dublin*		*Honolulu*		*Moscow*		*Nagasaki*		*Nottingham*		*Prague DOSMeD*		*Rochester*	
		N	%	N	%	N	%	N	%	N	%	N	%	N	%	N	%	N	%
Available	Months Retired																		
	. Inst.	0	0.0	0	0.0	0	0.0	0	0.0	0	0.0	1	1.8	0	0.0	0	0.0	0	0.0
	. Never	78	97.5	38	100.0	36	97.3	26	100.0	33	63.5	56	98.2	84	97.7	75	96.2	31	96.9
	≤ 12 Months	0	0.0	0	0.0	0	0.0	0	0.0	3	5.8	0	0.0	0	0.0	0	0.0	0	0.0
	13–23 Months	0	0.0	0	0.0	0	0.0	0	0.0	0	0.0	0	0.0	0	0.0	0	0.0	0	0.0
	24 Months	2	2.5	0	0.0	1	2.7	0	0.0	16	30.8	0	0.0	2	2.3	3	3.8	1	3.1
Missing	Unknown	0	—	0	—	0	—	0	—	0	—	0	—	0	—	1	100.0	1	100.0
Available		80	100.0	38	100.0	37	100.0	26	100.0	52	100.0	57	100.0	86	100.0	78	98.7	32	97.0
Missing		0	0.0	0	0.0	0	0.0	0	0.0	0	0.0	0	0.0	0	0.0	1	1.3	1	3.0
Total		80	100.0	38	100.0	37	100.0	26	100.0	52	100.0	57	100.0	86	100.0	79	100.0	33	100.0

		Agra		*Cali*		*Prague IPSS*		*Groningen*		*Mannheim*		*Sofia*		*Beijing*		*Hong Kong*		*Chennai (Madras)*	
		N	%	N	%	N	%	N	%	N	%	N	%	N	%	N	%	N	%
Available	Months Retired																		
	. Inst.	0	0.0	0	0.0	0	0.0	0	0.0	4	7.1	0	0.0	3	5.2	0	0.0	1	1.3
	. Never	56	91.8	70	97.2	33	76.7	63	100.0	37	66.1	48	90.6	31	53.4	67	95.7	76	98.7
	≤ 12 Months	2	3.3	1	1.4	0	0.0	0	0.0	1	1.8	0	0.0	2	3.4	0	0.0	0	0.0
	13–23 Months	0	0.0	0	0.0	0	0.0	0	0.0	0	0.0	0	0.0	1	1.7	1	1.4	0	0.0
	24 Months	3	4.9	1	1.4	10	23.3	0	0.0	14	25.0	5	9.4	21	36.2	2	2.9	0	0.0
Missing	Unknown	0	—	0	—	0	—	0	—	0	—	2	100.0	0	—	0	—	0	—
Available		61	100.0	72	100.0	43	100.0	63	100.0	56	100.0	53	96.4	58	100.0	70	100.0	77	100.0
Missing		0	0.0	0	0.0	0	0.0	0	0.0	0	0.0	2	3.6	0	0.0	0	0.0	0	0.0
Total		61	100.0	72	100.0	43	100.0	63	100.0	56	100.0	55	100.0	58	100.0	70	100.0	77	100.0

TABLE B.22 Disability Benefits, Psychiatric: Past 2 Years Alive Cohort—by Center

		Chandigarh Urban		*Chandigarh Rural*		*Dublin*		*Honolulu*		*Moscow*		*Nagasaki*		*Nottingham*		*Prague DOSMeD*		*Rochester*	
		N	%	N	%	N	%	N	%	N	%	N	%	N	%	N	%	N	%
Available	Months Received Dis. for Mental Cond.																		
	. Inst.	0	0.0	0	0.0	0	0.0	0	0.0	0	0.0	1	1.8	0	0.0	0	0.0	0	0.0
	. Never	79	98.8	37	97.4	18	48.6	12	46.2	42	80.8	44	77.2	50	58.1	31	39.7	18	58.1
	* Other Disability	1	1.2	1	2.6	0	0.0	2	7.7	2	3.8	0	0.0	4	4.7	0	0.0	1	3.2
	≤ 12 Months	0	0.0	0	0.0	0	0.0	1	3.8	0	0.0	3	5.3	0	0.0	2	2.6	0	0.0
	13–23 Months	0	0.0	0	0.0	0	0.0	0	0.0	0	0.0	1	1.8	1	1.2	2	2.6	0	0.0
	24 Months	0	0.0	0	0.0	19	51.4	11	42.3	8	15.4	8	14.0	31	36.0	43	55.1	12	38.7
Missing	Unknown	0	—	0	—	0	—	0	—	0	—	0	—	0	—	1	100.0	2	100.0
Available		80	100.0	38	100.0	37	100.0	26	100.0	52	100.0	57	100.0	86	100.0	78	98.7	31	93.9
Missing		0	0.0	0	0.0	0	0.0	0	0.0	0	0.0	0	0.0	0	0.0	1	1.3	2	6.1
Total		80	100.0	38	100.0	37	100.0	26	100.0	52	100.0	57	100.0	86	100.0	79	100.0	33	100.0

		Agra		*Cali*		*Prague IPSS*		*Groningen*		*Mannheim*		*Sofia*		*Beijing*		*Hong Kong*		*Chennai (Madras)*	
		N	%	N	%	N	%	N	%	N	%	N	%	N	%	N	%	N	%
Available	Months Received Dis. for Mental Cond.																		
	. Inst.	0	0.0	0	0.0	0	0.0	0	0.0	4	7.1	0	0.0	3	5.2	0	0.0	1	1.3
	. Never	61	100.0	69	95.8	19	44.2	29	46.0	45	80.4	25	46.3	44	75.9	49	70.0	76	98.7
	* Other Disability	0	0.0	0	0.0	5	11.6	0	0.0	0	0.0	0	0.0	0	0.0	2	2.9	0	0.0
	≤ 12 Months	0	0.0	0	0.0	0	0.0	2	3.2	0	0.0	2	3.7	1	1.7	2	2.9	0	0.0
	13–23 Months	0	0.0	0	0.0	0	0.0	0	0.0	0	0.0	2	3.7	1	1.7	2	2.9	0	0.0
	24 Months	0	0.0	3	4.2	19	44.2	32	50.8	7	12.5	25	46.3	9	15.5	15	21.4	0	0.0
Missing	Unknown	0	—	0	—	0	—	0	—	0	—	1	100.0	0	—	0	—	0	—
Available		61	100.0	72	100.0	43	100.0	63	100.0	56	100.0	54	98.2	58	100.0	70	100.0	77	100.0
Missing		0	0.0	0	0.0	0	0.0	0	0.0	0	0.0	1	1.8	0	0.0	0	0.0	0	0.0
Total		61	100.0	72	100.0	43	100.0	63	100.0	56	100.0	55	100.0	58	100.0	70	100.0	77	100.0

TABLE B.23 Student: Past 2 Years Alive Cohort—by Center

		Chandigarh Urban		*Chandigarh Rural*		*Dublin*		*Honolulu*		*Moscow*		*Nagasaki*		*Nottingham*		*Prague DOSMeD*		*Rochester*	
		N	%	N	%	N	%	N	%	N	%	N	%	N	%	N	%	N	%
Available	Ever a Student																		
	0: No	78	100.0	38	100.0	37	100.0	25	96.2	52	100.0	57	100.0	86	100.0	75	97.4	29	96.7
	1: Yes	0	0.0	0	0.0	0	0.0	1	3.8	0	0.0	0	0.0	0	0.0	2	2.6	1	3.3
Missing	. : Not Supplied	2	100.0	0	—	0	—	0	—	0	—	0	—	0	—	2	100.0	3	100.0
Available		78	97.5	38	100.0	37	100.0	26	100.0	52	100.0	57	100.0	86	100.0	77	97.5	30	90.9
Missing		2	2.5	0	0.0	0	0.0	0	0.0	0	0.0	0	0.0	0	0.0	2	2.5	3	9.1
Total		80	100.0	38	100.0	37	100.0	26	100.0	52	100.0	57	100.0	86	100.0	79	100.0	33	100.0

		Agra		*Cali*		*Prague IPSS*		*Groningen*		*Mannheim*		*Sofia*		*Beijing*		*Hong Kong*		*Chennai (Madras)*	
		N	%	N	%	N	%	N	%	N	%	N	%	N	%	N	%	N	%
Available	Ever a Student																		
	0: No	57	100.0	72	100.0	43	100.0	61	96.8	54	96.4	53	100.0	57	100.0	70	100.0	76	98.7
	1: Yes	0	0.0	0	0.0	0	0.0	2	3.2	2	3.6	0	0.0	0	0.0	0	0.0	1	1.3
Missing	. : Not Supplied	4	100.0	0	—	0	—	0	—	0	—	2	100.0	1	100.0	0	—	0	—
Available		57	93.4	72	100.0	43	100.0	63	100.0	56	100.0	53	96.4	57	98.3	70	100.0	77	100.0
Missing		4	6.6	0	0.0	0	0.0	0	0.0	0	0.0	2	3.6	1	1.7	0	0.0	0	0.0
Total		61	100.0	72	100.0	43	100.0	63	100.0	56	100.0	55	100.0	58	100.0	70	100.0	77	100.0

TABLE B.24 Global Work or Household Performance: Past 2 Years Alive Cohort—by Center

		Chandigarh Urban		*Chandigarh Rural*		*Dublin*		*Honolulu*		*Moscow*		*Nagasaki*		*Nottingham*		*Prague DOSMeD*		*Rochester*	
		N	%	N	%	N	%	N	%	N	%	N	%	N	%	N	%	N	%
Available	Global Performance																		
	1: Good	44	60.3	24	63.2	6	42.9	3	37.5	1	14.3	14	29.8	35	41.2	30	41.7	10	62.5
	2: Fair	21	28.8	10	26.3	4	28.6	3	37.5	4	57.1	8	17.0	15	17.6	26	36.1	2	12.5
	3: Poor	8	11.0	4	10.5	4	28.6	2	25.0	2	28.6	25	53.2	35	41.2	16	22.2	4	25.0
Missing	. : Not Supplied	3	42.9	0	—	20	87.0	10	55.6	45	100.0	6	60.0	0	0.0	0	0.0	16	94.1
	8: Not Applic.	3	42.9	0	—	3	13.0	8	44.4	0	0.0	3	30.0	0	0.0	2	28.6	0	0.0
	9: Unknown	1	14.3	0	—	0	0.0	0	0.0	0	0.0	1	10.0	1	100.0	5	71.4	1	5.9
Available		73	91.3	38	100.0	14	37.8	8	30.8	7	13.5	47	82.5	85	98.8	72	91.1	16	48.5
Missing		7	8.8	0	0.0	23	62.2	18	69.2	45	86.5	10	17.5	1	1.2	7	8.9	17	51.5
Total		80	100.0	38	100.0	37	100.0	26	100.0	52	100.0	57	100.0	86	100.0	79	100.0	33	100.0

		Agra		*Cali*		*Prague IPSS*		*Groningen*		*Mannheim*		*Sofia*		*Beijing*		*Hong Kong*		*Chennai (Madras)*	
		N	%	N	%	N	%	N	%	N	%	N	%	N	%	N	%	N	%
Available	Global Performance																		
	1: Good	21	72.4	38	61.3	22	55.0	22	37.3	0	—	10	32.3	10	18.2	9	30.0	11	30.6
	2: Fair	4	13.8	19	30.6	11	27.5	18	30.5	0	—	9	29.0	23	41.8	16	53.3	11	30.6
	3: Poor	4	13.8	5	8.1	7	17.5	19	32.2	0	—	12	38.7	22	40.0	5	16.7	14	38.9
Missing	. : Not Supplied	25	78.1	0	0.0	0	0.0	0	0.0	0	0.0	22	91.7	2	66.7	1	2.5	0	0.0
	8: Not Applic.	5	15.6	10	100.0	2	66.7	4	100.0	0	0.0	0	0.0	1	33.3	39	97.5	41	100.0
	9: Unknown	2	6.3	0	0.0	1	33.3	0	0.0	56	100.0	2	8.3	0	0.0	0	0.0	0	0.0
Available		29	47.5	62	86.1	40	93.0	59	93.7	0	0.0	31	56.4	55	94.8	30	42.9	36	46.8
Missing		32	52.5	10	13.9	3	7.0	4	6.3	56	100.0	24	43.6	3	5.2	40	57.1	41	53.2
Total		61	100.0	72	100.0	43	100.0	63	100.0	56	100.0	55	100.0	58	100.0	70	100.0	77	100.0

TABLE B.25 Work Performance by Highest Employment Status Held: Past 2 Years Alive Cohort—by Center

		Chandigarh Urban		*Chandigarh Rural*		*Dublin*		*Honolulu*		*Moscow*		*Nagasaki*		*Nottingham*		*Prague DOSMeD*		*Rochester*	
		N	%	N	%	N	%	N	%	N	%	N	%	N	%	N	%	N	%
Likely "Employment" Category	Global Performance																		
1: Employed	. : Not Supplied	0	0.0	0	0.0	7	53.8	5	35.7	29	87.9	0	0.0	0	0.0	0	0.0	6	46.2
	8: Not Applic.	0	0.0	0	0.0	0	0.0	4	28.6	0	0.0	0	0.0	0	0.0	0	0.0	0	0.0
	9: Unknown	0	0.0	0	0.0	0	0.0	0	0.0	0	0.0	1	4.3	1	2.6	3	6.8	0	0.0
	1: Good	32	62.7	8	47.1	3	23.1	2	14.3	1	3.0	11	47.8	29	74.4	21	47.7	7	53.8
	2, 3: Not Good	19	37.3	9	52.9	3	23.1	3	21.4	3	9.1	11	47.8	9	23.1	20	45.5	0	0.0
2: Housework	8: Not Applic.	0	0.0	0	0.0	0	0.0	0	0.0	0	0.0	0	0.0	0	0.0	1	5.6	0	0.0
	9: Unknown	0	0.0	0	0.0	0	0.0	0	0.0	0	0.0	0	0.0	0	0.0	0	0.0	0	0.0
	1: Good	12	57.1	16	76.2	3	50.0	1	50.0	0	0.0	3	42.9	6	46.2	8	44.4	2	66.7
	2, 3: Not Good	9	42.9	5	23.8	3	50.0	1	50.0	1	100.0	4	57.1	7	53.8	9	50.0	1	33.3
3: Retired	. : Not Supplied	1	50.0	0	—	1	100.0	0	—	14	100.0	0	—	0	0.0	0	—	0	—
	8: Not Applic.	1	50.0	0	—	0	0.0	0	—	0	0.0	0	—	0	0.0	0	—	0	—
	9: Unknown	0	0.0	0	—	0	0.0	0	—	0	0.0	0	—	0	0.0	0	—	0	—
	1: Good	0	0.0	0	—	0	0.0	0	—	0	0.0	0	—	0	0.0	0	—	0	—
	2, 3: Not Good	0	0.0	0	—	0	0.0	0	—	0	0.0	0	—	1	100.0	0	—	0	—
4: Mental Condition Disability	. : Not Supplied	0	—	0	—	11	78.6	3	42.9	1	33.3	2	25.0	0	0.0	0	0.0	9	81.8
	8: Not Applic.	0	—	0	—	1	7.1	4	57.1	0	0.0	1	12.5	0	0.0	1	6.3	0	0.0
	9: Unknown	0	—	0	—	0	0.0	0	0.0	0	0.0	0	0.0	0	0.0	1	6.3	0	0.0
	1: Good	0	—	0	—	0	0.0	0	0.0	0	0.0	0	0.0	0	0.0	1	6.3	0	0.0
	2, 3: Not Good	0	—	0	—	2	14.3	0	0.0	2	66.7	5	62.5	26	100.0	13	81.3	2	18.2
5: Other Condition Disability	8: Not Applic.	1	100.0	0	—	0	—	0	—	0	—	0	—	0	0.0	0	—	0	0.0
	1: Good	0	0.0	0	—	0	—	0	—	0	—	0	—	0	0.0	0	—	1	100.0
	2, 3: Not Good	0	0.0	0	—	0	—	0	—	0	—	0	—	3	100.0	0	—	0	0
6: Student	9: Unknown	0	—	0	—	0	—	0	—	0	—	0	—	0	—	0	—	0	—

7: Institution, 2 Years:	. : Not Supplied	0	0.0	0	—	0	—	2	100.0	0	—	3	33.3	0	—	0	—	1	100.0
	Not Applic.	0	0.0	0	—	0	—	0	0.0	0	—	2	22.2	0	—	0	—	0	0.0
	9: Unknown	1	100.0	0	—	0	—	0	0.0	0	—	0	0.0	0	—	0	—	0	0.0
	2, 3: Not Good	0	0.0	0	—	0	—	0	0.0	0	—	4	44.4	0	—	0	—	0	0.0
8: Unemployed	. : Not Supplied	2	50.0	0	—	1	33.3	0	0.0	1	100.0	1	10.0	0	0.0	0	—	0	0.0
	8: Not Applic.	1	25.0	0	—	2	66.7	0	0.0	0	0.0	0	0.0	0	0.0	0	—	0	0.0
	9: Unknown	0	0.0	0	—	0	0.0	0	0.0	0	0.0	0	0.0	0	0.0	0	—	0	0.0
	2, 3: Not Good	1	25.0	0	—	0	0.0	1	100.0	0	0.0	9	90.0	4	100.0	0	—	2	100.0
9: Unknown	8: Not Applic.	0	—	0	—	0	—	0	—	0	—	0	—	0	—	0	0.0	0	0.0
	9: Unknown	0	—	0	—	0	—	0	—	0	—	0	—	0	—	1	100.0	1	50.0
	2, 3: Not Good	0	—	0	—	0	—	0	—	0	—	0	—	0	—	0	0.0	1	50.0
1: Employed		51	100.0	17	100.0	13	100.0	14	100.0	33	100.0	23	100.0	39	100.0	44	100.0	13	100.0
2: Housework		21	100.0	21	100.0	6	100.0	2	100.0	1	100.0	7	100.0	13	100.0	18	100.0	3	100.0
3: Retired		2	100.0	0	—	1	100.0	0	—	14	100.0	0	—	1	100.0	0	—	0	—
4: Mental Condition Disability		0	—	0	—	14	100.0	7	100.0	3	100.0	8	100.0	26	100.0	16	100.0	11	100.0
5: Other Condition Disability		1	100.0	0	—	0	—	0	—	0	—	0	—	3	100.0	0	—	1	100.0
6: Student		0	—	0	—	0	—	0	—	0	—	0	—	0	—	0	—	0	—
7: Institution, 2 Years		1	100.0	0	—	0	—	2	100.0	0	—	9	100.0	0	—	0	—	1	100.0
8: Unemployed		4	100.0	0	—	3	100.0	1	100.0	1	100.0	10	100.0	4	100.0	0	—	2	100.0
9: Unknown		0	—	0	—	0	—	0	—	0	—	0	—	0	—	1	100.0	2	100.0
Total		80	100.0	38	100.0	37	100.0	26	100.0	52	100.0	57	100.0	86	100.0	79	100.0	33	100.0

(*continued*)

TABLE B.25 (*continued*)

Likely "Employment" Category	Global Performance	Agra N	Agra %	Cali N	Cali %	Prague IPSS N	Prague IPSS %	Groningen N	Groningen %	Mannheim N	Mannheim %	Sofia N	Sofia %	Beijing N	Beijing %	Hong Kong N	Hong Kong %	Chennai (Madras) N	Chennai (Madras) %
1: Employed	.: Not Supplied	19	70.4	0	0.0	0	0.0	0	0.0	0	0.0	4	16.7	0	0.0	1	2.6	0	0.0
	8: Not Applic.	0	0.0	0	0.0	0	0.0	0	0.0	0	0.0	0	0.0	0	0.0	19	48.7	31	86.1
	9: Unknown	1	3.7	0	0.0	0	0.0	0	0.0	27	100.0	0	0.0	0	0.0	0	0.0	0	0.0
	1: Good	4	14.8	28	57.1	15	68.2	16	84.2	0	0.0	7	29.2	7	43.8	6	15.4	2	5.6
	2, 3: Not Good	3	11.1	21	42.9	7	31.8	3	15.8	0	0.0	13	54.2	9	56.3	13	33.3	3	8.3
2: Housework	8: Not Applic.	0	0.0	0	0.0	1	7.1	0	0.0	0	0.0	0	0.0	0	0.0	0	0.0	0	0.0
	9: Unknown	0	0.0	0	0.0	1	7.1	0	0.0	1	100.0	0	0.0	0	0.0	0	0.0	0	0.0
	1: Good	17	81.0	10	76.9	6	42.9	6	42.9	0	0.0	3	60.0	3	16.7	3	27.3	9	32.1
	2, 3: Not Good	4	19.0	3	23.1	6	42.9	8	57.1	0	0.0	2	40.0	15	83.3	8	72.7	19	67.9
3: Retired	.: Not Supplied	1	33.3	0	0.0	0	0.0	0	—	0	0.0	2	100.0	1	8.3	0	0.0	0	—
	8: Not Applic.	1	33.3	1	100.0	0	0.0	0	—	0	0.0	0	0.0	0	0.0	1	100.0	0	—
	9: Unknown	1	33.3	0	0.0	0	0.0	0	—	13	100.0	0	0.0	0	0.0	0	0.0	0	—
	1: Good	0	0.0	0	0.0	1	100.0	0	—	0	0.0	0	0.0	0	0.0	0	0.0	0	—
	2, 3: Not Good	0	0.0	0	0.0	0	0.0	0	—	0	0.0	0	0.0	11	91.7	0	0.0	0	—
4: Mental	.: Not Supplied	0	—	0	0.0	0	0.0	0	0.0	0	—	15	75.0	0	0.0	0	0.0	0	—
Condition	8: Not Applic.	0	—	2	100.0	1	16.7	2	8.7	0	—	0	0.0	0	0.0	11	100.0	0	—
Disability	9: Unknown	0	—	0	0.0	0	0.0	0	0.0	0	—	0	0.0	0	0.0	0	0.0	0	—
	1: Good	0	—	0	0.0	0	0.0	0	0.0	0	—	0	0.0	0	0.0	0	0.0	0	—
	2, 3: Not Good	0	—	0	0.0	5	83.3	21	91.3	0	—	5	25.0	5	100.0	0	0.0	0	—
5: Other	8: Not Applic.	0	—	0	—	0	—	0	—	0	—	0	—	0	—	1	100.0	0	—
Condition	1: Good	0	—	0	—	0	—	0	—	0	—	0	—	0	—	0	0.0	0	—
Disability	2, 3: Not Good	0	—	0	—	0	—	0	—	0	—	0	—	0	—	0	0.0	0	—
6: Student	9: Unknown	0	—	0	—	0	—	0	—	2	100.0	0	—	0	—	0	—	0	—

7: Institution, 2 Years	.: Not Supplied	0	—	0	—	0	—	0	0.0	0	0.0	0	—	1	33.3	0	0.0	0	0.0
	8: Not Applic.	0	—	0	—	0	—	0	0.0	0	0.0	0	—	1	33.3	1	100.0	1	100.0
	9: Unknown	0	—	0	—	0	—	0	0.0	8	100.0	0	—	0	0.0	0	0.0	0	0.0
	2, 3: Not Good	0	—	0	—	0	—	1	100.0	0	0.0	0	—	1	33.3	0	0.0	0	0.0
8: Unemployed	.: Not Supplied	5	83.3	0	0.0	0	—	0	0.0	0	0.0	1	50.0	0	0.0	0	0.0	0	0.0
	8: Not Applic.	1	16.7	7	100.0	0	—	2	33.3	0	0.0	0	0.0	0	0.0	6	100.0	9	75.0
	9: Unknown	0	0.0	0	0.0	0	—	0	0.0	5	100.0	0	0.0	0	0.0	0	0.0	0	0.0
	2, 3: Not Good	0	0.0	0	0.0	0	—	4	66.7	0	0.0	1	50.0	3	100.0	0	0.0	3	25.0
9: Unknown	8.: Not Applic.	3	75.0	0	—	0	—	0	—	0	—	0	0.0	0	0.0	0	—	0	—
	9.: Unknown	0	0.0	0	—	0	—	0	—	0	—	2	100.0	0	0.0	0	—	0	—
	2, 3: Not Good	1	25.0	0	—	0	—	0	—	0	—	0	0.0	1	100.0	0	—	0	—
1: Employed		27	100.0	49	100.0	22	100.0	19	100.0	27	100.0	24	100.0	16	100.0	39	100.0	36	100.0
2: Housework		21	100.0	13	100.0	14	100.0	14	100.0	1	100.0	5	100.0	18	100.0	11	100.0	28	100.0
3: Retired		3	100.0	1	100.0	1	100.0	0	—	13	100.0	2	100.0	12	100.0	1	100.0	0	—
4: Mental Condition Disability		0	—	2	100.0	6	100.0	23	100.0	0	—	20	100.0	5	100.0	11	100.0	0	—
5: Other Condition Disability		0	—	0	—	0	—	0	—	0	—	0	—	0	—	1	100.0	0	—
6: Student		0	—	0	—	0	—	0	—	2	100.0	0	—	0	—	0	—	0	—
7: Institution, 2 Years		0	—	0	—	0	—	1	100.0	8	100.0	0	—	3	100.0	1	100.0	1	100.0
8: Unemployed		6	100.0	7	100.0	0	—	6	100.0	5	100.0	2	100.0	3	100.0	6	100.0	12	100.0
9: Unknown		4	100.0	0	—	0	—	0	—	0	—	2	100.0	1	100.0	0	—	0	—
Total		61	100.0	72	100.0	43	100.0	63	100.0	56	100.0	55	100.0	58	100.0	70	100.0	77	100.0

TABLE B.26 Assaults: Past 2 Years Alive Cohort—by Center

		Chandigarh Urban		*Chandigarh Rural*		*Dublin*		*Honolulu*		*Moscow*		*Nagasaki*		*Nottingham*		*Prague DOSMeD*		*Rochester*	
		N	%	N	%	N	%	N	%	N	%	N	%	N	%	N	%	N	%
Available	Assaults: Past 2 yrs																		
	0: No	72	90.0	34	91.9	35	100.0	21	95.5	46	88.5	44	78.6	66	91.7	60	85.7	26	89.7
	1: Yes	8	10.0	3	8.1	0	0.0	1	4.5	6	11.5	12	21.4	6	8.3	10	14.3	3	10.3
Missing	. : Not Supplied	0	—	0	0.0	0	0.0	2	50.0	0	—	0	0.0	0	0.0	0	0.0	1	25.0
	8: Not Applicable	0	—	1	100.0	0	0.0	2	50.0	0	—	0	0.0	0	0.0	0	0.0	0	0.0
	9: Unknown	0	—	0	0.0	2	100.0	0	0.0	0	—	1	100.0	14	100.0	9	100.0	3	75.0
Available		80	100.0	37	97.4	35	94.6	22	84.6	52	100.0	56	98.2	72	83.7	70	88.6	29	87.9
Missing		0	0.0	1	2.6	2	5.4	4	15.4	0	0.0	1	1.8	14	16.3	9	11.4	4	12.1
Total		80	100.0	38	100.0	37	100.0	26	100.0	52	100.0	57	100.0	86	100.0	79	100.0	33	100.0

		Agra		*Cali*		*Prague IPSS*		*Groningen*		*Mannheim*		*Sofia*		*Beijing*		*Hong Kong*		*Chennai (Madras)*	
		N	%	N	%	N	%	N	%	N	%	N	%	N	%	N	%	N	%
Available	Assaults: Past 2 yrs																		
	0: No	55	91.7	72	100.0	40	95.2	44	91.7	14	100.0	48	94.1	47	81.0	59	92.2	67	89.3
	1: Yes	5	8.3	0	0.0	2	4.8	4	8.3	0	0.0	3	5.9	11	19.0	5	7.8	8	10.7
Missing	. : Not Supplied	0	0.0	0	—	0	0.0	0	0.0	0	0.0	0	0.0	0	—	0	0.0	0	0.0
	8: Not Applicable	0	0.0	0	—	0	0.0	12	80.0	0	0.0	0	0.0	0	—	6	100.0	2	100.0
	9: Unknown	1	100.0	0	—	1	100.0	3	20.0	42	100.0	4	100.0	0	—	0	0.0	0	0.0
Available		60	98.4	72	100.0	42	97.7	48	76.2	14	25.0	51	92.7	58	100.0	64	91.4	75	97.4
Missing		1	1.6	0	0.0	1	2.3	15	23.8	42	75.0	4	7.3	0	0.0	6	8.6	2	2.6
Total		61	100.0	72	100.0	43	100.0	63	100.0	56	100.0	55	100.0	58	100.0	70	100.0	77	100.0

TABLE B.27 Suicide Attempts: Past 2 Years Alive Cohort—by Center

		Chandigarh Urban		*Chandigarh Rural*		*Dublin*		*Honolulu*		*Moscow*		*Nagasaki*		*Nottingham*		*Prague DOSMeD*		*Rochester*	
		N	%	N	%	N	%	N	%	N	%	N	%	N	%	N	%	N	%
Available	Suicide Attempts: Past 2 yrs																		
	0: No	77	96.3	37	100.0	34	97.1	25	96.2	52	100.0	55	98.2	69	89.6	66	93.0	29	96.7
	1: Yes	3	3.8	0	0.0	1	2.9	1	3.8	0	0.0	1	1.8	8	10.4	5	7.0	1	3.3
Missing	. : Not Supplied	0	—	0	0.0	0	0.0	0	—	0	—	0	0.0	0	0.0	0	0.0	0	0.0
	8: Not Applicable	0	—	1	100.0	0	0.0	0	—	0	—	0	0.0	1	11.1	1	12.5	0	0.0
	9: Unknown	0	—	0	0.0	2	100.0	0	—	0	—	1	100.0	8	88.9	7	87.5	3	100.0
Available		80	100.0	37	97.4	35	94.6	26	100.0	52	100.0	56	98.2	77	89.5	71	89.9	30	90.9
Missing		0	0.0	1	2.6	2	5.4	0	0.0	0	0.0	1	1.8	9	10.5	8	10.1	3	9.1
Total		80	100.0	38	100.0	37	100.0	26	100.0	52	100.0	57	100.0	86	100.0	79	100.0	33	100.0

		Agra		*Cali*		*Prague IPSS*		*Groningen*		*Mannheim*		*Sofia*		*Beijing*		*Hong Kong*		*Chennai (Madras)*	
		N	%	N	%	N	%	N	%	N	%	N	%	N	%	N	%	N	%
Available	Suicide Attempts: Past 2 yrs																		
	0: No	60	100.0	71	98.6	42	100.0	59	98.3	50	90.9	48	92.3	57	98.3	68	97.1	70	93.3
	1: Yes	0	0.0	1	1.4	0	0.0	1	1.7	5	9.1	4	7.7	1	1.7	2	2.9	5	6.7
Missing	. : Not Supplied	0	0.0	0	—	0	0.0	0	0.0	0	0.0	1	33.3	0	—	0	—	0	0.0
	8: Not Applicable	0	0.0	0	—	0	0.0	1	33.3	0	0.0	0	0.0	0	—	0	—	2	100.0
	9: Unknown	1	100.0	0	—	1	100.0	2	66.7	1	100.0	2	66.7	0	—	0	—	0	0.0
Available		60	98.4	72	100.0	42	97.7	60	95.2	55	98.2	52	94.5	58	100.0	70	100.0	75	97.4
Missing		1	1.6	0	0.0	1	2.3	3	4.8	1	1.8	3	5.5	0	0.0	0	0.0	2	2.6
Total		61	100.0	72	100.0	43	100.0	63	100.0	56	100.0	55	100.0	58	100.0	70	100.0	77	100.0

TABLE B.28 Assaults: Since First Contact Alive Cohort—by Center

		Chandigarh Urban		*Chandigarh Rural*		*Dublin*		*Honolulu*		*Moscow*		*Nagasaki*		*Nottingham*		*Prague DOSMeD*		*Rochester*	
		N	%	N	%	N	%	N	%	N	%	N	%	N	%	N	%	N	%
Available	Assaults: Since 1st																		
	0: No	61	76.3	30	78.9	31	91.2	14	63.6	42	80.8	33	58.9	56	77.8	56	76.7	22	78.6
	1: Yes	19	23.7	8	21.1	3	8.8	8	36.4	10	19.2	23	41.1	16	22.2	17	23.3	6	21.4
Missing	. : Not Supplied	0	—	0	—	0	0.0	2	50.0	0	—	0	0.0	0	0.0	0	0.0	0	0.0
	8: Not Applicable	0	—	0	—	0	0.0	1	25.0	0	—	0	0.0	0	0.0	0	0.0	0	0.0
	9: Unknown	0	—	0	—	3	100.0	1	25.0	0	—	1	100.0	14	100.0	6	100.0	5	100.0
Available		80	100.0	38	100.0	34	91.9	22	84.6	52	100.0	56	98.2	72	83.7	73	92.4	28	84.8
Missing		0	0.0	0	0.0	3	8.1	4	15.4	0	0.0	1	1.8	14	16.3	6	7.6	5	15.2
Total		80	100.0	38	100.0	37	100.0	26	100.0	52	100.0	57	100.0	86	100.0	79	100.0	33	100.0
		Agra		*Cali*		*Prague IPSS*		*Groningen*		*Mannheim*		*Sofia*		*Beijing*		*Hong Kong*		*Chennai (Madras)*	
		N	%	N	%	N	%	N	%	N	%	N	%	N	%	N	%	N	%
Available	Assaults: Since 1st																		
	0: No	52	86.7	72	100.0	36	83.7	39	76.5	16	100.0	43	86.0	39	67.2	43	66.2	61	79.2
	1: Yes	8	13.3	0	0.0	7	16.3	12	23.5	0	0.0	7	14.0	19	32.8	22	33.8	16	20.8
Missing	. : Not Supplied	0	0.0	0	—	0	—	0	0.0	0	0.0	0	0.0	0	—	0	0.0	0	—
	8: Not Applicable	1	100.0	0	—	0	—	10	83.3	0	0.0	0	0.0	0	—	5	100.0	0	—
	9: Unknown	0	0.0	0	—	0	—	2	16.7	40	100.0	5	100.0	0	—	0	0.0	0	—
Available		60	98.4	72	100.0	43	100.0	51	81.0	16	28.6	50	90.9	58	100.0	65	92.9	77	100.0
Missing		1	1.6	0	0.0	0	0.0	12	19.0	40	71.4	5	9.1	0	0.0	5	7.1	0	0.0
Total		61	100.0	72	100.0	43	100.0	63	100.0	56	100.0	55	100.0	58	100.0	70	100.0	77	100.0

TABLE B.29 Suicide Attempts: Since First Contact Alive Cohort—by Center

		Chandigarh Urban		*Chandigarh Rural*		*Dublin*		*Honolulu*		*Moscow*		*Nagasaki*		*Nottingham*		*Prague DOSMeD*		*Rochester*	
		N	%	N	%	N	%	N	%	N	%	N	%	N	%	N	%	N	%
Available	Suicide Attempts: Since 1st																		
	0: No	65	81.3	33	89.2	30	85.7	18	72.0	51	98.1	44	78.6	47	58.8	56	80.0	26	89.7
	1: Yes	15	18.8	4	10.8	5	14.3	7	28.0	1	1.9	12	21.4	33	41.3	14	20.0	3	10.3
Missing	8: Not Applicable	0	—	1	100.0	0	0.0	0	0.0	0	—	0	0.0	0	0.0	1	11.1	0	0.0
	9: Unknown	0	—	0	0.0	2	100.0	1	100.0	0	—	1	100.0	6	100.0	8	88.9	4	100.0
Available		80	100.0	37	97.4	35	94.6	25	96.2	52	100.0	56	98.2	80	93.0	70	88.6	29	87.9
Missing		0	0.0	1	2.6	2	5.4	1	3.8	0	0.0	1	1.8	6	7.0	9	11.4	4	12.1
Total		80	100.0	38	100.0	37	100.0	26	100.0	52	100.0	57	100.0	86	100.0	79	100.0	33	100.0

		Agra		*Cali*		*Prague IPSS*		*Groningen*		*Mannheim*		*Sofia*		*Beijing*		*Hong Kong*		*Chennai (Madras)*	
		N	%	N	%	N	%	N	%	N	%	N	%	N	%	N	%	N	%
Available	Suicide Attempts Since 1st																		
	0: No	58	95.1	70	97.2	42	97.7	41	68.3	39	72.2	38	74.5	52	89.7	60	87.0	62	82.7
	1: Yes	3	4.9	2	2.8	1	2.3	19	31.7	15	27.8	13	25.5	6	10.3	9	13.0	13	17.3
Missing	8: Not Applicable	0	—	0	—	0	—	1	33.3	0	0.0	0	0.0	0	—	1	100.0	2	100.0
	9: Unknown	0	—	0	—	0	—	2	66.7	2	100.0	4	100.0	0	—	0	0.0	0	0.0
Available		61	100.0	72	100.0	43	100.0	60	95.2	54	96.4	51	92.7	58	100.0	69	98.6	75	97.4
Missing		0	0.0	0	0.0	0	0.0	3	4.8	2	3.6	4	7.3	0	0.0	1	1.4	2	2.6
Total		61	100.0	72	100.0	43	100.0	63	100.0	56	100.0	55	100.0	58	100.0	70	100.0	77	100.0

TABLE B.30 Neuroleptic Medication: Past 2 Years Alive Cohort—by Center

		Chandigarh Urban		*Chandigarh Rural*		*Dublin*		*Honolulu*		*Moscow*		*Nagasaki*		*Nottingham*		*Prague DOSMeD*		*Rochester*	
		N	%	N	%	N	%	N	%	N	%	N	%	N	%	N	%	N	%
Available	Neuroleptics: Past 2 yrs																		
	0: Never	43	53.8	30	78.9	4	11.1	10	40.0	25	48.1	4	7.1	36	42.4	17	22.4	15	48.4
	1: Sometimes	11	13.8	5	13.2	5	13.9	2	8.0	12	23.1	5	8.9	6	7.1	18	23.7	1	3.2
	2: Most	26	32.5	3	7.9	27	75.0	13	52.0	15	28.8	47	83.9	43	50.6	41	53.9	15	48.4
Missing	. : Not Supplied	0	—	0	—	0	0.0	1	100.0	0	—	0	0.0	0	0.0	0	0.0	0	0.0
	8: Not Applicable	0	—	0	—	0	0.0	0	0.0	0	—	0	0.0	0	0.0	1	33.3	0	0.0
	9: Unknown	0	—	0	—	1	100.0	0	0.0	0	—	1	100.0	1	100.0	2	66.7	2	100.0
Available		80	100.0	38	100.0	36	97.3	25	96.2	52	100.0	56	98.2	85	98.8	76	96.2	31	93.9
Missing		0	0.0	0	0.0	1	2.7	1	3.8	0	0.0	1	1.8	1	1.2	3	3.8	2	6.1
Total		80	100.0	38	100.0	37	100.0	26	100.0	52	100.0	57	100.0	86	100.0	79	100.0	33	100.0

		Agra		*Cali*		*Prague IPSS*		*Groningen*		*Mannheim*		*Sofia*		*Beijing*		*Hong Kong*		*Chennai (Madras)*	
		N	%	N	%	N	%	N	%	N	%	N	%	N	%	N	%	N	%
Available	Neuroleptics: Past 2 yrs																		
	0: Never	40	72.7	46	64.8	9	21.4	26	42.6	19	33.9	12	22.2	17	29.3	1	1.4	38	49.4
	1: Sometimes	9	16.4	3	4.2	10	23.8	6	9.8	6	10.7	7	13.0	19	32.8	3	4.3	12	15.6
	2: Most	6	10.9	22	31.0	23	54.8	29	47.5	31	55.4	35	64.8	22	37.9	65	94.2	27	35.1
Missing	. : Not Supplied	0	0.0	0	0.0	0	0.0	0	0.0	0	—	0	0.0	0	—	0	0.0	0	—
	8: Not Applicable	5	83.3	0	0.0	0	0.0	2	100.0	0	—	0	0.0	0	—	1	100.0	0	—
	9: Unknown	1	16.7	1	100.0	1	100.0	0	0.0	0	—	1	100.0	0	—	0	0.0	0	—
Available		55	90.2	71	98.6	42	97.7	61	96.8	56	100.0	54	98.2	58	100.0	69	98.6	77	100.0
Missing		6	9.8	1	1.4	1	2.3	2	3.2	0	0.0	1	1.8	0	0.0	1	1.4	0	0.0
Total		61	100.0	72	100.0	43	100.0	63	100.0	56	100.0	55	100.0	58	100.0	70	100.0	77	100.0

TABLE B.31 Neuroleptic Medication: Since First Contact Alive Cohort—by Center

		Chandigarh Urban		*Chandigarh Rural*		*Dublin*		*Honolulu*		*Moscow*		*Nagasaki*		*Nottingham*		*Prague DOSMeD*		*Rochester*	
		N	%	N	%	N	%	N	%	N	%	N	%	N	%	N	%	N	%
Available	Neuroleptics: Since 1st																		
	0: Never	0	0.0	2	5.3	0	0.0	4	17.4	1	1.9	0	0.0	6	7.1	5	6.5	4	12.1
	1: Sometimes	53	66.3	34	89.5	8	21.6	7	30.4	36	69.2	8	14.0	43	50.6	27	35.1	16	48.5
	2: Most	27	33.8	2	5.3	29	78.4	12	52.2	15	28.8	49	86.0	36	42.4	45	58.4	13	39.4
Missing	. : Not Supplied	0	—	0	—	0	—	2	66.7	0	—	0	—	0	0.0	0	0.0	0	—
	8: Not Applicable	0	—	0	—	0	—	0	0.0	0	—	0	—	0	0.0	0	0.0	0	—
	9: Unknown	0	—	0	—	0	—	1	33.3	0	—	0	—	1	100.0	2	100.0	0	—
Available		80	100.0	38	100.0	37	100.0	23	88.5	52	100.0	57	100.0	85	98.8	77	97.5	33	100.0
Missing		0	0.0	0	0.0	0	0.0	3	11.5	0	0.0	0	0.0	1	1.2	2	2.5	0	0.0
Total		80	100.0	38	100.0	37	100.0	26	100.0	52	100.0	57	100.0	86	100.0	79	100.0	33	100.0

		Agra		*Cali*		*Prague IPSS*		*Groningen*		*Mannheim*		*Sofia*		*Beijing*		*Hong Kong*		*Chennai (Madras)*	
		N	%	N	%	N	%	N	%	N	%	N	%	N	%	N	%	N	%
Available	Neuroleptics: Since 1st																		
	0: Never	34	63.0	37	52.9	2	4.7	0	0.0	5	8.9	0	0.0	5	8.6	0	0.0	0	0.0
	1: Sometimes	14	25.9	14	20.0	15	34.9	37	58.7	20	35.7	22	40.0	30	51.7	3	4.3	33	42.9
	2: Most	6	11.1	19	27.1	26	60.5	26	41.3	31	55.4	33	60.0	23	39.7	67	95.7	44	57.1
Missing	.: Not Supplied	0	0.0	0	0.0	0	—	0	—	0	—	0	—	0	—	0	—	0	—
	8: Not Applicable	5	71.4	1	50.0	0	—	0	—	0	—	0	—	0	—	0	—	0	—
	9: Unknown	2	28.6	1	50.0	0	—	0	—	0	—	0	—	0	—	0	—	0	—
Available		54	88.5	70	97.2	43	100.0	63	100.0	56	100.0	55	100.0	58	100.0	70	100.0	77	100.0
Missing		7	11.5	2	2.8	0	0.0	0	0.0	0	0.0	0	0.0	0	0.0	0	0.0	0	0.0
Total		61	100.0	72	100.0	43	100.0	63	100.0	56	100.0	55	100.0	58	100.0	70	100.0	77	100.0

TABLE B.32 Trend of Medication Use: Since First Contact Alive Cohort—by Center

		Chandigarh Urban		Chandigarh Rural		Dublin		Honolulu		Moscow		Nagasaki		Nottingham		Prague DOSMeD		Rochester	
		N	%	N	%	N	%	N	%	N	%	N	%	N	%	N	%	N	%
Available	Trend of Medications																		
	XXX	25	31.6	13	35.1	0	0.0	0	0.0	7	13.5	0	0.0	3	3.5	3	4.0	0	0.0
	XX1[a]	2	2.5	2	5.4	0	0.0	6	23.1	0	0.0	6	10.5	8	9.3	5	6.7	0	0.0
	X1X	0	0.0	1	2.7	0	0.0	2	7.7	1	1.9	0	0.0	1	1.2	2	2.7	0	0.0
	X11	0	0.0	0	0.0	1	2.9	5	19.2	1	1.9	4	7.0	9	10.5	1	1.3	0	0.0
	1XX	38	48.1	21	56.8	5	14.3	8	30.8	24	46.2	7	12.3	26	30.2	40	53.3	18	54.5
	1X1	5	6.3	0	0.0	0	0.0	3	11.5	0	0.0	3	5.3	2	2.3	2	2.7	5	15.2
	11X	0	0.0	0	0.0	1	2.9	0	0.0	0	0.0	2	3.5	4	4.7	2	2.7	3	9.1
	111	9	11.4	0	0.0	28	80.0	2	7.7	19	36.5	35	61.4	33	38.4	20	26.7	7	21.2
Missing	MMM	1	100.0	1	100.0	2	100.0	0	—	0	—	0	—	0	—	4	100.0	0	—
Available		79	98.8	37	97.4	35	94.6	26	100.0	52	100.0	57	100.0	86	100.0	75	94.9	33	100.0
Missing		1	1.2	1	2.6	2	5.4	0	0.0	0	0.0	0	0.0	0	0.0	4	5.1	0	0.0
Total		80	100.0	38	100.0	37	100.0	26	100.0	52	100.0	57	100.0	86	100.0	79	100.0	33	100.0

		Agra		Cali		Prague IPSS		Groningen		Mannheim		Sofia		Beijing		Hong Kong		Chennai (Madras)	
		N	%	N	%	N	%	N	%	N	%	N	%	N	%	N	%	N	%
Available	Trend of Medications																		
	XXX	3	7.3	18	25.0	0	0.0	19	30.2	0	—	0	0.0	4	6.9	8	11.4	0	0.0
	XX1	2	4.9	11	15.3	2	4.8	3	4.8	0	—	1	1.8	0	0.0	7	10.0	0	0.0
	X1X	4	9.8	3	4.2	1	2.4	3	4.8	0	—	1	1.8	1	1.7	4	5.7	0	0.0
	X11	0	0.0	7	9.7	0	0.0	1	1.6	0	—	1	1.8	0	0.0	5	7.1	0	0.0
	1XX	27	65.9	30	41.7	31	73.8	16	25.4	0	—	21	38.2	35	60.3	22	31.4	64	86.5
	1X1	0	0.0	1	1.4	0	0.0	3	4.8	0	—	3	5.5	3	5.2	5	7.1	5	6.8
	11X	1	2.4	0	0.0	1	2.4	1	1.6	0	—	4	7.3	2	3.4	3	4.3	0	0.0
	111	4	9.8	2	2.8	7	16.7	17	27.0	0	—	24	43.6	13	22.4	16	22.9	5	6.8
Missing	MMM	20	100.0	0	—	1	100.0	0	—	56	100.0	0	—	0	—	0	—	3	100.0
Available		41	67.2	72	100.0	42	97.7	63	100.0	0	0.0	55	100.0	58	100.0	70	100.0	74	96.1
Missing		20	32.8	0	0.0	1	2.3	0	0.0	56	100.0	0	0.0	0	0.0	0	0.0	3	3.9
Total		61	100.0	72	100.0	43	100.0	63	100.0	56	100.0	55	100.0	58	100.0	70	100.0	77	100.0

[a]The number "1" designates that third of the entire period when variable was most prominent (where the leftmost position represents the earliest third). Where it appears in more than one time slot, the variable was considered to be equally prominent in the designated periods.

TABLE B.33 Trend of Hospitalization: Since First Contact Alive Cohort—by Center

		Chandigarh Urban		*Chandigarh Rural*		*Dublin*		*Honolulu*		*Moscow*		*Nagasaki*		*Nottingham*		*Prague DOSMeD*		*Rochester*	
		N	%	N	%	N	%	N	%	N	%	N	%	N	%	N	%	N	%
Available	Trend of Hospitalizations																		
	XXX	9	30.0	2	50.0	0	0.0	0	0.0	4	7.7	3	5.4	4	4.7	2	2.7	0	0.0
	XX1[a]	1	3.3	1	25.0	1	2.9	5	19.2	0	0.0	11	19.6	1	1.2	4	5.3	0	0.0
	X1X	0	0.0	0	0.0	1	2.9	3	11.5	0	0.0	2	3.6	1	1.2	5	6.7	5	15.2
	X11	0	0.0	0	0.0	0	0.0	1	3.8	1	1.9	6	10.7	0	0.0	1	1.3	0	0.0
	1XX	17	56.7	1	25.0	16	45.7	13	50.0	33	63.5	21	37.5	69	80.2	54	72.0	25	75.8
	1X1	2	6.7	0	0.0	2	5.7	1	3.8	3	5.8	3	5.4	3	3.5	6	8.0	2	6.1
	11X	0	0.0	0	0.0	5	14.3	3	11.5	6	11.5	5	8.9	3	3.5	3	4.0	1	3.0
	111	1	3.3	0	0.0	10	28.6	0	0.0	5	9.6	5	8.9	5	5.8	0	0.0	0	0.0
Missing	MMM	50	100.0	34	100.0	2	100.0	0	—	0	—	1	100.0	0	—	4	100.0	0	—
Available		30	37.5	4	10.5	35	94.6	26	100.0	52	100.0	56	98.2	86	100.0	75	94.9	33	100.0
Missing		50	62.5	34	89.5	2	5.4	0	0.0	0	0.0	1	1.8	0	0.0	4	5.1	0	0.0
Total		80	100.0	38	100.0	37	100.0	26	100.0	52	100.0	57	100.0	86	100.0	79	100.0	33	100.0

		Agra		*Cali*		*Prague IPSS*		*Groningen*		*Mannheim*		*Sofia*		*Beijing*		*Hong Kong*		*Chennai (Madras)*	
		N	%	N	%	N	%	N	%	N	%	N	%	N	%	N	%	N	%
Available	Trend of Hospitalizations																		
	XXX	1	5.0	9	13.0	0	0.0	18	28.6	0	—	0	0.0	32	55.2	15	21.4	1	1.6
	XX1	2	10.0	2	2.9	4	9.8	3	4.8	0	—	2	4.0	1	1.7	9	12.9	1	1.6
	X1X	1	5.0	3	4.3	5	12.2	3	4.8	0	—	3	6.0	0	0.0	8	11.4	0	0.0
	X11	0	0.0	0	0.0	0	0.0	1	1.6	0	—	0	0.0	0	0.0	2	2.9	1	1.6
	1XX	16	80.0	51	73.9	27	65.9	29	46.0	0	—	38	76.0	18	31.0	28	40.0	58	92.1
	1X1	0	0.0	2	2.9	0	0.0	3	4.8	0	—	1	2.0	3	5.2	2	2.9	2	3.2
	11X	0	0.0	1	1.4	4	9.8	0	0.0	0	—	3	6.0	1	1.7	6	8.6	0	0.0
	111	0	0.0	1	1.4	1	2.4	6	9.5	0	—	3	6.0	3	5.2	0	0.0	0	0.0
Missing	MMM	41	100.0	3	100.0	2	100.0	0	—	56	100.0	5	100.0	0	—	0	—	14	100.0
Available		20	32.8	69	95.8	41	95.3	63	100.0	0	0.0	50	90.9	58	100.0	70	100.0	63	81.8
Missing		41	67.2	3	4.2	2	4.7	0	0.0	56	100.0	5	9.1	0	0.0	0	0.0	14	18.2
Total		61	100.0	72	100.0	43	100.0	63	100.0	56	100.0	55	100.0	58	100.0	70	100.0	77	100.0

[a] The number "1" designates that third of the entire period when variable was most prominent (where the leftmost position represents the earliest third). Where it appears in more than one time slot, the variable was considered to be equally prominent in the designated periods.

TABLE B.34 Present Day Rediagnosis of Subject at First Contact Alive Cohort—by Center

		Chandigarh Urban		*Chandigarh Rural*		*Dublin*		*Honolulu*		*Moscow*		*Nagasaki*		*Nottingham*		*Prague DOSMeD*		*Rochester*	
		N	%	N	%	N	%	N	%	N	%	N	%	N	%	N	%	N	%
Available	Grouped First Contact Rediagnosis																		
	Schizophrenia	26	32.5	10	26.3	20	54.1	12	50.0	29	55.8	39	68.4	48	55.8	36	47.4	15	45.5
	Schizoaffective	0	0.0	0	0.0	4	10.8	1	4.2	0	0.0	1	1.8	2	2.3	14	18.4	5	15.2
	Acute Schizo-like	27	33.8	19	50.0	1	2.7	4	16.7	0	0.0	11	19.3	4	4.7	7	9.2	6	18.2
	Bipolar/Depression	17	21.2	8	21.1	7	18.9	5	20.8	5	9.6	0	0.0	22	25.6	2	2.6	5	15.2
	Other Psychotic	5	6.3	1	2.6	5	13.5	1	4.2	15	28.8	4	7.0	9	10.5	13	17.1	1	3.0
	Other Nonpsychotic	5	6.3	0	0.0	0	0.0	1	4.2	3	5.8	2	3.5	1	1.2	4	5.3	1	3.0
Missing	Missing/Unknown	0	—	0	—	0	—	2	100.0	0	—	0	—	0	—	3	100.0	0	—
Available		80	100.0	38	100.0	37	100.0	24	92.3	52	100.0	57	100.0	86	100.0	76	96.2	33	100.0
Missing		0	0.0	0	0.0	0	0.0	2	7.7	0	0.0	0	0.0	0	0.0	3	3.8	0	0.0
Total		80	100.0	38	100.0	37	100.0	26	100.0	52	100.0	57	100.0	86	100.0	79	100.0	33	100.0

		Agra		*Cali*		*Prague IPSS*		*Groningen*		*Mannheim*		*Sofia*		*Beijing*		*Hong Kong*		*Chennai (Madras)*	
		N	%	N	%	N	%	N	%	N	%	N	%	N	%	N	%	N	%
Available	Grouped First Contact Rediagnosis																		
	Schizophrenia	25	41.0	0	—	9	22.0	30	47.6	0	—	34	61.8	58	100.0	67	95.7	77	100.0
	Schizoaffective	7	11.5	0	—	12	29.3	0	0.0	0	—	4	7.3	0	0.0	0	0.0	0	0.0
	Acute Schizo-like	5	8.2	0	—	5	12.2	2	3.2	0	—	1	1.8	0	0.0	1	1.4	0	0.0
	Bipolar/Depression	19	31.1	0	—	12	29.3	6	9.5	0	—	7	12.7	0	0.0	0	0.0	0	0.0
	Other Psychotic	3	4.9	0	—	3	7.3	24	38.1	0	—	9	16.4	0	0.0	2	2.9	0	0.0
	Other Nonpsychotic	2	3.3	0	—	0	0.0	1	1.6	0	—	0	0.0	0	0.0	0	0.0	0	0.0
Missing	Missing/Unknown	0	—	72	100.0	2	100.0	0	—	56	100.0	0	—	0	—	0	—	0	—
Available		61	100.0	0	0.0	41	95.3	63	100.0	0	0.0	55	100.0	58	100.0	70	100.0	77	100.0
Missing		0	0.0	72	100.0	2	4.7	0	0.0	56	100.0	0	0.0	0	0.0	0	0.0	0	0.0
Total		61	100.0	72	100.0	43	100.0	63	100.0	56	100.0	55	100.0	58	100.0	70	100.0	77	100.0

TABLE B.35 Baseline Diagnoses: Converted to ICD-10 Alive Cohort—by Center

		Chandigarh Urban		*Chandigarh Rural*		*Dublin*		*Honolulu*		*Moscow*		*Nagasaki*		*Nottingham*		*Prague DOSMeD*		*Rochester*	
		N	%	N	%	N	%	N	%	N	%	N	%	N	%	N	%	N	%
Available	Grouped Baseline Diagnoses Converted to ICD-10																		
	Schzophrenia	27	33.8	10	26.3	20	54.1	13	52.0	37	71.2	52	91.2	54	62.8	40	53.3	7	21.2
	Schizoaffective	0	0.0	0	0.0	11	29.7	1	4.0	0	0.0	1	1.8	3	3.5	13	17.3	3	9.1
	Acute Schizo-like	28	35.0	18	47.4	5	13.5	5	20.0	8	15.4	3	5.3	3	3.5	4	5.3	17	51.5
	Bipolar/Depression	15	18.8	8	21.1	1	2.7	4	16.0	0	0.0	0	0.0	18	20.9	0	0.0	4	12.1
	Other Psychotic	5	6.3	2	5.3	0	0.0	1	4.0	0	0.0	0	0.0	5	5.8	13	17.3	2	6.1
	Other Nonpsychotic	5	6.3	0	0.0	0	0.0	1	4.0	7	13.5	1	1.8	3	3.5	5	6.7	0	0.0
Missing	Missing/Unknown	0	—	0	—	0	—	1	100.0	0	—	0	—	0	—	4	100.0	0	—
Available		80	100.0	38	100.0	37	100.0	25	96.2	52	100.0	57	100.0	86	100.0	75	94.9	33	100.0
Missing		0	0.0	0	0.0	0	0.0	1	3.8	0	0.0	0	0.0	0	0.0	4	5.1	0	0.0
Total		80	100.0	38	100.0	37	100.0	26	100.0	52	100.0	57	100.0	86	100.0	79	100.0	33	100.0

		Agra		*Cali*		*Prague IPSS*		*Groningen*		*Mannheim*		*Sofia*		*Beijing*		*Hong Kong*		*Chennai (Madras)*	
		N	%	N	%	N	%	N	%	N	%	N	%	N	%	N	%	N	%
Available	Grouped Baseline Diagnosis Converted to ICD-10																		
	Schizophrenia	27	44.3	44	61.1	13	30.2	12	19.4	44	78.6	40	74.1	58	100.0	69	98.6	77	100.0
	Schizoaffective	6	9.8	5	6.9	5	11.6	1	1.6	6	10.7	4	7.4	0	0.0	0	0.0	0	0.0
	Acute Schizo-like	6	9.8	20	27.8	4	9.3	2	3.2	1	1.8	0	0.0	0	0.0	1	1.4	0	0.0
	Bipolar/Depression	21	34.4	0	0.0	15	34.9	0	0.0	0	0.0	2	3.7	0	0.0	0	0.0	0	0.0
	Other Psychotic	0	0.0	0	0.0	5	11.6	46	74.2	2	3.6	8	14.8	0	0.0	0	0.0	0	0.0
	Other Nonpsychotic	1	1.6	3	4.2	1	2.3	1	1.6	3	5.4	0	0.0	0	0.0	0	0.0	0	0.0
Missing	Missing/Unknown	0	—	0	—	0	—	1	100.0	0	—	1	100.0	0	—	0	—	0	—
Available		61	100.0	72	100.0	43	100.0	62	98.4	56	100.0	54	98.2	58	100.0	70	100.0	77	100.0
Missing		0	0.0	0	0.0	0	0.0	1	1.6	0	0.0	1	1.8	0	0.0	0	0.0	0	0.0
Total		61	100.0	72	100.0	43	100.0	63	100.0	56	100.0	55	100.0	58	100.0	70	100.0	77	100.0

Appendix C

Deceased Subjects

TABLE C.1 Age at Death Dead Cohort—by Center

		Chandigarh Urban		*Chandigarh Rural*		*Dublin*		*Honolulu*		*Moscow*		*Nagasaki*		*Nottingham*		*Prague DOSMeD*		*Rochester*	
		N	%	N	%	N	%	N	%	N	%	N	%	N	%	N	%	N	%
Available	Age at Death																		
	09–19	0	0.0	0	0.0	0	0.0	0	0.0	0	0.0	0	0.0	0	0.0	0	0.0	0	—
	20–29	5	35.7	1	11.1	3	37.5	1	25.0	0	0.0	3	42.9	1	11.1	2	18.2	0	—
	30–39	6	42.9	1	11.1	2	25.0	1	25.0	3	30.0	2	28.6	1	11.1	5	45.5	0	—
	40–49	2	14.3	3	33.3	2	25.0	1	25.0	3	30.0	2	28.6	6	66.7	0	0.0	0	—
	50–59	1	7.1	4	44.4	1	12.5	1	25.0	2	20.0	0	0.0	1	11.1	4	36.4	0	—
	60–69	0	0.0	0	0.0	0	0.0	0	0.0	2	20.0	0	0.0	0	0.0	0	0.0	0	—
	70–79	0	0.0	0	0.0	0	0.0	0	0.0	0	0.0	0	0.0	0	0.0	0	0.0	0	—
Missing	Unknown	0	—	1	100.0	0	—	0	—	0	—	0	—	0	—	0	—	0	—
Available		14	100.0	9	90.0	8	100.0	4	100.0	10	100.0	7	100.0	9	100.0	11	100.0	0	—
Missing		0	0.0	1	10.0	0	0.0	0	0.0	0	0.0	0	0.0	0	0.0	0	0.0	0	—
Total		14	100.0	10	100.0	8	100.0	4	100.0	10	100.0	7	100.0	9	100.0	11	100.0	0	—

		Agra		*Cali*		*Prague IPSS*		*Groningen*		*Mannheim*		*Sofia*		*Beijing*		*Hong Kong*		*Chennai (Madras)*	
		N	%	N	%	N	%	N	%	N	%	N	%	N	%	N	%	N	%
Available	Age at Death																		
	09–19	0	0.0	0	0.0	0	0.0	0	0.0	0	0.0	0	0.0	0	0.0	1	9.1	0	0.0
	20–29	6	15.0	0	0.0	5	10.9	5	55.6	2	33.3	1	50.0	0	0.0	6	54.5	3	37.5
	30–39	9	22.5	2	16.7	11	23.9	2	22.2	3	50.0	0	0.0	3	15.0	1	9.1	3	37.5
	40–49	7	17.5	5	41.7	9	19.6	2	22.2	0	0.0	1	50.0	2	10.0	2	18.2	1	12.5
	50–59	12	30.0	3	25.0	16	34.8	0	0.0	1	16.7	0	0.0	4	20.0	1	9.1	1	12.5
	60–69	6	15.0	2	16.7	5	10.9	0	0.0	0	0.0	0	0.0	7	35.0	0	0.0	0	0.0
	70–79	0	0.0	0	0.0	0	0.0	0	0.0	0	0.0	0	0.0	4	20.0	0	0.0	0	0.0
Missing	Unknown	3	100.0	0	—	0	—	0	—	1	100.0	0	—	0	—	0	—	1	100.0
Available		40	93.0	12	100.0	46	100.0	9	100.0	6	85.7	2	100.0	20	100.0	11	100.0	8	88.9
Missing		3	7.0	0	0.0	0	0.0	0	0.0	1	14.3	0	0.0	0	0.0	0	0.0	1	11.1
Total		43	100.0	12	100.0	46	100.0	9	100.0	7	100.0	2	100.0	20	100.0	11	100.0	9	100.0

TABLE C.2 Year of Death Dead Cohort—by Center

		Chandigarh Urban		*Chandigarh Rural*		*Dublin*		*Honolulu*		*Moscow*		*Nagasaki*		*Nottingham*		*Prague DOSMeD*		*Rochester*	
		N	%	N	%	N	%	N	%	N	%	N	%	N	%	N	%	N	%
Available	Year of Death																		
	1965–1969	0	0.0	0	0.0	0	0.0	0	0.0	0	0.0	0	0.0	0	0.0	0	0.0	0	—
	1970–1974	0	0.0	0	0.0	0	0.0	0	0.0	0	0.0	0	0.0	0	0.0	0	0.0	0	—
	1975–1979	0	0.0	0	0.0	0	0.0	0	0.0	0	0.0	0	0.0	0	0.0	0	0.0	0	—
	1980–1984	5	35.7	5	55.6	3	37.5	1	25.0	6	60.0	1	14.3	2	22.2	6	54.5	0	—
	1985–1989	5	35.7	4	44.4	5	62.5	2	50.0	3	30.0	4	57.1	5	55.6	3	27.3	0	—
	1990–1994	4	28.6	0	0.0	0	0.0	0	0.0	1	10.0	2	28.6	2	22.2	2	18.2	0	—
	1995–1996	0	0.0	0	0.0	0	0.0	1	25.0	0	0.0	0	0.0	0	0.0	0	0.0	0	—
Missing	Unknown	0	—	1	100.0	0	—	0	—	0	—	0	—	0	—	0	—	0	—
Available		14	100.0	9	90.0	8	100.0	4	100.0	10	100.0	7	100.0	9	100.0	11	100.0	0	—
Missing		0	0.0	1	10.0	0	0.0	0	0.0	0	0.0	0	0.0	0	0.0	0	0.0	0	—
Total		14	100.0	10	100.0	8	100.0	4	100.0	10	100.0	7	100.0	9	100.0	11	100.0	0	—

		Agra		*Cali*		*Prague IPSS*		*Groningen*		*Mannheim*		*Sofia*		*Beijing*		*Hong Kong*		*Chennai (Madras)*	
		N	%	N	%	N	%	N	%	N	%	N	%	N	%	N	%	N	%
Available	Year of Death																		
	1965–1969	0	0.0	1	8.3	3	6.5	0	0.0	0	0.0	0	0.0	0	0.0	0	0.0	0	0.0
	1970–1974	9	22.5	0	0.0	8	17.4	0	0.0	0	0.0	0	0.0	0	0.0	0	0.0	0	0.0
	1975–1979	5	12.5	1	8.3	11	23.9	1	11.1	2	33.3	1	50.0	0	0.0	3	27.3	0	0.0
	1980–1984	4	10.0	2	16.7	7	15.2	5	55.6	0	0.0	1	50.0	3	15.0	3	27.3	0	0.0
	1985–1989	7	17.5	3	25.0	13	28.3	3	33.3	3	50.0	0	0.0	10	50.0	4	36.4	4	44.4
	1990–1994	15	37.5	5	41.7	4	8.7	0	0.0	1	16.7	0	0.0	7	35.0	1	9.1	5	55.6
	1995–1996	0	0.0	0	0.0	0	0.0	0	0.0	0	0.0	0	0.0	0	0.0	0	0.0	0	0.0
Missing	Unknown	3	100.0	0	—	0	—	0	—	1	100.0	0	—	0	—	0	—	0	—
Available		40	93.0	12	100.0	46	100.0	9	100.0	6	85.7	2	100.0	20	100.0	11	100.0	9	100.0
Missing		3	7.0	0	0.0	0	0.0	0	0.0	1	14.3	0	0.0	0	0.0	0	0.0	0	0.0
Total		43	100.0	12	100.0	46	100.0	9	100.0	7	100.0	2	100.0	20	100.0	11	100.0	9	100.0

TABLE C.3 Nature of Death Dead Cohort—by Center

		Chandigarh Urban		*Chandigarh Rural*		*Dublin*		*Honolulu*		*Moscow*		*Nagasaki*		*Nottingham*		*Prague DOSMeD*		*Rochester*	
		N	%	N	%	N	%	N	%	N	%	N	%	N	%	N	%	N	%
Available	Nature of Death (Modified)																		
	1: Natural	4	44.4	6	75.0	3	37.5	1	25.0	2	33.3	2	28.6	3	42.9	5	45.5	0	—
	2: Suicide	4	44.4	1	12.5	5	62.5	2	50.0	1	16.7	4	57.1	4	57.1	6	54.5	0	—
	3: Homicide	0	0.0	0	0.0	0	0.0	1	25.0	0	0.0	0	0.0	0	0.0	0	0.0	0	—
	5: Accident	1	11.1	1	12.5	0	0.0	0	0.0	0	0.0	0	0.0	0	0.0	0	0.0	0	—
	6: Suspected Suicide	0	0.0	0	0.0	0	0.0	0	0.0	3	50.0	1	14.3	0	0.0	0	0.0	0	—
Missing	9: Unknown	5	100.0	2	100.0	0	—	0	—	4	100.0	0	—	2	100.0	0	—	0	—
Available		9	64.3	8	80.0	8	100.0	4	100.0	6	60.0	7	100.0	7	77.8	11	100.0	0	—
Missing		5	35.7	2	20.0	0	0.0	0	0.0	4	40.0	0	0.0	2	22.2	0	0.0	0	—
Total		14	100.0	10	100.0	8	100.0	4	100.0	10	100.0	7	100.0	9	100.0	11	100.0	0	—

		Agra		*Cali*		*Prague IPSS*		*Groningen*		*Mannheim*		*Sofia*		*Beijing*		*Hong Kong*		*Chennai (Madras)*	
		N	%	N	%	N	%	N	%	N	%	N	%	N	%	N	%	N	%
Available	Nature of Death (Modified)																		
	1: Natural	26	78.8	8	80.0	25	55.6	1	11.1	1	14.3	0	0.0	18	90.0	2	18.2	5	55.6
	2: Suicide	4	12.1	1	10.0	19	42.2	7	77.8	4	57.1	2	100.0	2	10.0	9	81.8	4	44.4
	3: Homicide	2	6.1	1	10.0	0	0.0	0	0.0	0	0.0	0	0.0	0	0.0	0	0.0	0	0.0
	5: Accident	1	3.0	0	0.0	1	2.2	0	0.0	0	0.0	0	0.0	0	0.0	0	0.0	0	0.0
	6: Suspected Suicide	0	0.0	0	0.0	0	0.0	1	11.1	2	28.6	0	0.0	0	0.0	0	0.0	0	0.0
Missing	9: Unknown	10	100.0	2	100.0	1	100.0	0	—	0	—	0	—	0	—	0	—	0	—
Available		33	76.7	10	83.3	45	97.8	9	100.0	7	100.0	2	100.0	20	100.0	11	100.0	9	100.0
Missing		10	23.3	2	16.7	1	2.2	0	0.0	0	0.0	0	0.0	0	0.0	0	0.0	0	0.0
Total		43	100.0	12	100.0	46	100.0	9	100.0	7	100.0	2	100.0	20	100.0	11	100.0	9	100.0

TABLE C.4 Mental Health Status at Death Dead Cohort—by Center

		Chandigarh Urban		*Chandigarh Rural*		*Dublin*		*Honolulu*		*Moscow*		*Nagasaki*		*Nottingham*		*Prague DOSMeD*		*Rochester*	
		N	%	N	%	N	%	N	%	N	%	N	%	N	%	N	%	N	%
Available	Mental Health Status at Death																		
	1: Well	6	54.5	6	60.0	1	33.3	1	100.0	0	—	0	0.0	1	12.5	0	0.0	0	—
	2: Partial Remission	1	9.1	3	30.0	1	33.3	0	0.0	0	—	1	16.7	2	25.0	4	66.7	0	—
	3: Illness Episode	4	36.4	1	10.0	1	33.3	0	0.0	0	—	5	83.3	5	62.5	2	33.3	0	—
Missing	. : Not Supplied	0	0.0	0	—	0	0.0	0	0.0	9	90.0	0	0.0	0	0.0	0	0.0	0	—
	9: Unknown	3	100.0	0	—	5	100.0	3	100.0	1	10.0	1	100.0	1	100.0	5	100.0	0	—
Available		11	78.6	10	100.0	3	37.5	1	25.0	0	0.0	6	85.7	8	88.9	6	54.5	0	—
Missing		3	21.4	0	0.0	5	62.5	3	75.0	10	100.0	1	14.3	1	11.1	5	45.5	0	—
Total		14	100.0	10	100.0	8	100.0	4	100.0	10	100.0	7	100.0	9	100.0	11	100.0	0	—

		Agra		*Cali*		*Prague IPSS*		*Groningen*		*Mannheim*		*Sofia*		*Beijing*		*Hong Kong*		*Chennai (Madras)*	
		N	%	N	%	N	%	N	%	N	%	N	%	N	%	N	%	N	%
Available	Mental Health Status at Death																		
	1: Well	15	45.5	6	60.0	2	8.0	1	12.5	3	60.0	0	0.0	4	21.1	2	20.0	3	33.3
	2: Partial Remission	5	15.2	0	0.0	8	32.0	5	62.5	1	20.0	0	0.0	11	57.9	3	30.0	2	22.2
	3: Illness Episode	13	39.4	4	40.0	15	60.0	2	25.0	1	20.0	2	100.0	4	21.1	5	50.0	4	44.4
Missing	. : Not Supplied	0	0.0	0	0.0	0	0.0	0	0.0	1	50.0	0	—	0	0.0	0	0.0	0	—
	9: Unknown	10	100.0	2	100.0	21	100.0	1	100.0	1	50.0	0	—	1	100.0	1	100.0	0	—
Available		33	76.7	10	83.3	25	54.3	8	88.9	5	71.4	2	100.0	19	95.0	10	90.9	9	100.0
Missing		10	23.3	2	16.7	21	45.7	1	11.1	2	28.6	0	0.0	1	5.0	1	9.1	0	0.0
Total		43	100.0	12	100.0	46	100.0	9	100.0	7	100.0	2	100.0	20	100.0	11	100.0	9	100.0

TABLE C.5 Standardized Mortality Ratio (SMR)** by Total and Gender

Center	Total	Gender	
		Male	*Female*
Rochester	0.00	0.00	0.00
Sofia	1.04	1.12	0.96
Cali	1.31	1.68	0.79
Moscow	1.41	0.99	1.98
Agra	1.86*	1.34	2.88*
Chandigarh Urban	1.88*	2.05	1.70
Chennai (Madras)	1.90	1.73	2.11
Prague DOSMeD	2.53*	1.44	3.55*
Beijing	2.97*	3.37*	2.59*
Chandigarh Rural	3.02*	4.71*	1.76
Honolulu	3.13*	4.22*	0.00
Nottingham	3.31*	2.45	5.93*
Prague IPSS	3.84*	1.59	6.30*
Dublin	4.10*	5.14*	2.55
Mannheim	5.55*	6.55*	3.15
Nagasaki	5.71*	5.06*	6.90*
Hong Kong	5.76*	7.16*	3.78
Groningen	8.88*	11.04*	5.27

*Statistically significantly different from 1 at 5% level.

**The standardized mortality ratio for a given group is the observed number of deaths in the group divided by the expected number of deaths that would have occurred in the group as computed using age-gender-year-specific mortality rate of the general population. In mathematical notation, $SMR=O/E$ where $E=S\ (qij)$ and the summation (S) is taken over all individuals and their follow-up years and qij denotes the age-gender probability with which individual i is expected to die during follow-up year j. The age-gender probability is computed using the corresponding rate in the general population mortality table.

TABLE C.6 Sources of Population Mortality Rates: By Year

Sources

1. WHO Census Database
2. *National Family Health Survey 1993* (of India)
3. U.S. Bureau of the Census International Data Base (on Columbia)
4. U.S. Bureau of the Census International Data Base (on Mainland China)
5. *Demographic Yearbook*, United Nations, 1993
6. *CDC-Vital and Health Statistics: Russian Federation and US, Selected Years 1980–93*
7. Recent Trends in Age-Specific Mortality in India. Mari Bhat, P. N. & Navaneetham, K. (1991). *Journal of Institute of Economic Research*, 26 (1&2).
8. *Germany: National Statistical Yearbooks, 1977–1995*

The source used for each center and year is given in the table below.*

	68	69	70	71	72	73	74	75	76	77	78	79	80	81	82	83	84	85	86	87	88	89	90	91	92	93	94
Agra	7	7	7	7	7	7	7	7	7	7	7	7	7	7	7	7	7	7	7	7	7	7	7	2	—	—	—
Beijing	—	—	—	—	—	4	4	4	4	4	4	4	4	4	4	4	4	1	1	1	1	1	1	—	1	—	—
Cali	1	1	1	1	1	1	1	1	1	1	1	1	—	—	—	—	3	3	3	3	3	3	3	1	—	—	—
Chandigarh Urban	7	7	7	7	7	7	7	7	7	7	7	7	7	7	7	7	7	7	7	7	7	7	7	2	—	—	—
Chandigarh Rural	7	7	7	7	7	7	7	7	7	7	7	7	7	7	7	7	7	7	7	7	7	7	7	2	—	—	—
Dublin	1	1	1	1	1	1	1	1	1	1	1	1	1	1	1	1	1	1	1	1	1	1	1	1	1	—	—
Groningen	1	1	1	1	1	1	1	1	1	1	1	1	1	1	1	1	1	1	1	1	1	1	1	1	1	1	—
Hong Kong	1	1	1	1	1	1	1	1	1	1	1	1	1	1	1	1	1	1	1	1	1	1	1	1	1	1	—
Honolulu	1	1	1	1	1	1	1	1	1	1	1	1	1	1	1	1	1	1	1	1	1	1	1	1	—	—	—
Madras	7	7	7	7	7	7	7	7	7	7	7	7	7	7	7	7	7	7	7	7	7	7	7	2	—	—	—
Mannheim	—	—	—	—	—	—	8	8	8	8	8	8	8	8	8	8	8	8	8	8	8	8	8	8	8	8	1
Moscow	—	—	—	—	—	—	—	—	—	—	—	—	—	6	—	—	—	1	1	1	1	1	1	1	1	1	1
Nagasaki	1	1	1	1	1	1	1	1	1	1	1	1	1	1	1	1	1	1	1	1	1	1	1	1	1	1	1
Nottingham	1	1	1	1	1	1	1	1	1	1	1	1	1	1	1	1	1	1	1	1	1	1	1	1	1	—	—
Prague-DOSMeD	—	—	5	5	5	5	5	5	5	5	5	5	5	5	5	5	5	1	1	1	1	1	1	1	1	1	—
Prague-IPSS	—	—	5	5	5	5	5	5	5	5	5	5	5	5	5	5	5	1	1	1	1	1	1	1	1	1	—
Rochester	1	1	1	1	1	1	1	1	1	1	1	1	1	1	1	1	1	1	1	1	1	1	1	1	—	—	—
Sofia	1	1	1	1	1	1	1	1	1	1	1	1	1	1	1	1	1	1	1	1	1	1	1	1	1	1	—

*The missing entries were filled in by using the source of the closest year or the closest earlier year in the presence of two closest years.

INDEX